Techniques in ACL Surgery

Techniques in ACL Surgery

Editor-in-Chief

Sachin Ramchandra Tapasvi
MS (Ortho) DNB (Ortho) FRCS (Glasg) MNAMS AFAOA (Australia)
Consultant Arthroscopy and Arthroplasty Surgeon
The Orthopaedic Speciality Clinic
Pune, Maharashtra, India

Co-Editors

Shantanu Patil MBBS MS (Ortho)
Head
Translational Medicine and Research
SRM Medical College
SRM University
Chennai, Tamil Nadu, India

Anshu Shekhar MBBS MS (Ortho)
Associate Consultant
The Orthopaedic Speciality Clinic
Pune, Maharashtra, India

Foreword

Professor Philippe Neyret

JAYPEE The Health Sciences Publisher
New Delhi | London | Panama

Jaypee Brothers Medical Publishers (P) Ltd

Headquarters
Jaypee Brothers Medical Publishers (P) Ltd.
4838/24, Ansari Road, Daryaganj
New Delhi 110 002, India
Phone: +91-11-43574357
Fax: +91-11-43574314
E-mail: jaypee@jaypeebrothers.com

Overseas Offices
J.P. Medical Ltd.
83, Victoria Street, London
SW1H 0HW (UK)
Phone: +44-20 3170 8910
Fax: +44(0)20 3008 6180
E-mail: info@jpmedpub.com

Jaypee-Highlights Medical Publishers Inc.
City of Knowledge, Bld. 235, 2nd Floor, Clayton
Panama City, Panama
Phone: +1 507-301-0496
Fax: +1 507-301-0499
E-mail: cservice@jphmedical.com

Jaypee Brothers Medical Publishers (P) Ltd.
17/1-B, Babar Road, Block-B, Shaymali
Mohammadpur, Dhaka-1207
Bangladesh
Mobile: +08801912003485
E-mail: jaypeedhaka@gmail.com

Jaypee Brothers Medical Publishers (P) Ltd.
Bhotahity, Kathmandu, Nepal
Phone: +977-9741283608
E-mail: kathmandu@jaypeebrothers.com

Website: www.jaypeebrothers.com
Website: www.jaypeedigital.com

Inquiries for bulk sales may be solicited at: jaypee@jaypeebrothers.com

Techniques in ACL Surgery

First Edition: **2017**

ISBN 978-93-5270-036-3

Printed in India

Dedicated to

My teachers who mentored me
All the patients who trusted me
All my peers whom I deeply respect
All the friends who stand by me
All the people who inspired me

Contributors

Marcio Albers MD
Research Fellow
Department of Orthopedic Surgery
University of Pittsburgh Medical Center
University of Pittsburgh
Pittsburgh, Pennsylvania, USA

Sadem Amer MS
Assistant Professor
Department of Arthroscopy & Sports Medicine
Sri Ramachandra University
Chennai, Tamil Nadu, India

Renato Andrade
Clínica do Dragão
Espregueira-Mendes Sports Centre
FIFA Medical Centre of Excellence
Porto
Portugal
Dom Henrique Research Centre
Porto
Portugal
Faculty of Sports
University of Porto
Porto, Portugal

Prakash Ayyadurai MS (Ortho)
Assistant Professor
Department of Arthroscopy and Sports Medicine
Sri Ramachandra University
Chennai, Tamil Nadu, India

Ricardo Bastos
Clínica do Dragão
Espregueira-Mendes Sports Centre
FIFA Medical Centre of Excellence
Porto, Portugal
Dom Henrique Research Centre
Porto, Portugal
Fluminense Federal University
Rio de Janeiro, Brazil

Charles H Brown Jr MD
Director
International Knee and Joint Centre
Abu Dhabi, United Arab Emirates

Deepak Chaudhary MS
Director
Sports Injury Centre
Safdarjung Hospital
New Delhi, India

Cheli AF MD
Orthopedic Surgeon
Orthopedic and Arthroscopic Surgery Unit
New Sassuolo Hospital
Modena, Italy

Lee Yee Han Dave MBBS MMed (Ortho) FRCS (Tr & Ortho)
Consultant Orthopedic Surgeon
Department of Orthopedic Surgery
Changi General Hospital
Singapore City, Singapore

Mao Weijia David MBBS BMed (Sci) MRCS
Staff Registrar
Department of Orthopedic Surgery
Changi General Hospital
Singapore City, Singapore

Andrew de Vlieg MBBCH FCS (SA) (Orthopaedics)
Gateway Private Hospital
Prime Human Performance Centre
Durban, South Africa

Patrick Djian MD
Department of Orthopedic Surgery
Cabinet Goethe
Paris, France

Raju Easwaran MBBS MS (Ortho)
Shree Meenakshi Orthopaedics and Sports Medicine Clinic
Max Healthcare
New Delhi, India

João Espregueira-Mendes
Orthopedics Department
Minho University
Minho, Portugal
Clínica do Dragão
Espregueira-Mendes Sports Centre
FIFA Medical Centre of Excellence
Porto, Portugal
Dom Henrique Research Centre
Porto, Portugal
3B's Research Group—Biomaterials, Biodegradables and Biomimetics
University of Minho
Headquarters of the European Institute of Excellence on Tissue Engineering and Regenerative Medicine
Parque de Ciência e Tecnologia
Guimarães, Portugal
ICVS/3B's—PT Government Associate Laboratory
Braga/Guimarães, Portugal

Wolfgang Franz MD
Medical Director, Lutrina Klinik
Kaiserslautern, Germany

Freddie H Fu MD DSc (Hon) DPs (Hon)
Distinguished Service Professor and Chairman
Department of Orthopedic Surgery
University of Pittsburgh Medical Center
University of Pittsburgh
Pittsburgh, Pennsylvania, USA

Prashanth Gorur MS (Ortho) DNB D (Ortho)
Consultant Arthroscopy and Sports Medicine
Bengaluru, Karnataka, India

Ankit Goyal DNB
Associate Professor, Sports Injury Centre
Safdarjung Hospital
New Delhi, India

Sunny Gugale DNB (Ortho)
Consultant Orthopedic Surgeon
Department of Arthroscopy and Arthroplasty
Sancheti Institute for Orthopaedics and Rehabilitation
Pune, Maharashtra, India

Thomas Harlem MD
Clinical Director of Surgery and Orthopedics
Haraldsplass Deaconess Hospital
Bergen, Norway

Jonathan Herald MBBS MsdMed FRACS (Ortho)
Orthoclinic Sydney
Western Sydney University
New South Wales, Australia

Eivind Inderhaug MD MPH PhD
Knee Research Fellow
Imperial College London
London, UK
Consultant Knee Surgeon
Haraldsplass Deaconess Hospital
Bergen, Norway

Amit Kumar Jha MS (Ortho)
Ganga Hospital
Coimbatore, Tamil Nadu, India

Lim Wei-an Joel
Orthopedic Resident
Department of Orthopedic Surgery
Changi General Hospital
Singapore City, Singapore

Anant Joshi MS (Ortho) D (Ortho) Master of Sports Science (USA)
Sportsmed Mumbai
Parel ST Depot
Mumbai, Maharashtra, India

Deepak Joshi MS
Senior Specialist
Sports Injury Centre
Safdarjung Hospital
New Delhi, India

Sagar Kakatkar MS DNB MNAMS D (Ortho) FAS AOAFAS
Dr Vasantrao Pawar Medical College and Hospital
Nashik, Maharashtra, India
Vivaan Clinic
Nashik, Maharashtra, India

Vikram Kakatkar MS (Ortho)
Clinical and Research Fellow
The Orthopaedic Speciality Clinic
Pune, Maharashtra, India

Nilesh Kamat DNB (Ortho) MNAMS MRCS (Edin.) Fellowship in Arthroscopy and Sports Medicine (Singapore)
Consultant Arthroscopy and Sports Medicine
Jehangir Hospital
Pune, Maharashtra, India
Sancheti Institute for Orthopaedics and Rehabilitation
Pune, Maharashtra, India

B Bhupesh Karthik MS
Associate Professor
Department of Arthroscopy & Sports Medicine
Sri Ramachandra University
Chennai, Tamil Nadu, India

Mininder S Kocher MD MPH
Department of Orthopaedic Surgery
Division of Sports Medicine
Boston Children's Hospital
Harvard Medical School
Boston, Massachusetts, USA

Jun Matsuno MS ATC
Head Athletic Trainer
Spalding University
Louisville, Kentucky, USA

Michael P McClincy MD
Department of Orthopaedic Surgery
Division of Sports Medicine
Boston Children's Hospital
Harvard Medical School
Boston, Massachusetts, USA

Abhay Narvekar MS (Ortho) D (Ortho)
Consultant
PD Hinduja Hospital
Consultant
Hinduja Healthcare
Consultant
Global Hospital
Mumbai, Maharashtra, India

Nicoletta F MD
Orthopedic Surgeon
Orthopedic and Arthroscopic Surgery Unit
New Sassuolo Hospital
Modena, Italy

John Nyland DPT SCS EdD ATC CSCS FACSM
Athletic Training Program Director and Professor
Kosair Charities College of
Health and Natural Sciences
Spalding University
Louisville, Kentucky, USA

Shantanu Patil MBBS MS (Ortho)
Head
Translational Medicine and Research
SRM Medical College
SRM University
Chennai, Tamil Nadu, India

Thierry Pauyo MD FRCSC
Sports Medicine Fellow
University of Pittsburgh
Pittsburgh, Pennsylvania, USA
UPMC Center for Sports Medicine
Pittsburgh, Pennsylvania, USA

Pederzini LA MD
Director
Orthopedic and Arthroscopic Surgery Unit
New Sassuolo Hospital
Modena, Italy

Hélder Pereira
Orthopedics Department
Centro Hospitalar Póvoa de Varzim
Vila do Conde, Portugal
3B's Research Group—Biomaterials, Biodegradables and Biomimetics
University of Minho
Headquarters of the European Institute of Excellence on Tissue Engineering and Regenerative Medicine AvePark
Parque de Ciência e Tecnologia, Portugal
ICVS/3B's—PT Government Associate Laboratory
Braga/Guimarães
Portugal
Ripoll y De Prado Sport Clinic
FIFA Medical Centre of Excellence
Madrid, Spain
Dom Henrique Research Centre
Porto, Portugal

Rogério Pereira
Clínica do Dragão
Espregueira-Mendes Sports Centre
FIFA Medical Centre of Excellence
Porto, Portugal
Dom Henrique Research Centre
Porto, Portugal
Faculty of Sports
University of Porto
Porto, Portugal
University Fernando Pessoa
Porto, Portugal

Suresh Perumal MS
Assistant Professor
Department of Arthroscopy and Sports Medicine
Sri Ramachandra University
Chennai, Tamil Nadu, India

Ernesto Pinho
SMIC Group
Portugal
School of Allied Health Sciences of Porto
Porto, Portugal

S Rajasekaran MS FRCS MCH PhD
Clinical Director and Head of Orthopedics
Ganga Hospital
Coimbatore, Tamil Nadu, India

Sérgio Rodrigues-Gomes
Clínica do Dragão
Espregueira-Mendes Sports Centre
FIFA Medical Centre of Excellence
Porto, Portugal
Dom Henrique Research Centre
Porto, Portugal
SMIC Group, Portugal

Arumugam S AB (IM) MS (Ortho) FRCS (Glasg)
Director
Sri Ramachandra Arthroscopy & Sports Sciences Center
Head of the Department
Department of Arthroscopy and Sports Medicine
Sri Ramachandra University
Chennai, Tamil Nadu, India

Bhushan Sabnis MS (Ortho) DNB (Ortho) MRCS FRCS (Tr & Ortho) Dip (CAOS)
Sportsmed Mumbai
Parel ST Depot
Mumbai, Maharashtra, India

Soheil Sabzevari MD
University of Pittsburgh Medical Center
Pittsburgh, Pennsylvania, USA
Mashhad University of Medical Sciences
Mashhad, Iran

Balaji Sambandam MS (Ortho)
Ganga Hospital
Coimbatore, Tamil Nadu, India

Parag Sancheti FRCS (Ed) MS (Orth) DNB (Ortho) MCh (UK)
Professor and Chairman
Sancheti Institute for Orthopaedics and Rehabilitation
Pune, Maharashtra, India

Serafini F MD
Orthopedic Surgeon
Orthopedic and Arthroscopic Surgery Unit
New Sassuolo Hospital
Modena, Italy

Humza Shaikh BA
Department of Orthopaedic Surgery
University of Pittsburgh Medical Center
University of Pittsburgh
Pittsburgh, Pennsylvania, USA

Anshu Shekhar MBBS MS (Ortho)
Associate Consultant
The Orthopaedic Speciality Clinic
Pune, Maharashtra, India

Miten Sheth MS DNB
The Knee Clinic
Mumbai, Maharashtra, India

Ashok Shyam MS (Ortho)
Director, The Arthritis Clinic
Mumbai, Maharashtra, India
Consultant
Sancheti Institute for Orthopaedics and Rehabilitation
Pune, Maharashtra, India

Bertrand Sonnery-Cottet MD
Centre Orthopédique Santy
FIFA Medical Center of Excellence
Groupe Ramsay-Générale de Santé
Lyon, France

SR Sundararajan MS (Ortho)
Senior Consultant
Ganga Hospital
Coimbatore, Tamil Nadu, India.

Sachin Tapasvi MS (Ortho) DNB (Ortho) FRCS (Glasg) MNAMS AFAOA (Australia)
Consultant Arthroscopy and Arthroplasty Surgeon
The Orthopaedic Speciality Clinic
Pune, Maharashtra, India

Chirag Thonse MS (Ortho)
Consultant Orthopedic and Arthroscopy Surgeon
St. Martha's Hospital
Bengaluru, Karnataka, India

Sanjay Trivedi MS (Ortho) ODTS (England)
Consultant Knee and Shoulder Arthroscopy and Sports Medicine Surgeon
Dr Trivedi's Arthroscopy Clinic
Ahmedabad, Gujarat, India and
Sterling Hospital and HCG Hospital
Ahmedabad, Gujarat, India

Sanesh Vijay Tuteja DNB MRCS
Centre Orthopédique Santy
FIFA Medical Center of Excellence
Groupe Ramsay-Générale de Santé
Lyon, France

Sajeer Usman MS (Ortho)
Sportsmed Mumbai
Parel ST Depot
Mumbai, Maharashtra, India

Roshan Wade MS DNB D (Ortho) FCPS
Arthroscopy and Sports Medicine Consultant
Assistant Professor
Department of Orthopedics
Seth GSMC & KEM Hospital
Mumbai, Maharashtra, India

Chaitanya Waghchoure MS (Ortho) DNB (Ortho)
Clinical Associate
Sir HN Reliance Foundation Hospital
Mumbai, Maharashtra, India

Weimin Zhu MD
Department of Orthopedic Surgery
University of Pittsburgh Medical Center
University of Pittsburgh
Pittsburgh, Pennsylvania, USA
Department of Sports Medicine
The First Affiliated Hospital of Shenzhen University
Guangdong Sheng, China

Foreword

Dear Reader,

You will find in this book the latest updates in techniques for ACL surgery.

There are different options to manage an ACL-deficient knee—to reconstruct, to repair or to augment the ACL. There are also different techniques to reconstruct the ACL— hamstrings, patellar tendon or other grafts can be used. The use of each graft may influence the fixation.

All chronic anterolateral instabilities cannot be reconstructed by isolated ACL reconstruction. In some cases, an extra-articular augmentation or tenodesis may have to be considered.

Familiarity with all techniques and procedures will allow the surgeon to optimize the operation depending on the clinical and radiological examinations and on the patient's expectation or previous surgeries.

Rehabilitation is an important part of the treatment and the general principles are summarized neatly at the end of the book.

The authors who have contributed to this book have a unique experience in the management of the ACL-deficient knee. They have dedicated their time and effort to share this experience. Dr Sachin Tapasvi brings together these talents in a comprehensive book.

So, enjoy and read the latest knowledge about the technical options of the treatment of an ACL insufficiency for the benefit of your patients.

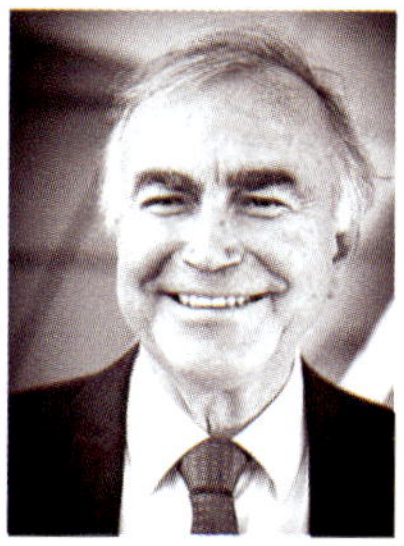

Professor Philippe Neyret
President of ISAKOS (2015-2017)
President of ACL Study Group (2014-2016)
Chairman of EFORT Fellowship
Health Point Consultant (Abu Dhabi, UAE)
Latilini Consultant (Barcelona, Spain)

Preface

The concept of the knee joint as an organ, where each of its elements—menisci, ligaments, cartilage and synovial lining—mutually enhance and affect each other's functioning and form, is still evolving. Enhanced understanding of the role of each of these elements has now contributed to better management options, surgical as well as conservative. We are gradually improving the outcome goals—return to pre-injury activity level, prevention of degenerative changes, elimination of laxity and greater patient satisfaction. New research continues to highlight previously unknown facts and also improve and update what we have known for the major part of the last century.

The anterior cruciate ligament plays a pivotal role in the functioning and stability of the knee joint. Treatment of injuries of this ligament continues to evolve and what was 'state of the art' a decade ago is passé today. The surgical modalities have continually improved with better techniques, better technology and better understanding of the patients' needs.

We have compiled this textbook, keeping in mind the need of the practicing surgeon today. Each critical step in performing ACL reconstruction surgery has been discussed in detail, covering the entire surgical technique. We were fortunate to get surgeons with tremendous expertise and phenomenal track record in treating this condition, to write each chapter and share their tips and tricks as well. Photographs and illustrations add to the clarity of the authors' intentions. Conservative management and rehabilitation after the surgery have also been addressed in detail at the end.

We hope this book will be a constant presence in the young arthroscopic specialists' career as well as for the more experienced discerning surgeons, who wish to update their knowledge and skills.

Sachin Tapasvi
Shantanu Patil
Anshu Shekhar

Acknowledgments

It would be a great travesty if we do not recognize the superhuman efforts of Dr Anshu Shekhar, who has been critical in the compilation of this book. Along with Dr Shantanu Patil, he has pored over each word and every illustration in this book—from the early drafts to each galley version, he has worked to ensure the success of this book, all the while working on a full surgical and clinical schedule. We must thank Mrs Asawari Bhende for managing the logistics involved and communicating with all the involved parties. The professional and meticulous Ms Neha Wadhwa Vaz has continued to be our shepherd, ensuring timely turnaround and adherence to deadlines.

A special note of thanks to Dr Philippe Neyret, a legend and stalwart of arthroscopic surgery, for writing the Foreword for our humble endeavor. His words of appreciation are a source of encouragement for us.

We would like to thank Dr Charles H Brown Jr for providing the images for the cover.

We also thank Shri Jitendar P Vij (Group Chairman), Mr Ankit Vij (Group President), and Ms Chetna Malhotra Vohra (Associate Director–Content Strategy) of Jaypee Brothers Medical Publishers (P) Ltd, New Delhi, India for kindly agreeing to publish this book, and the production team for their dedicated work.

Contents

CHAPTER

1

Placing Correct Portals for Transportal ACL Reconstruction

Nilesh Kamat

INTRODUCTION

Arthroscopic anterior cruciate ligament (ACL) reconstruction has been the standard of care for non-arthritic unstable ACL deficient knees in the recent past. The surgical technique of ACL reconstruction has undergone a major transition in the last decade with a shift from transtibial technique to transportal or the so called anatomic ACL reconstruction. The main difference in these two techniques being that the femoral tunnel was drilled through the tibial tunnel in the transtibial technique whereas it is drilled independent of the tibial tunnel in the transportal technique. The reasons for this transition of technique were twofold. Firstly, the graft position remains vertical in the transtibial technique which fails to provide adequate rotational control and may result in a residual positive pivot shift test.[1-4] Secondly, the transtibial technique fails to allow for anatomic positioning of the graft, allowing only anteromedial footprint coverage.[5-7] This chapter aims to describe the technique and the portals used for the anatomic arthroscopic ACL reconstruction.

TECHNIQUE

Positioning

The patient is positioned supine on a standard operating table under appropriate anesthesia. A well-padded high tourniquet is applied on the ipsilateral thigh. A heel support is placed at 90° flexion with a valgus side support along the thigh. This position should allow hyperflexion of the knee to up to 120–125°.[8] This is one of the prerequisites to performing a transportal ACL reconstruction. A thorough examination under anesthesia is performed to note and confirm the findings prior to the surgical incision. The limb is the painted using chlorhexidine solution and draped with sterile sheets allowing free access to the knee with lower end of the femur and upper end of the tibia (Fig. 1.1A). A sterile skin marker is used to make the surface markings along the patella, joint line, and the proposed portal sites. Surface marking is performed with the knee in 90° flexion. The lower pole of patella is the most prominent landmark and is outlined first. This is followed by identifying the tibial tuberosity and the patellar tendon. The medial and lateral joint lines are palpated on either side of the patella and are outlined accordingly (Fig. 1.1B). The operating limb is exsanguinated using a sterile Eschmarch bandage prior to the incision and the tourniquet is elevated to 100 mm Hg above the systolic blood pressure of the patient.

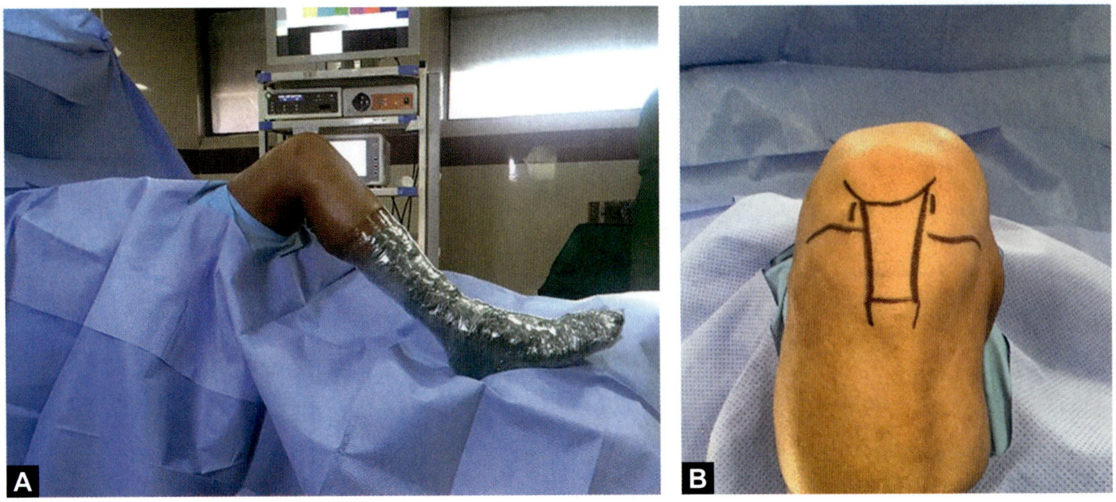

Figs. 1.1A and B: (A) Positioning and draping of the patient. (B) Skin marking of the joint line and proposed portals.

ESTABLISHING THE ANTEROLATERAL PORTAL

The soft spot along the lateral side of the patella is identified above the joint line. It is important to place this portal as high as possible to allow adequate visualization of the tibial footprint and secondly to avoid entering through the Hoffa's fat pad. A No. 11 scalpel blade is used to incise the skin, subcutaneous tissue, and the capsule. It is important to place the sharp edge of the blade pointing upward to prevent inadvertent damage to the articular surface of the lateral femoral condyle and to prevent a radial tear of the lateral meniscus. After incising the skin, the joint is then entered using a semi blunt trocar and cannula by extending the joint and entering the suprapatellar pouch. This can be confirmed by free side to side movement of the trocar in the suprapatellar pouch. The irrigation fluid is started using a Y connector. Routine use of an irrigation pump is not mandatory and gravity assisted irrigation is sufficient for adequate distension of the joint.

The trocar is replaced with a 30° arthroscope and a complete diagnostic round is performed examining the following structures in sequence:

- Suprapatellar pouch
- Trochlea
- Medial facet, central ridge, and lateral facet of patella
- Lateral and medial gutters
- Medial compartment including medial meniscus (roots, posterior horn, body, and anterior horn)
- Lateral compartment including lateral meniscus (roots, posterior horn body and anterior horn including popliteal hiatus and popliteus tendon).

ESTABLISHING THE STANDARD ANTEROMEDIAL PORTAL

After completion of a diagnostic round, the next step is to establish a standard anteromedial portal. This portal is used to probe the structures and to perform any therapeutic meniscal procedures. Keeping the knee in 30° flexion, an 18 FG spinal needle is used to determine the portal site by "outside in technique"

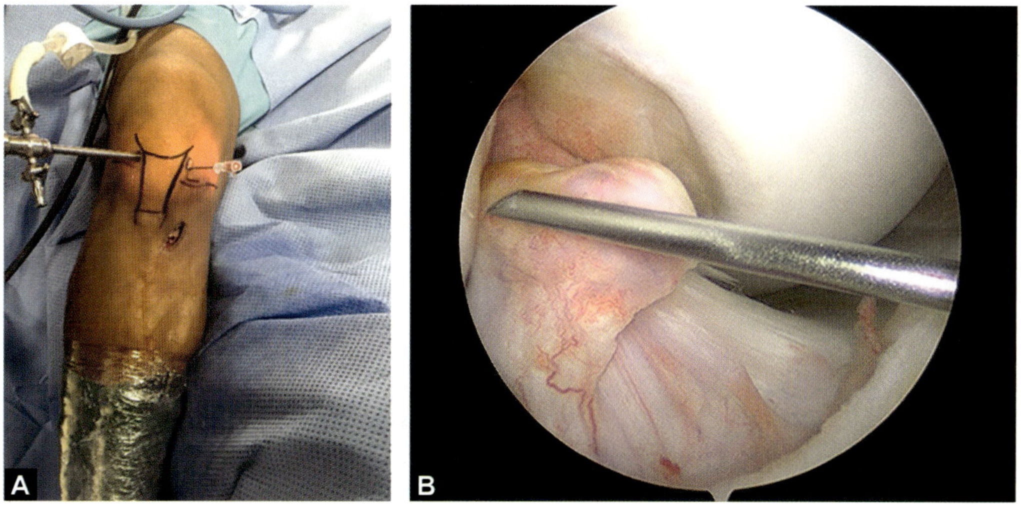

Figs. 1.2A and B: (A) Position of the knee hanging by the side of the operating table while establishing the anteromedial portal. (B) Arthroscopy image of the position of the 18 FG spinal needle.

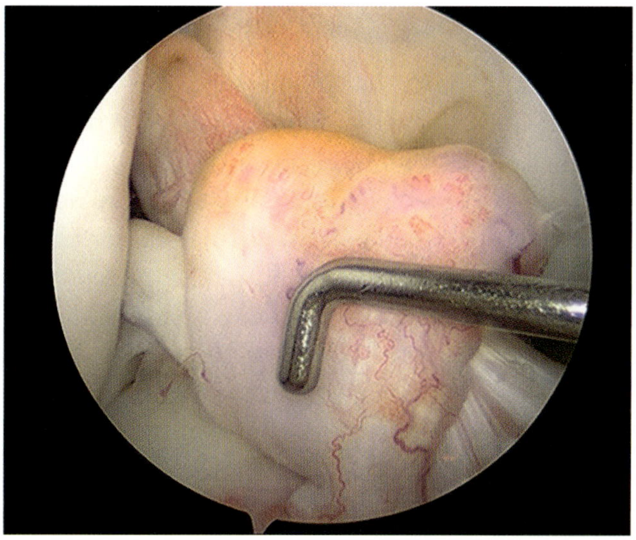

Fig. 1.3: Probing of torn ACL stump through the anteromedial portal.

(Figs. 1.2A and B). Care should be taken to place this portal above the medial meniscus and it should not be too close to the midline. This may cause crowding of instrumentation making maneuverability difficult. After establishing the anteromedial portal, a motorized shaver is used to clear up the fat pad and to trim the footprint of the ACL at the tibial and the femoral side (Fig. 1.3).

At this point it may be noted that the visualization of the femoral footprint from the anterolateral portal is not adequate. The main reason for this being that the anterolateral viewing portal is along the same visual axis of the femoral footprint. To improve visualization, the arthroscope can be shifted to the anteromedial portal. Before performing this step, it is important to establish the accessory medial portal which will be eventually used as a working portal (Figs. 1.4A and B).

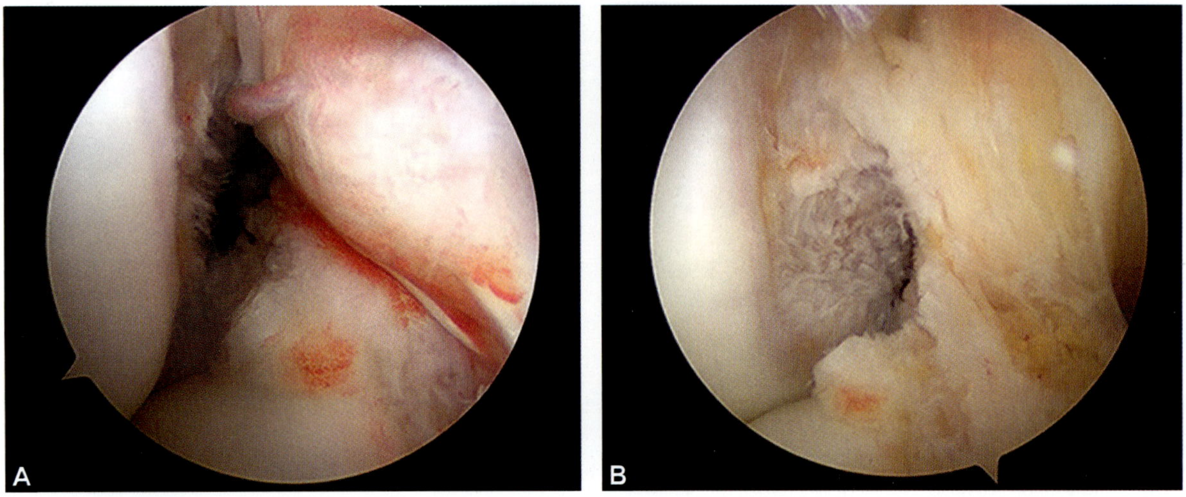

Figs. 1.4A and B: (A) Inadequate visualization of the femoral footprint of ACL from AL portal. (B) Complete visualization of the femoral footprint of ACL from AM portal.

ESTABLISHING THE ACCESSORY ANTEROMEDIAL PORTAL

Keeping the scope in the anterolateral portal the knee is hyperflexed to 125°. This allows the skin and subcutaneous tissue to move cranially along the anterior aspect of the knee. This allows the femoral footprint to move anteriorly in relation to its index position which in turn aids in better access and visualization. To establish the accessory medial portal an 18 FG spinal needle is used. In this technique the scope is kept in the anterolateral portal and accessory medial portal is established inferior and far medial to the anteromedial portal by "outside in" technique. The trajectory of the spinal needle is placed from inferior to superior from medial to lateral in such a manner that it would exit along the anterolateral aspect of femur (Fig. 1.5A). Medial placement of the accessory medial portal allows a longer and elliptical femoral tunnel.[8] Caution is to be taken to prevent inadvertent scuffing of the cartilage of the medial femoral condyle. In order to prevent this, the scope is directed toward the medial compartment and the spinal needle is inserted under direct vision. Also avoid too close placement of the accessory medial portal to the anteromedial portal as instrumentation eventually will become difficult. The next step is to switch the viewing portal from the anterolateral portal to anteromedial portal and using the accessory anteromedial portal as the working portal (Figs. 1.5B and 1.6).

Contraindications of using the Accessory Medial Portal

There are certain scenarios where using an accessory medial portal may not be possible. These are relative contraindications which may be overcome with some difficulties.

- Obese patients with high body mass index which prevents achieving hyperflexion due to contact of the posterior aspect of the calf and thigh. In these cases, the femoral tunnel is created using an outside-in technique *(described in Chapter 14)* or a flexible reamer system is used *(described in Chapter 13).* Alternatively, in these patients, it may be worthwhile to consider a transtibial technique *(described in Chapter 15)* over the accessory medial portal technique if the outside-in jig or flexible reamers are not available.

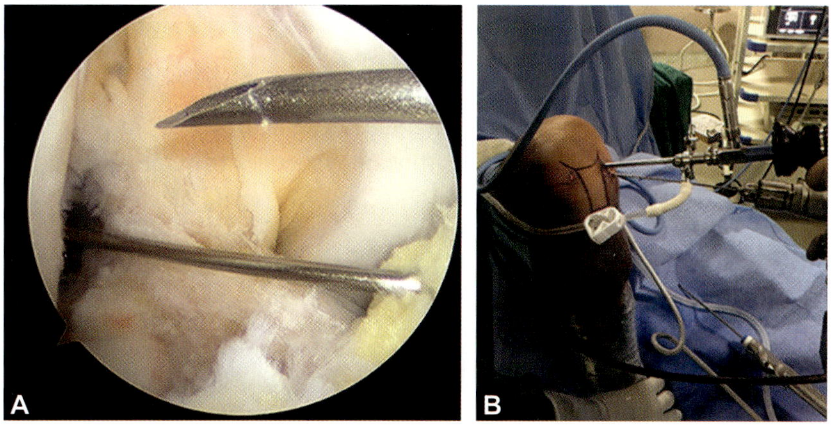

Figs. 1.5A and B: (A) Establishing accessory anteromedial portal medial and inferior to the anteromedial portal (Hypodermic needle in the AM portal and spinal needle in the AMP portal). (B) Using the anteromedial portal as the viewing portal and the accessory medial portal as the working portal.

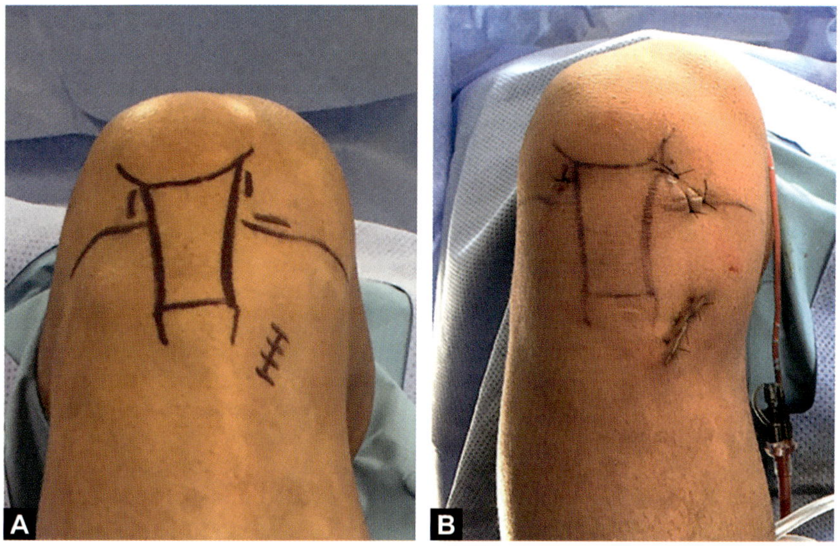

Figs. 1.6A and B: (A) Skin marking with proposed portal sites. (B) Final portals and skin incisions after closure.

- Type A or stenosed intercondylar notch which fails to allow access to the femoral footprint. Liberal notchplasty may have to be considered to allow access and visualization of the footprint *(described in Chapter 10)*.

Advantages of Accessory Medial Portal Technique[8]

Advantages of accessory medial portal technique are*:*

- Independent tunnel drilling allows optimal restoration of the femoral footprint due to better access and visualization.
- As the tibial tunnel is independent of femoral tunnel, it can be altered in length according to the nature and length of the graft and its placement in combined multiligament reconstruction surgeries.

- No specialized instrumentation is required for this technique.
- Placement of the interference screw, if needed is along the direction of the femoral tunnel avoiding screw tunnel divergence and preventing damage to the graft.

Literature has shown that inaccurate placement of the tunnels is the most common cause of failure of ACL reconstruction surgeries.[9-14] Adequate visualization is the key to successful outcome of all reconstructive arthroscopic procedures and the key to adequate visualization is optimal portal placement. As described above, the accessory medial portal technique offers several advantages over the conventional transtibial technique. Also, literature shows better functional outcome with anatomical placement of the graft with transportal technique over the transtibial technique.

PEARLS

- Hyperflexion of the knee to 120° is a prerequisite to transportal ACL reconstruction.
- High placement of anterolateral and anteromedial portal allows adequate visualization.
- Using the anteromedial portal allows better visualization of the femoral ACL footprint.
- Accessory medial portal should be placed medial and inferior to the anteromedial portal to avoid crowding of instruments.

REFERENCES

1. Kato Y, Ingham JM, Kramer S, et al. Effect of tunnel position for anatomic single-bundle ACL reconstruction on knee biomechanics in a porcine model. Knee Surg Sports Traumatol Arthrosc. 2010;18:2-10.
2. Driscoll MD, Isabell GP, Conditt MA, et al. Comparison of 2 femoral tunnel locations in anatomic single-bundle anterior cruciate ligament re-construction: a biomechanical study. Arthroscopy. 2012;28:1481-9.
3. Bedi A, Musahl V, Steuber V, et al. Transtibial versus anteromedial portal reaming in anterior cruciate ligament reconstruction: an anatomic and biomechanical evaluation of surgical technique. Arthroscopy. 2011;27:380-90.
4. Steiner ME, Battaglia TC, Heming JF, et al. Independent drilling outperforms conventional transtibial drilling in anterior cruciate ligament reconstruction. Am J Sports Med. 2009;37:1912-9.
5. Pearle AD, Shannon FJ, Granchi C, et al. Comparison of 3-dimensional obliquity and anisometric characteristics of anterior cruciate ligament graft positions using surgical navigation. Am J Sports Med. 2008;36:1534-41.
6. Kopf S, Pombo MW, Shen W, et al. The ability of 3 different approaches to restore the anatomic anteromedial bundle femoral insertion site during anatomic anterior cruciate ligament reconstruction. Arthroscopy. 2011;27(2):200-6.
7. Steiner ME, Battaglia TC, Heming JF, et al. Independent drilling outperforms conventional transtibial drilling in anterior cruciate ligament reconstruction. Am J Sports Med. 2009;37(10):1912-9.
8. Brown CH Jr, Spalding T, Robb C. Medial portal technique for single-bundle anatomical anterior cruciate ligament (ACL) reconstruction. Int Orthop. 2013;37:253-69.
9. Hensler D, Working Z, Illingworth K, et al. Medial portal drilling: effects on the femoral tunnel aperture morphology during anterior cruciate ligament reconstruction. J Bone Joint Surg Am. 2011;93:2063-71.
10. Kamath GV, Redfern JC, Greis PE, et al. Revision anterior cruciate ligament reconstruction. Am J Sports Med. 2011;39:199-217.
11. Marchant B, Noyes F, Barber-Westin S, et al. Prevalence of nonanatomical graft placement in a series of failed anterior cruciate ligament reconstruction. Am J Sports Med. 2010;38:1987-96.
12. George MS, Dunn WR, Spindler KP. Current concepts review: revision anterior cruciate ligament reconstruction. Am J Sports Med. 2006;34:2026-37.
13. Jaureguito JW, Paulos LE. Why grafts fail. Clin Orthop Relat Res. 1996;325:25-41.
14. Johnson DL, Fu FH. Anterior cruciate ligament reconstruction: why do failures occur? Instr Course Lect. 1995;44:391-406.

CHAPTER

2 Harvesting and Preparing an Ideal Bone Patella Tendon Bone Graft

Arumugam S, Prakash Ayyadurai, Suresh Perumal

INTRODUCTION

Bone patella tendon bone (BPTB) graft remains the "gold standard" for the choice of graft in primary anterior cruciate ligament (ACL) reconstruction[1]. Despite the shift toward the use of hamstring tendons as a graft choice, BPTB has regained its popularity.

The biggest advantage of BPTB graft is the osteointegration between the bone plug and the tibial and femoral tunnels and this gives an edge over other grafts in use. This provides faster healing potential and quick return to preoperative activity level through accelerated rehabilitation.[1]

The reported enduring donor site morbidity such as pain while kneeling down, less functional muscle strength and anterior knee pain can be successfully overcome by modified graft harvest technique.

INDICATIONS

The lead author (Arumugam S) has been the exponent of BPTB for the past two decades and his general indication for using BPTB for primary ACL reconstruction is young and active patients (after physeal closure) aged between 18 years and 35 years, which includes recreational as well professional athletes.

SURGICAL TECHNIQUE

Anesthesia and Patient Positioning

Patient undergoes surgery under general or regional anesthesia in supine position. The affected limb is fixed in a leg holder and the tourniquet is applied high on the thigh.

Preoperative Preparation

Thorough clinical examination of the patient with careful assessment of the laxity and the graft site for surrounding skin condition, scars, adhesions and features of tendinitis should be done.

Diagnostic arthroscopy is done through standard anterolateral and anteromedial portals, to confirm the diagnosis of ACL insufficiency and make thorough joint evaluation to identify associated joint lesions.

Harvesting Bone Patella Tendon Bone Graft through "Mobile Window Technique"

The knee is then positioned at 60°, a 4–5 cm oblique incision is made from a point just distal to the lower pole of patella to a point 2–3 cm medial to the tibial tuberosity (Fig. 2.1).

Exposure

The incision is then transformed into a rectangular window using parallel skin hooks (Figs. 2.2 and 2.3). The subcutaneous plane is vertically dissected to reach the peritenon. A small nick is made on the

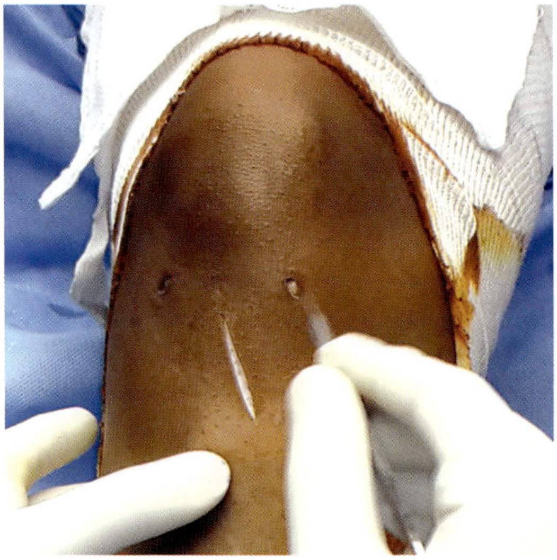

Fig. 2.1: Small oblique incision.

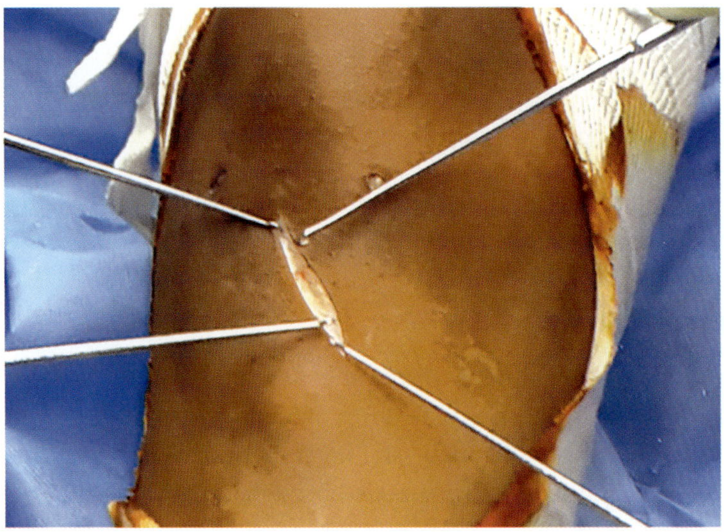

Fig. 2.2: Skin hook is placed in the incision.

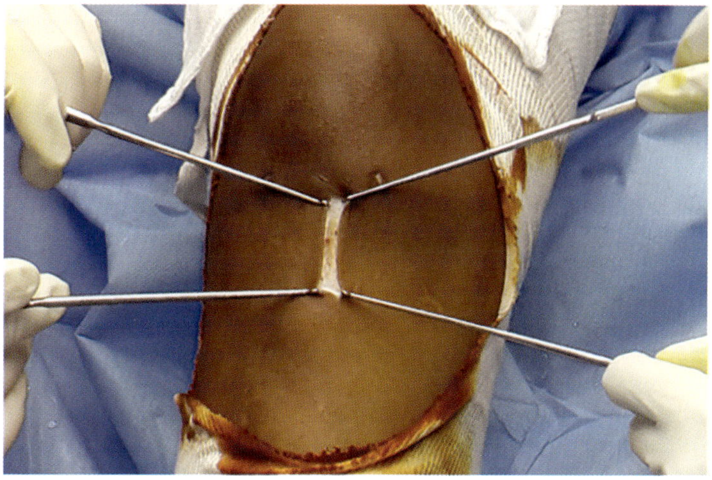

Fig. 2.3: Oblique incision made into a rectangular window.

peritenon and using a curved scissors the peritenon is reflected exposing the underlying patellar tendon. A mobile window is created and exposure superiorly up to the patella (with knee in full extension) and inferiorly about 1 cm below the tibial tuberosity (with knee in 60° flexion) is achieved.

Tendon Harvest

Knee is now positioned to 120° flexion to make the patellar tendon taut. The inferior pole of patella is palpated, and the medial and lateral borders of the patella tendon are identified (Fig. 2.4). Using an 11 No blade, 10 mm of the tendon from middle one-third of the patella tendon is incised vertically along the fibers of the patellar tendon (Fig. 2.5).

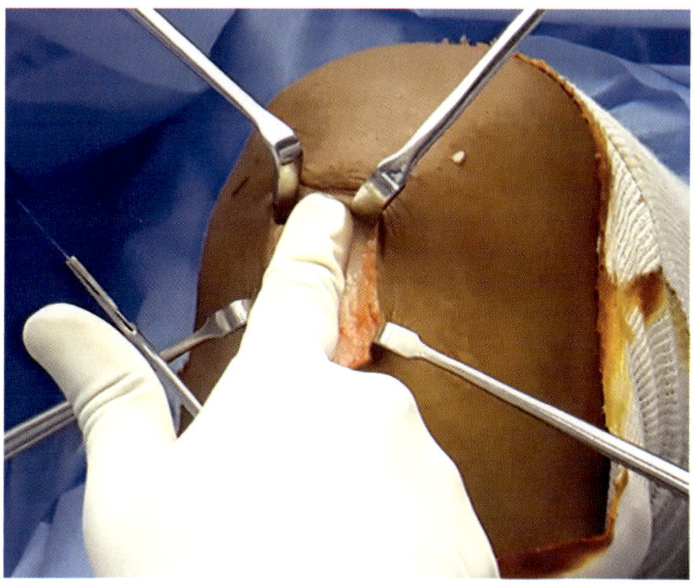

Fig. 2.4: Palpating inferior pole of patella.

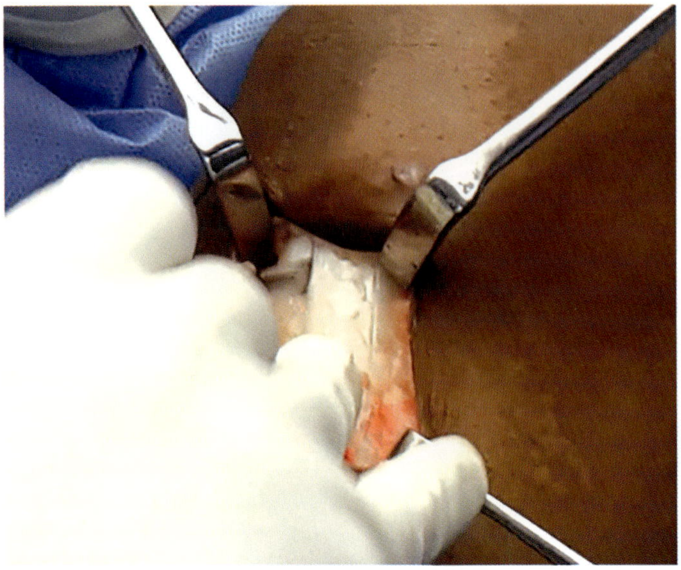

Fig. 2.5: 1 cm width of tendon strip incised along the fibers.

Tendon Bone Plug

The knee is now brought back to 60° flexion. The external tibial torsion, if present is corrected with internal rotation of the leg. The borders of the bone plug are marked using an 11 No blade in continuity with the patellar tendon extending just proximal to the tibial tuberosity. Using a 2 mm K-wire, three holes are drilled at equidistance from each other on the tibial bone plug before harvest (Fig. 2.6). Later, these holes will be used to pass No 5 Ethibond® (Ethicon LLC) sutures for tensioning the graft during fixation.

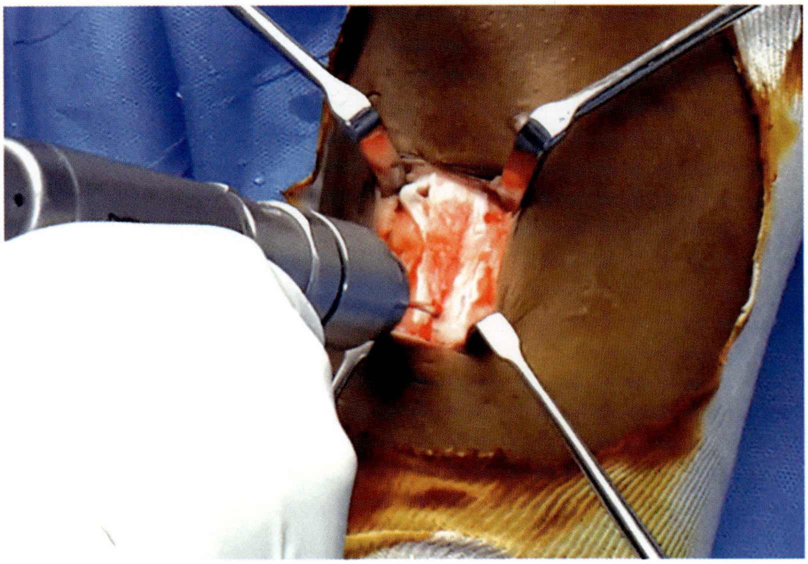

Fig. 2.6: Drill hole made in tibial plug.

Tibial bone plug of width 11 mm is carefully harvested using a sagittal oscillating saw at an angle of 60° to the anterior cortex to a depth of 10 mm on either side. The distal transverse cut is made perpendicular to the anterior cortex. Care is taken to harvest the bone plug from the anterior slope of tibia just below the joint line to obtain a good tibial tongue. The bone plug is lifted carefully from its bed using an osteotome (Fig. 2.7). The harvested bone plug is held using Kocher forceps (Fig. 2.8).

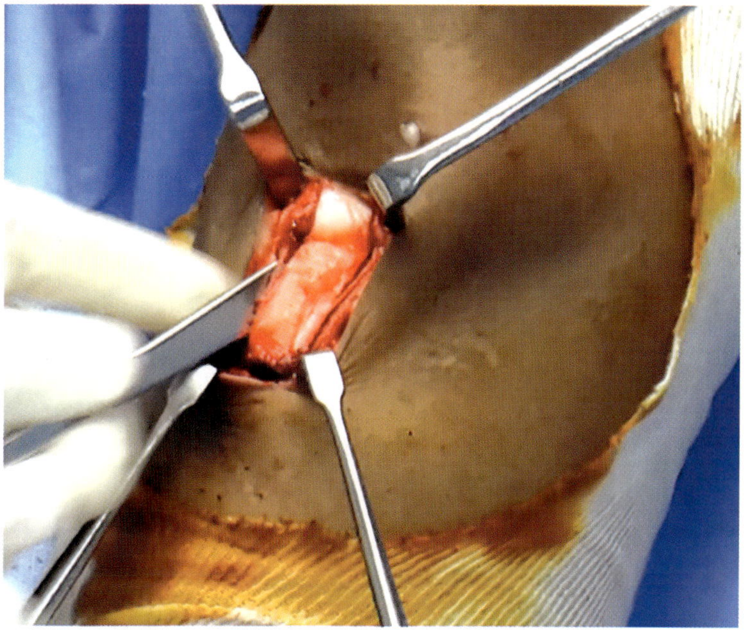

Fig. 2.7: Fine osteotome slid in to separate the bone plug from the tibia.

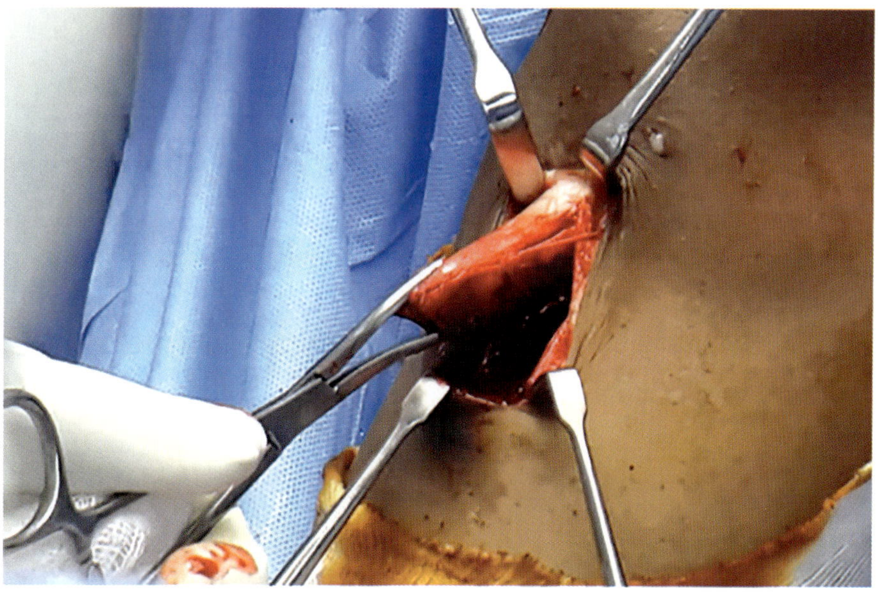

Fig. 2.8: Tibial bone plug is held with Kocher forceps and longitudinal traction is given to the graft.

Patella Bone Plug

The knee is then extended completely. The graft is held with constant longitudinal traction to bring the inferior pole of patella inside the mobile window (Fig. 2.9). The peritenon is reflected to expose the patella underneath. Patella bone plug is marked for a length of 25 mm. A single hole is predrilled in the proximal end with 2 mm K-wire. Patellar bone plug is harvested using the sagittal saw at angle of 45° to the anterior cortex to a depth of 10 mm on either side and a transverse cut at its proximal end is made perpendicular to the underlying bone. The proximal end of the bone plug is harvested in a conical fashion for ease of entry inside the femoral tunnel during graft passage.

Care should be taken to separate and retain the fat pad, which will be adherent to the patella tendon near the inferior pole of patella to avoid saline leakage (Figs. 2.10A and B).

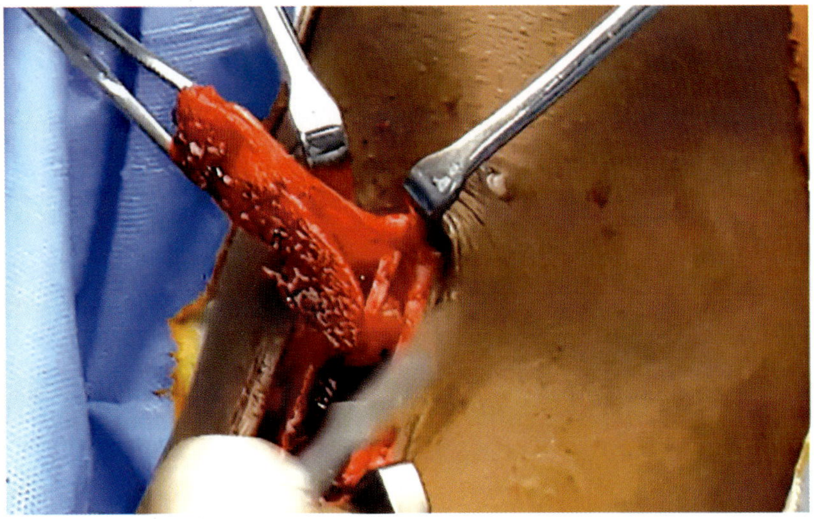

Fig. 2.9: The resultant tibial bone plug held with a bone tongue.

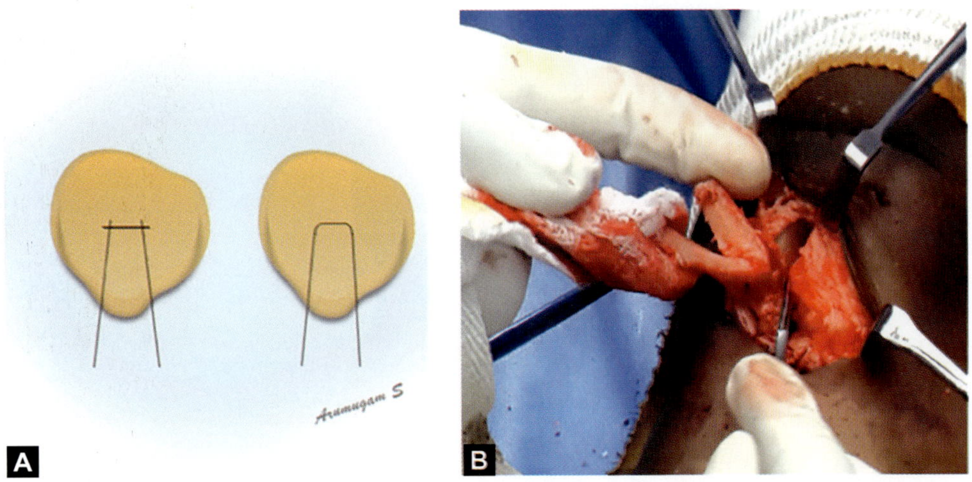

Figs. 2.10A and B: (A) Incorrect sharp edged and correct rounded patella bone plug. (B) Hoffa's fat pad separated from the patella bone plug.

Graft Preparation

The separated graft is placed in a kidney tray by the surgeon and carefully transferred, to be prepared on a separate trolley. The tendon is cleared off the fat and bone debris. The excess bone is removed off the bone plug using a bone nibbler and size measured using a standard graft sizer.

The author recommends a standard diameter of 10 mm patella bone plug and 11 mm tibial bone plug. This configuration is better for use with transtibial femoral tunnel technique, which will be discussed in chapter 15 "*Creating a Transtibial Femoral Tunnel*" No 5 Ethibond® sutures are passed through the predrilled holes in the patellar and tibial bone plugs and secured with straight small hemostat clamps. This configuration of sutures will provide reliable and solid traction during interference screw fixation. The patella bone plug-tendon junction is marked using a surgical marker to aid in visualization during femoral interference screw fixation.

Bone Patella Tendon Bone Graft

The resultant BPTB graft has a 25 mm patella bone plug (leading end), 10 mm width patella tendon and a tibial bone plug with a tibial tongue (trailing end). The entire length of the graft will be around 80–90 mm (Fig. 2.11).

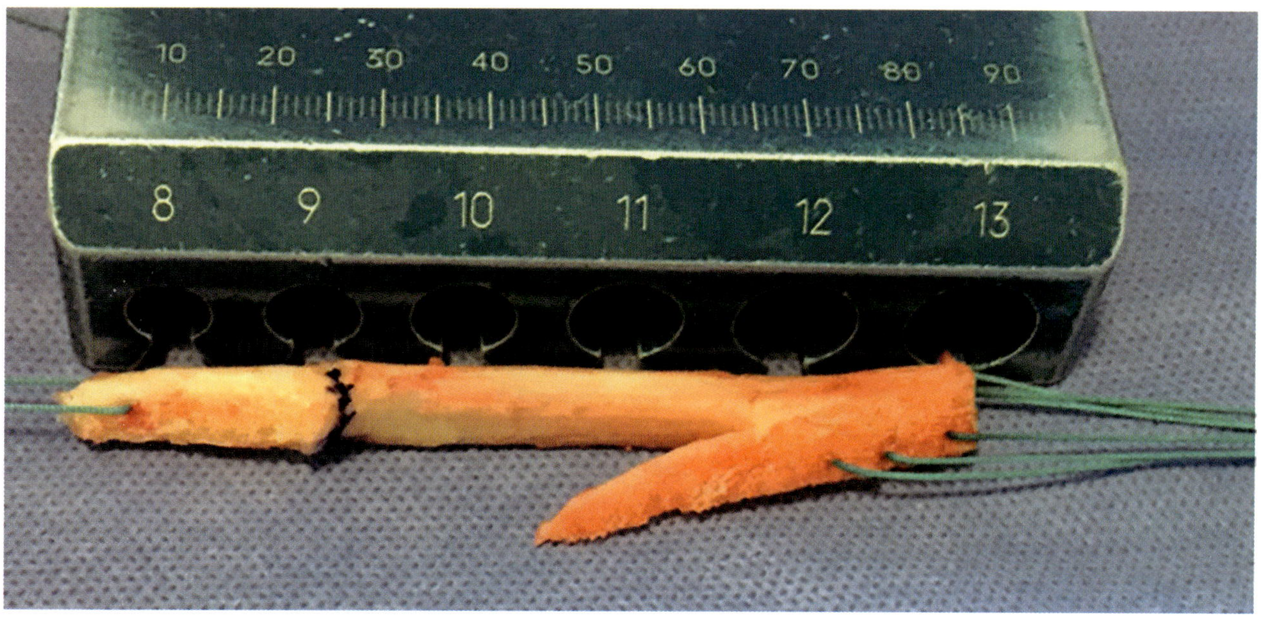

Fig. 2.11: Bone patella tendon bone graft after harvest.

Closure

Only the peritenon is closed using interrupted sutures with No 1.0 Vicryl®. Care is taken to avoid bites into the patellar tendon. Subcutaneous layer is closed with No. 1.0 Vicryl®. Skin is closed using subcuticular stich with No 3.0 Ethilon®.

ADVANTAGES OF BONE-PATELLA TENDON-BONE GRAFT TECHNIQUE

- A small oblique incision avoids the morbid knee pain while kneeling down.
- A good graft is obtained using a relatively small incision. The tibial tunnel can be made using the same incision.
- The tibial bone tongue reduces the effective length of the tendon and it is helpful in overcoming the tunnel-graft length mismatch.
- This technique is easily reproducible.

PEARLS AND PITFALLS

Patella fractures in postoperative period can be prevented by avoiding stress risers. This can be achieved by avoiding crossing the line of cut at the corners and rounding off the cut.

If inadvertently the bone plug is fractured intraoperatively, it can be overcome by "piggy backing" (fractured ends held with sutures) if the remaining portion is large. If the remaining portion is very small then it can be sacrificed and with whip stiches in the patellar tendon, the graft can be made into soft tissue graft (Fig. 2.12).

If care is not taken during tendon harvest, then there can be mismatch between tendon fibers and the bone plug. Either not all tendon fibers are attached to bone plug or fibers that are attached to bone plug are not present through the entire length (Fig.2.13). This can be avoided by incising the tendon in tension.

Graft-tunnel mismatch is another potential complication (Fig. 2.14). If the length of the graft is long then the entire bone plug will be out of the tunnel. This can be overcome by following ways:

- Creating a trough on tibia and fixing the plug with a screw.
- Advancing the bone plug into femoral tunnel and fixing it with a bio screw.
- Graft can be twisted to shorten it.[2]
- Flipping the bone plug on to graft and fixing it with bioabsorbable screw.[3]

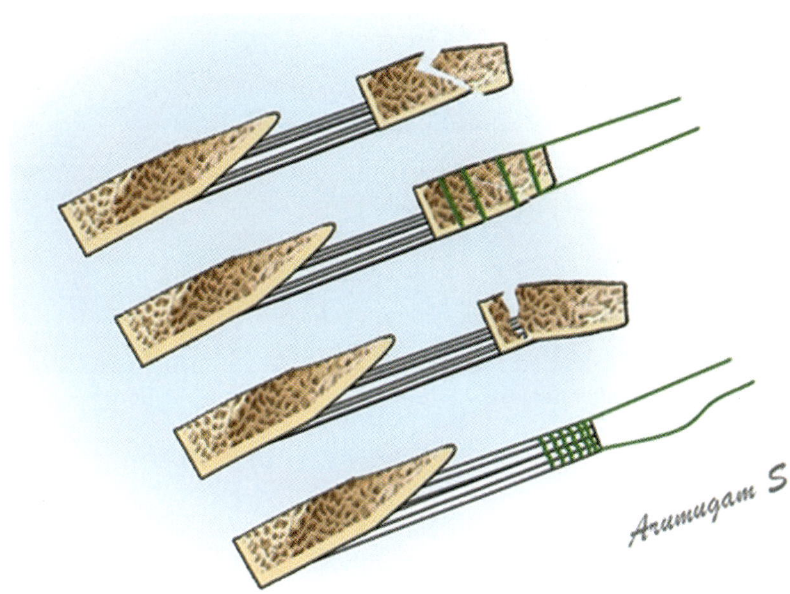

Fig. 2.12: Bail-out options when bone plug fractures.

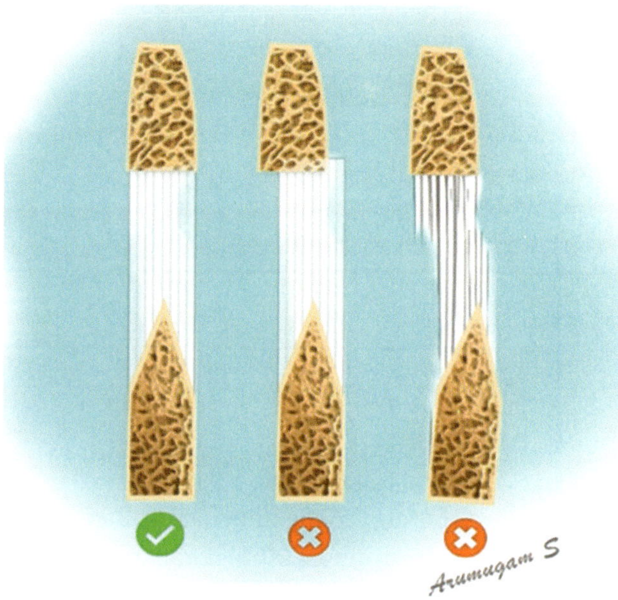

Fig. 2.13: Ideal bone patella tendon bone (BPTB) graft and illustrations of graft with tendon bone plug mismatch.

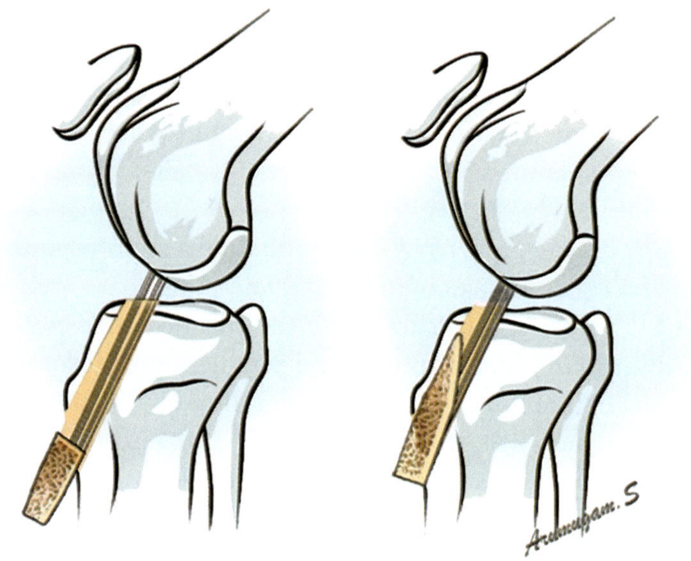

Fig. 2.14: Tibial bone tongue overcomes the graft-tunnel mismatch.

REFERENCES

1. Matteo D, Quaglia A, Randelli P. Arthroscopic anterior cruciate ligament reconstruction with bone-patellar tendon-bone. Arthroscopy. Berlin Heidelberg: Springer; 2016. pp. 223-7.
2. Augé WK 2nd, Yifan K. A Technique for resolution of graft-tunnel length mismatch in central third bone–patellar tendon–bone anterior cruciate ligament reconstruction. Arthroscopy. 1999;8:877-81.
3. Barber FA. Flipped patellar tendon autograft anterior cruciate ligament reconstruction. Arthroscopy. 2000;16:483-90.

CHAPTER

3 Harvesting Hamstring Tendons

Patrick Djian

INTRODUCTION

Among the various surgical procedures for correcting knee laxity after anterior cruciate ligament (ACL) rupture, the standard treatment is an intra-articular ACL reconstruction with autogenous tissues. The bone-patellar tendon-bone (BPTB) had been traditionally considered as the gold standard. Nowadays, hamstring tendons, gracilis tendons (GTs), and semitendinosus tendon (ST) are increasingly used for ACL reconstruction.

Harvesting of the hamstring tendons is associated with less graft-site morbidity and is less difficult technically than preparation of BPTB graft. They provide higher structural properties when folded to a tripled or quadrupled construct and replicate the nonisometric behavior of the intact ACL (with its anteromedial and posterolateral bundles) more closely than a single-stranded graft. Harvesting the hamstring tendons does not significantly compromise strength or function of the leg. Subsequently, the rehabilitation protocol for patients has been less aggressive after reconstruction using a hamstring graft.

Potential complications during graft harvest include inadvertent premature division of the tendons, damage to the medial collateral ligament (MCL), and neurologic injury. The STs and GTs have had a significant historical role in reconstructive procedures designed to treat the injured knee. In 1914, Phillips reported transplantation of the GT for augmentation of a ruptured MCL. Bosworth advocated anterior mobilization of the ST and its implantation on the medial femoral condyle for the treatment of medial collateral insufficiency.[1] Hey-Groves[2-4] and Macey pioneered the use of the ST in intra-articular cruciate ligament reconstruction. Previous reports included little mention of the complications related to tendon harvest. Selection of any technique for tendon harvest should include cognizance of this fact, and methods should be developed to avoid complications while obtaining high-quality tendon grafts.

We commonly use a combined semitendinosus-gracilis graft for the treatment of ACL insufficiency. While we recognize the inherent strength of the patellar tendon graft as well as the advantages of fixation with a bone-tendon-bone construction, there are disadvantages to using the patellar tendon, including risks of patellar fracture, patellar tendinitis, and patellar pain syndrome.[5]

Sometimes, we have used the ST to reconstruct the MCL in selected patients with combined anterior cruciate and MCL injuries and gross valgus instability. In addition, we have come to consider these tendons for use as free grafts in distant anatomic locations as ankle pathology for example.

We examined the anatomic relationships of the ST and GT to facilitate tendon harvest, to improve the quality of tendon grafts, and to reduce the risk of complications.

ANATOMIC CONSIDERATIONS

Tibial Insertion

Semitendinosus, gracilis, and sartorius have a common insertion into the anterior-medial aspect of the tibia, the *pes anserinus.*[6] These muscles act as flexors of the knee but also provide internal tibial rotation and act as rotatory and valgus constraints to the knee. Gracilis originates from the inferior ramus of the pubis and is a long fusiform muscle that gives rise to a cylindrical tendon, and is innervated by the obturator nerve. Semitendinosus originates from the ischial tuberosity, is a fusiform muscle that about halfway down the thigh gives rise to a tubular tendon, and is innervated by the tibial branch of the sciatic nerve. Sartorius originates form the anterior superior iliac spine and its tendon becomes thin and flat, like a fascial layer.[7] Gracilis and semitendinosus lie between layers I that includes the sartorius fascia and II that includes the MCL of the medial structures of the knee.[8] Although gracilis and semitendinosus are separate structures proximally, they converge prior to their insertion onto the tibia. The insertion of gracilis is superior to that of semitendinosus.

Apart from the main hamstring tendon insertion to the *pes anserinus* there may be accessory tendon insertions, particularly for semitendinosus. In addition, there are variable numbers of thick fascial bands that pass between semitendinosus and gracilis and also from these hamstring tendons to gastrocnemius, popliteal, pretibial, and superficial fascia.[9] Recognizing these accessory insertions and fascial bands and dividing them is essential. If these are not recognized and divided they can divert the tendon stripper from the main tendon leading to premature tendon amputation and short graft.[10]

Accessory Insertions and Fascial Bands

Cadaveric studies by Candal-Couto and Deehan[9] and Tuncay[11] reported the existence of several accessory bands of gracilis and semitendinosus. Tuncay et al. studied the anatomy of the fascial bands between semitendinosus and gastrocnemius in 23 cadaveric knees. They found that the mean width of the main band was 2.6 cm (1–4 cm) and the mean distance from the semitendinosus insertion to this fascial band was 7 cm (6–8 cm). However, Candal-Couto and Deehan in another cadaveric study, found that accessory bands originated at greater than 10 cm from the tibial insertion of 8/10 semitendinosus and 2/10 GTs, contrary to the common belief that 10 cm proximal to the insertion of pes anserinus is a safe distance to avoid encountering such a band. This has been confirmed more recently by Yasin et al.[12] in vivo. They studied the number of accessory bands and their location in 25 patients undergoing ACL reconstruction using hamstring tendons. For gracilis, the most common number of accessory bands was 2 (range 0–3). The average distance of the most proximal band from the common insertion was 5.14 cm with none of the gracilis accessory bands being more than 10 cm proximal to the tibial crest attachment. For ST, the most common number of accessory bands was 3 (range 1–4), the average distance of the most proximal band from the tibial crest insertion was 8.14 cm. However, five STs had accessory bands located more than 10 cm proximal to the tibial crest attachment. In a cadaveric study,

Sanders et al.[13] described three zones with the knee in 90° flexion and the femur parallel to the floor. Zone A included the area anterior-superior to gracilis, zone B between gracilis and semitendinosus, and zone C, posterior-inferior to semitendinosus. They described that proximally semitendinosus had variable slips inserting onto the crural fascia and gastrocnemius. Distally there were reproducible accessory tendon slips. In zone A, a membranous band originating from the medial epicondyle of the femur was found to insert on the intratendinous fascia of gracilis and semitendinosus. In zone B, fibrous bands existed between the two tendons, reproducibly found at 2.5 cm, 5.5 cm, and 6.5 cm from the distal tendon insertion. Zone C included the only true accessory insertional tendon from the semitendinosus at 5.1 cm which was preceded by a variable band at 3.8 cm.

Saphenous Nerve

After leaving the adductor canal, the saphenous nerve follows a posteromedial course toward the medial side of the knee where it emerges between the sartorius and GTs. The nerve is consistently found lying immediately superficial to the GT at the posteromedial joint line. When the knee is extended, the nerve is held taut against the tendon. With the knee flexed, tension on the nerve diminishes.

The infrapatellar branch of the saphenous nerve (IPBSN) may be described as posterior, penetrating, parallel, and anterior according to its relationship to sartorius.[14] The posterior type (nerve emerges under the posterior border of sartorius) is the most common, seen in 62% of cases. The infrapatellar branch passes between the inferior pole of the patella and the tibial tuberosity in 98.5% and distal to the tuberosity in 1.5% of cases. It passes as one branch in 25%, two branches in 62%, three branches in 10%, and four branches in 1.5% of cases.[15,16]

Sanders et al.[13] found that the saphenous nerve frequently ran parallel and closely to gracilis on the deep surface of sartorius crossing gracilis from lateral to medial at 11.8 cm (range 7–13.2 cm) from its distal insertion. It then continued distally on the posterior-medial side of the tendon. The sartorial branch left the sartorius fascia at a mean of 7.2 cm (range 6.4–9.3 cm) from the distal gracilis insertion to become subcutaneous, hence it was closely related to gracilis for 4.6 cm prior to leaving layer I of the knee.

Luo et al.[17] examined the relationship between skin incision and injury of the infrapatellar branch during ACL reconstruction. A vertical incision was used in 35 and an oblique incision in 25 cases. 23 (65.7%) in the vertical incision and 6 (24%) in the oblique incision group had evidence of infrapatellar nerve injury. The skin area of altered sensation was greater in the vertical as compared to the oblique incision group. Four cases developed medial lower leg paresthesia, suggestive of damage to the sartorial branch.

Papastergiou et al.[18] carried out a retrospective study of 230 ACL reconstructions using hamstring tendons. In one group harvesting was through a 3 cm vertical incision, and in a second group through a 3 cm horizontal incision. There was a 39.7% rate of sensory changes in the area innervated by the infrapatellar branch in the first group a 14.9% rate in the second group.

Boon et al.[19] tried to determine safe areas and angles for skin incisions for harvesting semitendinosus and gracilis by looking at 40 cadaveric knees. They reported that when the knee is placed in flexed position, a horizontal line was drawn on the plane of the tibial tuberosity. In the right knee the safe area was between 3.7 cm and 5.5 cm from the tibial tuberosity with a safe incision line at an angle of 51.6°. In left knee, the safe area was between 3.6 cm and 4.9 cm from the tibial tuberosity with the safe incision line being at an angle of 52.5°. However, such measurements may be difficult to reproduce intraoperatively.

Mochizuki et al.[6] reported that the incidence of altered sensitivity through harvesting of the flexor tendons was 58%, which was similar to the findings from our group in which both flexor tendons were harvested and the rate was 58.1%.

LITERATURE REVIEW

Incision

A literature review did not reveal a standard incision method for ST–GT harvest. Friedman[20] stated that the tendon harvest incision should be placed 1 inch (2.54 cm) medial to the tibial tuberosity and then a vertical incision should be placed 3 inches (7.62 cm) distal. Brown et al.[21] preferred an oblique incision placed along the lines of the creases at the superior aspect of the pes anserinus because it allowed for the skin to be retracted parallel to the orientation of the ST and GT, providing better exposure and a more cosmetic scar. Marder et al.[22] recommended making a 4-cm oblique incision over the pes anserinus insertion, approximately 3 finger breadths below the medial joint line to adequately identify the ST and GT.

Yasuda et al.[23] used a 4-cm long incision through the pes anserinus insertion, then split the membranous insertion of the sartorius parallel with its fiber orientation and detached the ST and GT from their tibial insertions through this slit before harvest. Pagnani et al.[24] measured the insertion point of the conjoined structure and the anteromedial tibial surface and reported a mean location 1.9 cm distal to and 2.25 cm medial to the apex of the tibial tuberosity. They also reported that the ST and GT became distinct structures at 1.8 cm proximal to their combined insertion site.

Tillet et al.[25] have described a diagonal surgical incision created between a proximal point placed 3 cm medial to the tibial tuberosity and at 3 cm distal and 5 cm medial to the tibial tuberosity would provide consistent ST and GT identification for graft harvest.

Prodromos[26] has described a posterior approach. The posterior mini-incision graft harvest technique provides safe and reliable graft harvest, virtually eliminates the risk of cutting hamstring grafts short, and provides excellent cosmetic.

Damage to the IPBSN is a well-known complication of knee surgery.[6,15,16,27-35] Many patients are not advised of this preoperatively because the nerve is purely sensory.[35] Injury can result in postoperative numbness, dysesthesia, painful neuroma, and possibly reflex sympathetic dystrophy.[29,34] Furthermore, anterior knee pain and difficulty kneeling have been directly attributed to damage of these branches. The course of the IPBSN has been well described.[35-37] Care should be taken to prevent injury to the IPBSN if possible. The incidence rate of IPBSN injury in one recent study was 22.2%.[30] In a study Portland et al.[38] have compared horizontal and vertical incisions. They have shown that horizontal incision leads to less complications with the IPBSN 43% (18 patients) for the horizontal incision versus 59% (20 patients) for the vertical incision.

Sanders et al.[13] found a 19% prevalence of isolated injury to the infrapatellar branch after hamstring harvest with a mini-incision and a 32% injury rate to both the IPBSN and sartorial branch, which is comparable to reported rates of sensory disturbance ranging from 22% to 58%. However, they found an increased isolated injury rate of 23% to the sartorial branch of the saphenous nerve (SBSN), which has not been previously reported. In all, 55% of our patients had sartorial branch injury with or without IPBSN injury. Similar to prior authors, they found that the nerve damage was present after 6 months and likely be permanent in most cases (80%).[18,39-41] Slocum and Larson noted sensory loss in the distribution of the saphenous nerve in three patients after pes anserinus transplantation.[42] Zarins and Rowe observed similar changes after reoperation in two patients who had previously undergone pes anserinus transfer.[43] Sgaglione et a1. reported a 37% incidence of infrapatellar paresthesia in patients who had undergone primary repair of a torn ACL with ST augmentation.[44] This procedure was performed by an open technique, and this finding may be a result of the arthrotomy rather than the tendon harvest.

Harvesting

The technique of harvest has varied in previous reports, but most authors identified the tendons at their musculotendinous junction in the thigh and then proceeded to free the grafts in a proximal-to-distal direction.[45-48] In our experience, current technical advances favor the isolation of these tendons from a distal-to-proximal direction, using an antero medial incision over the proximal tibia. In ACL reconstruction-augmentation procedures, this same incision may be used for subsequent intra-articular placement of a distally based graft through a tibial drill hole.

SURGICAL PERSONAL TECHNIQUE

The patient is placed in a supine position with a tourniquet high on the thigh to allow for full knee flexion. The knee is placed at 90° flexion, and the pes anserinus tendons are located manually under the skin; then a vertical incision is used (Fig. 3.1). An incision at the level of the musculotendinous junction in the medial thigh has not been needed.

The tendons are identified at a point proximal to where they blend into a conjoined structure. The interval between the tendons is palpable through the skin incision. The sartorius (layer I) is incised along the course of the ST and GT—either along the superior border of the GT (Fig. 3.2). The knee is flexed, to minimize the tension on the saphenous nerve. A curved clamp is passed into the interval between the sartorius and the ST and the GT (Fig. 3.3). A traction force is applied to the tendon via the clamp while fascial connections are meticulously freed in a distal-to-proximal direction using scissors (Fig. 3.4). When performing this dissection, it is helpful to remember that the saphenous nerve crosses just superficial to the GT at the posteromedial joint line. At this point, with the second tendon still largely undissected and the first tendon freed for several centimeters proximally, a right-angled retractor is used to apply counter traction while a Linvatec tendon stripper (Conmed, Utica, NY) is used to carefully ensnare the delivered tendon (Fig. 3.5). The knee remains flexed to protect the saphenous nerve, and a firm, continuous force is delivered in a proximal and medial direction to strip the remainder of the tendon while avoiding deeper neurovascular structures (Fig. 3.6). If the tendon stripper cannot be passed because of a great deal of resistance, it is prudent to remove the stripper and search for the cause of the resistance. The second tendon then may be delivered in a similar manner. At the end of the procedure, we detach from the tibia the conjoint tendon to get a free graft (Fig. 3.7).

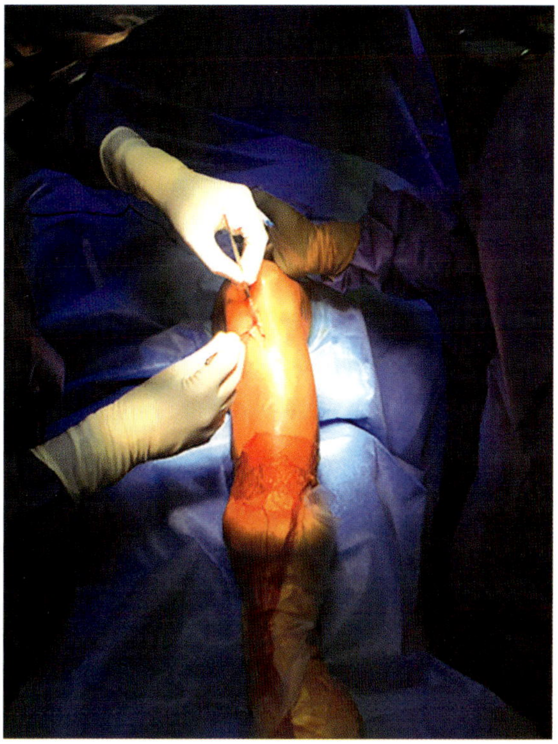

Fig. 3.1: Cutaneous incision.

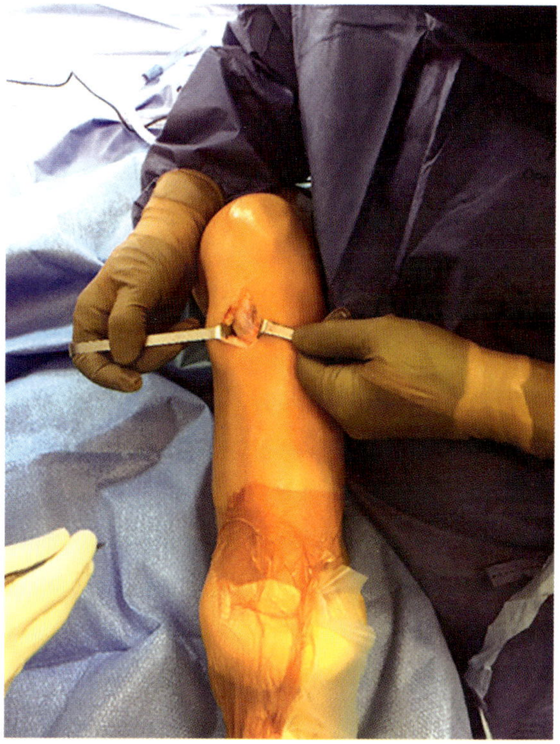

Fig. 3.2: Incision of the sartorius fascia.

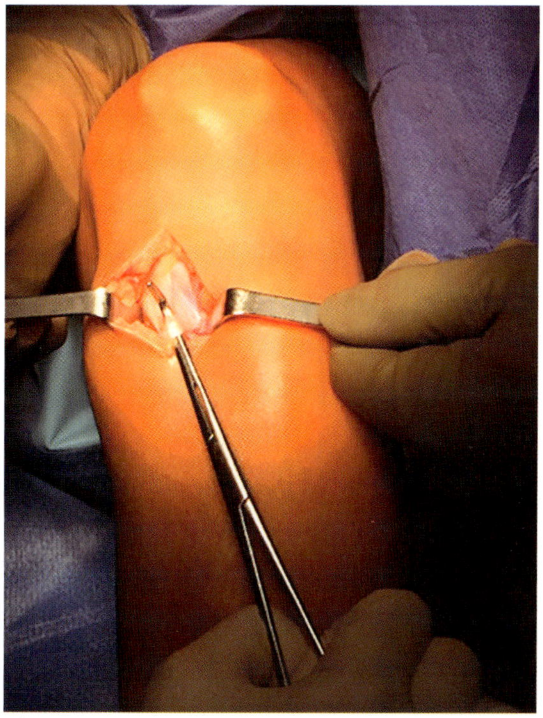

Fig. 3.3: Curved clamp passed into the interval between the sartorius and the semitendinosus and gracilis tendons.

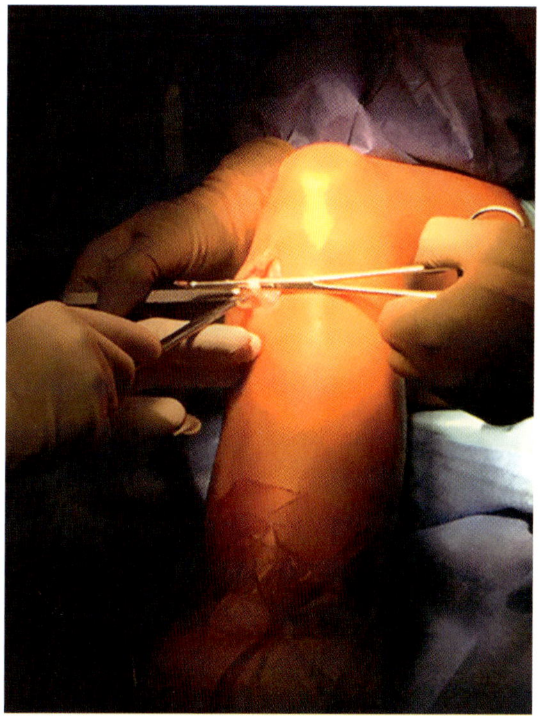

Fig. 3.4: Section of the fascial band.

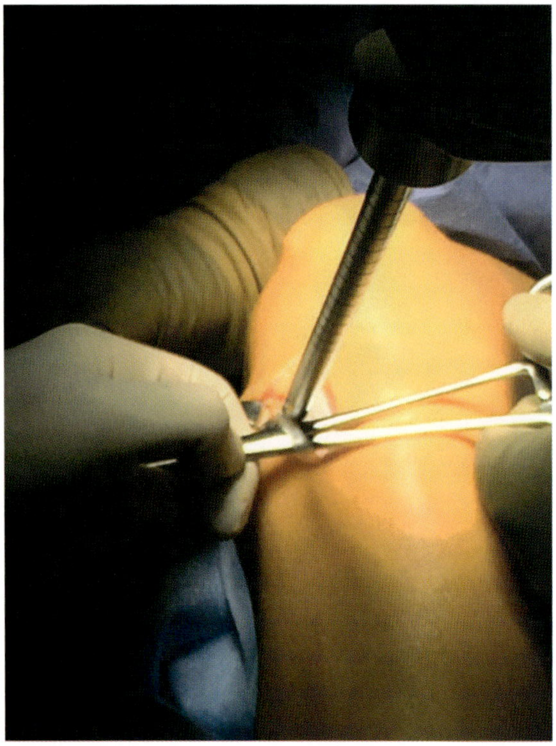

Fig. 3.5: Tendon stripper being harvested.

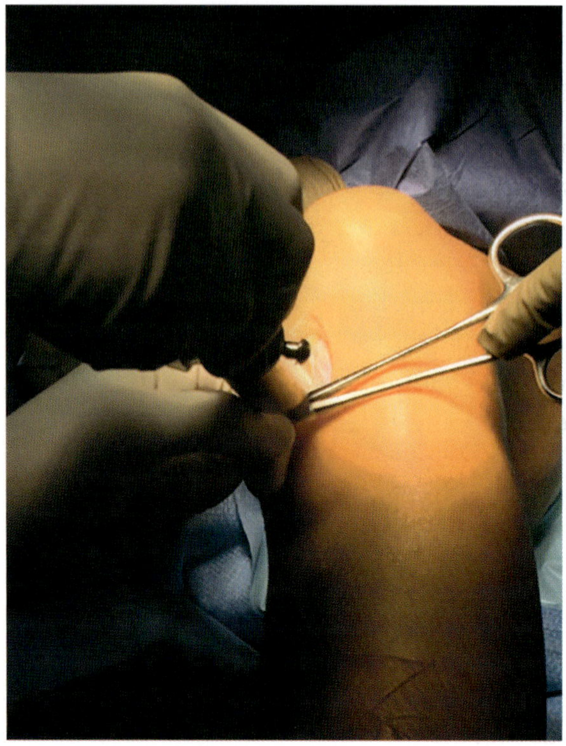

Fig. 3.6: Aspect of the stripper at the end of the procedure.

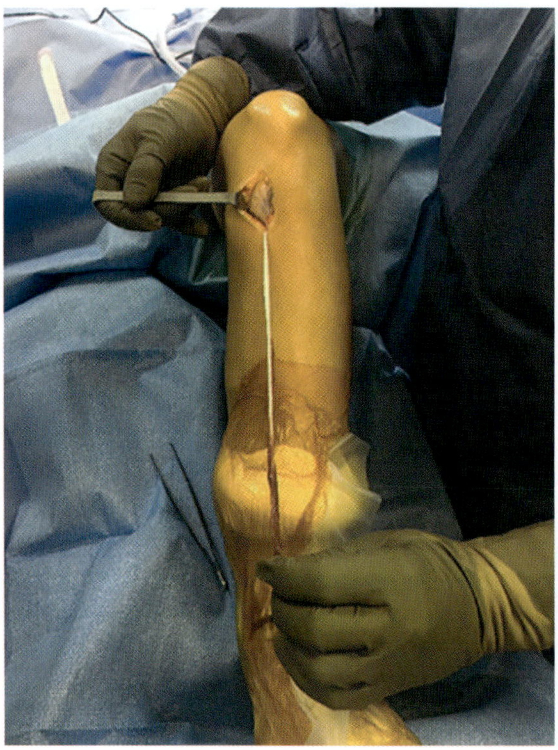

Fig. 3.7: Aspect of the tendon harvested.

COMPLICATIONS

Premature Graft Amputation

A potential disadvantage of the use of hamstring tendons is inconsistency in the graft obtained. There are two main reasons for this inconsistency: It could be due to anatomical small tendons or difficulties with the harvest that results in suboptimal grafts. To successfully harvest the maximal amount of graft available, however, it is imperative to pay strict attention to the anatomy and the potential variations.

Insufficient tendon length can be avoided by a strict and precise surgical technique. If there is a resistance when using the stripper, it could be caused by fascial band or accessory attachment and may cause the stripper to be misdirected and transect the tendon prematurely. The first step is to clearly identify each tendon. The tendons must be separated before harvesting.

The second step is to section with a scissor all the inferior bands to the tendon. Premature division of the tendon graft is the potential disadvantage of this technique, resulting in a shorter graft and possibly necessitating an alternative graft choice.[24,49] The fascial band from ST to GT is one of the reasons for this complication. Studies concerning this fascial band show that this anatomical structure is variable both in size and placement.[8,24,25,49,50]

Prodromos et al.[26] suggested a posterior mini-incision technique that aided in visualizing and releasing a posterior accessory insertion of the semitendinosus. A 2 cm incision in the popliteal crease is used to dissect the hamstring tendons in a proximal-to-distal direction before the harvest to ensure all attachments are released.

Donor Site Pain

Harvesting graft around the knee can lead to donor site pain. We know this problem with the central third of the patellar tendon. However, donor site pain also can occur after hamstring tendon harvest but appears to be transient.

Corry et al.[51] reported only 6% of patients with pain on kneeling after 2 years follow-up with hamstring as compared with 31% after using patellar tendon graft. Yasuda et al. found that activity related at the donor site was rarely restricting and solved by 3 months.[23]

Medial Collateral Ligament Injury

There are no case reports of injury to the superficial MCL during tendon harvesting, but, given the anatomy, the danger is obvious.

The MCL is just deep (layer III) to the gracilis end STs at the point where they become distinct structures. Care must be taken to avoid problem with the scalpel when incising the sartorius fascia or when releasing the GT and ST from their tibial insertion.

Hamstring Strength

There is a lot of debate in the literature regarding the effects of hamstring tendon harvest on tendons strength. It seems intuitive, as BPTB harvesting, that hamstring strength would be reduced after harvesting of GT and ST, but most studies suggest that the deficit is minimal. Lipscomb et al.[47] found no significant deficit with isokinetic testing. Yasuda et al.[23] found that hamstring strength in the reconstructed knee was significantly reduced 1 month after the surgery. Soon et al.[41] found that hamstring strength recovered to preoperative levels by 6 months after surgery. Simonian et al.[52] reported that hamstring strength in the operative side was 95.3% of the nonoperative knee. However, in contrast, Marder et al.[22] reported a significant decrease in hamstring peak torque at 60° per second in knee reconstructed with hamstring compared with knee reconstructed with patellar tendon autograft.

The return of the strength of the hamstring could be caused by regeneration of the hamstring. In 1992, Cross et al.[53] were the first to describe the potential of hamstring tendons to regenerate after harvesting for ACL reconstruction.

Several predictive factors have been identified for tendon regeneration in general. Some examples of determinants that may negatively influence tendon regeneration are the use of nonsteroidal anti-inflammatory drugs,[54] the use of nicotine,[55] and diabetes mellitus.[50,56] However, only one systematic review has described determinants for hamstring tendon regeneration.[57]

Multiple radiologic studies have demonstrated that hamstring tendons regenerate and frequently insert at a more proximal site. Nakamae et al.[58] reported the presence of tendons with more proximal sites insertion on computed tomography scans at 6 months and 12 months; there is a study on strength and there is no effect after tendon harvesting on hamstring peak torque ratios 12 months after surgery.

Other studies have demonstrated the regeneration of the harvested hamstring tendons on postoperative magnetic resonance imaging (MRI) scans. Simonian et al.[52] have measured the precise site: ST and GT inserted in average of 26.7 mm and 47.1 mm more proximal than those on the nonoperative side. Eriksson et al.[50] demonstrated regeneration to the level of the tibial plateau in 8 of 11 patients at 6–12 months postoperatively. They also noted less atrophy in patients with normalized distal hamstring insertions. Rispoli et al.[5] have demonstrated that tendons appeared to regenerate in a proximal-to-distal direction to a level 1–2 cm above the original attachment by 32 months after surgery.

These studies showed that the process of regeneration took place in the 1st year after harvesting and that the regeneration rate could be 100% after 1 year. However, none of these studies reported a clearly defined time period of regeneration. Other studies, with only one evaluation moment, reported regeneration rates for the semitendinosus ranging from 64% to 97%.[58,59]

CONCLUSION

A thorough understanding of the anatomy of the medial side of the knee facilitates hamstring tendon harvest and minimizes the injuries to the saphenous nerve because of proximity to the site of harvest. An oblique incision could reduce injury to the IPBSN.

A good dissection of any accessory fascial bands is required before using the stripper to ensure an adequate graft can be obtained. While hamstring strength reduces, this is not a common long-term functional problem because of the regrowth of the tendons. A careful harvesting technique is mandatory.

REFERENCES

1. Bosworth DM. Transplantation of the semitendinosus for repair of laceration of medial collateral ligament of the knee. J Bone Joint Surg Am. 1952;34-A(1):196-202.
2. Hey-Groves EW. Operation for the repair of the crucial ligaments. Lancet. 1917;190(4914):674-76.

3. Hey-Groves EW. The crucial ligaments of the knee-joint: Their function, rupture, and the operative treatment of the same. Br J Surg. 1919;7(28):505-15.
4. Hey-Groves EW. The use of fascial and tendon grafts in certain fractures and dislocations. Ann Surg. 1934;100(1):20-9.
5. Rispoli DM, Sanders TG, Miller MD, et al. Magnetic resonance imaging at different time periods following hamstring harvest for anterior cruciate ligament reconstruction. Arthroscopy. 2001;17(1):2-8.
6. Mochizuki T, Akita K, Muneta T, et al. Pes anserinus: layered supportive structure on the medial side of the knee. Clin Anat. 2003;17(1):50-4.
7. Ellis H. "Last's Anatomy. 9th ed. R. M. H. McMinn (ed). 245 × 190 mm. Pp 705. Illustrated. 1994. Edinburgh: Churchill Livingstone. £37.50." (Book Review). Br J Surg. 1995;82(2):285.
8. Warren LF, Marshall JL. The supporting structures and layers on the medial side of the knee. J Bone Joint Surg Am. 1979;61(1):56-62.
9. Candal-Couto JJ, Deehan DJ. The accessory bands of Gracilis and Semitendinosus: an anatomical study. Knee. 2003;10(4):325-8.
10. Charalambous CP, Kwaees TA. Anatomical considerations in hamstring tendon harvesting for anterior cruciate ligament reconstruction. Muscles, Ligaments Tendons J. 2013;2(4):253-7.
11. Tuncay I, Kucuker H, Uzun I, et al. The fascial band from semitendinosus to gastrocnemius: the critical point of hamstring harvesting An anatomical study of 23 cadavers. Acta Orthop. 2007;78(3):361-3.
12. Yasin MN, Charalambous CP, Mills SP, et al. Accessory bands of the hamstring tendons: A clinical anatomical study. Clin Anat. 2010;23(7):862-5.
13. Sanders B, Rolf R, McClelland W, et al. Prevalence of saphenous nerve injury after autogenous hamstring harvest: an anatomic and clinical study of sartorial branch injury. Arthroscopy. 2007;23(9):956-63.
14. Arthornthurasook A, Gaew-Im K. The sartorial nerve: Its relationship to the medial aspect of the knee. Am J Sports Med. 1990;18(1):41-2.
15. Kartus J, Ejerhed L, Eriksson BI, et al. The localization of the infrapatellar nerves in the anterior knee region with special emphasis on central third patellar tendon harvest: a dissection study on cadaver and amputated specimens. Arthroscopy. 1999;15(6):577-86.
16. Kartus J, Ejerhed L, Sernert N, et al. Comparison of traditional and subcutaneous patellar tendon harvest. A prospective study of donor site-related problems after anterior cruciate ligament reconstruction using different graft harvesting techniques. Am J Sports Med. 2000;28(3):328-35.
17. Luo H, Yu JK, Ao YF, et al. Relationship between different skin incisions and the injury of the infrapatellar branch of the saphenous nerve during anterior cruciate ligament reconstruction. Chin Med J (Engl). 2007;120(13):1127-30.
18. Papastergiou SG, Voulgaropoulos H, Mikalef P, et al. Injuries to the infrapatellar branch(es) of the saphenous nerve in anterior cruciate ligament reconstruction with four-strand hamstring tendon autograft: vertical versus horizontal incision for harvest. Knee Surg Sports Traumatol Arthrosc. 2006;14(8):789-93.
19. Boon JM, Van Wyk MJ, Jordaan D. A safe area and angle for harvesting autogenous tendons for anterior cruciate ligament reconstruction. Surg Radiol Anat. 2004;26(3):167-71.
20. Friedman MJ. Arthroscopic semitendinosus (gracilis) reconstruction for anterior cruciate ligament deficiency. Tech Orthop. 1988;2(4):74-80.
21. Brown CH Jr, Steiner ME, Carson EW. The use of hamstring tendons for anterior cruciate ligament reconstruction. Technique and results. Clin Sports Med. 1993;12(4):723-56.
22. Marder RA, Raskind JR, Carroll M. Prospective evaluation of arthroscopically assisted anterior cruciate ligament reconstruction. Am J Sports Med. 1991;19(5):478-84.
23. Yasuda K, Tsujino J, Ohkoshi Y, et al. Graft site morbidity with autogenous semitendinosus and gracilis tendons. Am J Sports Med. 1995;23(6):706-14.
24. Pagnani MJ, Warner JJP, O'Brien SJ, et al. Anatomic considerations in harvesting the semitendinosus and gracilis tendons and a technique of harvest. Am J Sports Med. 1993;21(4):565-71.
25. Tillet E, Madsen R, Rogers R, et al. Localization of the semitendinosus-gracilis tendon bifurcation point relative to the tibial tuberosity: an aid to hamstring tendon harvest. Arthroscopy. 2004;20(1):51-4.
26. Prodromos CC, Han YS, Keller BL, et al. Posterior mini-incision technique for hamstring anterior cruciate ligament reconstruction graft harvest. Arthroscopy. 2005;21(2):130-7.

27. Liden M, Ejerhed L, Sernert N, et al. Patellar tendon or semitendinosus tendon autografts for anterior cruciate ligament reconstruction: a prospective, randomized study with a 7-year follow-up. Am J Sports Med. 2007;35(5):740-8.
28. Mochida H, Kikuchi S. Injury to infrapatellar branch of saphenous nerve in arthroscopic knee surgery. Clin Orthop Relat Res. 1995;(320):88-94.
29. Poehling GG, Pollock FE, Koman LA. Reflex sympathetic dystrophy of the knee after sensory nerve injury. Arthroscopy. 1988;4(1):31-5.
30. Sherman OH, Fox JM, Snyder SJ, et al. Arthroscopy--'no-problem surgery'. An analysis of complications in two thousand six hundred and forty cases. J Bone Joint Surg Am. 1986;68(2):256-65.
31. Small NC. Complications in arthroscopic surgery performed by experienced arthroscopists. Arthroscopy. 1988;4(3): 215-21.
32. Small NC. Complications in arthroscopic meniscal surgery. Clin Sports Med. 1990;9(3):609-17.
33. Swanson AJ. The incidence of prepatellar neuropathy following medial meniscectomy. Clin Orthop Relat Res. 1983;(181):151-3.
34. Tennent TD, Birch NC, Holmes MJ, et al. Knee pain and the infrapatellar branch of the saphenous nerve. J R Soc Med. 1998;91(11):573-5.
35. Tifford CD, Spero L, Luke T, et al. The relationship of the infrapatellar branches of the saphenous nerve to arthroscopy portals and incisions for anterior cruciate ligament surgery. An anatomic study. Am J Sports Med. 2000;28(4):562-7.
36. Ebraheim NA, Mekhail AO. The Infrapatellar Branch of the Saphenous Nerve: An Anatomic Study. J Orthop Trauma. 1997;11(3):195-9.
37. Hunter LY, Louis DS, Ricciardi JR, et al. The saphenous nerve: its course and importance in medial arthrotomy. Am J Sports Med. 1979;7(4):227-30.
38. Portland GH, Martin D, Keene G, et al. Injury to the infrapatellar branch of the saphenous nerve in anterior cruciate ligament reconstruction: Comparison of horizontal versus vertical harvest site incisions. Arthroscopy. 2005;21(3): 281-5.
39. Bertram C, Porsch M, Hackenbroch MH, et al. Saphenous neuralgia after arthroscopically assisted anterior cruciate ligament reconstruction with a semitendinosus and gracilis tendon graft. Arthroscopy. 2000;16(7):763-6.
40. Spicer DD, Blagg SE, Unwin AJ, et al. Anterior knee symptoms after four-strand hamstring tendon anterior cruciate ligament reconstruction. Knee Surg Sports Traumatol Arthrosc. 2000;8(5):286-9.
41. Soon M, Neo CP, Mitra AK, et al. Morbidity following anterior cruciate ligament reconstruction using hamstring autograft. Ann Acad Med Singapore. 2004;33(2):214-9.
42. Slocum DB, Larson RL. Rotatory instability of the knee. J Bone Joint Surg Am. 2002;84(5):868.
43. Zarins B, Rowe CR. Combined anterior cruciate-ligament reconstruction using semitendinosus tendon and iliotibial tract. J Bone Joint Surg Am. 1986;68(2):160-77.
44. Sgaglione NA, Warren RF, Wickiewicz TL, et al. Primary repair with semitendinosus tendon augmentation of acute anterior cruciate ligament injuries. Am J Sports Med. 1990;18(1):64-73.
45. Ellera Gomes JL, Marczyk LR. Anterior cruciate ligament reconstruction with a loop or double thickness of semitendinosus tendon. Am J Sports Med. 1984;12(3):199-203.
46. Lipscomb AB, Johnston RK, Snyder RB. The technique of cruciate ligament reconstruction. Am J Sports Med. 1981;9(2):77-81.
47. Lipscomb AB, Johnston RK, Snyder RB, et al. Evaluation of hamstring strength following use of semitendinosus and gracilis tendons to reconstruct the anterior cruciate ligament. Am J Sports Med. 1982;10(6):340-2.
48. McMaster JH, Weinert CR, Scranton P. Diagnosis and management of isolated anterior cruciate ligament tears. J Trauma. 1974;14(3):230-5.
49. Solman CG, Pagnani MJ. Hamstring tendon harvesting. Orthop Clin North Am. 2003;34(1):1-8.
50. Eriksson K, Larsson H, Wredmark T, et al. Semitendinosus tendon regeneration after harvesting for ACL reconstruction. Knee Surg Sports Traumatol Arthrosc. 1999;7(4):220-5.
51. Corry IS, Webb JM, Clingeleffer AJ, et al. Arthroscopic reconstruction of the anterior cruciate ligament. A comparison of patellar tendon autograft and four-strand hamstring tendon autograft. Am J Sports Med. 1999;27(4):444-54.
52. Simonian PT, Harrison SD, Cooley VJ, et al. Assessment of morbidity of semitendinosus and gracilis tendon harvest for ACL reconstruction. Am J Knee Surge. 1997;10(2):54-9.

53. Cross MJ, Roger G, Kujawa P, et al. Regeneration of the semitendinosus and gracilis tendons following their transection for repair of the anterior cruciate ligament. Am J Sports Med. 1992;20(2):221-3.
54. O' Connor JP, Lysz T. Celecoxib, NSAIDs and the skeleton. Drugs Today (Barc). 2008;44(9):693-709.
55. Nho SJ, Yadav H, Shindle MK, et al. Basic Science Update: Rotator Cuff Degeneration. Am J Sports Med. 2008;36(5): 987-93.
56. Eriksson K, Kindblom LG, Hamberg P, et al. The semitendinosus tendon regenerates after resection: A morphologic and MRI analysis in 6 patients after resection for anterior cruciate ligament reconstruction. Acta Orthop. 2001;72(4):379-84.
57. Suijkerbuijk MA, Reijman M, Lodewijks SJ, et al. Hamstring Tendon Regeneration After Harvesting. Am J Sports Med. 2015;43(10):2591-8.
58. Nakamae A, Deie M, Yasumoto M, et al. Three-dimensional computed tomography imaging evidence of regeneration of the semitendinosus tendon harvested for anterior cruciate ligament reconstruction. J Comput Assist Tomogr. 2005;29(2):241-5.
59. Janssen RP, van der Velden MJ, Pasmans HL, et al. Regeneration of hamstring tendons after anterior cruciate ligament reconstruction. Knee Surg Sports Traumatol Arthrosc. 2013;21(4):898-905.

CHAPTER

4

Cosmetic Harvesting of the Hamstring Tendons

Wolfgang Franz

INTRODUCTION

Arthroscopic anterior cruciate ligament (ACL) reconstruction has become a routine elective procedure in sports medicine. The most commonly used grafts for ACL reconstruction are the bone-patellar tendon-bone graft, the quadriceps tendon, and the hamstring tendon (HT) graft.[1-4] But harvesting the tendon graft is one of the most challenging aspects of hamstring ACL reconstruction.

Several reports have demonstrated fewer donor-site-related problems, so HT reconstruction has gained increasing popularity in recent years.[5-7] However, some studies have reported permanent postoperative paresthesia in the distribution of the saphenous nerve with the use of HT grafts.[6,8,9] HT harvest is commonly performed with a longitudinal anterior skin incision directly over the pes anserinus on the proximal tibia.[9] Paraesthesia over the anterolateral aspect of the leg postoperatively due to an injury to the saphenous nerve is a well-known complication linked to this approach.[10] Sanders et al. found that up to 74% of their patients reported reduced sensation in the distribution of the saphenous nerve with the anteromedial approach.[10] Identifying and releasing the HTs at their distal insertion can be technically demanding sometimes.[11]

To avoid these issues related to the anteromedial approach we have been using a minimal invasive technique for harvesting the HTs from a posteromedial incision in the popliteal fossa since 2001 and have performed this procedure in over 5,000 patients. The surgical technique was first published in 2004 and has subsequently been described by Kodkani and later, with an additional anterior incision, by Prodromos.[12-14]

Last but not least, it yields superior cosmetic results, since the scar will be nearly invisible in the backside of the knee.

SURGICAL TECHNIQUE

With the help of an assistant, the knee is flexed to approximately 40° and the hip maximally externally rotated (Fig. 4.1). The assistant must not hold the leg at the calf but only at the foot and thigh. A small transverse incision about 20–30 mm, in line with the skin crease, is made directly over the semitendinosus (ST) tendon in the posteromedial aspect of the popliteal fossa. At this location, the tendon lies subcutaneous and can easily be palpated. The site of the incision is visible as a small dimple overlying the tendon—this landmark has previously been named "Jobert's groove" in Pernkopf's topographical anatomy atlas.[15] Subcutaneous tissue overlying the tendon is usually scarce, even in obese patients.

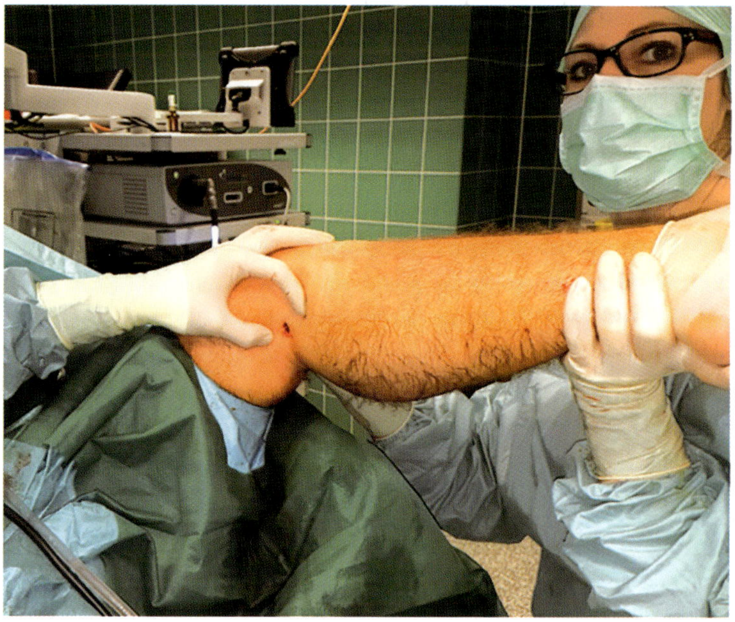

Fig. 4.1: Positioning of the leg and skin incision.

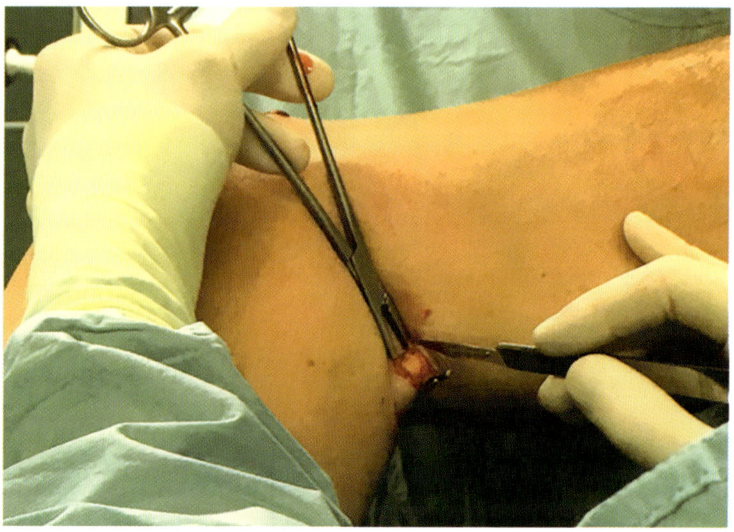

Fig. 4.2: Hooking the tendon and releasing surrounding tissue.

Once the skin incision is made, the fascia covering the tendon is cut longitudinally over the tendon under direct vision. A curved artery clip is hooked around the tendon and a FiberTape® (Arthrex, Naples, FL) suture is pulled through and looped around the tendon to grip the graft (Fig. 4.2).

With the knee flexed to 90° the tendon is mobilized and pulled out with a quite powerful motion to distal and proximal.

An open tendon stripper is threaded over the tendon and pushed proximally to release the tendon of its muscular attachment. The stripper has to go forward with minimum force. Otherwise there will be an

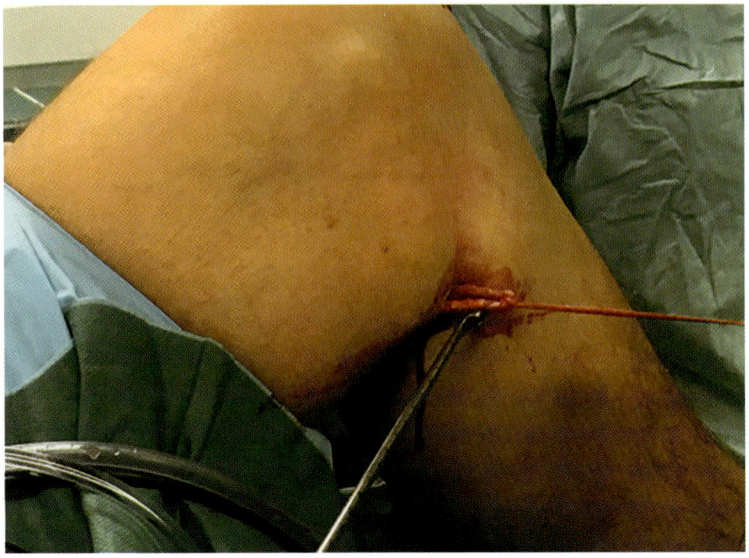

Fig. 4.3: Pulling out the tendon and applying the open stripper.

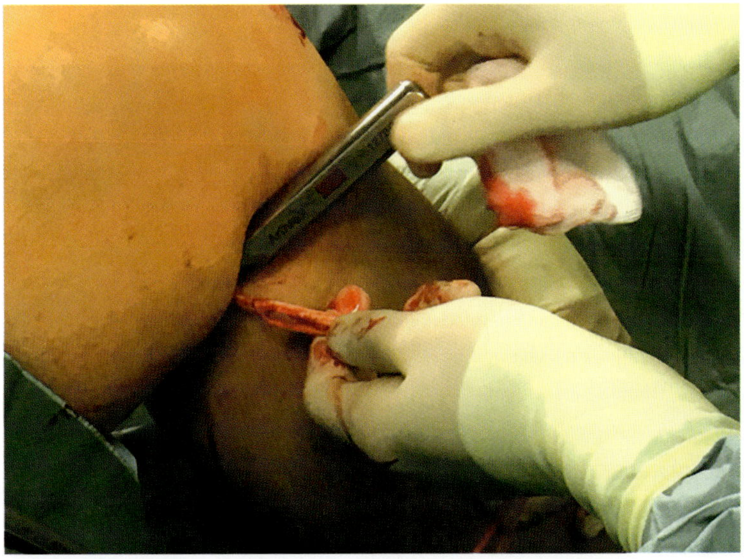

Fig. 4.4: Releasing the tendon proximally.

obstacle by the fascia and the fascial incision should be slightly increased (Fig. 4.3). It must also be ensured that there are no fascial bands which may lead to premature tendon amputation.

The free end of the tendon is then delivered out of the wound. At this point we scrape remaining muscular tissue off the proximal tendon to facilitate passage of a closed tendon stripper (Fig. 4.4).

The closed tendon stripper is then advanced distally while a controlled pull on the tendon is maintained. With slow careful twisting motions the tendon harvester is pushed further distal to release the tendon from its insertion on the tibia. Distally, the stripper can be seen through the skin over the medial aspect of the proximal tibial crest (Fig. 4.5).

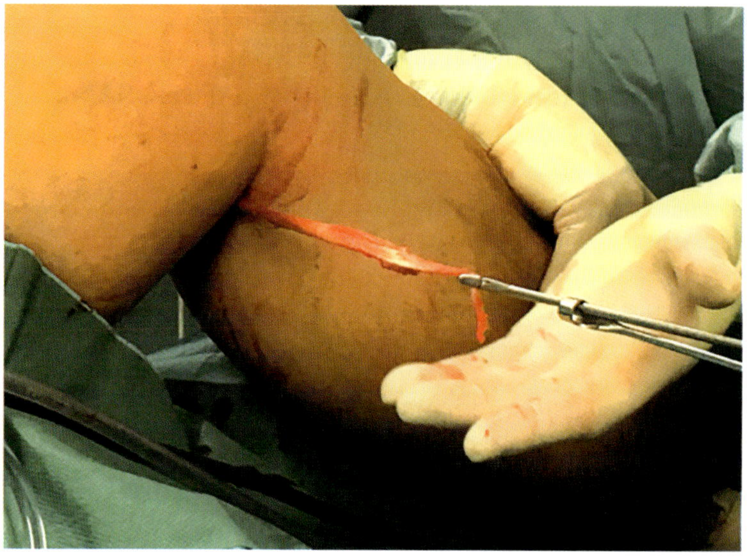

Fig. 4.5: Applying the closed stripper.

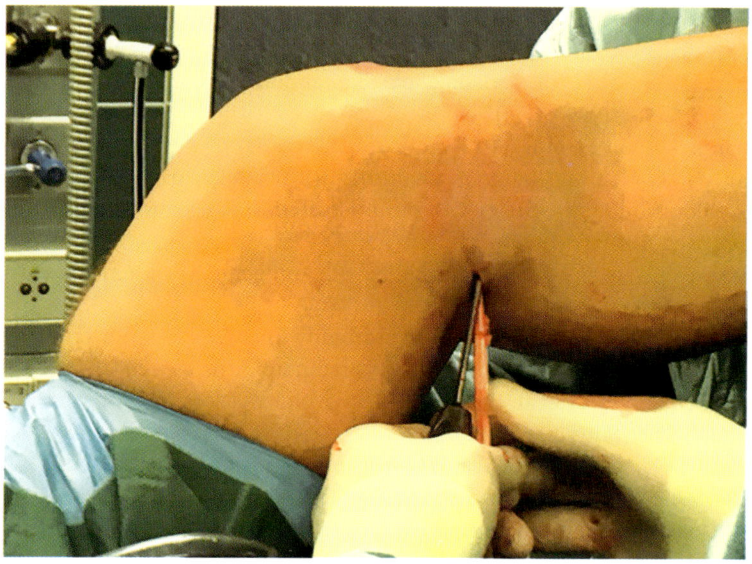

Fig. 4.6: Releasing the tendon distally.

If required, the gracilis tendon can be harvested in the same way. It lies approximately 10 mm medial to the ST tendon and can be delivered through the same skin incision.[14] The skin is closed with interrupted nonabsorbable sutures. Care has to be taken not to catch deeper tissues with the needle (Fig. 4.6). It is not necessary to close the sartorius fascia.

In a study published in 2016, we assessed the incidence of iatrogenic injury to branches of the saphenous nerve, the length of the harvested ST tendon and the time needed to harvest the tendon graft comparing our posteromedial approach to the conventional anteromedial approach.[16] This study confirmed our hypothesis that ST tendon harvesting through a small incision in the popliteal fossa is quicker, needs a smaller incision, and avoids the risk of injury to the saphenous nerve. We, therefore, recommend its routine use for hamstring graft harvesting.

https://www.arthrex.com/resources/video/5C9KtJqFiUW5uAFGkEs1lA/minimally-invasive-posteromedial-hamstring-graft-harvesting

PEARLS AND PITFALLS

The positioning of the leg is essential for this technique. The assistant should hold the foot and the distal thigh, but not any soft tissues. If the tendon cannot be palpated through the skin, especially in obese patients, the skin incision should be made right over the medial dimple of the fossa. By this way the tendon always can be found. Then it is important to cut the fascia over the tendon in parallel. This incision should be large enough to prevent the stripper from adhering there. Finally, when using the closed stripper to release the tendon from the pes anserinus, it should be done with controlled force. First the closed stripper should go ahead with the tendon and then the pulling force should be slightly increased while turning the stripper back and forth and by this way approaching to the tibial attachment of the tendon.

REFERENCES

1. Eichhorn HJ, Birkner W. Aktuelle Trends zur Rekonstruktion des vorderen Kreuzbandes. SFA Arthroskopie Aktuell. 2006;19:5-8.
2. Aglietti P, Buzzi R, Zaccherotti G, et al. Patellar tendon versus doubled semitendinosus and gracilis tendons for anterior cruciate ligament reconstruction. Am J Sports Med. 1994;22(2):211-7;discussion 217-8.
3. Feller JA, Webster KE. A randomized comparison of patellar tendon and hamstring tendon anterior cruciate ligament reconstruction. Am J Sports Med. 2003;31(4):564-73.
4. Pinczewski LA, Lyman J, Salmon LJ, et al. A 10-year comparison of anterior cruciate ligament reconstructions with hamstring tendon and patellar tendon autograft: a controlled, prospective trial. Am J Sports Med. 2007;35(4):564-74.
5. Rubinstein RA Jr, Shelbourne KD, VanMeter CD, et al. Isolated autogenous bone-patellar tendon-bone graft site morbidity. Am J Sports Med. 1994;22(3):324-7.
6. Yasuda K, Tsujino J, Ohkoshi Y, et al. Graft site morbidity with autogenous semitendinosus and gracilis tendons. Am J Sports Med. 1995;23(6):706-14.
7. Feller JA, Webster KE, Gavin B. Early post-operative morbidity following anterior cruciate ligament reconstruction: patellar tendon versus hamstring graft. Knee Surg Sports Traumatol Arthrosc. 2001;9(5):260-6.
8. Simonian PT, Harrison SD, Cooley VJ, et al. Assessment of morbidity of semitendinosus and gracilis tendon harvest for ACL reconstruction. Am J Knee Surg. 1997;10(2):54-9.
9. Brown CH Jr, Steiner ME, Carson EW. The use of hamstring tendons for anterior cruciate ligament reconstruction. Technique and results. Clin Sports Med. 1993;12(4):723-56.
10. Sanders B, Rolf R, McClelland W, et al. Prevalence of saphenous nerve injury after autogenous hamstring harvest: an anatomic and clinical study of sartorial branch injury. Arthroscopy. 2007;23(9):956-63.
11. Pagnani MJ, Warner JJ, O'Brien SJ, et al. Anatomic considerations in harvesting the semitendinosus and gracilis tendons and a technique of harvest. Am J Sports Med. 1993;21(4):565-71.
12. Franz W, Ulbrich J. Eine neue Technik zur Entnahme der Semitendinosussehne für den Kreuzbandersatz. Arthroskopie. 2004;17(2):104-7.
13. Kodkani PS, Govekar DP, Patankar HS. A new technique of graft harvest for anterior cruciate ligament reconstruction with quadruple semitendinosus tendon autograft. Arthroscopy. 2004;20(8):e101-4.
14. Prodromos CC, Han YS, Keller BL, et al. Posterior mini-incision technique for hamstring anterior cruciate ligament reconstruction graft harvest. Arthroscopy. 2005;21(2):130-7.
15. Pernkopf E. Topographische Anatomie des Menschen. Lehrbuch und Atlas, II. Urban und Schwarzenberg. 1941.
16. Franz W, Baumann A. Minimally invasive semitendinosus tendon harvesting from the popliteal fossa versus conventional hamstring tendon harvesting for ACL reconstruction: A prospective, randomised controlled trial in 100 patients. Knee. 2016;23(1):106-10.

CHAPTER 5

Preparation of 5- and 6-Strand Hamstring Tendon Grafts for Single-Bundle Hamstring Anterior Cruciate Ligament Reconstruction

Charles H Brown Jr

INTRODUCTION

Single-bundle hamstring anterior cruciate ligament (ACL) reconstruction is most commonly performed using a doubled gracilis and doubled semitendinosus, 4-strand hamstring tendon autograft (Fig. 5.1). Hamner et al.[1] demonstrated that the initial tensile strength of a 4-strand hamstring tendon graft increases linearly with the cross-sectional area of the graft. Larger diameter hamstring tendon grafts are stronger than smaller diameter grafts. Since the diameter of the gracilis and semitendinosus tendons is variable from patient-to-patient, there is concern amongst knee surgeons that ACL reconstructions performed using smaller diameter hamstring tendon grafts may have inadequate initial tensile strength. A recent systematic review demonstrated a 6.8 times greater relative risk of failure for hamstring ACL reconstructions performed with hamstring tendon graft diameters less than 8 mm[2]. This information and other clinical studies support the concept of achieving a minimum hamstring tendon ACL graft diameter of 8 mm when performing a single-bundle hamstring ACL reconstruction.[3-6] In some patients the goal of achieving an 8 mm diameter hamstring tendon ACL graft may be accomplished using a doubled gracilis and semitendinosus, 4-strand graft. However, in other patients it may be necessary to add additional hamstring tendon graft strands to increase the diameter of the hamstring tendon graft. This chapter describes a simple, cost-effective technique using materials commonly available in the operating room to increase the diameter of hamstring tendon ACL

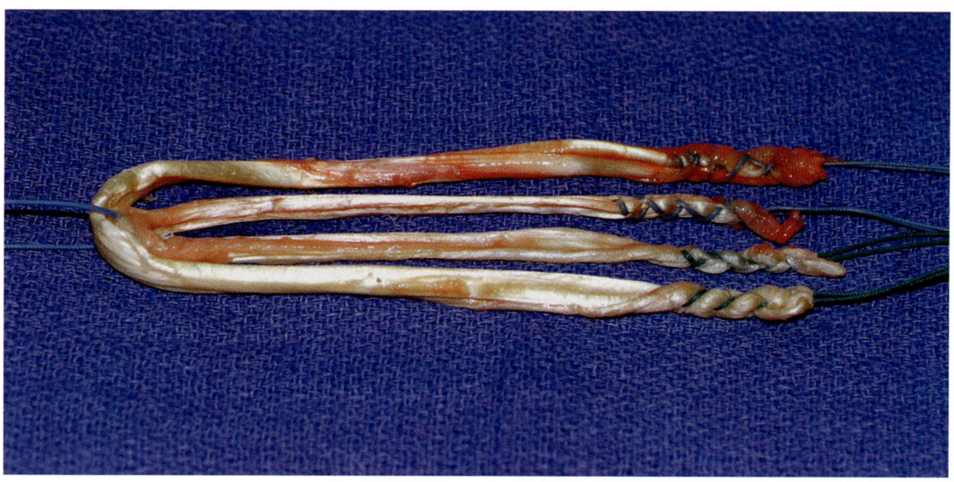

Fig. 5.1: Doubled gracilis and doubled semitendinosus, 4-strand hamstring tendon graft.

grafts. The technique described in this chapter was developed by the author in 2006 and has been used in over 2,000 cases at the author's institution.

HAMSTRING TENDON HARVEST

To prepare a 5- or 6-strand hamstring tendon ACL graft, the gracilis and semitendinosus tendons must be detached from the tibia. The distal end of each tendon is sutured with 5 throws of a running baseball type whip-stitch using a #2 FiberWire® suture (Arthrex, Naples, FL). It is important to use a high strength suture material such as FiberWire since this allows the connecting knots used in the preparation of the graft to be tied firmly. A #1 or #2 polyester suture may break when tied with firm tension. After whip-stitching the distal end of each tendon with a #2 FiberWire suture, the two tendons are harvested with a tendon stripper. Preparation of the hamstring tendon grafts is facilitated by the use of a graft preparation board (Graft Master III, Smith and Nephew Advanced Surgical Devices, Andover, MA). Residual muscle fibers on the proximal end of both tendons are removed using blunt dissection with a metal ruler, a large curette or a Cushing type periosteal elevator.

PREPARATION OF 5-STRAND HAMSTRING TENDON GRAFT

A 5-strand hamstring tendon graft is prepared by tripling the semitendinosus tendon and doubling the gracilis tendon (Fig. 5.2). A minimum length of 240 mm after pretensioning the whip-stitches is required to triple the semitendinosus tendon. A semitendinosus tendon of this length will result in a graft length of 75–80 mm when tripled. A 75–80 mm long tripled semitendinosus graft will allow 20–25 mm of tendon graft to be inserted into the ACL femoral socket, 25–30 mm across the joint for the intra-articular length of the ACL, and 20–35 mm for insertion into the ACL tibial tunnel. The proximal ends of the gracilis and semitendinosus tendons are whip-stitched with a #2 FiberWire® suture (Arthrex, Naples, FL). It is important to use a high strength suture as this allows the connecting knots used to tie the semitendinosus tendon to the polyester loop of the ACL femoral implant and the Dacron tape to be tied with firm tension. A minimum of 5 whip-stitch throws in each tendon are required to achieve adequate strength and security.

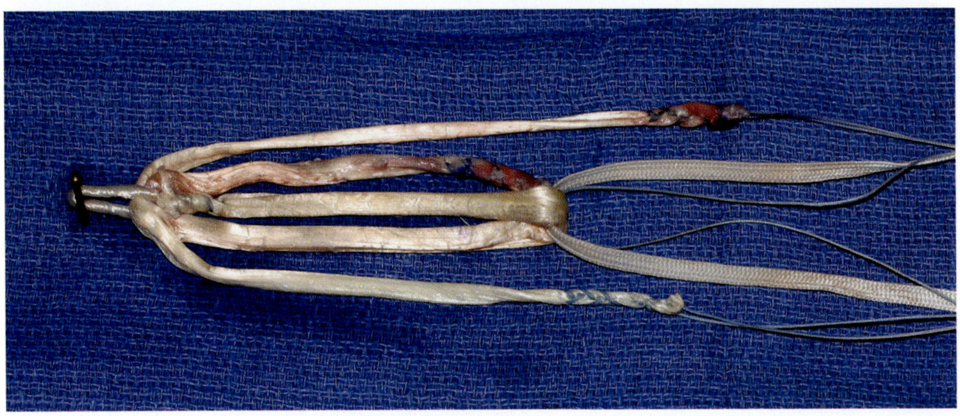

Fig. 5.2: A 5-strand hamstring tendon ACL graft is prepared by tripling the semitendinosus tendon and doubling the gracilis tendon.

Thinner tendons will require more suture throws. Slack in the whip-stitches is removed and the ends of each tendon compressed by applying tension to the FiberWire sutures at both ends of the tendon using a back and forth "cinching" motion. This is a very important step as it removes slack from the suture-tendon construct and compresses the ends of the two tendons. Cinching the whip-stitch sutures will often shorten the total length of the two tendons by 5–10 mm.

A 15 mm ENDOBUTTON CL® fixed loop implant (Smith & Nephew Advanced Surgical Devices, Andover, MA) is most commonly used for femoral fixation of the ACL graft. Using a 3-portal surgical technique and drilling the ACL femoral tunnel through an accessory anteromedial (AAM) portal typically results in a femoral tunnel length of 35–45 mm. When used in ACL femoral tunnels in this length range, a 15 mm ENDOBUTTON CL® implant will allow 20–30 mm of graft to be inserted into the ACL femoral socket. A 15 mm ENDOBUTTON CL® implant is inserted into the ENDOBUTTON Holder (Smith and Nephew Advanced Surgical Devices, Andover, MA) and the #2 FiberWire sutures from the proximal end of the semitendinosus tendon are tied to the polyester loop of the ENDOBUTTON CL® implant (Fig. 5.3). The knots should be tied as firmly as possible. It is important that the proximal and not the distal end of the semitendinosus tendon be tied to the polyester loop of the ENDOBUTTON CL® implant. Tying the proximal end of the semitendinosus tendon to the ENDOBUTTON CL® polyester loop will usually produce a 5-stranded graft in which the tibial end of the graft is 0.5–1 mm larger in diameter than the femoral end of the graft. Since the native ACL tibial attachment site is larger than the ACL femoral attachment site, an ACL graft with a larger diameter on the tibial end of the graft will increase the percentage of the native ACL tibial attachment site that is restored.

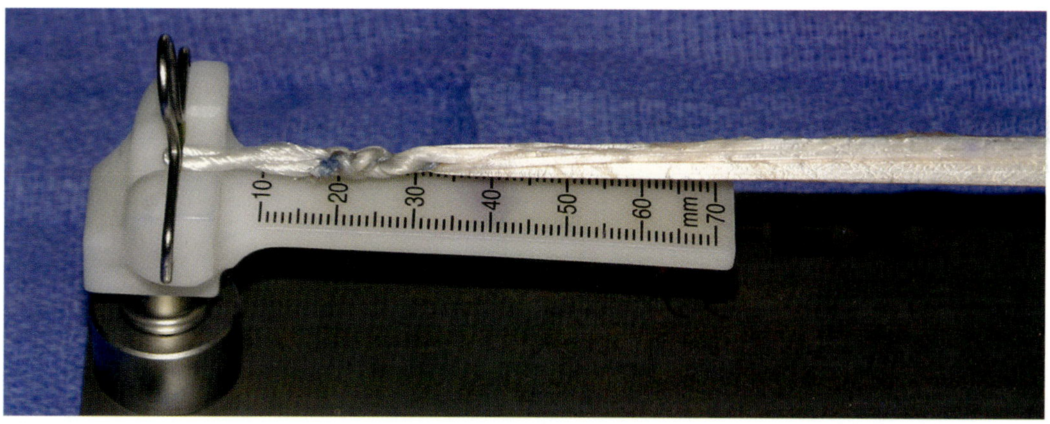

Fig. 5.3: The #2 FiberWire sutures from the proximal end of the semitendinosus tendon graft are tied to the polyester loop of the ENDOBUTTON implant. This step connects the semitendinosus tendon graft to the polyester loop of the ENDOBUTTON implant.

Using a tapered free needle the #2 FiberWire sutures from the distal end of the semitendinosus tendon are passed 5 mm apart through the midpoint of a 5-mm Dacron tape, creating a horizontal mattress suture configuration. The FiberWire sutures are tied firmly against the Dacron tape. This step connects the distal end of the semitendinosus tendon to the Dacron tape (Figs. 5.4A to C). Although it is possible to create a 5-strand hamstring tendon graft without using Dacron tape, the Dacron tape locks the middle strand of the graft into the axilla of the looped end of the semitendinosus tendon and helps prevent the

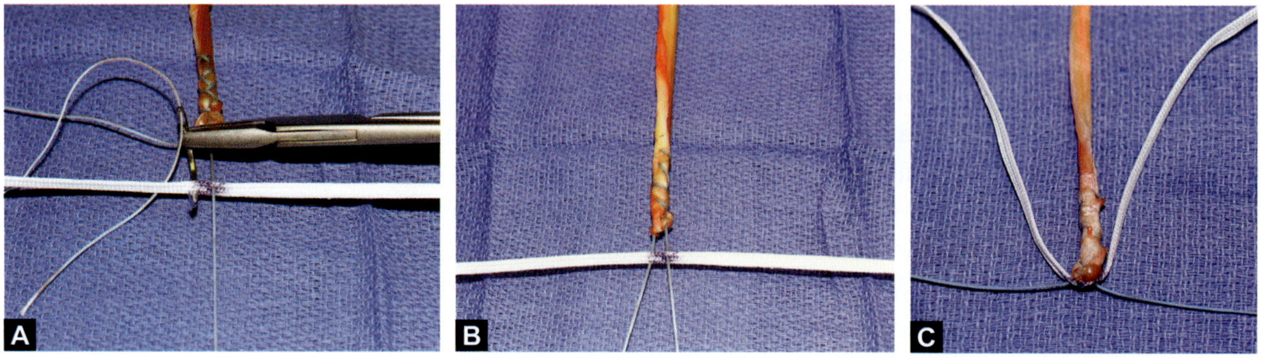

Figs. 5.4A to C: (A and B) The FiberWire sutures from the distal end of the semitendinosus graft are passed through the middle of the 5 mm Dacron tape using a tapered free needle. This step creates a horizontal mattress suture. (C) The FiberWire sutures are tied together firmly, connecting the distal end of the semitendinosus tendon to the 5 mm Dacron tape.

middle strand from slipping out of the looped end of the tripled semitendinosus graft. Securing the middle strand of the semitendinosus graft inside the axilla of the looped end of the semitendinosus grafts allows more uniform tension to be applied to the 3 graft strands (Figs. 5.5A and B). Using a small curved clamp, the FiberWire sutures and both ends of the Dacron tape and the distal end of the semitendinosus tendon graft are passed through the polyester loop of the ENDOBUTTON CL® implant. The distal end of the semitendinosus tendon is passed through the polyester loop of the ENDOBUTTON CL® implant using the Dacron tape and the FiberWire sutures. The ends of the Dacron tape and the FiberWire sutures are

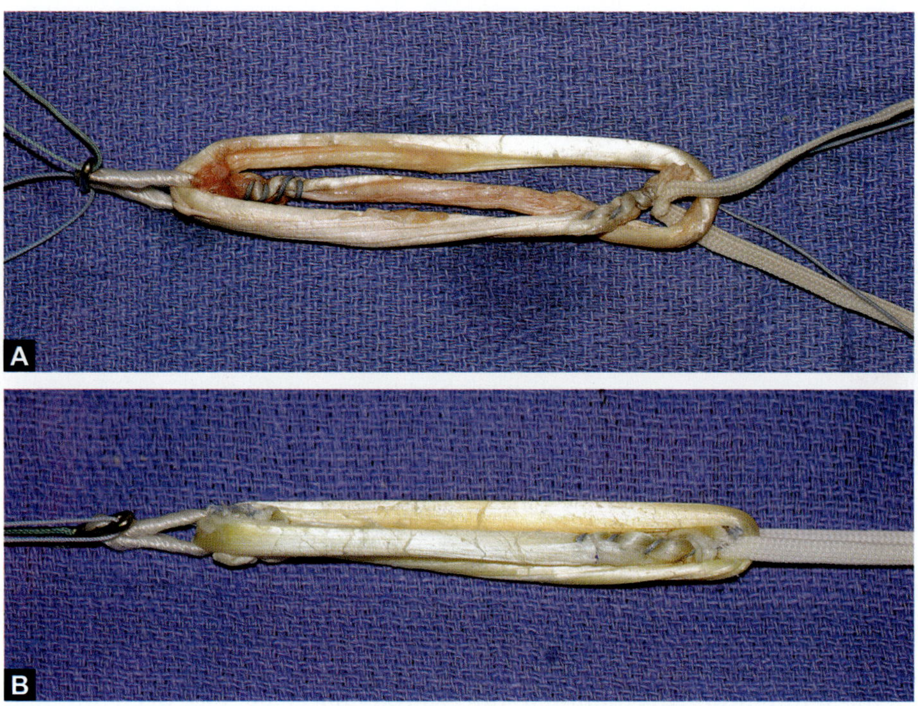

Figs. 5.5A and B: (A) Tripled-semitendinosus graft. The distal end of the semitendinosus graft is passed into the axilla of the looped end of the graft. (B) Tensioning both ends of the 5 mm Dacron tape locks the middle strand of the semitendinosus tendon inside the axilla of the looped end of the semitendinosus tendon graft.

separated and one end of the Dacron tape and one of the #2 FiberWire sutures are passed on each side of the loop of semitendinosus tendon. This step results in the looped part of the semitendinosus tendon being straddled on either side by the Dacron tape and FiberWire sutures. Tension is applied to both ends of the Dacron tape and the FiberWire sutures, pulling the distal end of the semitendinosus tendon into the axilla of the looped part of the semitendinosus tendon, creating a tripled semitendinosus tendon graft in the process. Tension is applied to the Dacron tape and FiberWire sutures. This step aligns and locks the distal end of the semitendinosus tendon inside the looped end of the semitendinosus tendon and equally tensions all 3 strands of the tripled semitendinosus tendon graft (Figs. 5.6A to E).

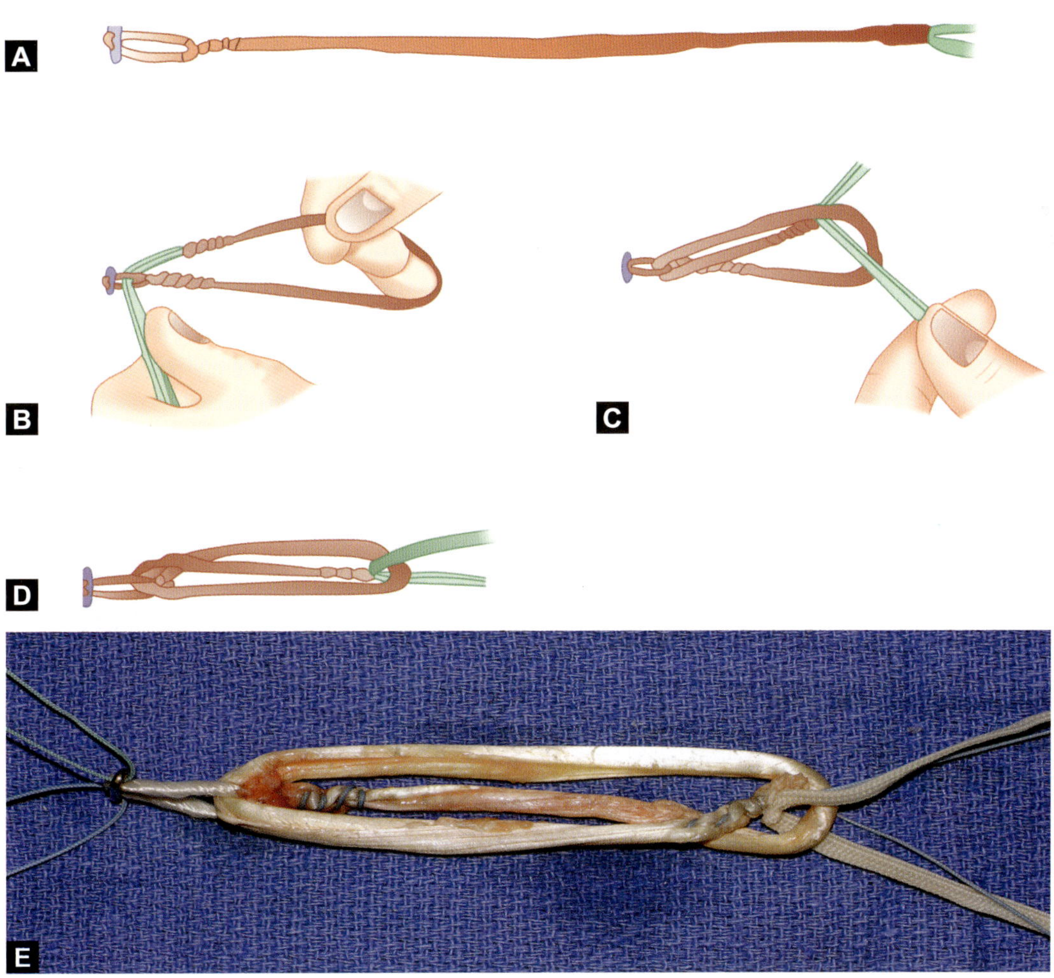

Figs. 5.6A to E: Steps in preparing a tripled-semitendinosus anterior cruciate ligament (ACL) graft. (A) The proximal end of the semitendinosus graft is tied to the polyester loop of the ENDOBUTTON CL® implant, and the distal end to 5 mm Dacron tape. (B) The #2 FiberWire sutures, both ends of the Dacron tape and the distal end of the semitendinosus tendon are passed through the polyester loop of the ENDOBUTTON CL® implant. (C) One side of the Dacron tape and one of the #2 FiberWire sutures are passed on each side of the distal loop of semitendinosus tendon. (D) The distal end of the semitendinosus graft, which becomes the middle strand of the tripled graft, is pulled into the axilla of the looped end of the semitendinosus, creating a tripled semitendinosus graft. The looped end of the semitendinosus tendon is straddled by the 5 mm Dacron tape and #2 FiberWire sutures, which helps lock the middle strand of the semitendinosus graft inside the axilla of the looped end of the graft. (E) Final appearance of the tripled semitendinosus tendon graft.

Although it is possible to use other techniques to triple the semitendinosus tendon, one of the advantages of the above technique is that the suture connections on each end of the semitendinosus tendon graft are stress shielded by the looped part of the semitendinosus tendon.

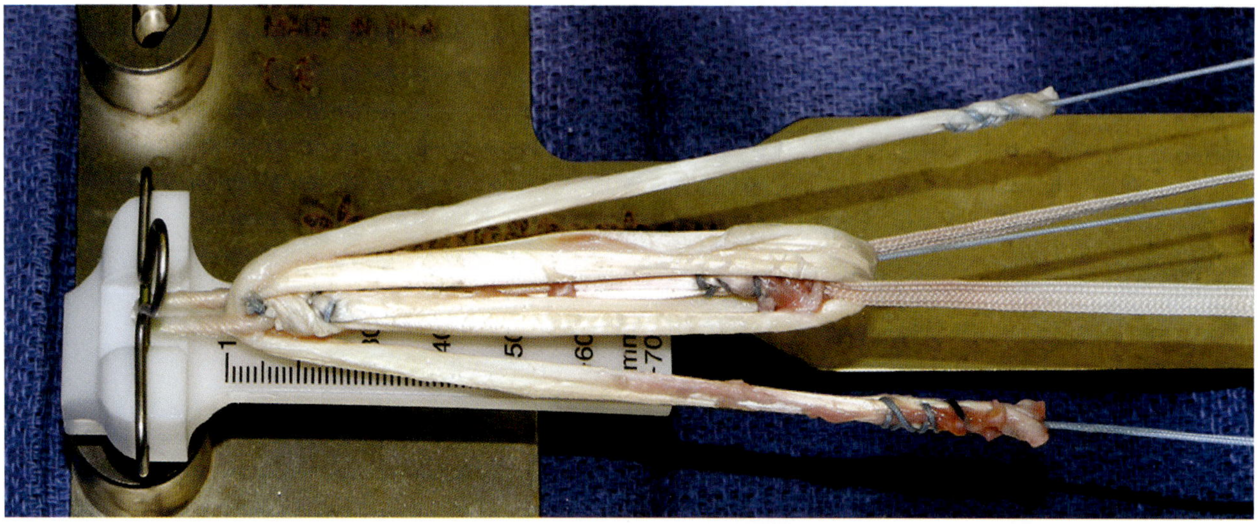

Fig. 5.7: The gracilis tendon is passed through the polyester loop of the ENDOBUTTON implant creating a 5-strand hamstring tendon graft.

The gracilis tendon is passed through the polyester loop of the ENDOBUTTON CL® implant, and the ends of the gracilis tendon adjusted such that they are equal in length. This step creates a 5-strand hamstring tendon graft (Fig. 5.7). The FiberWire sutures from one end of the gracilis and one of the FiberWire sutures and one end of the Dacron tape on the same side of the semitendinosus graft are tied together at a distance of 120–150 mm from the end of the graft using a single throw. The Dacron tape and FiberWire sutures on the opposite side of the graft are marked with a surgical marker at the same distance as the previously tied knot on the opposite side of the graft. The Dacron tape and FiberWire sutures on this side of the graft are tied together at the marked location. This step creates 2 equal length suture/tape loops on each side of the 5-strand graft. It is important not to suture the 5 graft strands together, as this will prevent equal tensioning of the 5 graft strands. At the time of final graft fixation, the two Dacron tape/suture loops are looped around the opposite sides of a graft tensioning device. This step applies equal tension to all 5 graft strands (Figs. 5.8A and B).

The diameter of each end of the 5-strand graft is measured to the nearest 0.5 mm using a sizing block. If the 5-strand graft has been prepared as described, the tibial end of the graft is usually 0.5–1 mm larger in diameter than the femoral end of the graft. The 5-strand graft is pretensioned to 10 lbs. using a suture vise with tensiometer (Smith and Nephew Advanced Surgical Devices, Andover, MA). This step allows stress relaxation of the Dacron tape, FiberWire sutures and tendon graft strands (Fig. 5.9). The prepared 5-strand hamstring tendon graft is wrapped in a 4" × 4" sponge that has been soaked in 500 mg of vancomycin mixed with 100 cc of normal saline (Figs. 5.10A and B). The use of this "vancomycin wrap" technique has been shown to significantly decrease the infection rate after ACL reconstruction.[7-9]

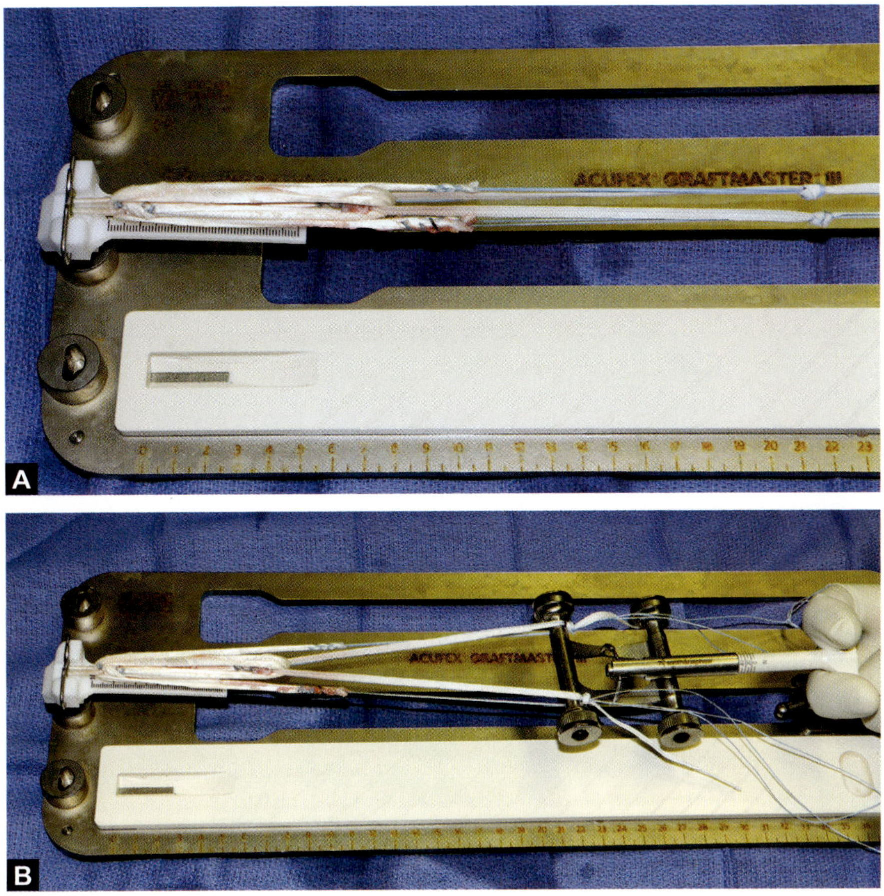

Figs. 5.8A and B: (A) The Dacron tape and one of the attached FiberWire sutures on one side of the semitendinosus graft and the two #2 FiberWire sutures on one side of the gracilis tendon are tied together at an equal length on each side of the 5-strand graft. (B) A spring loaded tensioning device is connected to the two suture/Dacron tape loops on each side of the 5-strand graft at the time of final graft tensioning and fixation.

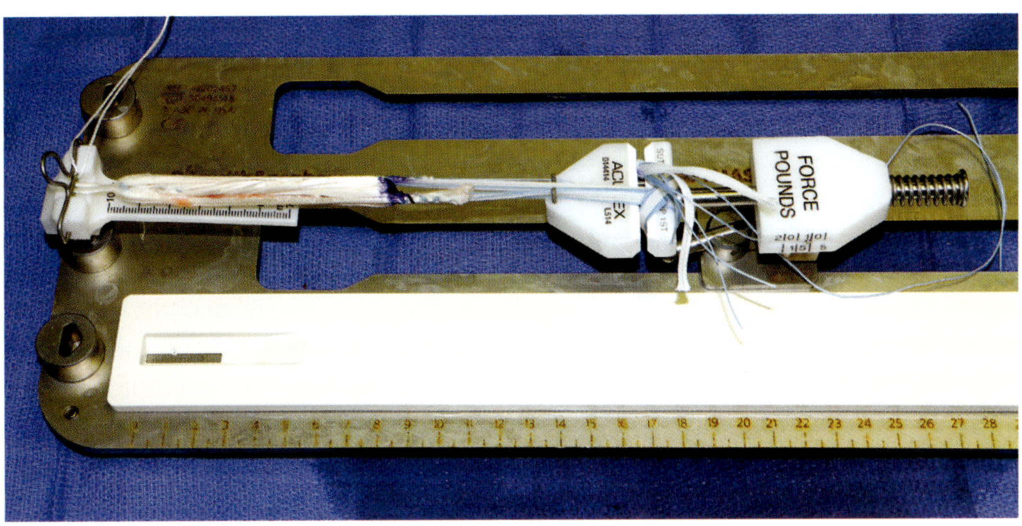

Fig. 5.9: The 5-strand hamstring anterior cruciate ligament (ACL) graft is pretensioned on the graft preparation board.

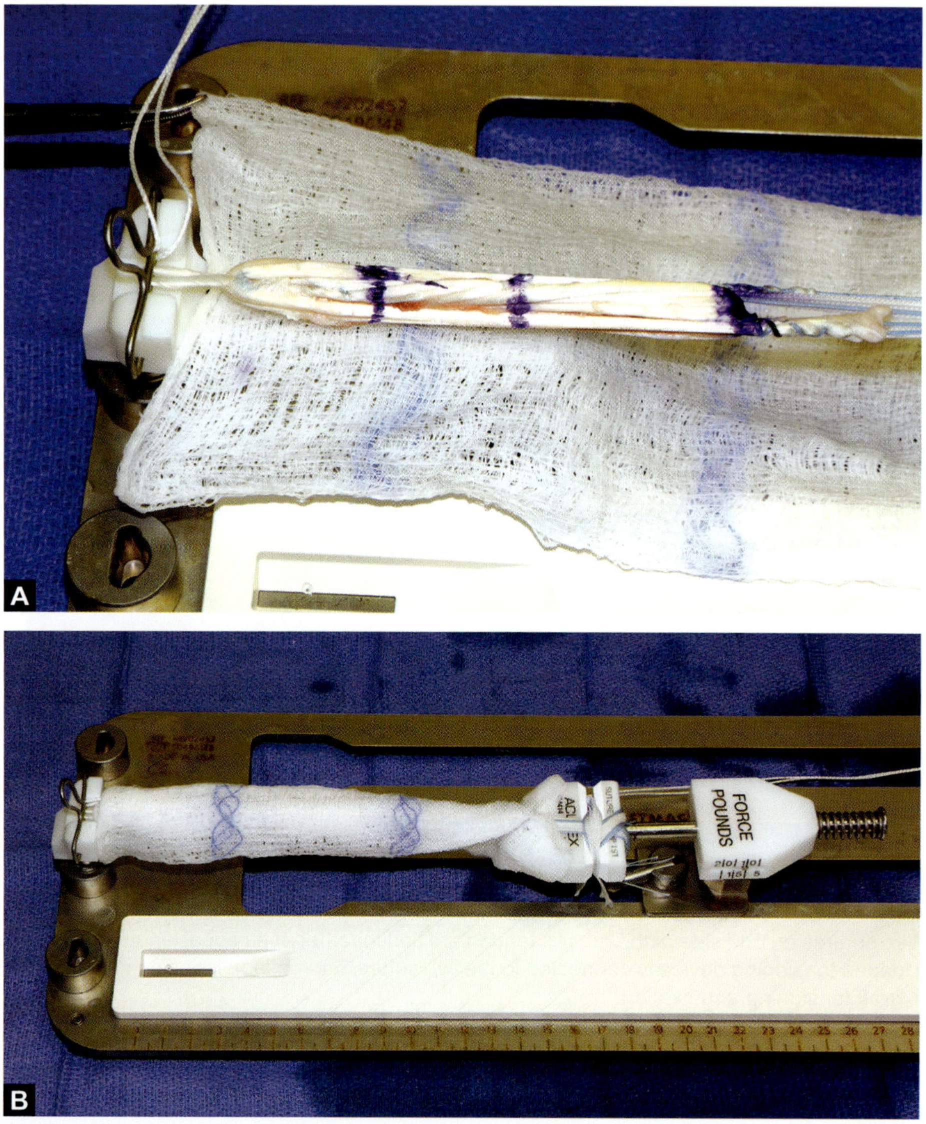

Figs. 5.10A and B: The prepared hamstring anterior cruciate ligament (ACL) graft is wrapped with a surgical sponge soaked in a Vancomycin solution.

PREPARATION OF 6-STRAND HAMSTRING TENDON GRAFT

A 6-strand hamstring tendon graft is prepared by tripling the semitendinosus and gracilis tendons (Fig. 5.11). The proximal end of the gracilis tendon is whip-stitched with a #2 FiberWire suture. The tendon is compressed and slack in the whip-stitch sutures is removed by applying tension to the sutures using a "cinching" motion. The length of the gracilis tendon is then measured. The minimum length for tripling the gracilis tendon is 230 mm. A tendon length less than 230 mm will result in less than 20 mm of tendon graft being inserted into the ACL femoral socket and less than 30 mm of graft in the tibial tunnel, when a 35–40 mm length femoral tunnel is drilled and a 15 mm ENDOBUTTON CL® implant is used. If the gracilis tendon is less than 230 mm in length, preparation of a 5-strand hamstring tendon graft is recommended.

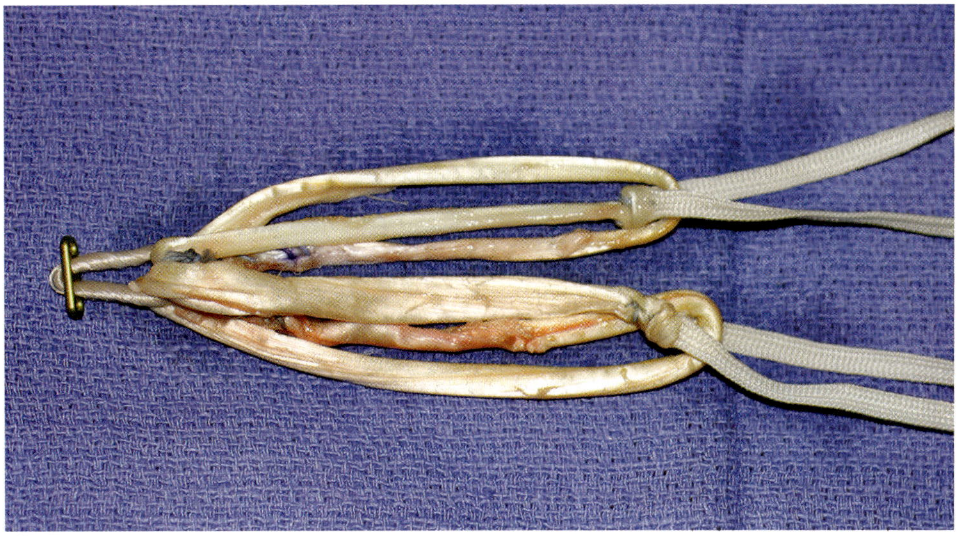

Fig. 5.11: A 6-strand hamstring anterior cruciate ligament (ACL) graft is prepared by tripling both the semitendinosus and gracilis tendons.

The semitendinosus tendon is cut to a length of 10 mm longer than the final length of the gracilis tendon and the proximal end of the semitendinosus tendon whip-stitched with a #2 FiberWire suture. The two tendons will end up being the same length as the semitendinosus tendon will typically shorten by 10 mm after the ends of the graft have been compressed.

A 15 mm ENDOBUTTON CL® implant is placed in the ENDOBUTTON Holder and the thinner, proximal ends of both tendons are individually tied to the polyester loop of the ENDOBUTTON CL® implant using the FiberWire sutures. After tying each tendon to the polyester loop of the ENDOBUTTON CL® implant, one of the FiberWire sutures from the semitendinosus tendon and one from the gracilis tendon are tied together. This step is repeated for the remaining two FiberWire sutures. This step connects the two tendons together and provides additional strength and security to the construct. The gracilis and semitendinosus tendon grafts are individually tripled as previously described for a 5-strand graft. The distal end of each tendon is passed through the polyester loop of the ENDOBUTTON CL® implant from inside the axilla of the two tendons to an outside direction. Passing the tendons in this direction will bury the connecting knots inside the looped tendons, decreasing the bulk on the femoral side of the graft (Figs. 5.12A to F). The tripled gracilis and semitendinosus grafts are combined to create a 6-stranded graft (Fig. 5.13). A loop is created by tying the ends of the Dacron tape together with a single throw, 120–150 mm from the end of tripled semitendinosus graft. The tape on the end of the tripled gracilis tendon is marked at the same location as the knot on the semitendinosus tendon and Dacron tape is tied together with a single throw. These steps create two equal length Dacron tape loops. The #2 FiberWire sutures on each tendon are left untied. The untied FiberWire sutures can be tied around a screw/washer or small staple to provide supplemental tibial fixation if required. Equal tension is applied to the 6 graft strands by looping the two tape loops around the opposite ends of a spring loaded graft tension device at the time of final tensioning and tibial fixation of the graft (Figs. 5.14A and B). The diameter of each end of the graft is measured to the nearest 0.5 using a sizing block. The 6-strand graft is pretensioned to 10 lbs. using a suture vise with tensiometer and wrapped with a "vancomycin wrap" as previously described.

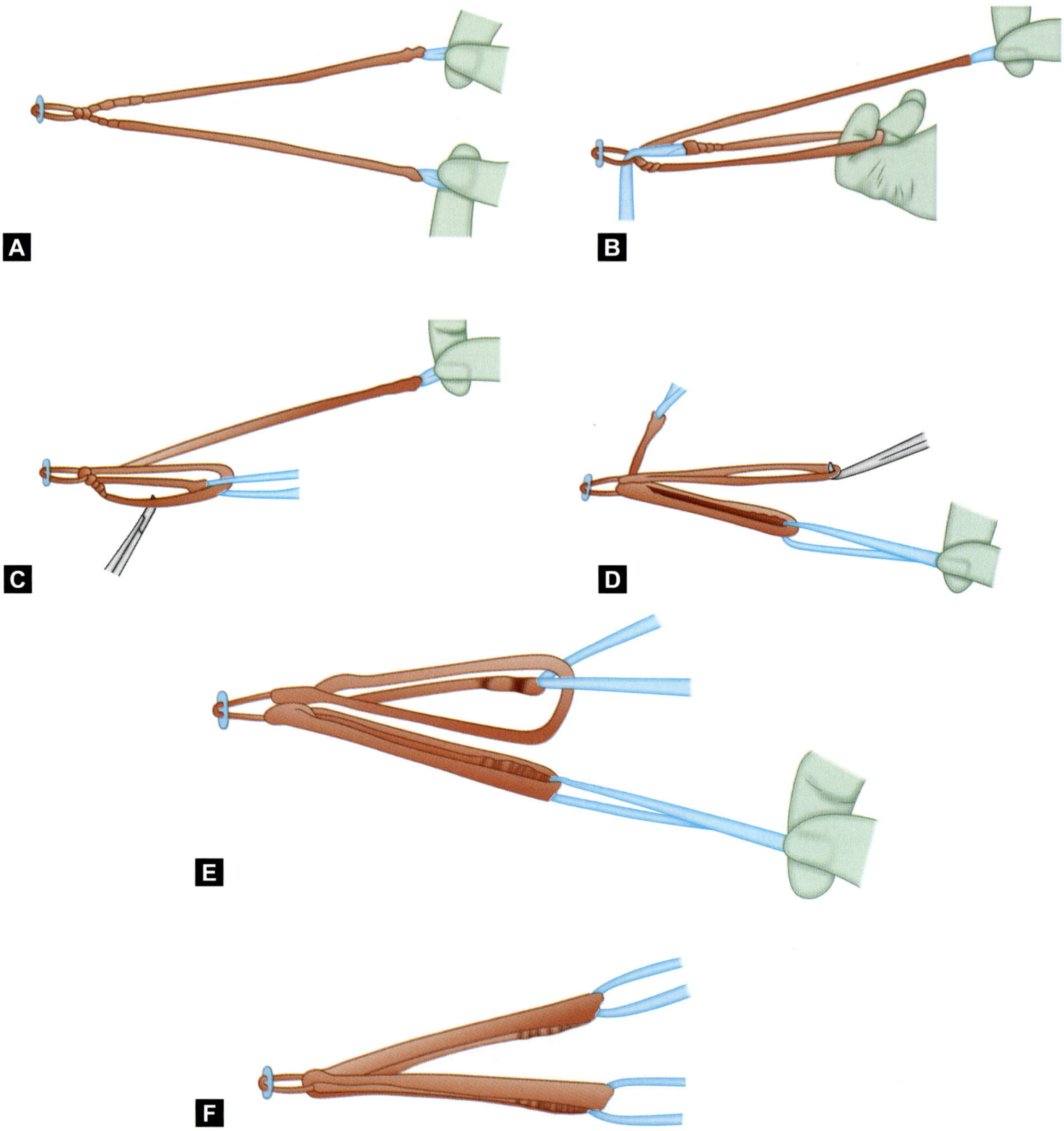

Figs. 5.12A to F: Steps in preparing a 6-strand hamstring anterior cruciate ligament (ACL) graft. (A) The proximal ends of the gracilis and semitendinosus tendons are individually tied to the polyester loop of the ENDOBUTTON implant. This step connects the polyester loop and the ends of the two tendons together. (B) The distal end of one tendon and attached Dacron tape and FiberWire sutures are passed through the polyester loop of the ENDOBUTTON CL® implant from inside the axilla of the anchored tendons to an outside direction. (C) One side of the Dacron tape and one of the #2 FiberWire sutures are passed on each side of the distal loop of the tendon graft. The distal end of the tendon graft which becomes the middle strand of the tripled graft is pulled into the axilla of the looped end of the tendon, tripling the graft. (D) The distal end of the second tendon and attached Dacron tape and FiberWire sutures is passed in an inside-out direction through the polyester loop of the ENDOBUTTON CL® implant as in step B. (E) One side of the Dacron tape and one of the #2 FiberWire sutures are passed on each side of the distal loop of the tendon graft. The distal end of the tendon graft which becomes the middle strand of the tripled graft is pulled into the axilla of the looped end of the tendon, tripling the second graft. (F) Final appearance of the 6-strand hamstring tendon ACL graft.

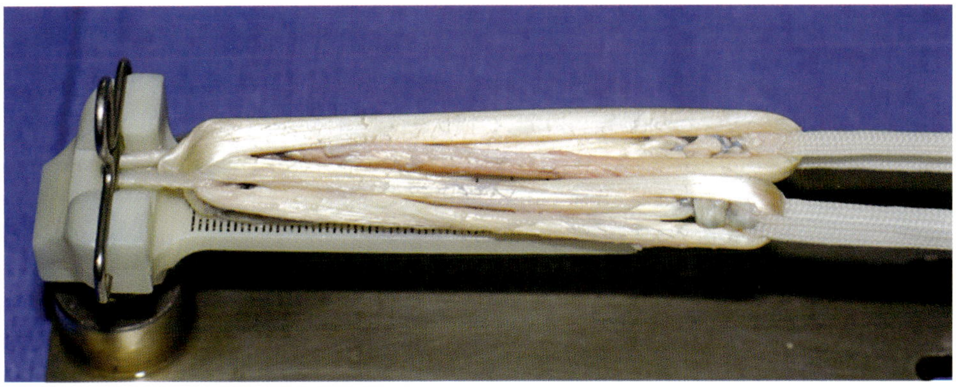

Fig. 5.13: 6-strand hamstring tendon graft.

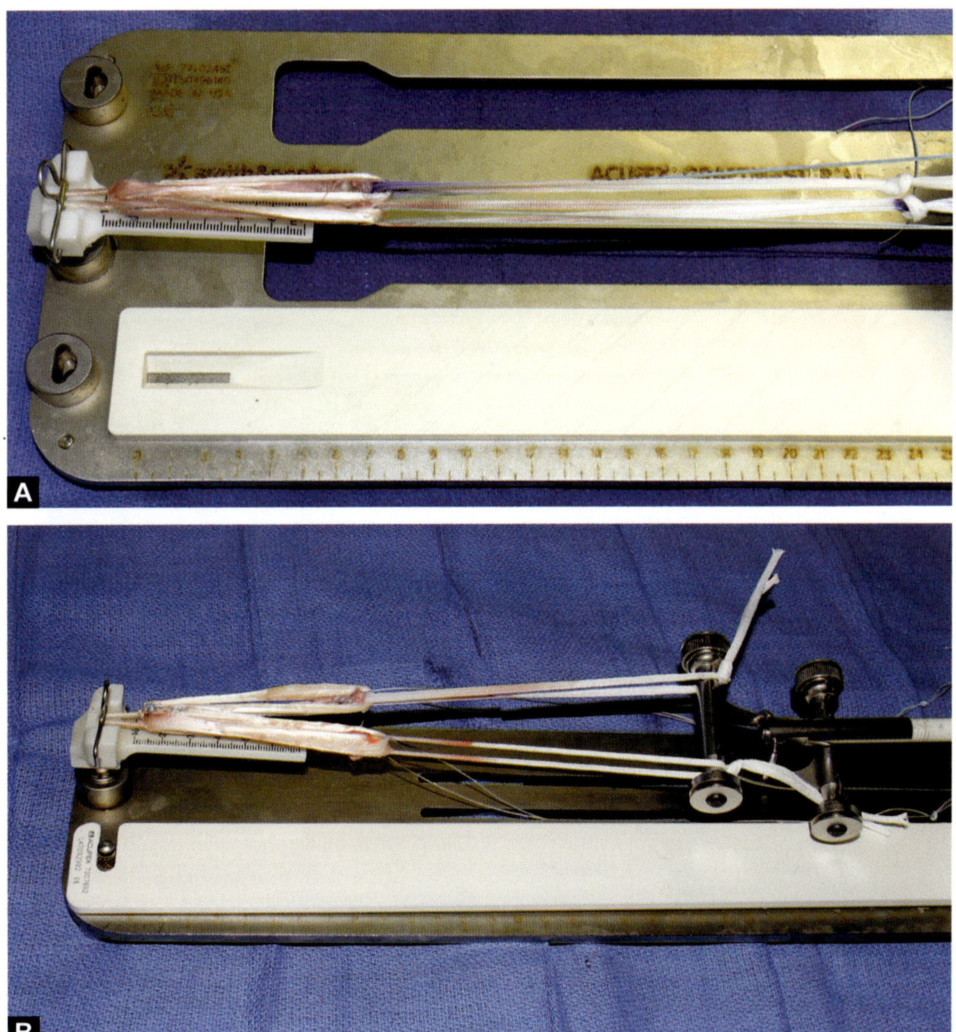

Figs. 5.14A and B: (A) Equal length Dacron tape loops at the end of a 6-strand hamstring tendon graft. (B) A spring loaded tensioning device is connected to the Dacron tape loops on each side of the 5-strand graft at the time of final graft tensioning and fixation.

CALCULATION OF THE TIBIAL TUNNEL LENGTH

The final step after preparing a 5- or 6-strand hamstring tendon ACL graft involves estimating the femoral and tibial tunnel lengths that need to be drilled to avoid a graft-tunnel mismatch. A sterile surgical marking pen is used to mark the prepared graft at the estimated femoral tunnel length from the ENDOBUTTON CL ULTRA implant. Usually, this distance is 40 mm when a 3-portal surgical technique with drilling of the ACL femoral tunnel through a low AMM portal is used. From the mark on the hamstring tendon graft representing the estimated ACL femoral tunnel length, the estimated intra-articular length of the ACL (25–28 mm for patients from the Gulf States, India and the Far East and 28–30 mm for Western populations) is then marked on the hamstring tendon graft. Thus, for the typical patient from the Gulf States, India or the Far East, the hamstring tendon graft would be marked at 40 mm (femoral tunnel length) and at 65 mm (40 mm femoral tunnel length + 25 mm for the length of the intra-articular part of the ACL graft) from the ENDOBUTTON implant. The length of tendon graft which lies beyond the 65 mm mark represents the amount of tendon graft to be inserted into the tibial tunnel (Figs. 5.15A to D). Typically, this distance is 30–35 mm, in which case a 40 mm length tibial tunnel would be drilled.

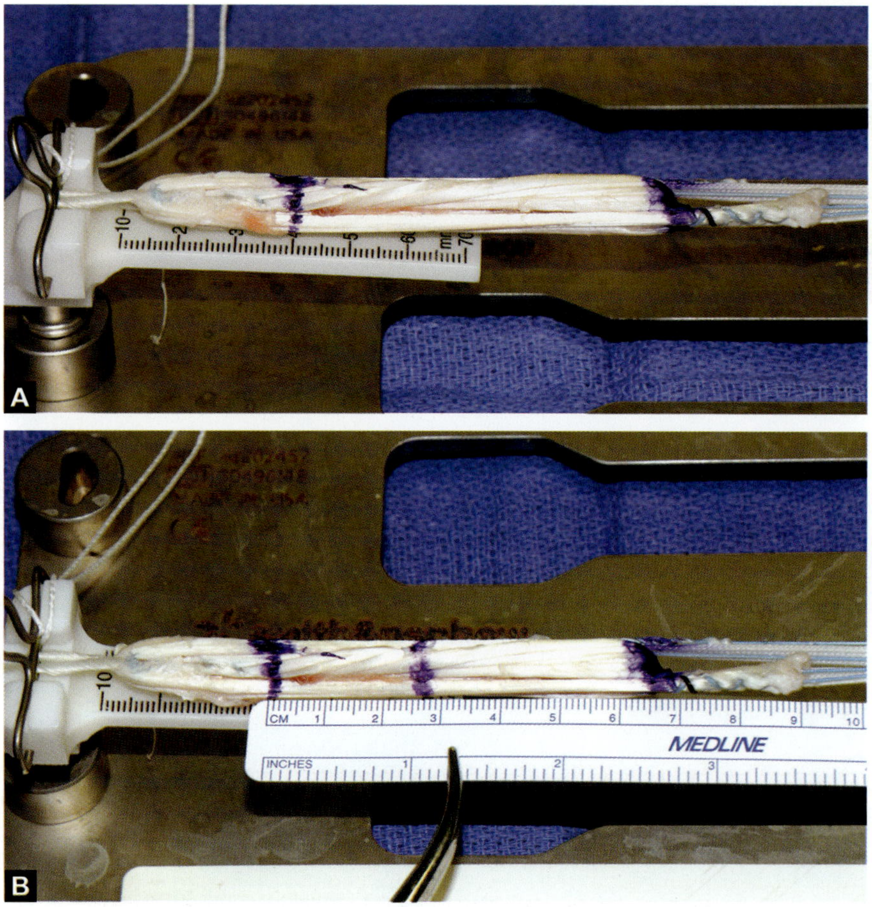

Figs. 5.15A and B: (A) 5-strand hamstring tendon graft marked at the estimated anterior cruciate ligament (ACL) femoral tunnel length (40 mm). (B) 5-strand hamstring tendon graft marked at the estimated intra-articular length of the ACL (27 mm).

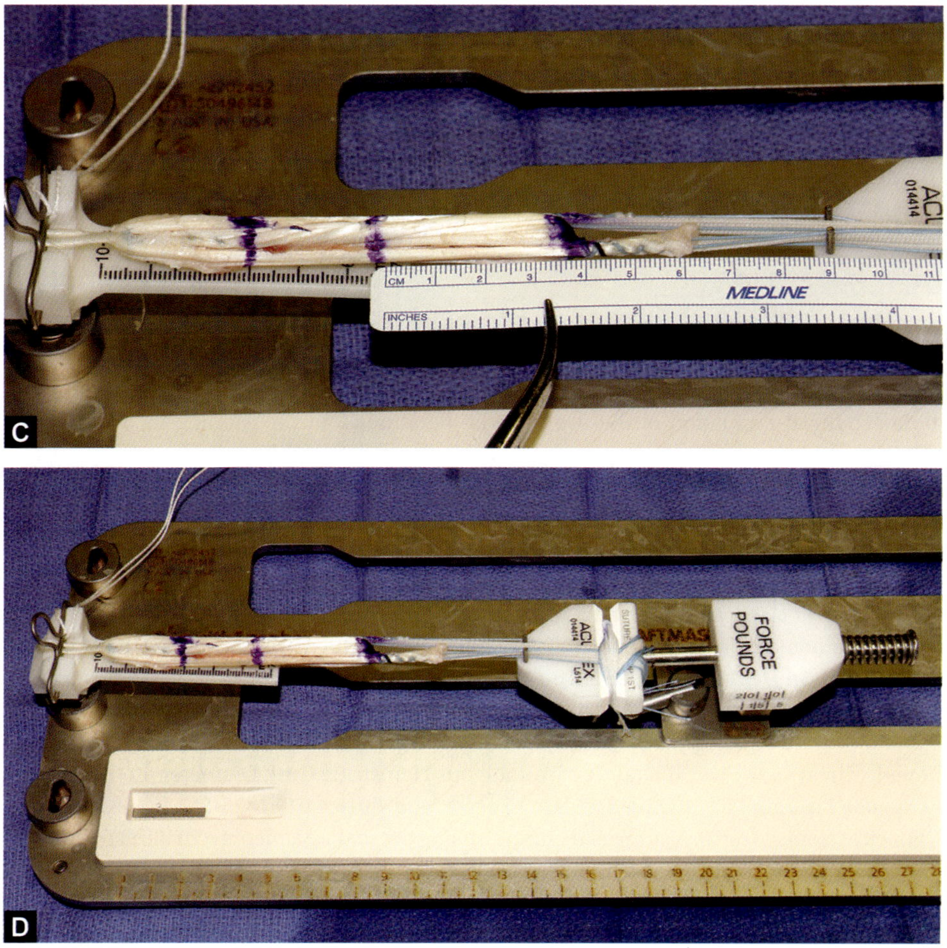

Figs. 5.15C and D: (C) Distance between the second mark and the end of the graft (38 mm) represents the length of graft that will lie in the tibial tunnel. (D) Pretensioning of the 6-strand graft. The distance from the ENDOBUTTON CL® implant to the first mark on the graft represents the length of graft that will be inserted in a 40 mm femoral tunnel. The graft lying between the first and second marks represents the intra-articular length of the ACL. The graft between the second mark and the end of the graft represents the length of graft in the tibial tunnel.

An extra #5 polyester suture is passed through the end hole of the ENDOBUTTON implant containing the white passing suture. This provides an additional traction suture in case of suture breakage when passing the graft.

PEARLS AND PITFALLS

- It is important to whip-stitch the tendons using a high-strength non-absorbable suture material with a tapered needle such as #2 FiberWire.
- Avoid suturing the tendons with polyester sutures as these may break when tied firmly during graft preparation.
- The proximal end of the tendons should be tied to the polyester loop of the ENDOBUTTON CL® implant.
- When tripling a tendon, tie the distal end of the tendon to a 5-mm Dacron tape.
- When preparing a 6-strand graft, the Dacron tape, sutures and the distal end of the graft should be passed from and inside to outside direction to decrease the bulk on the femoral side of the graft.
- To achieve more uniform tensioning of the graft strands, it is important to not suture the graft limbs together.

SUMMARY

Recent studies have shown that hamstring tendon graft diameter less than 8 mm is a potential risk factor for hamstring ACL reconstruction failure. A hamstring tendon graft diameter of 8 mm may not always be achieved using a 4-strand doubled semitendinosus and gracilis tendon autograft. In these situations, it may be necessary to add additional graft strands and create a 5- or 6-strand hamstring tendon autograft to achieve an ACL graft with a minimum diameter of 8 mm. This chapter describes a simple, cost-effective technique using commonly available materials in the operating room to prepare 5- and 6-strand hamstring tendon ACL grafts.

REFERENCES

1. Hamner DL, Brown CH Jr, Steiner ME, et al. Hamstring tendon grafts for reconstruction of the anterior cruciate ligament: biomechanical evaluation of the use of multiple strands and tensioning techniques. J Bone Joint Surg. 1999;81(4):549-57.
2. Conte EJ, Hyatt AE, Gatt CJ, et al. Hamstring autograft size can be predicted and is a potential risk factor for anterior cruciate ligament reconstruction failure. Arthroscopy. 2014;30(7):882-90.
3. Magnussen RA, Lawrence JTR, West RL, et al. Graft size and patient age are predictors of early revision after anterior cruciate ligament reconstruction with hamstring autograft. Arthroscopy. 2012;28(4):526-31.
4. Park SY, Oh H, Park S, et al. Factors predicting hamstring tendon autograft diameters and resulting failure rates after anterior cruciate ligament reconstruction. Knee Surg Sports Traumatol Arthrosc. 2012;21(5):1111-8.
5. Mariscalco MW, Flanigan DC, Mitchell J, et al. The Influence of hamstring autograft size on patient-reported outcomes and risk of revision after anterior cruciate ligament reconstruction: a Multicenter Orthopaedic Outcomes Network (MOON) Cohort Study. Arthroscopy. 2013;29(12):1948-53.
6. Spragg L, Chen J, Mirzayan R, et al. The Effect of Autologous Hamstring Graft Diameter on the Likelihood for Revision of Anterior Cruciate Ligament Reconstruction. Am J Sports Med. 2016;44(6):1475-81.
7. Vertullo CJ, Quick M, Jones A, et al. A surgical technique using presoaked vancomycin hamstring grafts to decrease the risk of infection after anterior cruciate ligament reconstruction. Arthroscopy. 2012;28(3):337-42.
8. Pérez-Prieto D, Torres-Claramunt R, Gelber PE, et al. Autograft soaking in vancomycin reduces the risk of infection after anterior cruciate ligament reconstruction. Knee Surg Sports Traumatol Arthrosc. 2014;24(9):2724-28.
9. Phegan M, Grayson JE, Vertullo CJ. No infections in 1300 anterior cruciate ligament reconstructions with vancomycin pre-soaking of hamstring grafts. Knee Surg Sports Traumatol Arthrosc. 2015;24(9):2729-35.

CHAPTER

6

Quadriceps Tendon Autograft in ACL Reconstruction

Andrew de Vlieg

INTRODUCTION

Quadriceps tendon autograft use for anterior cruciate ligament (ACL) reconstruction was first described by Marshall et al. in 1979,[1] however, it has never been used as much as other autograft options despite having certain advantages. Recent literature would indicate an upswing in interest in quadriceps tendon usage and a predicted increase in its usage for ACL reconstruction.[2]

Quadriceps tendon grafts can be taken as a soft tissue graft only or a bone block from the patella can be included. If a bone block is preferred caution must be taken in harvesting to prevent potential patella fracture. Only soft tissue graft is preferable and a graft of 7–8 cm length and 10 mm width can be obtained.[3] This can also be taken as a full-thickness or partial-thickness graft where the deep layer is left to maintain integrity of the suprapatellar pouch.

Quadriceps tendon autograft offers advantages over other graft choices:

- Predictable size of graft
- Less anterior knee pain and numbness than bone-patellar tendon-bone (BPTB) graft[4]
- No residual hamstring cramping[4]
- Denser collagen matrix and 20% more collagen per unit volume than BPTB graft[5]
- Favorable structural properties versus BPTB graft[6]
- Almost double the cross-sectional area and increased load to failure and higher stiffness than BPTB.[6]

Disadvantages in comparison to other graft choices:

- Technically demanding and time-consuming procedure
- Limited length of available graft making it unsuitable for certain fixation methods
- Only one bone block available
- Unfamiliarity with graft harvest
- Best achieved with specialized instrumentation.

Indications would be the same as for other autograft options for ACL reconstruction including revision surgery. Contraindications are limited to chronic quadriceps tendinopathy, quadriceps tendon contracture or prior quadriceps tendon harvest.

Although the use of quadriceps tendon as an autograft for ACL reconstruction was first described in 1979, it has never gained widespread popularity despite it having excellent mechanical properties. Some of this reticence may be as a result of unfavorable findings in a paper by Noyes et al.[7] in 1984. The graft construct used in this study was significantly different to the free central quadriceps tendon grafts that have subsequently been studied by several authors,[3,6,8] with favorable outcomes. There is a relative paucity of literature regarding the use of quadriceps tendon autograft for ACL reconstruction and thus despite studies showing advantages over other graft choices, it still remains the least used of the available autografts. This is possibly due to lack of familiarity and therefore less exposure to the harvest and graft preparation techniques, rather than to inferior outcomes. Despite this, it may be that the central quadriceps free tendon autograft may be the least morbid of the available autografts currently used for ACL reconstruction.[3]

ANATOMY

The anatomy of the quadriceps tendon is variable, but is generally trilaminar. The most superficial fibers are from rectus femoris and the deepest are from vastus intermedius and these layers are separated by a fat stripe.[3,9] A partial-thickness graft would be separated from a full-thickness graft along this layer. Maximal tendon length without bone block is 7–9 cm (average 88 mm) and this length is found slightly lateral to the midpoint of the insertion.[9] The mean width of the insertion on to the patella is 43 mm and the maximum depth at the insertion is 11 mm.[9] Quadriceps tendon length correlates with patient height and a height of at least 5 feet is sufficient to provide graft lengths of 7–8 cm.[3,10] Preoperative magnetic resonance imaging (MRI) measurements of the thickness of the quadriceps tendon at 3 cm proximal to the patella in the mid-sagittal plane can help to determine if a full- or partial-thickness graft is to be harvested. A partial-thickness graft is taken, if the tendon is greater than 7 mm thick and a full-thickness graft, if the tendon is 6 mm or less.[10] The advantage of a partial-thickness graft is the preservation of the integrity of the suprapatellar pouch and less risk of damaging vascular structures which are more abundant in the deep layers.[3]

MY TECHNIQUE

My preference is to use quadriceps tendon autograft in conjunction with an all-inside surgical technique for ACL reconstruction. A graft length of 65–70 mm is required for this technique and this is readily available in a predictable diameter from the quadriceps tendon.

The knee is placed at 90° which tensions the quadriceps tendon. The skin is marked for the following:

- Superior patella border
- Medial aspect of vastus medialis obliquus (VMO)
- Lateral edge of quadriceps tendon
- Incision line which is 2-cm long starting 5 mm above the patella border and situated a few millimeters lateral to the midpoint of the quadriceps tendon
- A point on the skin at the desired length of the graft above the patella.

The incision is made and subcutaneous fat is dissected out and removed to expose the upper surface of the quadriceps tendon (Fig. 6.1). Bluntly dissect from the proximal patella to the point on the skin marking the desired graft length. It is useful to elevate the skin and insert the arthroscope along the tendon to visualize its course to plan the harvest. The Quad Tendon Graft Cutting Blade® (Arthrex, Naples, FL) is inserted and

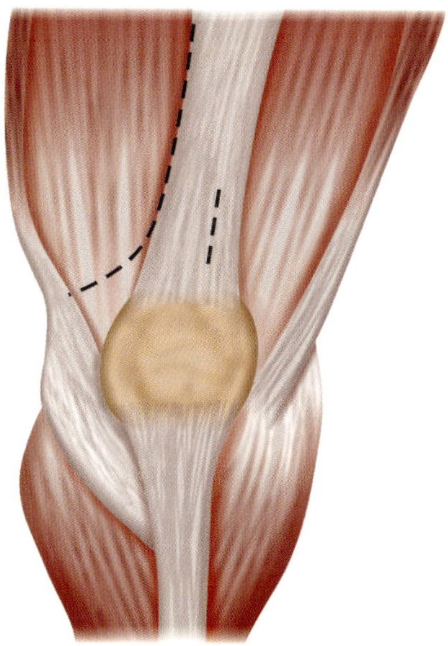

Fig. 6.1: Position of incision for left knee.

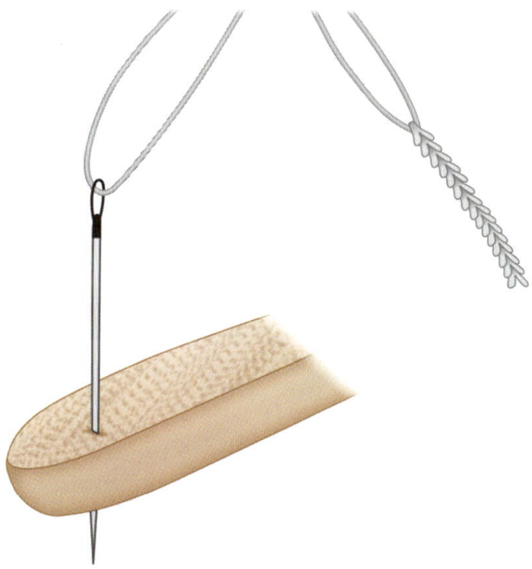

Fig. 6.2: First pass of FibreTag® through the quadriceps tendon graft.

pressed down so that the roof of the blade is in contact with the quadriceps tendon. This ensures a 7 mm thick graft. The width of the blade can be chosen but my preference is 10 mm. The blade is pushed proximally until the point marking the desired graft length is reached. The knee is then extended and a scalpel is used to continue the cuts down to the patella and dissect the tendon off the patella subperiosteally. The distal end of the harvested tendon is grasped and the dissection is continued proximally on the undersurface of the harvested tendon. The distal end is now whip-stitched using a Fibreloop w/FibreTag® (Arthrex, Naples, FL) to attach the TightRope® (Arthrex, Naples, FL) implant (Fig. 6.2). The initial pass of the suture

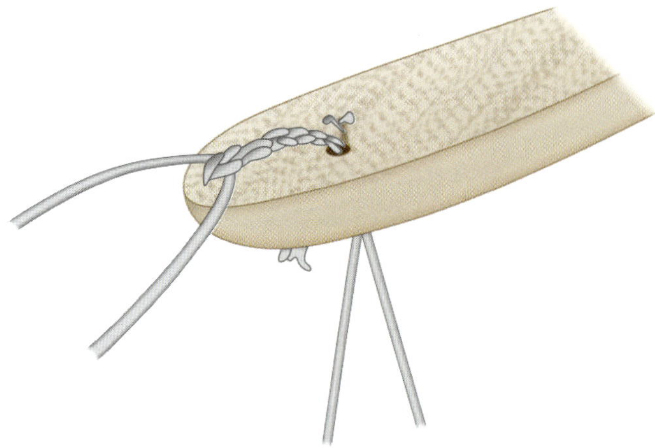

Fig. 6.3: First loop through graft with FibreTag® and with loop of TightRope® attached.

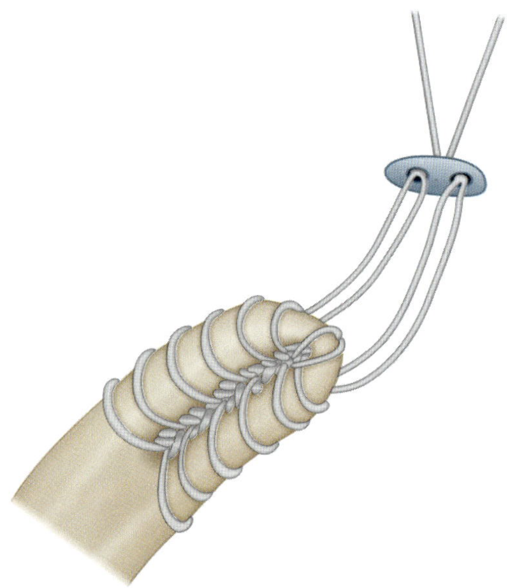

Fig. 6.4: Completed graft preparation with TightRope® attached.

is made 15 mm from the end of the graft leaving 3 mm of the FibreTag® protruding. The FibreTag® is held along the graft and a second pass is made a few millimeters from the tip of the graft. The FibreTag® is then looped through the TightRope® and the needle is passed back through the graft at the site of the initial pass incorporating the FibreTag® on both sides of the graft (Fig. 6.3). Multiple passes are made through the graft including the FibreTag® on each side of the tendon moving toward the distal end. At the distal end the Fibreloop® is passed through the TightRope® and sutured proximally through the FibreTag® again to create a locking construct. The TightRope® is thus attached with both the FibreTag and Fibreloop®. Once the proximal end is reached the Fibreloop® is cut, looped around the graft and tied. One end is cut and the other end passed through the graft to bury the knot (Fig. 6.4).

The Quad Tendon Stripper/Cutter® (Arthrex, Naples, FL) is passed over the TightRope® and along the graft (Figs. 6.5 and 6.6). The handle is locked to prevent premature amputation of the graft. Advance the

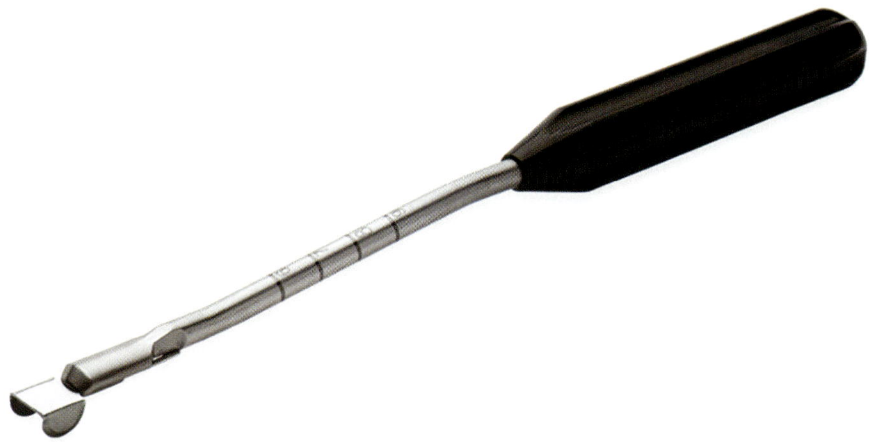

Fig. 6.5: Quads tendon graft cutting tool.

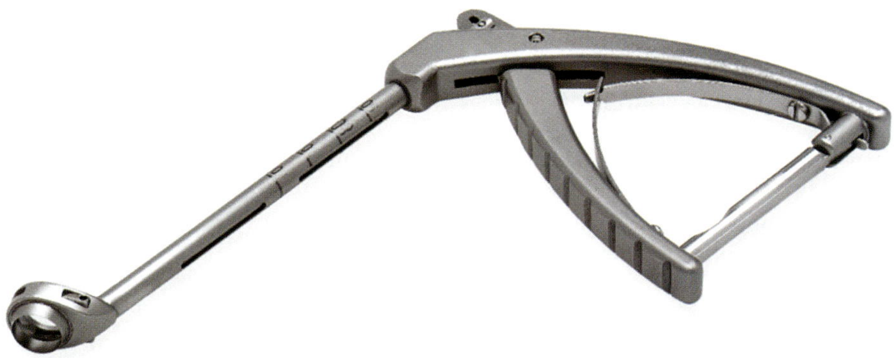

Fig. 6.6: Quads tendon graft cutter.

stripper proximally using a rotation action. Once it reaches the desired graft length as indicated on the shaft and by the skin marking, the handle is unlocked and squeezed to cut the proximal tendon. The graft is retrieved and the same process is followed to attach the TightRope® device at the proximal end.

The arthroscope can be reinserted into the graft harvest site to check for any violation of the suprapatellar pouch. If there is any found, this should be sutured. The tendon defect is not closed as this may cause quadriceps contracture. The skin is then closed leaving a small scar.

PEARLS

- Centre the graft harvest a few millimeters lateral to the midpoint of the quadriceps tendon insertion onto the patella as this will allow for maximum length, if needed.
- The described technique attaches the button fixation devices in a strong construct but the graft is very suitable for normal whip stitching as well.
- Violation of the suprapatellar pouch can be avoided by harvesting a partial-thickness graft of around 7 mm. There is a thin fatty layer that lies at this depth, along which the tendon can be dissected without disturbing the suprapatellar pouch.

PITFALLS

- If the suprapatellar pouch is violated, it should be sutured securely to prevent fluid extravasation during the subsequent ligament reconstruction.
- Hematoma formation can be avoided by obtaining hemostasis after removal of the harvested tendon. The tendon is relatively hypovascular distally and proximally the vasculature is usually superficial.
- Very short grafts (6 cm) may still be used for an all-inside reconstruction technique, but grafts of 7–8 cm can be reliably harvested with a careful approach.

REFERENCES

1. Marshall JL, Warren RF, Wickiewicz TL, et al. The anterior cruciate ligament: a technique of repair and reconstruction. Clin Orthop Relat Res. 1979;(143):97-106.
2. Lubowitz JH. Editorial Commentary: Quadriceps Tendon Autograft Use for Anterior Cruciate Ligament Reconstruction Predicted to Increase. Arthroscopy. 2016;32(1):76-7.
3. Slone HS, Romine SE, Premkumar A, et al. Quadriceps tendon autograft for anterior cruciate ligament reconstruction: a comprehensive review of current literature and systematic review of clinical results. Arthroscopy. 2015;31(3):541-54.
4. De Angelis JP, Fulkerson JP. Quadriceps tendon—a reliable alternative for reconstruction of the anterior cruciate ligament. Clin Sports Med. 2007;26(4):587-96.
5. MARS Group. Effect of graft choice on the outcome of revision anterior cruciate ligament reconstruction in the Multicenter ACL Revision Study (MARS) Cohort. Am J Sports Med. 2014;42(10):2301-10.
6. Shani RH, Umpierez E, Nasert M, et al. Biomechanical comparison of quadriceps and patella tendon grafts in anterior cruciate ligament reconstruction. Arthroscopy. 2016;32(1):71-5.
7. Noyes FR, Butler DL, Grood ES, et al. Biomechanical analysis of human ligament grafts used in knee ligament repairs and reconstructions. J Bone Joint Surg Am. 1984;66(3):344-52.
8. Lund B, Nielsen T, Fauno P, et al. Is quadriceps tendon a better graft choice than patella tendon? A prospective randomized study. Arthroscopy. 2014;30(5):593-8.
9. Lippe J, Armstrong A, Fulkerson JP. Anatomic guidelines for harvesting a quadriceps free tendon autograft for anterior cruciate ligament reconstruction. Arthroscopy. 2012;28(7):980-4.
10. Xerogeanes JW, Mitchell PM, Karasev PA, et al. Anatomic and morphological evaluation of quadriceps tendon using 3-dimensional magnetic resonance imaging reconstruction: applications for anterior cruciate ligament autograft choice and procurement. Am J Sports Med. 2013;41(10):2392-9.

CHAPTER

7

Harvesting Peroneus Longus Tendon

Sanjay Trivedi

INTRODUCTION

Ligament reconstruction is a routinely performed surgery by arthroscopy and sports injury surgeons. Most common of these is anterior cruciate ligament (ACL) reconstruction surgery. The graft choice for ligament reconstruction also has been shifting from bone patellar tendon to soft tissue grafts. Hamstring tendon is the most popular soft tissue graft currently and has become the most preferred choice as soft tissue graft.

There are some circumstances where hamstring graft is not available or unsuitable. These force a surgeon to look for other sources of soft tissue graft. In India, allografts are not readily available or not accessible. This makes us opt for other sources of autogenous soft tissue graft.

Peroneus longus (PL) is one such soft tissue graft which has generated immense interest and has been used successfully by me for the last 7 years. I first used it in 2010 for a revision anterior cruciate ligament reconstruction (ACLR) surgery where the patient had compound bony injury on the opposite upper tibia making graft harvest unsuitable and same side primary ACLR had failed, requiring revision. Earlier I used it sparingly, but for the past few years I have been able to refine the technique and define the indications to harvest the peroneus graft more clearly. I have done several cases of ligament reconstruction using PL tendon graft successfully, until now.

INDICATIONS

- Revision ACL or posterior cruciate ligament (PCL) reconstruction
- Multiligament reconstruction (ACL/medial collateral ligament, ACL/PCL, PCL/posterior lateral corner)
- Augmentation/replacement option for inadequate hamstring graft (graft amputation, thin or short graft)
- Rarely, primary graft choice in short stocky females for ligament reconstruction.

ANATOMY OF PERONEUS TENDONS

The two peroneus tendons arise from the fibula and course distally in peroneal compartment, cross the ankle laterally and terminate in the foot. The PL originates from the upper two-thirds of the lateral part of the fibula and passes underneath the lateral malleolus, enters the foot laterally and crosses the sole to go medially and insert at the medial cuneiform and base of the first metatarsal bone. The peroneus brevis (PB) also originates from the fibula but from the lower two-thirds of the same surface, courses down underneath PL laterally and behind lateral malleolus, to insert at the base of the fifth metatarsal bone. PL is more tendinous like semitendinosus tendon unlike brevis, which has a short tendon and big muscle belly.

Near the lateral part of the ankle, the tendons pass through the common synovial sheath underneath the smooth, slightly grooved tip of the lateral malleolus, longus on top of brevis, held in position by superior peroneal retinaculum (Fig. 7.1). This is a suitable area for their harvest incision. At the distal point in the lateral aspect of the foot where both tendons turn to the sole, PB and PL pass through the inferior peroneal retinaculum which holds them in a secure position.

SURGICAL TECHNIQUE OF PERONEUS HARVEST

- Patient is in a supine position with the table slightly tilted away from the surgeon while the surgeon stands facing the lateral part of the ankle and foot. The foot is painted and draped appropriately. The harvest is done under tourniquet. Keeping a rolled towel underneath the distal leg and lifting the ankle and foot off the table help in harvest of the graft.
- Bony landmark of the lateral malleolus is identified and marked with a marker pen. A skin knife is used to make approximately 4 cm long incision directly over superior peroneal retinaculum, curving slightly distally underneath the tip of lateral malleolus (Fig. 7.2). The incision should end slightly below the tip of the lateral malleolus (Fig. 7.3).
- The skin and subcutaneous tissue are incised, and by blunt dissection, superior peroneal retinaculum is exposed (Fig. 7.4). The retinaculum is incised in the line of the incision to expose the PL tendon. At this point, PL overlies the PB tendon.

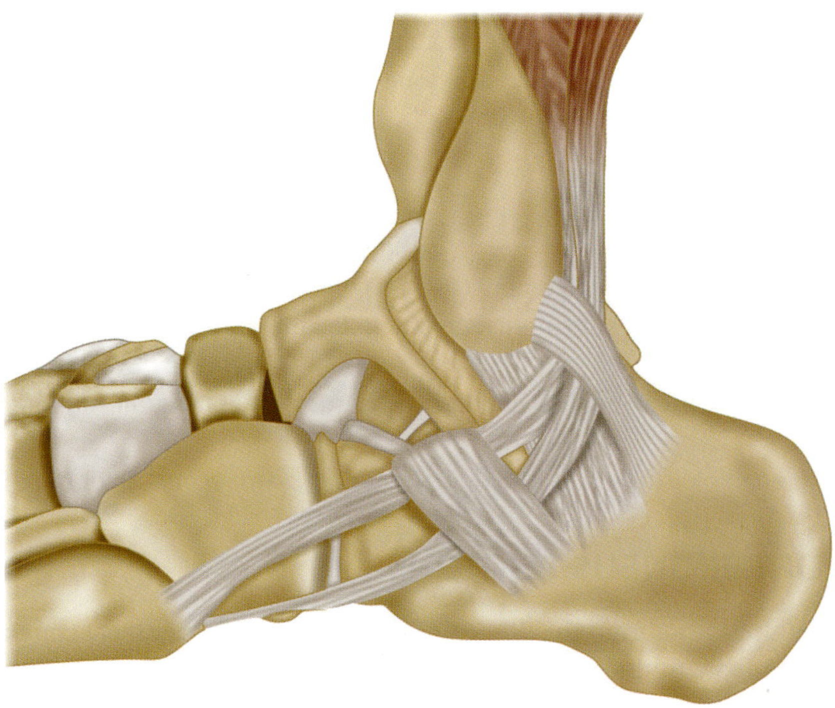

Fig. 7.1: Superior and inferior peroneal retinaculum.

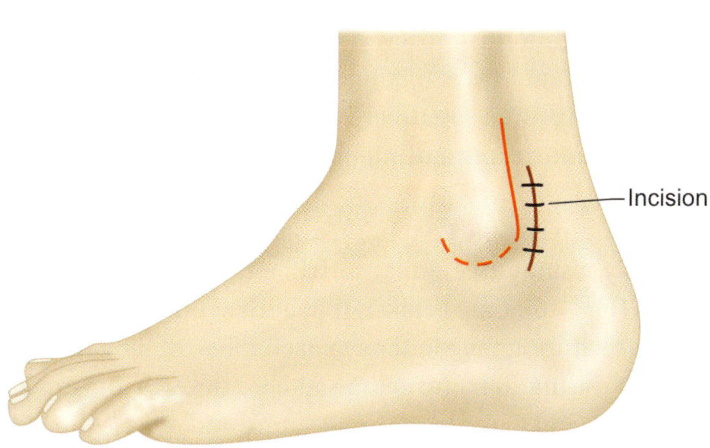

Fig. 7.2: Incision behind the lateral malleolus.

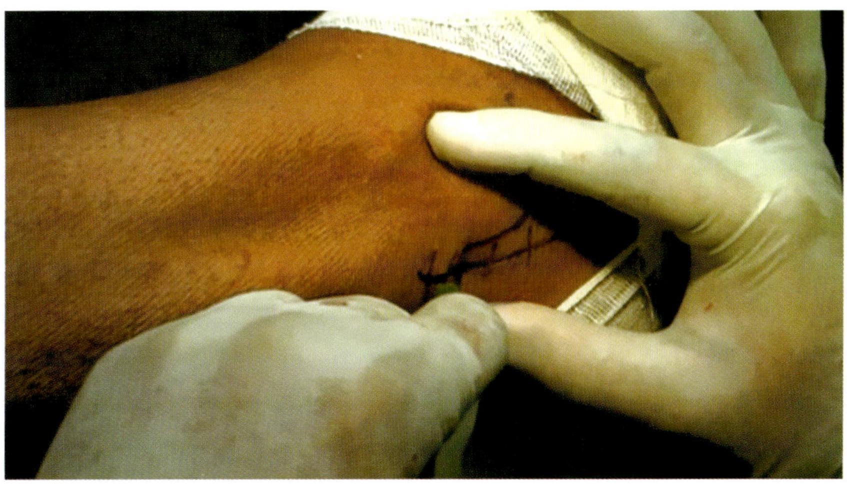

Fig. 7.3: Clinical picture of surgical incision.

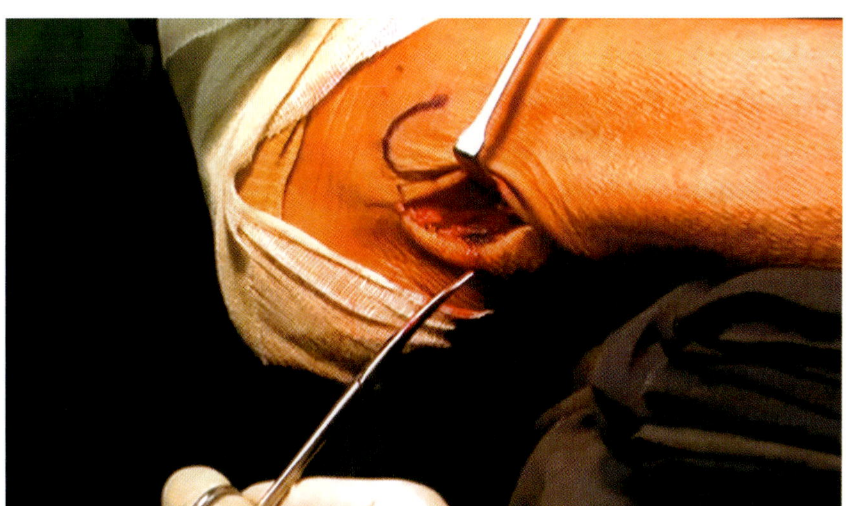

Fig. 7.4: Exposed superior peroneal retinaculum.

- Using the Mixter forceps, PL tendon is retrieved out of the groove and held with one No. 2 nonabsorbable suture (e.g. No. 2 Ethibond Excel®, Ethicon LLC) cinch loop (Fig. 7.5). The PB tendon is then retrieved from behind PL and secured separately with No. 2 nonabsorbable suture cinch loop. At this point, one can easily differentiate the primarily tendinous and superficial PL tendon from musculotendinous and deeper PB tendon.
- Peroneus longus tendon is sutured to the PB tendon distally starting from the level of tip of lateral malleolus progressing proximally, using three nonabsorbable doubly passed sutures, preferably Prolene® 1-0 (Ethicon Inc.) sutures (Fig. 7.6). Care is taken that each suture goes through and around both tendons with each pass. While suturing the tendons to each other, pulling hard on each cinch loop helps deliver both tendons out of the incision and get the stitches through and around more easily (Fig. 7.7).
- Cut the PL tendon 2 mm proximal to the last joining suture and release the PL tendon free (Fig. 7.8).

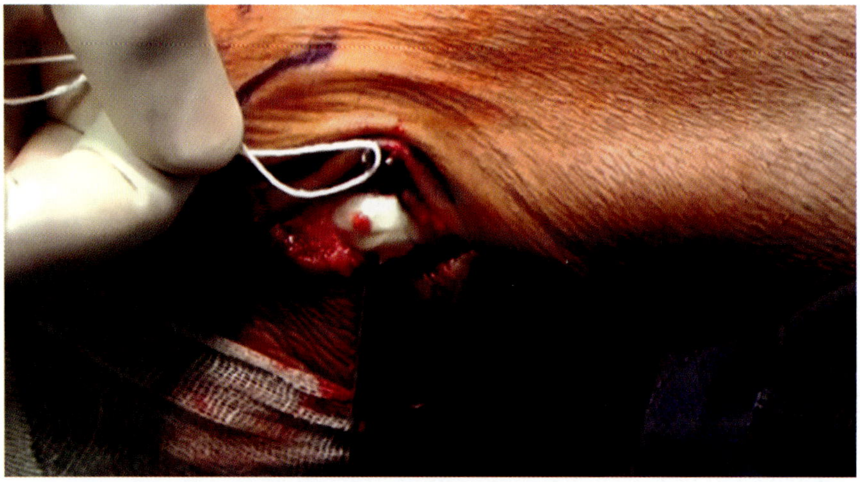

Fig. 7.5: Cinch loop being inserted around peroneus longus tendon.

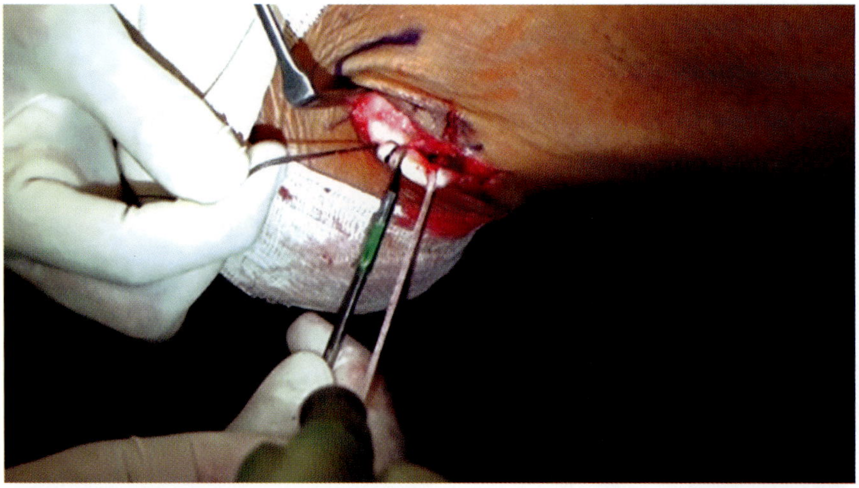

Fig. 7.6: Three Prolene® No. 1 stitches used to suture peroneus longus (PL) with brevis before cutting proximal part of PL tendon.

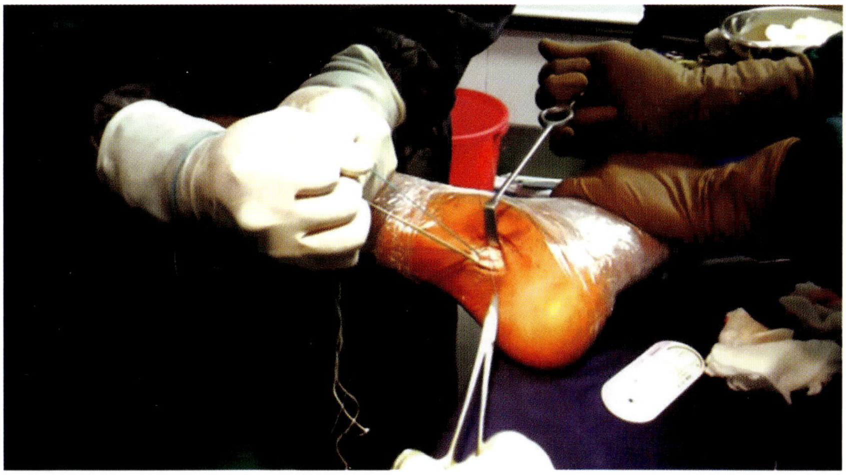

Fig. 7.7: Pulling both cinch loops out of the incision helps in suturing the tendons with each other.

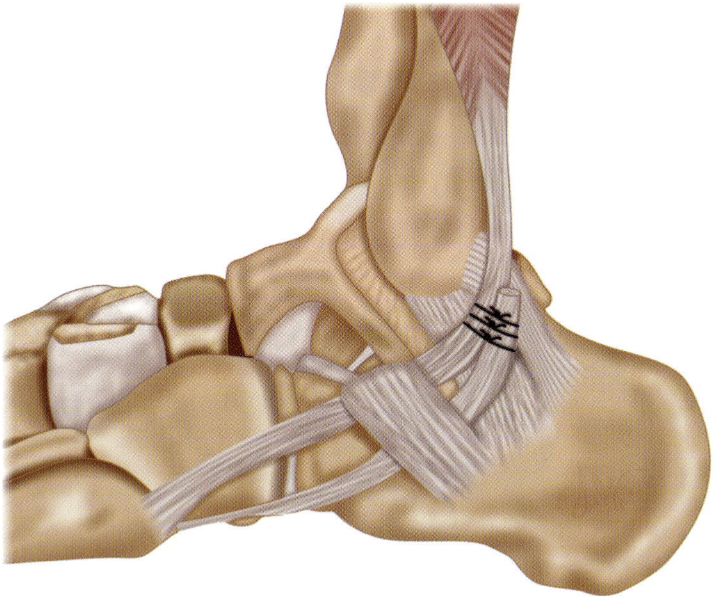

Fig. 7.8: View of peroneus longus (PL) tendon stump after suturing it with brevis and PL tendon harvest.

- Hold the PL tendon and pass a nonabsorbable holding suture in Bunnell-type fashion so that each suture tail comes out through the cut end face of the tendon. This makes threading of closed tendon stripper easier. Sometimes, due to thicker diameter of the PL, use of 7 mm size closed tendon stripper is necessitated.
- Pass a blunt dissector or surgeon's little finger all around the tendon in the proximal part of the wound to free up soft tissue adhesion around the PL tendon.
- Thread the close-ended tendon stripper at the free distal, sutured end of the PL tendon and surgeon shifts himself to the foot end of the patient, to be in line of the tendon (Fig. 7.9).
- Now the tendon stripper is advanced firmly yet steadily in prono-supination motion and at the same time pulling the suture at the distal end of the tendon in counter traction. Take care not to give undue

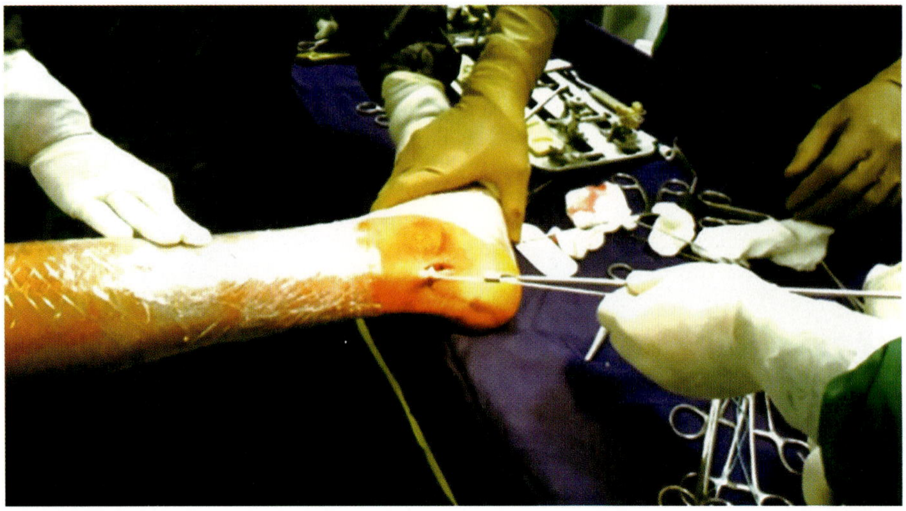

Fig. 7.9: For harvest of peroneus longus (PL) tendon, tendon stripper is inserted in straight line with PL tendon to avoid premature amputation.

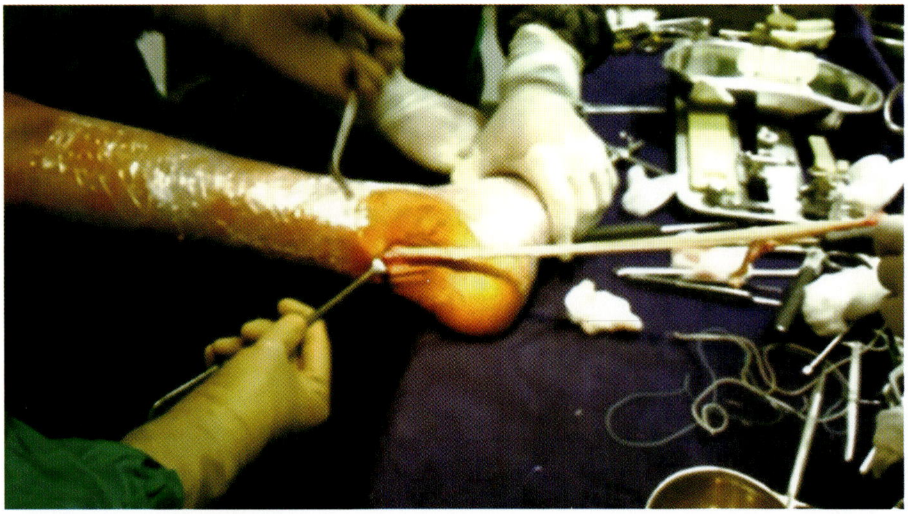

Fig. 7.10: Adequate harvested tendon length.

jerks or change the direction of the tendon stripper. Once the tendon stripper reaches the end of the musculotendinous junction, the surgeon feels sudden give way and tendon graft is ready to be pulled out of the wound (Fig. 7.10).

- Graft is transferred to the back table for length measurements. The average graft length of the PL tendon is 29 cm with the range being from 27 cm to 31.5 cm. The average tripled diameter of the graft is 9 mm, ranging between 8.5 mm and 10 mm in most of the cases. This length and diameter is adequate for any ligament reconstruction. I do not close the superior peroneal retinaculum as I feel that inferior retinaculum holds the tendons securely.
- Perform two layer closure using appropriate Vicryl® No. 1-0 followed by skin sutures and apply compression bandage.

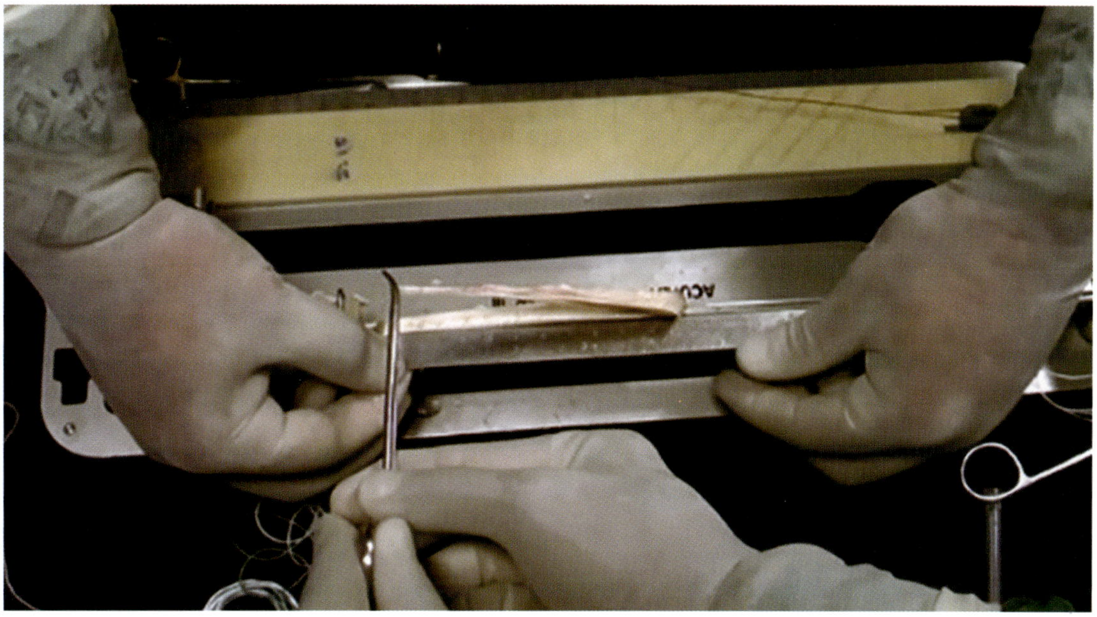

Fig. 7.11: Preparation of three-stranded peroneus longus tendon graft.

Graft Preparations

The graft is prepared in the same way as one would prepare a semitendinosus graft. I prefer to triple it for PCL reconstruction and triple or quadruple it for ACL reconstruction, depending upon the length and diameter of the tendon available and graft desired (Fig. 7.11).

POSTOPERATIVE CARE

The postoperative protocol is the same as any surgeon would do for his other soft tissue graft ligament reconstruction. The choice of PL graft does not alter the postoperative mobilization or rehabilitation of ligament reconstruction. No special splint or off-weight mobilization is necessary as far as PL graft harvest is concerned.

PEARLS AND PITFALLS

- The skin incision of 4 cm is usually sufficient to complete the procedure safely but if needed it can be extended distally to get more length of the graft.
- The separate nonabsorbable suture cinch loops help in delivering the tendons out of the incision for easy suturing of the distal end of the PL tendon to the PB tendon.
- Suturing the PL tendon to PB tendon before cutting it for harvest is easier than suturing the stump of PL tendon after harvest (Fig. 7.12).
- I normally take three stitches of No. 1 Prolene® (Ethicon LLC) suture to stitch the PL stump with PB so as to make the stump less bulky and thus facilitating its gliding under the groove of lateral malleolus.
- When in doubt about the length of the PL tendon harvest, open tendon stripper can be used to get desired length of the tendon distally (Fig. 7.13).
- Take care in identifying and protecting the sural nerve while dissecting the tendons as it passes very close to the area of dissection (Fig. 7.14).

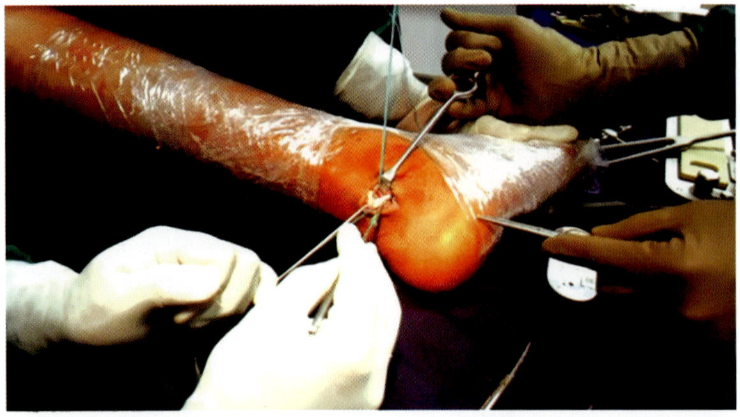

Fig. 7.12: Proximal part of peroneus longus tendon being cut after suturing the distal end with peroneus brevis.

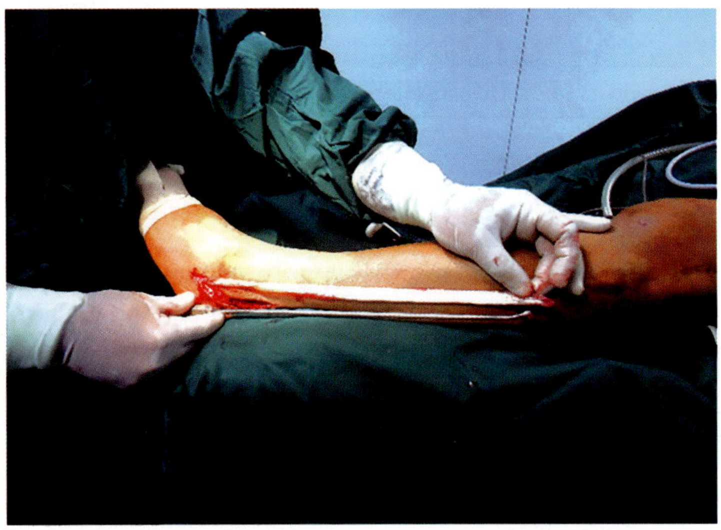

Fig. 7.13: Open tendon stripper helps to gain more length of the peroneus longus (PL) tendon by cutting PL tendon more distally.

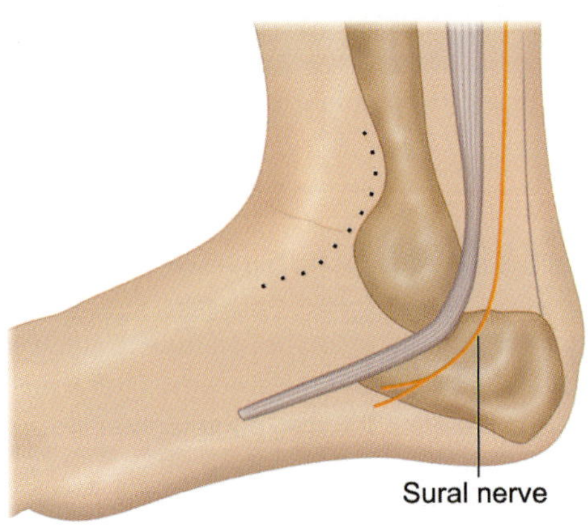

Fig. 7.14: Sural cutaneous nerve passes very close to the incision site.

COMPLICATIONS

The hypoesthesia and or paresthesia of the lateral border of foot and sole is often observed when sural nerve is injured during the harvest but the sensation usually returns in 6–8 months without any grave discomfort.

The transient weakness in eversion of foot is seldom observed early in the postoperative period up to 6 months but eversion weakness lasting beyond 6 months has not yet been observed. The brevis steps up to compensate for the PL muscle belly. The gait pattern remains normal in spite of transient weakness in eversion.

DISCUSSION

I have been using PL tendon graft since 2010 and have done significant number of cases using it. It is still not my primary choice of graft but I do not hesitate to harvest it, if need arises.

Its length and diameter is adequate to be used for either ACL or PCL. In revision ACL reconstruction surgery, I tend to quadruple it and make it thicker to accommodate in the wide femoral tunnel I encounter during surgery. In PCL reconstruction, I tend to use three strands to obtain the required length. The scar of PL graft harvest is hidden behind the lateral malleolus so cosmesis is not an issue with this graft. The gait pattern is not altered with usage of this graft and patient satisfaction in case of ligament reconstruction remains equal to hamstring graft in my experience. There is published data[1] to support the normalcy of the gait after harvest of PL harvest. In this published study, all the patients of PL graft harvest were evaluated at 6 months for gait pattern using 3D kinematics, kinetic of ankles and spatiotemporal walking parameters, which showed no difference in the gait.

CONCLUSION

The PL tendon as source of soft tissue graft can be used safely in ligament reconstruction without any hesitation, in specified indication as described earlier.[2] The use of PL tendon as primary source of graft as a routine needs further long-term evaluation of a larger number of patients.

REFERENCES

1. Nazem K, Barzegar M, Hosseini A, et al. Can we use peroneus longus in addition to hamstring tendons for anterior cruciate ligament reconstruction? Adv Biomed Res. 2014;3:115.
2. Zhao J, Huangfu X. The biomechanical and clinical application of using the anterior half of the peroneus longus tendon as an autograft source. Am J Sports Med. 2012;40(3):662-71.

CHAPTER

8

Clinical Evaluation and Imaging for a Patient with ACL Injury

Ricardo Bastos, Renato Andrade, Rogério Pereira, Ernesto Pinho, Sérgio Rodrigues-Gomes, Hélder Pereira, João Espregueira-Mendes

INTRODUCTION

Anterior cruciate ligament (ACL) injuries are among the most frequent morbidities of the knee and remains one of the most common causes of orthopedic surgery.[1,2] These injuries are often accompanied by meniscal and cartilage lesions, especially in the sporting population, which should be addressed concomitantly.[3-7] Despite the technological advances in terms of diagnostic imaging and manual instrumented devices, medical history and physical examination still constitute the most common tools for diagnosis. Unlike meniscal and cartilage injuries which elicit painful stimuli and can often result in false-positive or false-negative results, ligament injury tests are much more sensitive. On the other hand, conclusions depend exclusively on the tactile sensitivity, experience, and training of the surgeon.[8] Ligament manual testing leads to a satisfactory sensitivity and specificity in the diagnosis of the ACL tears but quantification of the instability currently relies on subjective impressions.[8] In this way, history and physical examination can provide the diagnosis in most of the patients,[9] and complementary exams (imaging and instrumented laxity devices) can aid in cases of limited instability (partial lesions or ACL partially healed), in the evaluation of associated lesions and specially when the quantification of instability is required.

MEDICAL HISTORY

Associating the patient's medical history and the physical examination has great diagnostic value in ACL ruptures, especially if performed by an experienced orthopedic surgeon.[9] In most cases, a history of sports activity accompanies the ACL injury. Nonetheless, low-energy mechanisms are also described. Most ACL ruptures (around 75%) occur with minimal or no contact at the time of injury.[10] Rotational indirect trauma is most commonly observed. The classic combination of valgus stress, tibial internal rotation, and flexion of the knee joint is reported. Other mechanisms are described as hyperextension (kick in the air), external rotation of the tibia or direct trauma applied to the posterior region of the knee. Sometimes the mechanism cannot be well-detailed due to the complexity of the movement and speed of the event. Rapid deceleration moments, including planting the injured leg to cut and rapidly change direction, landing from a jump twisting, and pivoting are often related.[11]

The feeling of a "clunk" may also be reported. This symptom is not pathognomonic of a ruptured ACL and might be related to other ligament injuries, meniscal tear or fractures. Still, this information must be taken into account.

The evaluation of joint effusion should be detailed. Time of onset, volume and characteristics of the effusion provide valuable information regarding the etiology of the injury. Bulky, hematic joint effusions which appear in the first few minutes have a great probability of ACL injury. The synovial membrane that covers ACL is richly vascularized and its rupture promotes bleeding. The existence of ACL injury without joint effusion may be present in situations as integrity of the synovial membrane or in cases of high energy trauma with posterior capsule rupture.

Patient's anatomical and demographic factors must also be registered since they can be considered as risk factors for ACL rupture. In this sense, several risk factors have been reported to predispose the individuals to a higher risk of injury, including anatomical and biomechanical risk factors.[12-14]

An increased medial and lateral tibial plateau slope are risk factors for ACL rupture.[12,15] The normal posterior tibial slope is usually within the range of 5–7°, depending on the measurement technique, and should be considered pathologic if it exceeds 12°.[16,17] An intercondylar notch stenosis and the shape of the femoral notch at the anterior outlet have also been associated with ACL injury.[12] In addition, the relationship of the lateral femoral condyle and lateral tibial plateau bone morphology also play a role in the ACL injury risk.[18] In this sense, a decreased anteroposterior distance of the lateral tibial plateau in relation to an increased distal anteroposterior flattened femoral surface may predispose to a higher risk of ACL injury—Porto ratio (Fig. 8.1).

In addition, some gender-specific factors are also considered. In this line, females have three times greater risk of ACL injury than males participating in the same sport. Hormonal factors are related to ligamentous laxity during the first half of menstrual cycle[19] and can be explained by the increased levels of relaxin, estrogen and reduction of procollagen. Moreover, there may be a genetic predisposition to an ACL

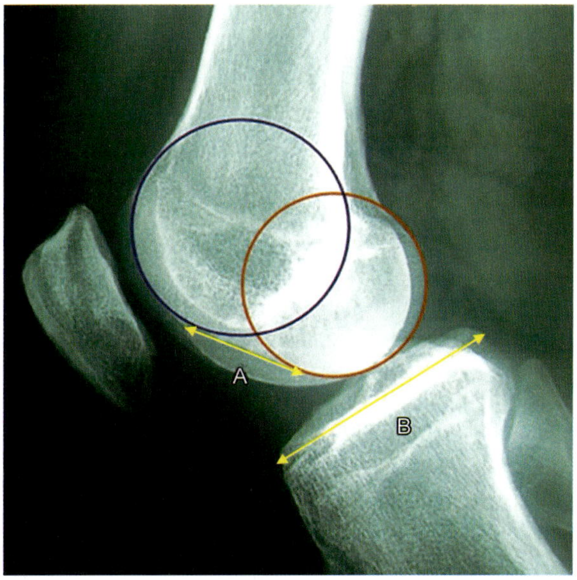

Fig. 8.1: Porto ratio—anteroposterior distance of the lateral tibial plateau by the distal anteroposterior flattened surface of the femoral condyle (B/A).

injury. Individuals who have a family history of ACL tears show twice the risk of ACL rupture. In fact, there is an association between collagen type 3 α1 and collagen type 1 α1 and ACL ruptures.[20]

CLINICAL EXAMINATION

Inspection

Patient's gait should be observed. Antalgic positions like flexed attitude of the knee is assumed to better accommodate the presence of joint effusion, relieve pain or could mean joint blocking.

Anatomical alignment of the lower limb is a fundamental factor to be measured. Although association between valgus of the knee and ACL tear is still controversial, this deviation affects the axial compressive force on the lateral side of the knee and may contribute to an internal rotation.[21] Moreover, in lateral knee evaluation, genu recurvatum should be observed. Increased knee hyperextension of 10° and hamstring flexibility are significantly associated with the risk of ACL tear.[22]

Previous scars in the knee region that indicate previous surgeries are important for future surgical procedure planning.

Palpation

Active and passive range of motion is measured and any limitation of extension and flexion must be recorded. General joint laxity should be evaluated on the non-injured side. Knee joint laxity is considered to be a risk factor for ACL injury and for failure of ACL reconstruction.[23-25]

Specific Physical Examination

Lachman-Noulis Test

Lachman test is considered the most sensitive test for ACL tear diagnosis.[26] It has high sensitivity and specificity (about 95%).[27]

The first description of the so-called Lachman test was given by George K Noulis in his doctoral thesis "Entorse du Genou" in 1875.[28] Indeed, Noulis' thesis appears to be the first full description of this important test for anterior cruciate function that almost a century later was attributed to John W Lachman by his student, Joseph S Torg.[29]

The test is performed with the patient in supine position. The knee is placed in 30° of flexion. ACL's greatest contribution occurs at this position[30] and when this ligament is sectioned, maximum anterior translation occurs at 30°. The tibia rests in neutral rotation. In neutral position, secondary stabilizers will be relaxed. The examiner stabilizes the anterolateral distal femur with one hand and applies pressure on the posterior aspect of proximal tibia with the other hand, in an attempt to produce posteroanterior (PA) translation (Fig. 8.2). The anterior tibial translation is noted in deficient ACL knees, but the most important finding is the feeling of a "soft" endpoint.[29] The result is described quantitatively and qualitatively in comparison with the contralateral knee. Anterior translation can be graduated in grade 1 (1–5 mm), grade 2 (6–10 mm) and grade 3 (more than 10 mm). The endpoint can be classified as firm, soft or absent.[31]

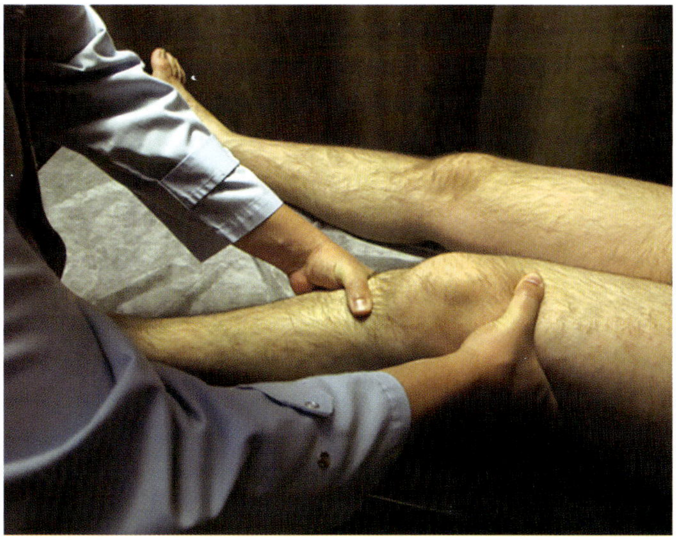

Fig. 8.2: Lachman-Noulis test for anterior cruciate ligament injury.

False-negative results may be seen in concomitant bucked-handle meniscal tears with anterior tibial translation.[29]

Anterior Drawer Test

The anterior drawer test has been widely used in the diagnosis of ACL ruptures and its origin remains unclear. Subject is lied supine with the hip flexed to 45°, knee flexed to 90°, and foot in a neutral position. The examiner is sitting on the subject's foot with both hands behind the subject's proximal tibia and thumbs on the tibial plateau. Then, a PA force is applied to the proximal tibia (Fig. 8.3). Increased anterior tibial displacement as compared by side-to-side difference is indicative of a partial or complete tear of the ACL.

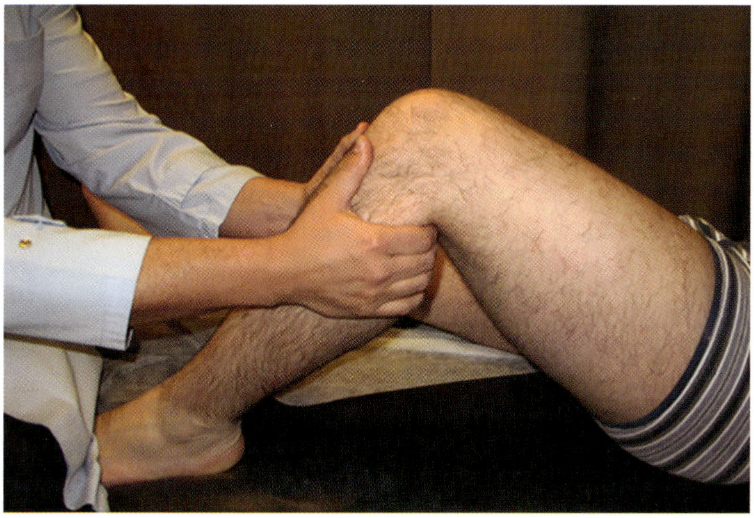

Fig. 8.3: Anterior drawer test for anterior cruciate ligament injury.

The test has relatively low sensitivity for detecting ACL tears in the acute setting. This should serve as a caution to examiners not to rule out an acute ACL injury solely on the basis of a negative anterior drawer test. Conversely, the specificity of the test is quite high, and therefore, a positive anterior drawer would strongly suggest ACL pathology.[32]

Pivot-shift Test

Pivot-shift test was described by Galway and Macintosh in 1972[33] and has been considered a better predictor of clinical outcomes than any uniplanar maneuver[27,34] and the "gold standard" for diagnosis of ACL injury. It is more specific than Lachman test.[35] In an ACL-deficient knee, it evaluates the combined tibial-femoral internal rotation (rotation of the tibia relative to the femur) and anterior tibial translation (the anterior subluxation of the lateral tibial plateau followed by its reduction).

The examiner applies an internal rotation and valgus force to the extended knee, and in ACL incompetence, an anterolateral tibia subluxation is observed. A flexion and valgus force is then applied to the knee and consequently, the iliotibial band changes its role from being an extender to a flexor of the knee and will visibly reduce the subluxation (Fig. 8.4). This signal is observed in the lateral compartment at about 20–30° of flexion. It is mandatory to perform the exam in the healthy knee to determine, if the patient may have some underlying laxity.

Limitations, particularly in awake patients, must be considered due to muscle guarding, and in patients with medial collateral ligament injury, this maneuver can be painful.

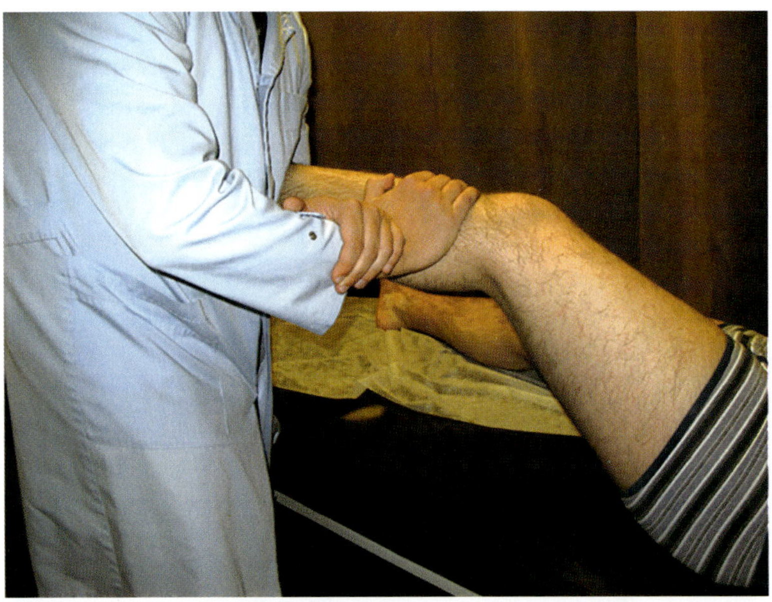

Fig. 8.4: Pivot-shift test for anterior cruciate ligament injury.

Manual Instrumented Testing Devices

Manual instrumented testing aims to provide a more objective evaluation in addition to the physical examination, which may be easily applied at the clinician's office. Nevertheless, these devices are often limited by the absence of bony landmarks, muscle guarding, or dependent on the operator.[36] In this sense,

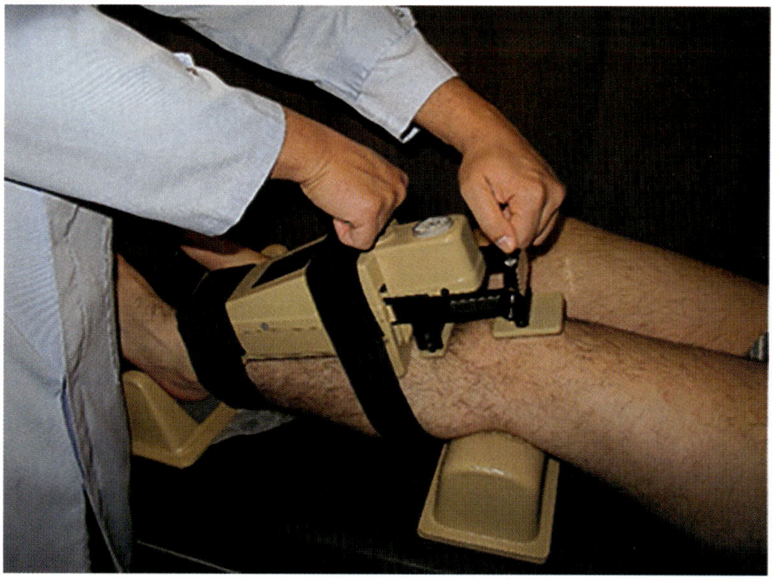

Fig. 8.5: KT-1000 assessment for PA knee laxity. (PA: Posteroanterior).

several arthrometers have been presented in the literature, including the KT-1000/2000 (Fig. 8.5), Genucom, Rolimeter and Rotameter.[37-41]

More recently, an iPad application (Apple Inc., Cupertino, CA) has been developed to overcome the difficulties in grading the pivot-shift test.[42-44] It has the advantage of being noninvasive, user-friendly, and is able to quantify the pivot shift by accurately assessing the acceleration, velocity, and rotation of the tibia in relation to the femur during the pivot shift maneuver.[44]

IMAGING

The examination of ACL tear on magnetic resonance imaging (MRI) plays an essential role in the preoperative planning. MRI is an accurate noninvasive tool that is widely used in the evaluation of intra-articular knee injuries and it has been proved to be useful in cases of diagnosis of uncertain or concomitant injuries, as well as for research purposes.[45] It is the most frequent diagnostic procedure for confirmation of suspected ACL injuries with reported rates of sensitivity of 86% to 94%, and specificity of 95% to 94%, respectively.[46,47]

A routine MRI protocol tries to offer the best visualization of the overall structures of the knee, including meniscus, ligaments, articular cartilage, subchondral bone and peripheral soft tissue. In the presence of clinical or imaging suspicion of ACL injury, a more comprehensive investigation protocol is needed. Although a routine MRI protocol would acceptably differentiate the normal from complete ACL rupture (Figs. 8.6A and B), it has lower accuracy for partial tears.[48]

The MRI study of ACL has evolved over time. The patient knee position in the MRI dedicated extremity coil is not consensual. The full knee extension or approximately 30° of flexion may impact the ACL evaluation and yield different outcomes. In this sense, some authors have described that with knee flexion, the femoral portion of the ACL moves away from the notch roof of intercondylar fossa and therefore, ruptures around proximal portion of ACL may be better detected.[49] Nevertheless, some authors

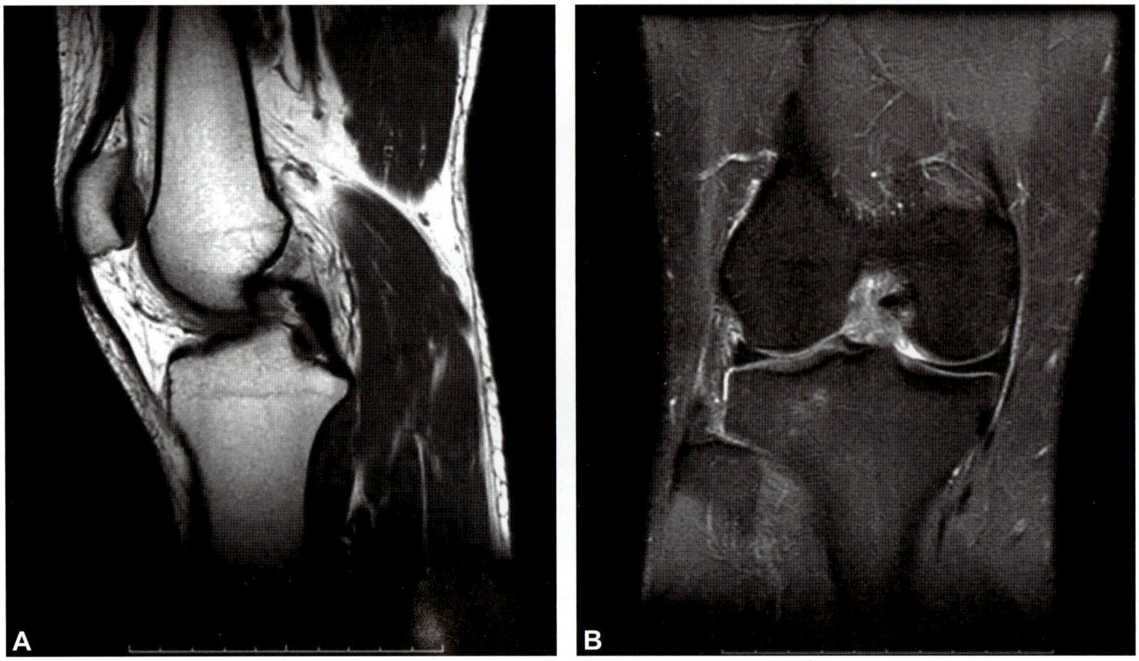

Figs. 8.6A and B: Magnetic resonance imaging of an ACL tear. (A) A sagittal view; (B) A coronal view. (ACL: Anterior cruiciate ligament).

have described the so-called "sagittal oblique plus oblique coronal sequences" at knee full extension, aiming to achieve images more similar to the long axis of the ACL, providing the same sensitivity of MRI acquisition as in knee flexion.

In addition to the knee position, another potential problem that may affect the diagnostic accuracy of MRI is related to the time elapsed from injury to image acquisition. An acute ACL tear may be accompanied by edema of surrounding tissues that may make the evaluation of ACL fibers difficult. Moreover, a partial ruptured ACL has the potential to heal. T2 and proton density (PD) with fat saturation weighted images, employing fast spin echo (FSE) sequences, are most relevant and widely used for the diagnosis of ACL ruptures. Nonetheless, in the acute setting which usually presents ACL tear with edema and effusion, the T2-weighted images may be preferable over PD images.

The hardware evolution at MRI systems has been continuously evolving, offering new imaging sequences, higher magnetic fields, and higher performance multichannel coils, among other technical factors. Hence, higher resolutions at two-dimensional FSE morphological images, and the possibility to use volumetric FSE T2 acquisitions (SPACE, CUBE, VISTA) can offer better accuracy and reliability.

In the presence of a patient with an ACL-reconstructed knee, the accuracy of the tunnel position, usually assessed by the tunnel angle, implant position and length, may be assessed by three-dimensional reconstructions of computed tomography (CT) scans with high reliability.[50,51]

Dynamic Imaging Evaluation of the Knee Instability

Measurement of sagittal knee laxity has been extensively reported for the diagnosis of ACL injuries,[52] but the objective measurement of rotational knee laxity has been recently in focus.[53,54] Knee rotatory instability will induce variations on the knee cartilage load distribution resulting in abnormal kinematics that will increase the risk of development of degenerative knee osteoarthritis.[55]

The Porto-knee testing device (PKTD) (Fig. 8.7) is a knee instrumented testing device designed to test the multiplanar knee instability. It is made of polyurethane compounds to allow compatibility with MRI and CT examinations. The PKTD is able to test the knee sagittal and rotational laxity concomitantly with the imaging examination, which allows the assessment of the ligament "anatomy" and "functionality" within the same exam.[13]

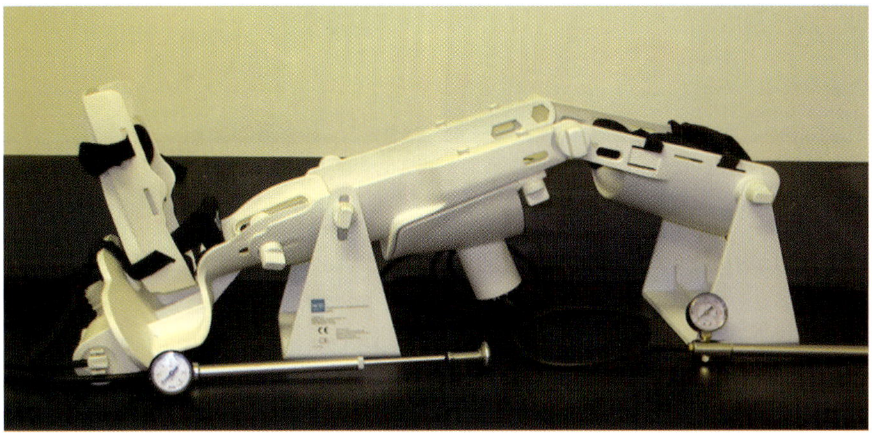

Fig. 8.7: Photograph of the Porto-knee testing device.

The PKTD assessment starts with the patient positioned in a supine position, with the knee flexed at 30°. Initially, with the knee at the rest position, the first MRI sequences are taken (Fig. 8.8A). Then, a PA pressure (4 Bar) is applied through a pressurized plunger platform at the proximal posterior calf region to assess sagittal laxity (Fig. 8.8B). By applying pressure at the footplate through the plunger, it is possible to perform tibial internal (Fig. 8.8C) and external rotation (Fig. 8.8D).

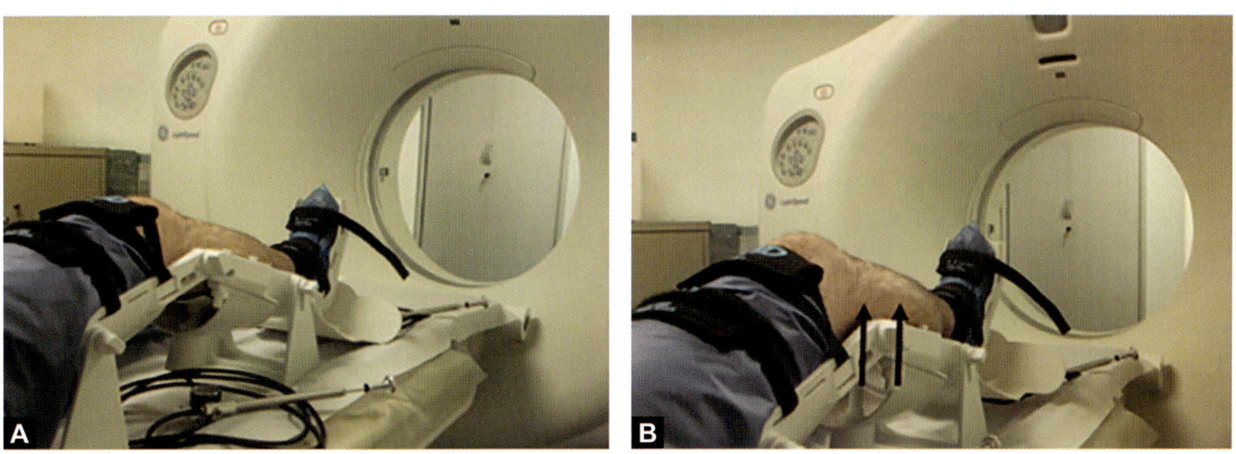

Figs. 8.8A and B: Porto-knee testing device setting for anterior cruciate ligament assessment. The mechanical axis of the device (set at 30° of flexion) is aligned with the knee joint line. (A) Lower limb at rest position (no pressure); (B) PA pressure (arrow shows tibial translation);

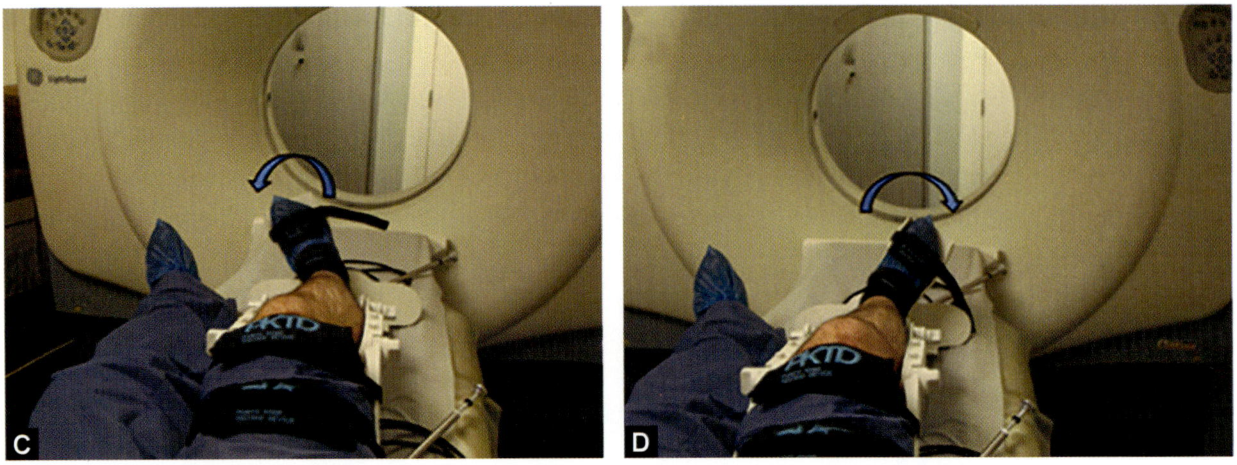

Figs. 8.8C and D: (C) Tibial internal rotation; (D) Tibial external rotation. (PA: Posteroanterior).

The PKTD measurements (in mm) are performed to quantify the lateral and medial tibial plateaus translation in relation to the distal femur. Thus, the first step is to set the tibial slope. Then, two perpendicular lines are made, one crossing the most posterior point of the tibial plateau and other crossing the most posterior point of the femoral condyle, and the distance between the two lines is calculated. This process of measurement is replicated for sequences without pressure (Figs. 8.9A and B) and with PA pressure (Figs. 8.9C and D), and for the rotation measurements (Figs. 8.9E and F). By this approach, it is possible to measure the knee sagittal and rotational laxity.

The PKTD is able to identify partial ruptures by placing stress at the ACL during MRI examination. By combining the sagittal and rotational laxity measurements, the PKTD is able to assess the ligament anatomy and test the functional competence of the remnant bundle.[56]

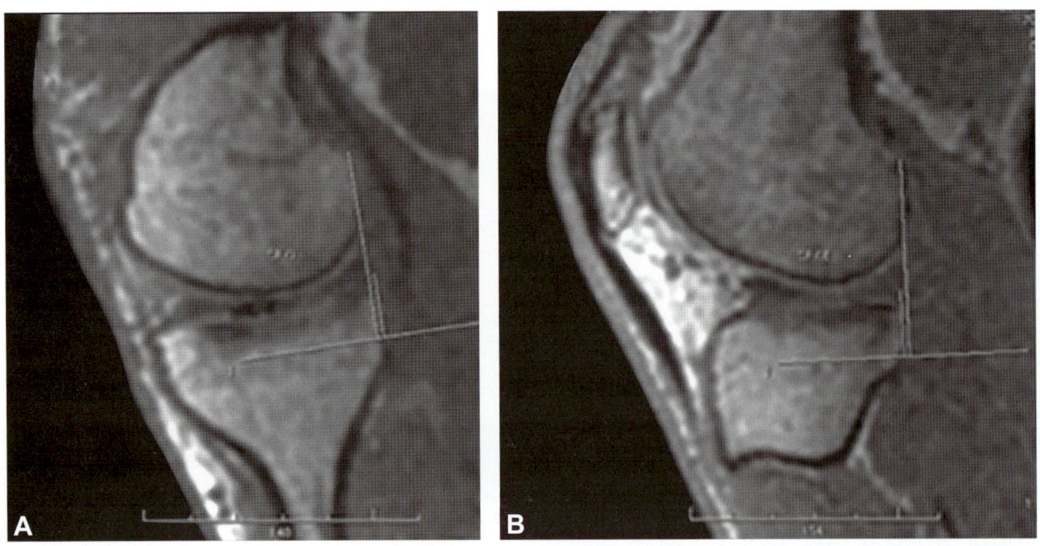

Figs. 8.9A and B: Magnetic resonance imaging measurements of an anterior cruciate ligament-ruptured patient who underwent Porto-knee testing device examination. (A) Medial plateau, no stress (1 mm); (B) Lateral plateau, no stress (1 mm);

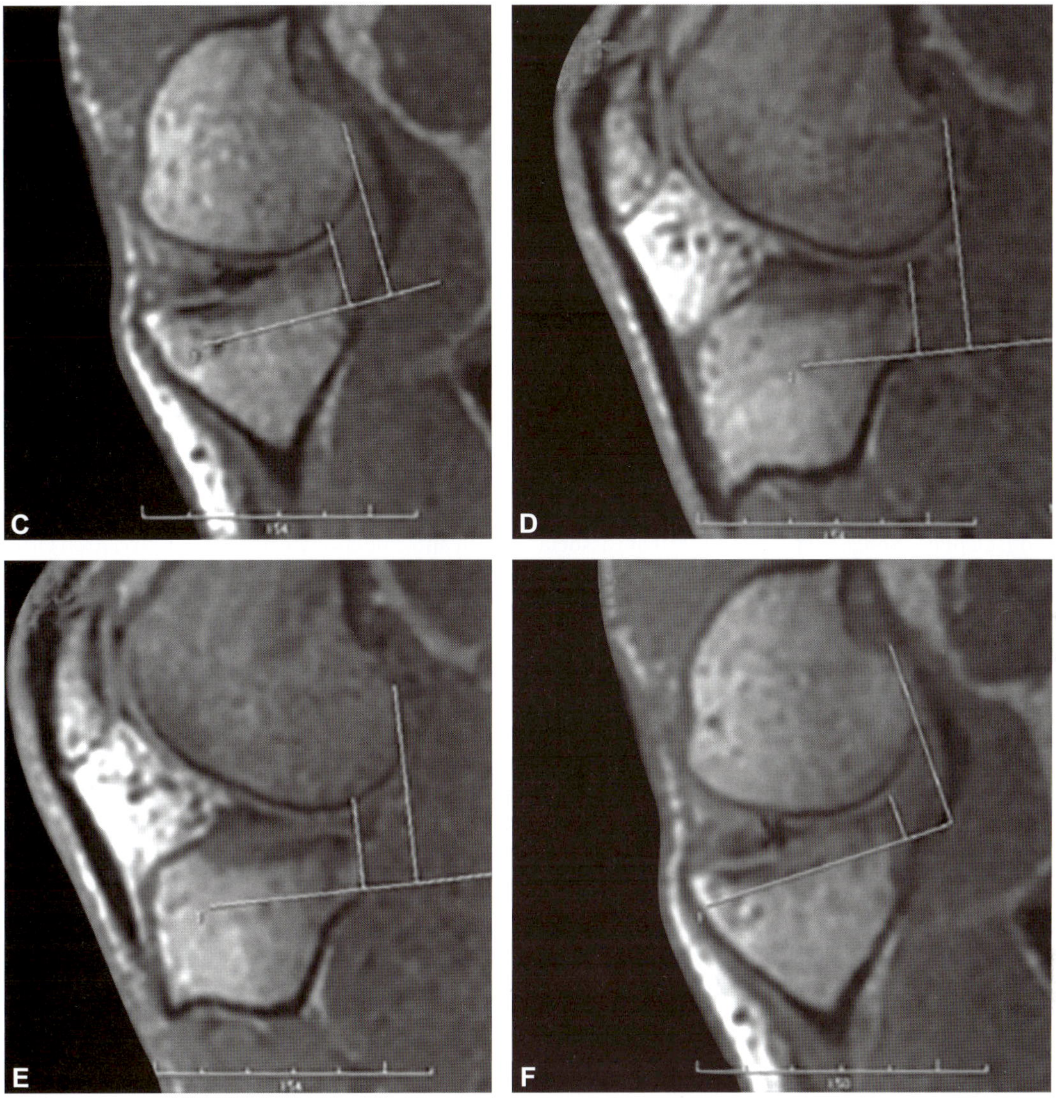

Figs. 8.9C to F: (C) Medial plateau, PA stress (9 mm); (D) Lateral plateau, PA stress (11 mm); (E) Lateral plateau, maximum internal rotation (12 mm); (F) Medial plateau, maximum external rotation (13 mm). (PA: Posteroanterior).

Previous studies have shown that the PKTD is a reliable tool for measuring the knee sagittal (correlation with KT-1000 for PA translation, correlation coefficient = 0.73; $p < 0.05$) and rotational laxity (correlation with lateral pivot-shift test for rotatory laxity under anesthesia, correlation coefficient = 0.8; $p < 0.05$).[57,58] In addition, it has the advantage of adjusting the knee flexion at any angle and combine the rotational measurements with different angles of knee flexion.

More recently, two PKTD calculated measures showed high sensitivity and specificity in identifying total ACL ruptures—the anterior global translation and the global rotation. The anterior global translation (PA translation of both medial and lateral tibial plateaus) has shown to be highly specific (94%), with a cut-off point of 11.1 mm. The global rotation (internal rotation at the lateral tibial plateau plus external rotation at the medial tibial plateau) has shown high sensitivity (93%) with a cut-off point of 15.1 mm.[57]

SUMMARY

The medical history and physical examination are still the most used methods for diagnosing an ACL tear. The MRI assessment provides morphological evaluation of the knee structures, including the ACL, with good reported sensitivity and sensibility figures. The PKTD assessment within MRI allows high sensitivity and specificity in identifying total ACL ruptures, allowing the evaluation of the ligament's functional competence.

REFERENCES

1. Griffin LY, Agel J, Albohm MJ, et al. Noncontact anterior cruciate ligament injuries: risk factors and prevention strategies. J Am Acad Orthop Surg. 2000;8(3):141-50.
2. Chadwick C, Rogowski J, Joyce B. The economics of anterior cruciate ligament reconstruction. In: Prodromos C, Brown C, Fu F, et al. (Eds). The anterior Cruciate Ligament: Reconstruction and Basic Science, 1st Edition. Philadelphia: Saunders Elsevier; 2008. pp. 79-83.
3. Andrade R, Vasta S, Papalia R, et al. Prevalence of articular cartilage lesions and surgical clinical outcomes in football (soccer) players' knees: a systematic review. Arthroscopy. 2016;32(7):1466-77.
4. Hagino T, Ochiai S, Senga S, et al. Meniscal tears associated with anterior cruciate ligament injury. Arch Orthop Trauma Surg. 2015;135(12):1701-6.
5. Andrade R, Pereira H, Espregueira-Mendes J. ACL treatment in 2016–controversy and consensus. Asian Journal of Arthroscopy. 2016;1(1):3-10.
6. Heijink A, Gomoll AH, Madry H, et al. Biomechanical considerations in the pathogenesis of osteoarthritis of the knee. Knee Surg Sports Traumatol Arthrosc. 2012;20(3):423-35.
7. Vannini F, Spalding T, Andriolo L, et al. Sport and early osteoarthritis: the role of sport in aetiology, progression and treatment of knee osteoarthritis. Knee Surg Sports Traumatol Arthrosc. 2016;24(6):1786-96.
8. Branch TP, Mayr HO, Browne JE, et al. Instrumented examination of anterior cruciate ligament injuries: minimizing flaws of the manual clinical examination. Arthroscopy. 2010;26(7):997-1004.
9. Geraets SE, Meuffels DE, van Meer BL, et al. Diagnostic value of medical history and physical examination of anterior cruciate ligament injury: comparison between primary care physician and orthopaedic surgeon. Knee Surg Sports Traumatol Arthrosc. 2015;23(4):968-74.
10. Boden BP, Dean GS, Feagin JA, et al. Mechanisms of anterior cruciate ligament injury. Orthopedics. 2000;23(6):573-8.
11. Shimokochi Y, Shultz SJ. Mechanisms of noncontact anterior cruciate ligament injury. J Athl Train. 2008;43(4):396-408.
12. Andrade R, Vasta S, Sevivas N, et al. Notch morphology is a risk factor for ACL injury: a systematic review and meta-analysis. J ISAKOS. 2016;1(2):70-81.
13. Pereira HFC, Fernandes M, Pereira R, et al. ACL Injuries identifiable for pre-participation imagiological analysis: risk factors. In: Doral MN, Karlsson J (Eds). Sports Injuries: Prevention, Diagnosis, Treatment and Rehabilitation. Springer; 2013. pp. 1-15.
14. Alentorn-Geli E, Mendiguchia J, Samuelsson K, et al. Prevention of anterior cruciate ligament injuries in sports. Part I: systematic review of risk factors in male athletes. Knee Surg Sports Traumatol Arthrosc. 2014;22(1):3-15.
15. Zeng C, Yang T, Wu S, et al. Is posterior tibial slope associated with noncontact anterior cruciate ligament injury? Knee Surg Sports Traumatol Arthrosc. 2014;24(3):830-7.
16. Hohmann E, Bryant A, Reaburn P, et al. Is there a correlation between posterior tibial slope and non-contact anterior cruciate ligament injuries? Knee Surg Sports Traumatol Arthrosc. 2011;19(1): 109-14.
17. Li Y, Hong L, Feng H, et al. Posterior tibial slope influences static anterior tibial translation in anterior cruciate ligament reconstruction a minimum 2-year follow-up study. Am J Sports Med. 2014;42(4):927-33.
18. Fernandes MS, Pereira R, Andrade R, et al. Is the femoral lateral condyle's bone morphology the trochlea of the ACL? Knee Surg Sports Traumatol Arthrosc. 2017;25(1):207-14.
19. Collins M, Posthumus M. Type V collagen genotype and exercise-related phenotype relationships: a novel hypothesis. Exerc Sport Sci Rev. 2011;39(4):191-8.
20. Stępień-Słodkowska M, Ficek K, Eider J, et al. The +1245G/T polymorphisms in the collagen type I alpha I (*Coliai*) gene in polish skiers with anterior cruciate ligament injury. Biol Sport. 2013;30:57-60.
21. Boden BP, Sheehan FT, Torg JS, et al. Non-contact ACL injuries: mechanisms and risk factors. J Am Acad Orthop Surg. 2010;18(9):520.

22. Posthumus M, Collins M, September AV, et al. The intrinsic risk factors for ACL ruptures: an evidence-based review. Phys Sportsmed. 2011;39(1):62-73.
23. Ramesh R, Von Arx O, Azzopardi T, et al. The risk of anterior cruciate ligament rupture with generalised joint laxity. Bone Joint J. 2005;87(6):800-3.
24. Uhorchak JM, Scoville CR, Williams GN, et al. Risk factors associated with noncontact injury of the anterior cruciate ligament a prospective four-year evaluation of 859 west point cadets. Am J Sports Med. 2003;31(6):831-42.
25. Kim SJ, Kim TE, Lee DH, et al. Anterior cruciate ligament reconstruction in patients who have excessive joint laxity. J Bone Joint Surg Am. 2008;90(4):735-41.
26. Prins M. The Lachman test is the most sensitive and the pivot shift the most specific test for the diagnosis of ACL rupture. Aust J Physiother. 2006;52(1):66.
27. Katz JW, Fingeroth RJ. The diagnostic accuracy of ruptures of the anterior cruciate ligament comparing the Lachman test, the anterior drawer sign, and the pivot shift test in acute and chronic knee injuries. Am J Sports Med. 1986;14(1): 88-91.
28. Noulis G. Entorse du genou. Fac Med Paris (PhD Thesis). 1875:1-53.
29. Torg JS, Conrad W, Kalen V. Clinical I diagnosis of anterior cruciate ligament instability in the athlete. Am J Sports Med. 1976;4(2):84-93.
30. Butler D, Noyes F, Grood E. Ligamentous restraints to anterior-posterior drawer in the human knee. J Bone Joint Surg Am. 1980;62(2):259-70.
31. Lubowitz JH, Bernardini BJ, Reid JB. Current concepts review comprehensive physical examination for instability of the knee. Am J Sports Med. 2008;36(3):577-94.
32. Malanga GA, Andrus S, Nadler SF, et al. Physical examination of the knee: a review of the original test description and scientific validity of common orthopedic tests. Arch Phys Med Rehabil. 2003;84(4):592-603.
33. Galway R, Beaupre A, MacIntosh D. Pivot shift: a clinical sign of symptomatic anterior cruciate insufficiency. J Bone Joint Surg Br. 1972;54(4):763-4.
34. Citak M, Suero EM, Rozell JC, et al. A mechanized and standardized pivot shifter: technical description and first evaluation. Knee Surg Sports Traumatol Arthrosc. 2011;19(5):707-11.
35. Benjaminse A, Gokeler A, van der Schans CP. Clinical diagnosis of an anterior cruciate ligament rupture: a meta-analysis. J Orthop Sports Phys Ther. 2006;36(5):267-88.
36. Pereira H, Sevivas N, Pereira R, et al. New tools for diagnosis, assessment of surgical outcome and follow-up. In: Hermoso JAH, Monllau JC (Eds). Lesiones ligamentosas de la rodilla. Barcelona: Marge Medica Books; 2012. pp. 185-97.
37. Daniel DM, Stone ML, Sachs R, et al. Instrumented measurement of anterior knee laxity in patients with acute anterior cruciate ligament disruption. Am J Sports Med. 1985;13(6):401-7.
38. Myrer JW, Schulthies SS, Fellingham GW. Relative and absolute reliability of the KT-2000 arthrometer for uninjured knees testing at 67, 89, 134, and 178 n and manual maximum forces. Am J Sports Med. 1996;24(1):104-8.
39. Oliver JH, Coughlin LP. Objective knee evaluation using the Genucom knee analysis system clinical implications. Am J Sports Med. 1987;15(6):571-8.
40. Balasch H, Schiller M, Friebel H, et al. Evaluation of anterior knee joint instability with the Rolimeter A test in comparison with manual assessment and measuring with the KT-1000 arthrometer. Knee Surg Sports Traumatol Arthrosc. 1999;7(4):204-8.
41. Lorbach O, Wilmes P, Maas S, et al. A non-invasive device to objectively measure tibial rotation: verification of the device. Knee Surg Sports Traumatol Arthrosc. 2009;17(7):756-62.
42. Hoshino Y, Musahl V, Irrgang JJ, et al. Quantitative evaluation of the pivot shift-relationship to clinical pivot shift grade. A prospective international multicenter study. Orthop J Sports Med. 2015;3(7 suppl 2):2325967115S00108.
43. Hoshino Y, Araujo P, Ahldén M, et al. Quantitative evaluation of the pivot shift by image analysis using the iPad. Knee Surg Sports Traumatol Arthrosc. 2013;21(4):975-80.
44. Zaffagnini S, Signorelli C, Grassi A, et al. Assessment of the pivot shift using inertial sensors. Curr Rev Musculoskelet Med. 2016;9(2):160-3.
45. Meuffels DE, Poldervaart MT, Diercks RL, et al. Guideline on anterior cruciate ligament injury: a multidisciplinary review by the Dutch Orthopaedic Association. Acta Orthop. 2012;83(4):379-86.
46. Crawford R, Walley G, Bridgman S, et al. Magnetic resonance imaging versus arthroscopy in the diagnosis of knee pathology, concentrating on meniscal lesions and ACL tears: a systematic review. Br Med Bull. 2007;84(1):5-23.
47. Oei EH, Nikken JJ, Verstijnen AC, et al. MR imaging of the menisci and cruciate ligaments: A systematic review 1. Radiology. 2003;226(3):837-48.
48. Nenezić D, Kocijancic I. The value of the sagittal-oblique MRI technique for injuries of the anterior cruciate ligament in the knee. Radiol Oncol. 2013;47(1):19-25.

49. Chang MJ, Chang CB, Choi JY, et al. How useful is MRI in diagnosing isolated bundle ACL injuries? Clin Orthop Relat Res. 2013;471(10):3283-90.
50. Meuffels DE, Potters JW, Koning AH, et al. Visualization of postoperative anterior cruciate ligament reconstruction bone tunnels: reliability of standard radiographs, CT scans, and 3D virtual reality images. Acta Orthop. 2011;82(6):699-703.
51. Pereira H, Sevivas N, Pereira R, et al. Systematic Approach from Porto School. In: Siebold R, Dejour D, Zaffagnini S (Eds). Anterior Cruciate Ligament Reconstruction. Berlin: Springer; 2014. pp. 367-86.
52. van Eck CF, Loopik M, van den Bekerom MP, et al. Methods to diagnose acute anterior cruciate ligament rupture: a meta-analysis of instrumented knee laxity tests. Knee Surg Sports Traumatol Arthrosc. 2013;21(9):1989-97.
53. Branch T, Siebold R, Freedberg H, et al. Double-bundle ACL reconstruction demonstrated superior clinical stability to single-bundle ACL reconstruction: a matched-pairs analysis of instrumented tests of tibial anterior translation and internal rotation laxity. Knee Surg Sports Traumatol Arthrosc. 2011;19(3):432-40.
54. Lorbach O, Brockmeyer M, Kieb M, et al. Objective measurement devices to assess static rotational knee laxity: focus on the rotameter. Knee Surg Sports Traumatol Arthrosc. 2012;20(4):639-44.
55. Chung JH, Ryu KJ, Lee DH, et al. An analysis of normative data on the knee rotatory profile and the usefulness of the rotatometer, a new instrument for measuring tibiofemoral rotation: the reliability of the knee rotatometer. Knee Surg Sports Traumatol Arthrosc. 2015;23(9):2727-33.
56. Ohashi B, Ward J, Araujo P, et al. Partial anterior cruciate ligament ruptures: knee laxity measurements and pivot shift. In: Doral MN, Karlsson J (Eds). Sports Injuries: Prevention, Diagnosis, Treatment and Rehabilitation. Berlin: Springer; 2015. pp. 1245-58.
57. Espregueira-Mendes J, Andrade R, Leal A, et al. Global rotation has high sensitivity in ACL lesions within stress MRI. Knee Surg Sports Traumatol Arthrosc. 2016 Aug 16. (Ahead of Print)
58. Espregueira-Mendes J, Pereira H, Sevivas N, et al. Assessment of rotatory laxity in anterior cruciate ligament-deficient knees using magnetic resonance imaging with Porto-knee testing device. Knee Surg Sports Traumatol Arthrosc. 2012;20(4):671-8.

CHAPTER

9

Arthroscopic Diagnosis and Injury Patterns of Anterior Cruciate Ligament

Anshu Shekhar, Sachin Tapasvi, Chirag Thonse, Vikram Kakatkar

INTRODUCTION

Clinical diagnosis of an anterior cruciate ligament (ACL) injury is based on relevant history and performance of standard tests for its insufficiency. During the physical examination, a positive result for the pivot shift test is the best for ruling in an ACL rupture, whereas a negative result to the Lachman test is the best for ruling out an ACL rupture. It can also be concluded that, solely using sensitivity and specificity values, the Lachman test is better overall for both ruling in and ruling out ACL ruptures.[1] Suggestive tears can be reliably confirmed on an MRI scan. Both clinical examination and MRI are reliable and reproducible methods of diagnosing chronic ACL tears with great accuracy.[2,3] However, MR evaluation of partial ACL tears is not sufficiently sensitive to establish the diagnosis without arthroscopy.[4] Arthroscopy can be considered the "gold standard" for diagnosis and its high diagnostic accuracy allows it to be used as a benchmark when assessing the usefulness and sensitivity of other diagnostic methods.[5] Arthroscopy provides information that other tests do not, which is derived by probing the ACL (e.g. ACL elongation, occult tears, and intrasubstance partial tears). Arthroscopy provides the tactile information by probing the ACL tissue and evaluation by direct visualization. In this chapter, we discuss the technique and nuances of accurate diagnosis of an ACL tear and the tear patterns that have been described.

ARTHROSCOPIC DIAGNOSIS

After induction with appropriate anesthesia, the patient must be carefully examined clinically to confirm the diagnosis. The leg can be positioned in a leg holder or with the table flat and a thigh side-post and this is our preferred technique. A high thigh tourniquet is applied. The positioning is rechecked to ensure that the leg can be drawn into valgus against the side-post and brought into a figure-of-4 position freely before skin preparation and draping. Marking of the portals is a good practice prior to joint distension when landmarks become obscured (Fig. 9.1). Though every operator can have his own method of performing a diagnostic arthroscopy amongst the several described, it is essential to learn and develop a specific routine to perform the procedure in a consistent and reproducible manner.[6] The technique of correct portal placement avoiding the fat pad and performing a diagnostic arthroscopy has been described in Chapter 1 (*Placing correct portals for Transportal ACL Reconstruction*). The ACL is

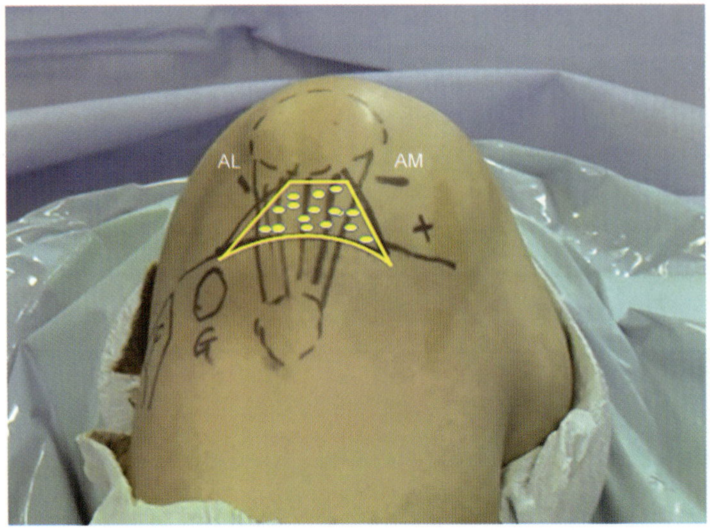

Fig. 9.1: Skin marking of the two basic portals for arthroscopy of the right knee. The yellow dotted area marks the extent of infrapatellar fat-pad which must be avoided to obtain a good view and hassle-free instrumentation. (AL: Anterolateral; AM: Anteromedial).

visualized through the anterolateral (AL) portal in the intercondylar notch with the knee at about 60–90 degrees flexion (Fig. 9.2). There are various tear patterns described as discussed in the next section. A sound knowledge of these patterns helps identify the tears and different scars patterns. Careful probing using a hook probe inserted from the anteromedial (AM) portal is essential, especially when there is a large remnant attached at some point proximally, for example to the posterior cruciate ligament (PCL). A note must also be made of the intercondylar notch morphology because patients with a stenotic notch are prone to ACL tears and require a notchplasty to prevent graft impingement.

The ACL consists of two bundles, the AM and posterolateral (PL) based on the tibial insertion.[7] The PL bundle is tight in extension, whereas the AM bundle is tight in flexion, which correlates with increased

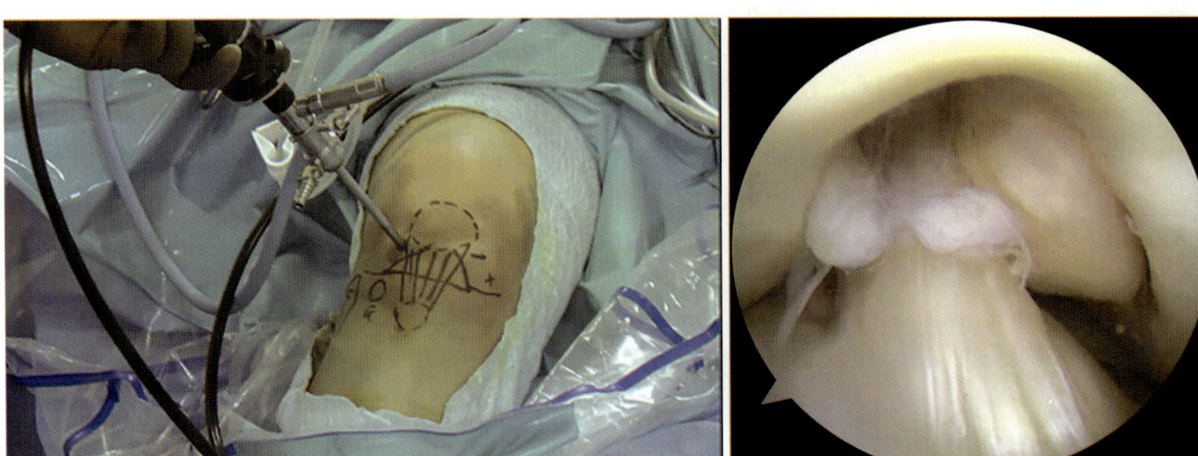

Fig. 9.2: The anterior cruciate ligament (ACL) as visualized with the arthroscope in the anterolateral portal (right knee). Note the knee is at about 60 degrees of flexion.

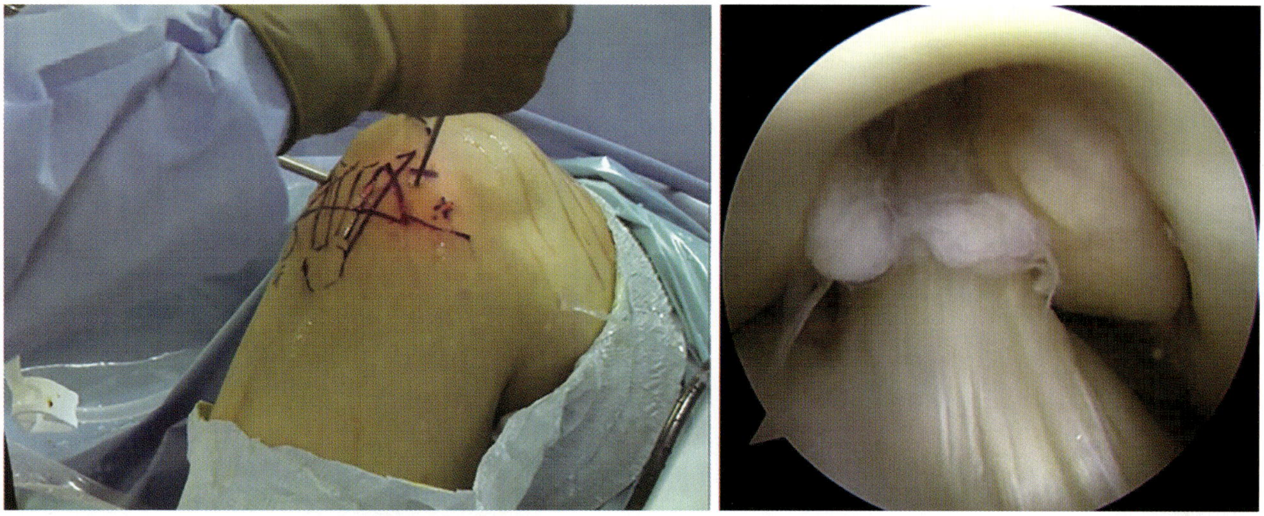

Fig. 9.3: The anteromedial (AM) bundle as seen from the anterolateral (AL) portal (right knee) at a flexion of 90 degrees. The tension and continuity of this bundle is assessed using a hook probe inserted from the AM portal.

contributions to knee stability and the likelihood of partial ruptures in these positions.[8] The AM bundle lies anteriorly when viewing from the AL portal and must be thoroughly probed using an arthroscopic hook probe from the AM portal with the knee in 90 degrees flexion (Fig. 9.3). This is essential, so as not to miss an AM bundle tear when the ACL otherwise looks intact on inspection only. The PL bundle lies posteriorly and can be visualized by retracting the AM bundle with a probe. It is best visualized in a figure-of-4 position while viewing from the AL portal (Fig. 9.4) with bleeding or discontinuity as features of a PL bundle tear. There is a caveat however; the PL bundle is normally lax in 90 degrees of flexion and demonstration of such a laxity on probing must not drive one to diagnose it as an isolated PL bundle tear or even an elongated, dysfunctional ACL.[9] This laxity would disappear when the knee is brought into extension but then, the PL bundle itself cannot be visualized!

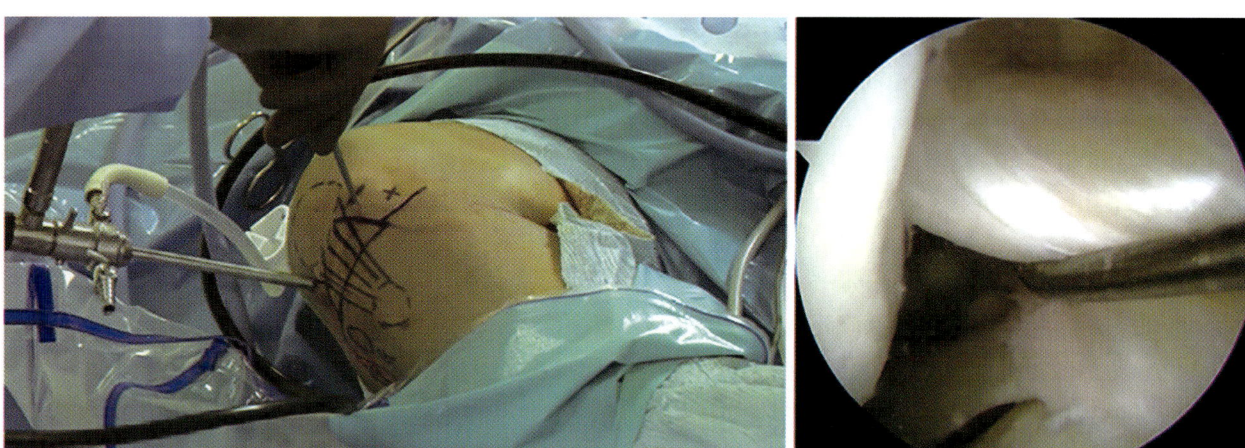

Fig. 9.4: The posterolateral bundle of anterior cruciate ligament (ACL) is best visualized within the figure-of-4 position and viewing from the anterolateral (AL) portal (right knee). A hook probe is inserted through the anteromedial (AM) portal for confirming the tension in this bundle.

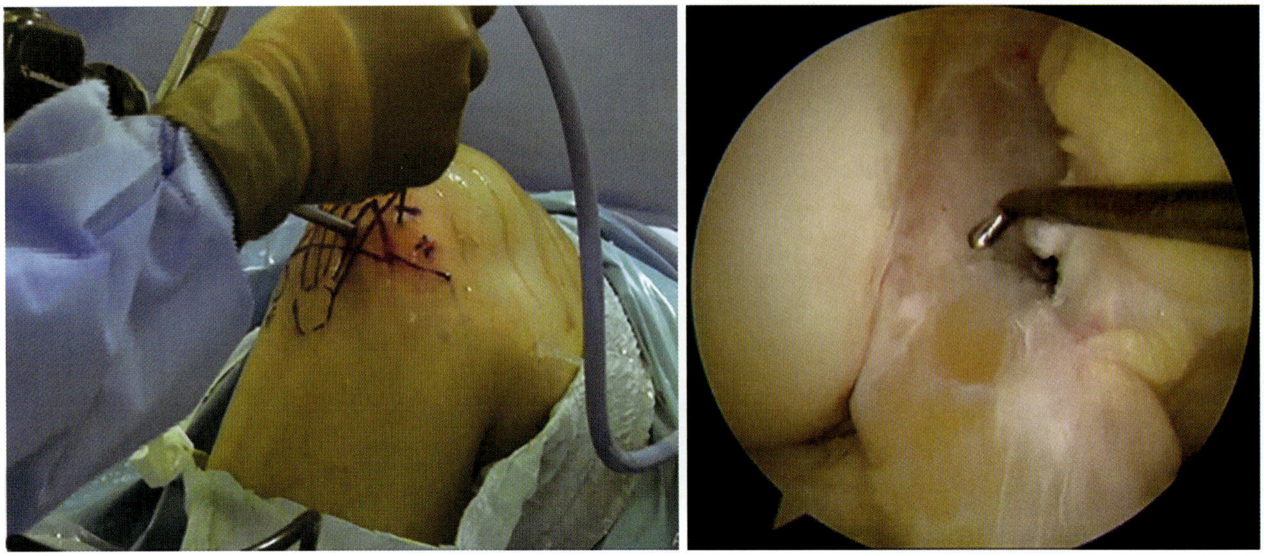

Fig. 9.5: The anterior cruciate ligament (ACL) femoral insertion site is visualized "end-on" when viewed from the central portal with the knee in 90 degrees flexion (right knee). A direct visualization is helpful in locating the anatomic insertion site and assessment of femoral avulsion injuries.

Another dilemma arises when diagnosing avulsions from the femoral insertion site (FIS) of the ACL on the lateral femoral condyle. It may sometimes be difficult to completely visualize the FIS with the arthroscope in the AL portal as is provides a side view instead of an end-on picture. In such a scenario, one must shift the scope to the AM portal or create an additional central portal (CP) through the medial third of patella tendon, which allows excellent visualization of the FIS (Fig. 9.5).[10]

INJURY PATTERNS OF ANTERIOR CRUCIATE LIGAMENT

An awareness of the injury patterns of the ACL is necessary when performing diagnostic arthroscopy for an unstable knee. The simplest classification is either a complete or a partial ACL tear, which may further be divided into an isolated AM or PL bundle tear. Several authors have studied tear and scarring patterns encountered during arthroscopy, though the clinical significance of such classifications are not well established.

Sherman et al. classified tears of the ACL based on location with respect to the femur and tibia.[11] They also classified the tissue quality of the torn ACL as *excellent*—broad stump with no interstitial tearing and intact synovium; *good*—mild degree of interstitial tearing and *fair*—thin ligament with shredding and interstitial tearing (Fig. 9.6 and Table 9.1). This classification system was devised to determine which ACL tears are most amenable to repair. With a resurgence of interest in primary ACL repairs, this classification assumes significance.[12,13] Basically, type 1 tears with excellent tissue quality are candidates for primary suture repair [discussed in detail in Chapter 26 (*Primary ACL Repair*)].

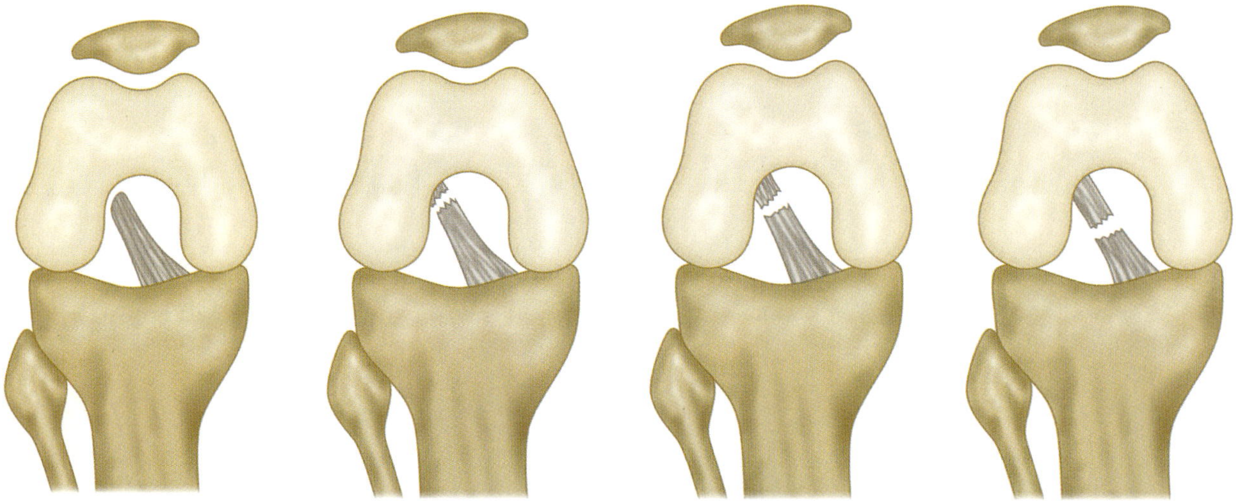

Fig. 9.6: Sherman's classification of anterior cruciate ligament (ACL) tears based on location of the tear with respect to the femur and tibia (Modified from Sherman[11]).

Table 9.1: Sherman classification of anterior cruciate ligament (ACL) tears—based on location of tear.

Type 1	Avulsion of the entire ligament off the femoral insertion, without a major bone fragment, leaving no remnant of proximal tissue
Type 2	Tear with proximal femoral stump of 20% and distal tibial stump of 80%
Type 3	Tear with proximal femoral stump of 33% and distal tibial stump of 67%
Type 4	True midsubstance tear with 50% ligament remaining on both ends

Gachter et al. formulated an extensive classification of the arthroscopic morphology of a torn ACL into seven classes (Figs. 9.7A to G and Table 9.2).[14] This was modified by Lo et al. who added a class H to include those in whom the morphology resembled more than one type.[15] Further, they divided these variants into two categories:

1. With intra-articular reattachments (class B, E, and G) suggesting possible scarring or healing of the ACL remnants
2. Without intra-articular reattachments (class A, C, D, and F) suggesting the absence of a scarring or healing response.

They concluded that even in chronic situations in which the knee remains functionally unstable, human ACLs rarely resorb and that torn ACLs commonly reattach in the knee, mainly to the PCL via a process that is consistent with scarring. While the function of these reattachments is clearly inadequate in people with unstable knees because of a combination of reattachment location, scar quantity, or quality, they believed that the intra-articular environment in humans often maintains ACL stumps and it is not totally inhibitory to ACL reattachment via some biological process.

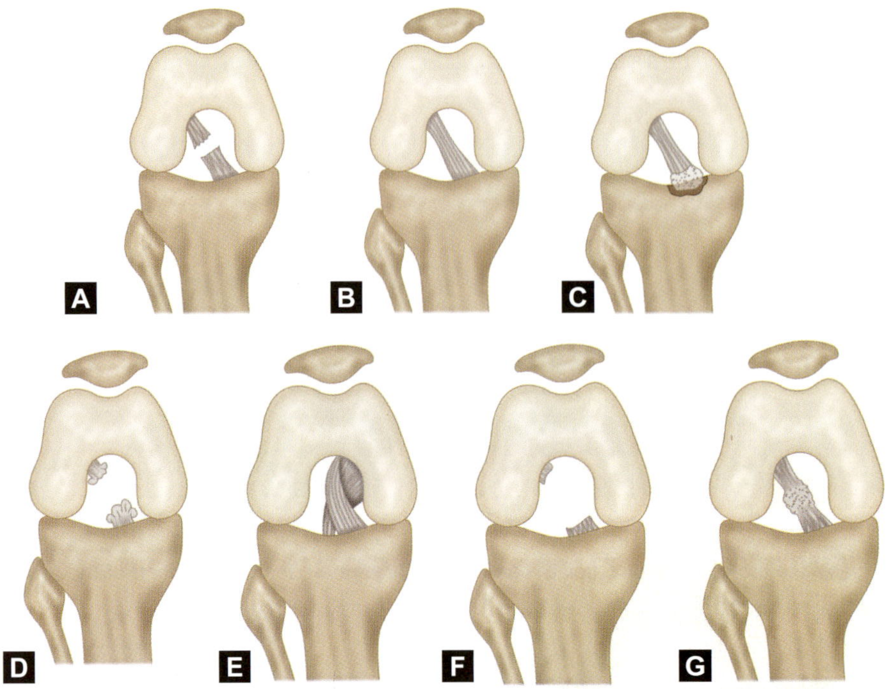

Figs. 9.7A to G: Gachter classification of anterior cruciate ligament (ACL) tears based on morphology of the tear.[14]

Table 9.2: Gachter classification of anterior cruciate ligament (ACL) tears—based on morphology.	
Class A	Frayed torn ends resembling a mop
Class B	Intrasynovial or intrasubstance tear with intact synovium and elongated ACL
Class C	Bony avulsion from tibial insertion
Class D	Retracted ACL tear with club-head like distension of torn ends
Class E	Scarring or reattachment of the ACL to posterior cruciate ligament (PCL)—anterior/posterior or both
Class F	Complete resorption of the ACL with small tibial remnant
Class G	Scarring of the torn ends to each other with elongation

Crain et al. described patterns of scar formation after ACL tears encountered on arthroscopy.[16] This was done to test the hypothesis whether certain scar patterns provide stability after a tear as was reported by some investigators and whether such patients could be managed without a reconstruction.[17,18] They classified four types of scar:

1. *Scarring to the PCL*: The ACL fibers are retracted and became matted down to the PCL. The ligament scarring to the PCL was either along the anterior margin of the PCL or wrapped around the ligament along the tibial surface (Fig. 9.8A).
2. *Attachment to roof of the intercondylar notch*: The stump is attached to the femur usually near the 12 o'clock position and anterior to the femoral attachment of the ACL (Fig. 9.8B).
3. *Attachment to lateral wall of notch*: At a position anterior and distal to the ACL anatomic footprint (Fig. 9.8C).

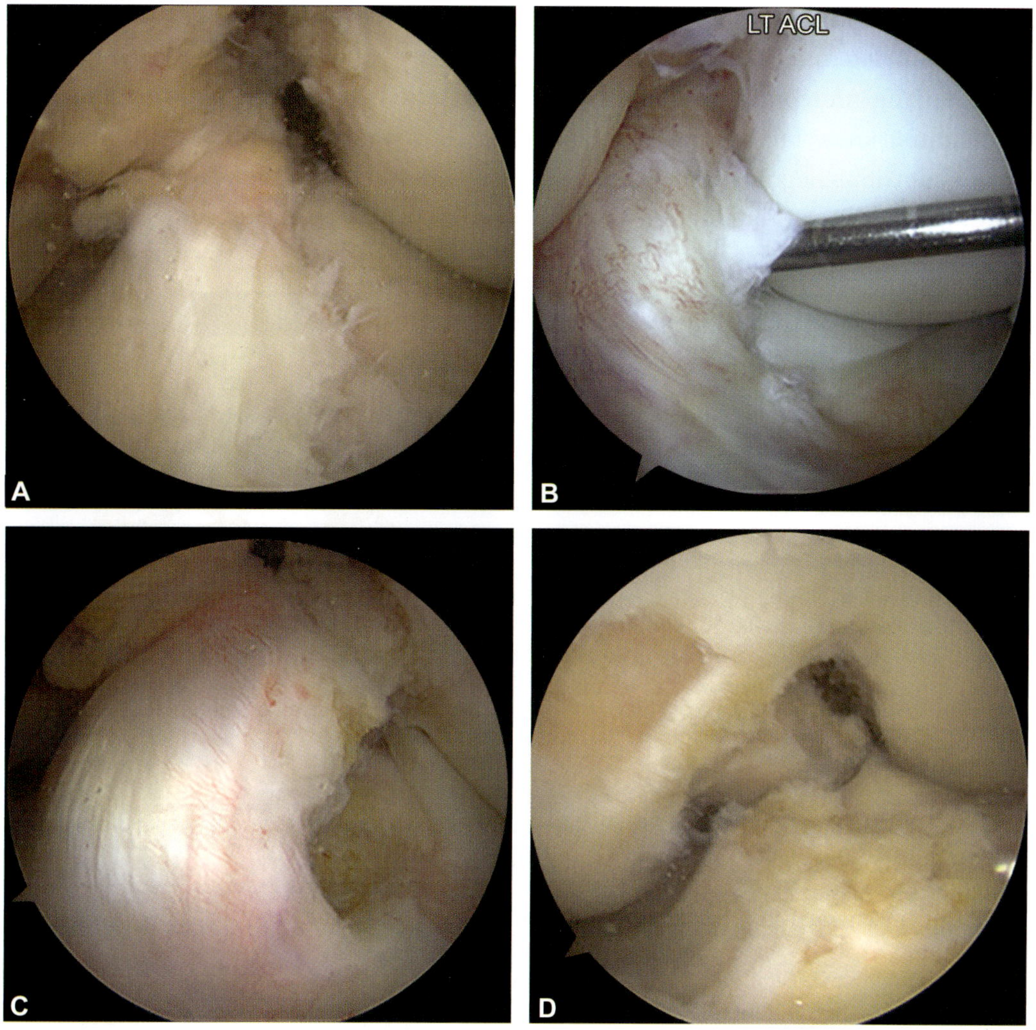

Figs. 9.8A to D: Patterns of scarring of the anterior cruciate ligament (ACL) following a tear as described by Crain.[16] (A) Stump attached to the posterior cruciate ligament (PCL). (B) Stump attached to the roof of intercondylar notch near 12 o'clock position. (C) Stump attached to the lateral condyle anterior to the anatomic insertion. (D) Absence of a stump.

4. *No identified ligament tissue:* Presence of a small stump on the tibial side with empty lateral wall (Fig. 9.8D).

Crain et al. found that when the ACL healed to the roof of the notch or along the lateral wall, measurable control of anterior translation did exist and this subset of patients could potentially cope without a surgery. Further, they advocated preserving the remnant in such cases for its mechanical properties.[16] However, more recent studies using objective assessment tools to validate this conclusion have found conflicting results. Maeda et al. assessed anterior tibial translation (ATT) and range of tibial internal/external rotation using a navigation system before and after resection of ACL remnants.[19] The results showed that the mean ATT significantly increased after resection in knees with ACL remnants bridging to the lateral wall of intercondylar notch. They concluded that ACL remnants bridging to the lateral wall of the intercondylar notch significantly decreased ATT only, but the knee stability provided by ACL remnants was not significant. Nagai quantitatively evaluated the biomechanical function of ACL remnants by measuring the

ATT with KT-1000 and during the Lachman test with an electromagnetic measurement system (EMS) and tibial acceleration during the pivot shift test with EMS system.[20] They found that ACL remnants attached to the lateral wall of the intercondylar notch partially contributed to anterior-posterior stability but did not contribute to dynamic knee stability. They concluded that ACL remnants attached to non-anatomic insertion sites do not contribute significantly to knee stabilization and recommended that ACL augmentation procedures would be inappropriate, but ACL reconstruction would be appropriate from a biomechanical perspective.

PEARLS AND PITFALLS

- Arthroscopy is the "gold standard" for diagnosis of ACL tear especially when the clinical laxity is subtle and MRI is equivocal or if there is a mismatch between inferences of the two.
- Creation of accurate AL and AM portals is essential to allow performance of a smooth diagnostic round prior to proceeding with any surgery. The fat pad must be avoided for clear visualization and hassle free instrumentation.
- Diagnosing on inspection only is fallacious. Through probing with a hook probe is essential to check the continuity and tension of the ligament remnant.
- Anteromedial bundle is visualized best with the knee at 90 degrees of flexion and its tension is relatively constant in mid-flexion range. The PL bundle in best visualized in a figure-of-4 position and in lax in flexion and taut in extension.
- Knowledge of scar patterns improves the accuracy of diagnosing a tear when there is a large remnant. Presence of such scarred tissue does not provide adequate stability to the knee and an ACL reconstruction must be performed, preserving the remnant for both, its biological and mechanical value.

REFERENCES

1. Ostrowski JA. Accuracy of 3 Diagnostic Tests for Anterior Cruciate Ligament Tears. J Athl Train. 2006;41:120-1.
2. Felli L, Garlaschi G, Muda A, et al. Comparison of clinical, MRI and arthroscopic assessments of chronic ACL injuries, meniscal tears and cartilage defects. Musculoskelet Surg. 2016;100:231-8.
3. Orlando Júnior N, de Souza Leão MG, de Oliveira NHC. Diagnosis of knee injuries: comparison of the physical examination and magnetic resonance imaging with the findings from arthroscopy. Rev Bras Ortop (English Edition). 2015;50:712-9.
4. Umans H, Wimpfheimer O, Haramati N, et al. Diagnosis of partial tears of the anterior cruciate ligament of the knee: value of MR imaging. AJR Am J Roentgenol. 1995;165:893-7.
5. Nickinson R, Darrah C, Donell S. Accuracy of clinical diagnosis in patients undergoing knee arthroscopy. Int Orthop. 2010;34:39-44.
6. Frank RM, McCormick F, Harris J, et al. Diagnostic knee arthroscopy: surgical technique. OKOJ. 2014;12:1.
7. Zantop T, Petersen W, Fu FH. Anatomy of the anterior cruciate ligament. Op Tech Orthop. 2005;15:20-8.
8. Amis AA, Dawkins GP. Functional anatomy of the anterior cruciate ligament. Fibre bundle actions related to ligament replacements and injuries. J Bone Joint Surg Br. 1991;73:260-7.
9. Petersen W, Zantop T. Partial rupture of the anterior cruciate ligament. Arthroscopy. 2006;22:1143-5.
10. Araujo PH, van Eck CF, Macalena JA, et al. Advances in the three-portal technique for anatomical single- or double-bundle ACL reconstruction. Knee Surg Sports Traumatol Arthrosc. 2011;19:1239-42.
11. Sherman MF, Lieber L, Bonamo JR, et al. The long-term follow-up of primary anterior cruciate ligament repair: Defining a rationale for augmentation. Am J Sports Med. 1991;19:243-55.
12. DiFelice GS, Villegas C, Taylor S. Anterior Cruciate Ligament Preservation: Early Results of a Novel Arthroscopic Technique for Suture Anchor Primary Anterior Cruciate Ligament Repair. Arthroscopy. 2015;31:2162-71.
13. Achtnich A, Herbst E, Forkel P, et al. Acute Proximal Anterior Cruciate Ligament Tears: Outcomes After Arthroscopic Suture Anchor Repair Versus Anatomic Single-Bundle Reconstruction. Arthroscopy. 2016;32:2562-9.
14. Jakob RP, Stäubli HU. The Knee and the Cruciate Ligaments. In: Gächter A (Ed) The Various Faces of Anterior Cruciate Ligament Tears During Arthroscopic Examination. Berlin Heidelberg: Springer Nature; 1992. pp. 190-2.
15. Lo IK, de Maat GH, Valk JW, et al. The gross morphology of torn human anterior cruciate ligaments in unstable knees. Arthroscopy. 1999;15:301-6.

16. Crain EH, Fithian DC, Paxton EW, et al. Variation in anterior cruciate ligament scar pattern: does the scar pattern affect anterior laxity in anterior cruciate ligament-deficient knees? Arthroscopy. 2005;21:19-24.
17. Ihara H, Miwa M, Deya K, et al. MRI of anterior cruciate ligament healing. J Comput Assist Tomogr. 1996;20:317-21.
18. Fujimoto E, Sumen Y, Ochi M, et al. Spontaneous healing of acute anterior cruciate ligament (ACL) injuries—conservative treatment using an extension block soft brace without anterior stabilization. Arch Orthop Trauma Surg. 2002;122:212-6.
19. Maeda S, Ishibashi Y, Tsuda E, et al. Intraoperative navigation evaluation of tibial translation after resection of anterior cruciate ligament remnants. Arthroscopy. 2011;27:1203-10.
20. Nagai K, Araki D, Matsushita T, et al. Biomechanical Function of Anterior Cruciate Ligament Remnants: Quantitative Measurement With a 3-Dimensional Electromagnetic Measurement System. Arthroscopy. 2016;32:1359-66.

CHAPTER

10 How to Perform Notchplasty during ACL Surgery?

Parag Sancheti, Sunny Gugale, Ashok Shyam

INTRODUCTION

The anterior cruciate ligament (ACL) plays a key role in knee stability and therefore has gained significance in orthopedic surgical practice. The numbers of ACL reconstruction are increasing every year. The mechanism of ACL injury is multifactorial and hence several factors need to be considered in order to prevent the occurrence of ACL tear. While traumatic ACL injuries are a majority of the volume of ACL injured patients, nontraumatic ACL injuries are a matter of concern. The bony anatomy and morphological parameters that are of prime importance in relation to ACL tear are the femoral intercondylar notch (ICN) and femoral condyles' shape and dimensions, notch width index (NWI) and tibial slopes. The ICN is filled with the cruciates and the intimate relationship of the cruciates with the notch results in impingement of the ACL ligament resulting in tear. The pathological association between the ICN and the ACL tear was first described by Palmer in 1938 when he noticed that as the knee was flexed and supinated, that the ACL was placed in a vulnerable position by being stretched over the inner margin of the lateral femoral condyle (Fig. 10.1).

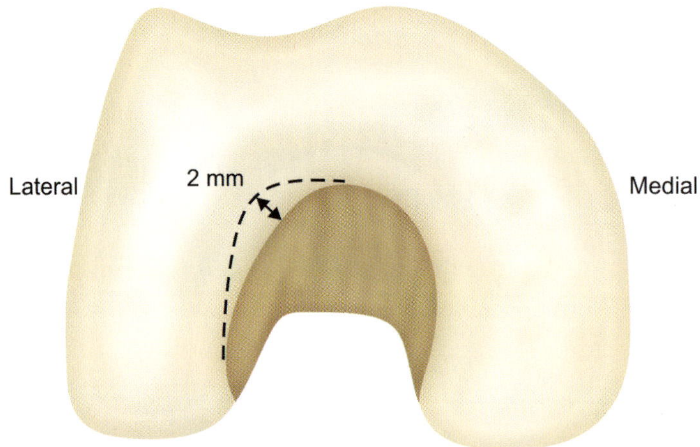

Fig. 10.1: Schematic view of the knee which shows notch.
Source: Koga H, Muneta T, Yagishita K, et al. Effect of Notchplasty in Anatomic Double-Bundle Anterior Cruciate Ligament Reconstruction. Am J Sports Med. 2014;42:1813.

DIAGNOSIS OF A NARROW NOTCH

The shape of the ICN cannot be well assessed on the standard views of plain radiographs of the knee. When ICN impingement is suspected, special views at specific knee flexion angles such as the Rosenberg notch view and prone knee view are used to assess the stenotic notch radiologically.

Radiology

- *Rosenberg notch view of the knee joint:* It is a posteroanterior (PA) weight-bearing view with the knee flexed to 45° with both patellae touching the image receptor and the X-ray beam directed perpendicular to the knee joint (Fig. 10.2). The Rosenberg view is more sensitive and specific for joint space narrowing, the anatomy of the ICN and hence is useful for the assessment of morphology of the ICN (Fig. 10.3).
- *Holmblad knee intercondylar prone view of knee joint:* It is a PA prone view of the knee joint with the knee flexed to 45° with beam perpendicular to the leg directed to the popliteal fossa (Fig. 10.4). It gives an elaborate anatomy of the knee joint intercondylar area.

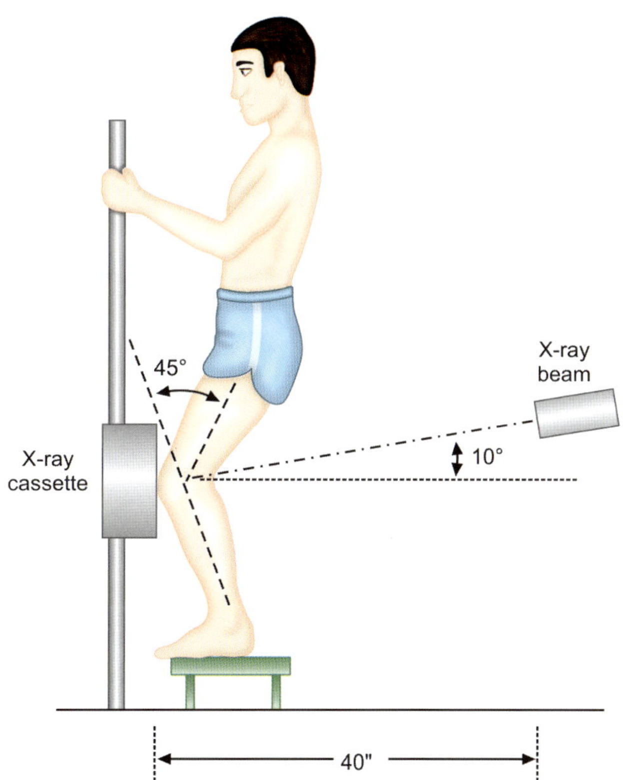

Fig. 10.2: Technique for Rosenberg notch view.
Source: Hobbs DL. Osteoarthritis and the Rosenberg method. Radiol Technol. 2006;77(3):179.

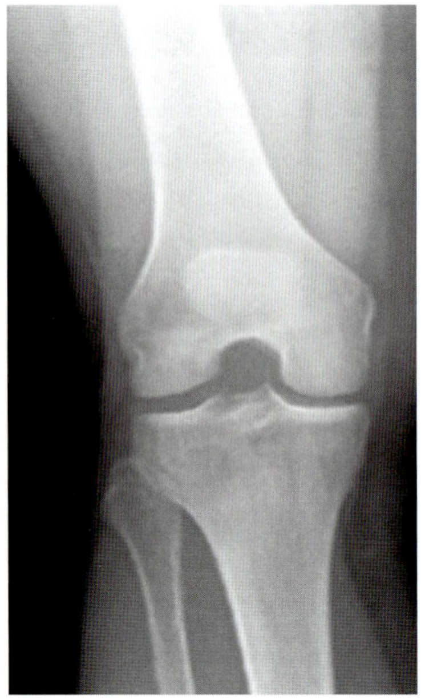

Fig. 10.3: Rosenberg PA notch view.

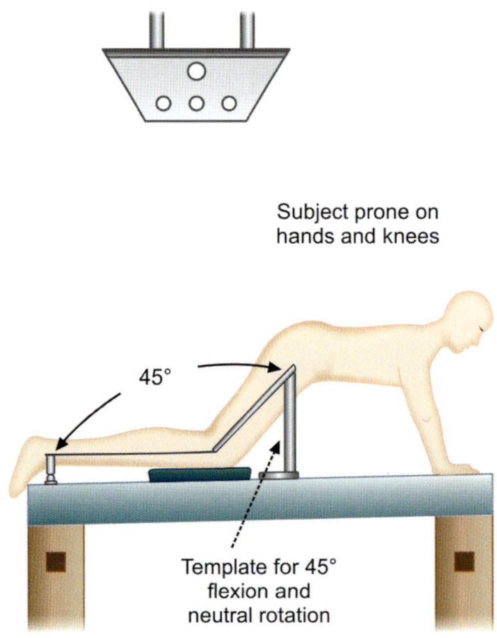

Fig. 10.4: Technique of Holmblad knee intercondylar prone view.
Source: Lombardo S, Sethi PM, Starkey C. Intercondylar notch stenosis is not a risk factor for anterior cruciate ligament tears in professional male basketball players an 11-year prospective study. Am J Sports Med. 2005;33(1):29-34.

Computed Tomography Scan of the Knee Joint

The CT scan images are more accurate in showing the ICN bony anatomy, but has a disadvantage of exposure to radiation dose (Fig. 10.5).

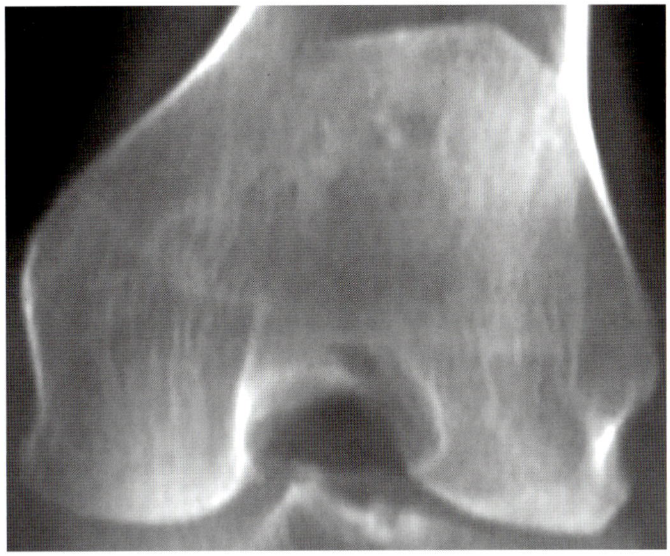

Fig. 10.5: Computed tomography notch view.

Magnetic Resonance Imaging of the Knee

It is the most accurate and least hazardous in terms of radiation exposure to identify the bony ICN and the NWI. It is a routinely performed investigation for internal derangement of knee joint and is readily available for screening for all the patients (Fig. 10.6).

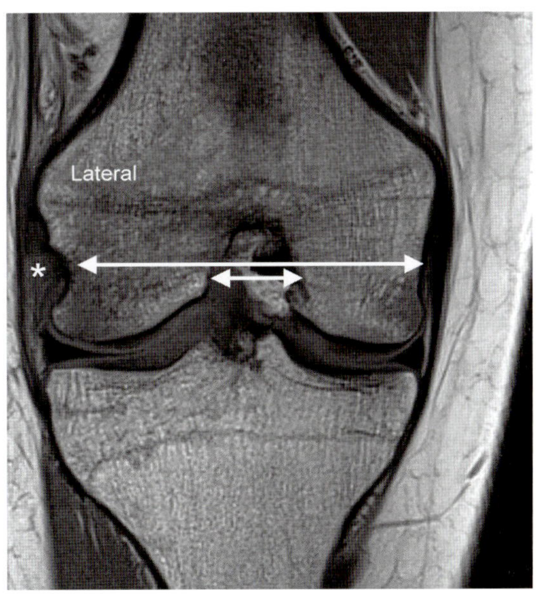

Fig. 10.6: Magnetic resonance imaging view in frontal plane showing the notch view.

Notch width index: The two-dimensional measurement of the notch size is the notch width index. This method was described by Souryal and Freeman in 1988 and is defined as the width of the ICN at the level of the popliteal groove divided by the bicondylar width at the same level. The average NWI varies in the population studied and the age group. Though Carola F et al. in their paper show the average NWI to be 0.31, Souryal et al. described a mean NWI of 0.23. An NWI of less than 0.20 is considered to be critical stenosis and it is advised to do notchplasty in such cases (Fig. 10.7).

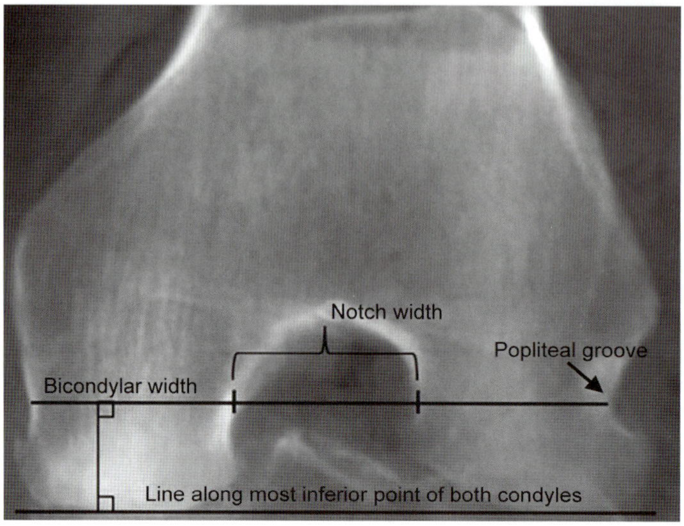

Fig. 10.7: Notch width index at the level of popliteal fossa.

WHAT IS NOTCHPLASTY?

A surgical procedure to enlarge the ICN and space available for an ACL graft during knee reconstruction. The lateral wall of the notch, which is the medial portion of the lateral femoral condyle, may be removed by various means to enlarge the notch.

Indications for Notchplasty

- It is required to be done in cases with critical narrowing of the notch with NWI of less than 0.20. It helps to widen the space required by the structures of the ICN, i.e. the ACL and the posterior cruciate ligament and reduce the impingement.
- Notchplasty needs to be done in patients with V-shaped notch, especially in females with narrow NWI; the minimum ACL graft thickness of 8 mm should be accommodated in order to give stability to the knee joint.
- It needs to be done in cases where we need to see the posterior end of the medial wall of the lateral femoral condyle to ensure that the femoral tunnel for ACL reconstruction is placed adequately posterior at an anatomic footprint, so that it prevents elongation of the graft.
- It is also important to do notchplasty in cases with revision ACL reconstruction where we have to augment the ACL with a thicker graft.

Surgical Technique of Notchplasty

Notchplasty involves not only removal of the bone from the medial wall of the lateral femoral condyle but also smoothening of the edges so as to avoid impingement. It can be done with the help of motorized arthroscopy burr, sharp curved thin osteotomes and with bone curette. Whatever may be the technique

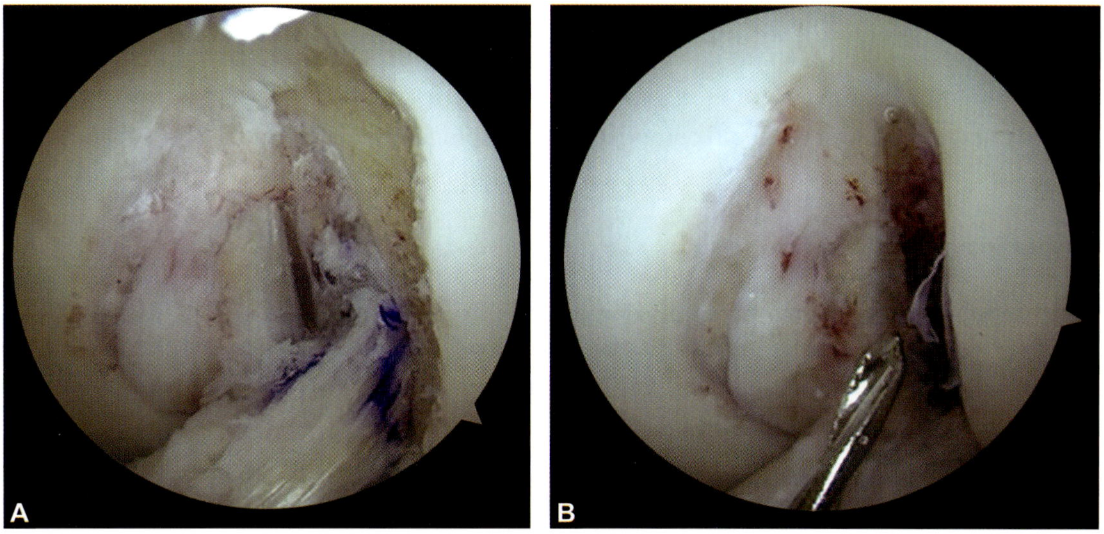

Figs. 10.8A and B: (A) A female patient with a stenotic intercondylar notch with complete anterior cruciate ligament (ACL) tear; (B) Notchplasty done with arthroscopic ACL reconstruction.

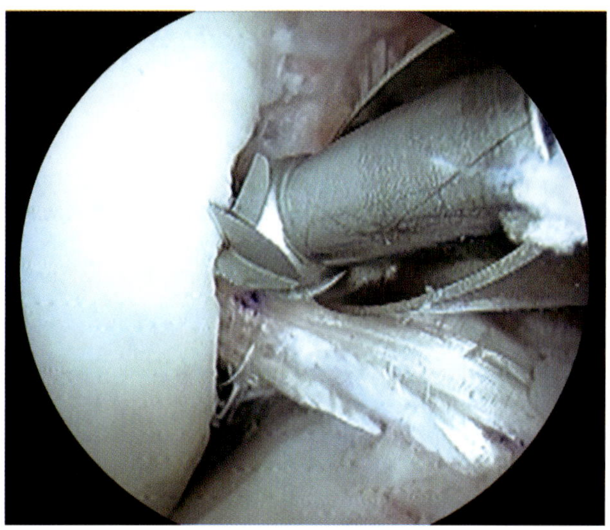

Fig. 10.9: Notchplasty technique using an arthroscopic motorized burr.

used, smoothening of the edges is a critical step in performing notchplasty. The resultant osteochondral fragments need to be removed completely one by one so as not to leave any fragment in the joint which can be a potential loose body.

Complete clearance of the notch is important; it has to be done in mid flexion and extension so as to ensure that there is no impingement on the ACL ligament either in complete extension of the knee joint as well as in deep flexion (Figs. 10.8 and 10.9).

Notchplasty in Revision ACL Reconstruction

Notchplasty to enlarge the ICN is an important step as in revision ACL cases, there are two issues. One is with the thickness of the ACL graft and second is with the placement of the femoral tunnel and position of the tibial tunnel. All these issues can have a bearing on the ACL graft impingement due to narrow notch. The terminal restriction of movement can occur, if the graft is placed too anteriorly, in such cases notchplasty is done to remove the bone from the roof of the notch, so as to avoid impingement. So in revision cases, notchplasty is done initially only to avoid complication of impingement of the graft. Though later on after the tunnels are made and the graft is passed, if at all there is any impingement, additional notchplasty can be done.

Complications of Notchplasty

Though notchplasty is beneficial so as to reduce impingement of the ACL graft, it is associated with numerous complications. Complications such as excess removal causing reduction in the thickness of the lateral femoral condyle, damage to the adjacent articular cartilage while performing the procedure and keeping loose osteochondral fragments in the joint.

LITERATURE REVIEW

Berg E et al., in their study, showed that errors in femoral tunnel placement in ACL reconstruction can cause excessive length changes in the graft during knee flexion and extension, resulting in graft elongation during the postoperative period. To improve the accuracy of tunnel placement and to avoid graft impingement, a notchplasty is commonly performed. Aglietti et al. in their study noted that there was graft tightening with knee in flexion from approximately 20° to 90° after a 2 mm femoral notchplasty had been performed. In addition, Tanzer et al. demonstrated that notch stenosis is a relative phenomenon, dependent on the size of the cruciate ligament graft. The larger the graft, the greater the degree of notch impingement in terminal knee extension. Thus, a wide notchplasty to prevent abrasive graft attrition has become a critical element of ACL reconstructive surgery.

PEARLS AND PITFALLS

- Correlation of the ICN stenosis and the incidence of nontraumatic ACL injuries are higher.
- Patients with unilateral ACL injuries with ICN stenosis are more predisposed to have injury in the other leg also.
- Widening the space in the ICN with removal of the osteochondral fragment from the medial wall of the lateral femoral condyle is known as notchplasty.
- The role of notchplasty in widening of the ICN is important, so as to accommodate a minimum graft size of 8 mm while doing arthroscopic ACL reconstruction.
- Critical notch stenosis is in cases where the NWI is less than 0.20. Arthroscopic equipment like motorized burr or curette or an osteotome can also be used for doing notchplasty. Notchplasty is essential while performing revision ACL reconstruction surgeries, so as to accommodate a larger graft thickness.

BIBLIOGRAPHY

1. Aglietti P, Buzzi R, Giron F, et al. Arthroscopic-assisted anterior cruciate ligament reconstruction with the central third patellar tendon: A 5-8 year follow-up. Knee Surg Sports Traumatol Arthrosc. 1997;5:138-44.
2. Andrade R, Vasta S, Sevivas N, et al. Notch morphology is a risk factor for ACL injury: a systematic review and meta-analysis. J ISAKOS. 2016;1:70-81.
3. Bents RT, Jones RC, May DA, et al. Intercondylar notch encroachment following anterior cruciate ligament reconstruction: A prospective study. Am J Knee Surg. 1998;11:81-8.
4. Berg EE. Assessing arthroscopic notchplasty. Arthroscopy. 1991;7:275-7.
5. Chandrashekar N, Slauterbeck J, Hashemi J. Sex-based differences in the anthropometric characteristics of the anterior cruciate ligament and its relation to intercondylar notch geometry: a cadaveric study. Am J Sports Med. 2005;33:1492-8.
6. Davis TJ, Shelbourne KD, Klootwyk TE. Correlation of the intercondylar notch width of the femur to the width of the anterior and posterior cruciate ligaments. Knee Surg Sports Traumatol Arthrosc. 1999;7:209-14.

7. Feagin JA Jr, Cabaud HE, Curl WW, et al. The anterior cruciate ligament: radiologic and clinical signs of successful and unsuccessful repairs. Clin Orthop. 1982;164:54-8.
8. Fu FH, Bennett CH, Ma B, et al. Current trends in anterior cruciate ligament reconstruction: Part II. Operative procedures and clinical correlations. Am J Sports Med. 2000;28:124-30.
9. Grossman MG, ElAttrache NS, Shields CL, et al. Revision anterior cruciate ligament reconstruction: three-to nine-year follow-up. Arthroscopy. 2005;21(4):418-23.
10. Hame SL, Markolf KL, Hunter DM, et al. Effects of notchplasty and femoral tunnel position on excursion patterns of an anterior cruciate ligament graft. Arthroscopy. 2003;19(4):340-5.
11. Harner CD, Giffin JR, Dunteman RC, et al. Evaluation and treatment of recurrent instability after anterior cruciate ligament reconstruction. J Bone Joint Surg Am. 2000;82:1651-64.
12. Hernigou P, Garabedian JM. Intercondylar notch width and the risk for anterior cruciate ligament rupture in the osteoarthritic knee: evaluation by plain radiography and CT scan. Knee. 2002;9:313-6.
13. Herzog RJ, Silliman JF, Hutton K, et al. Measurements of the intercondylar notch by plain film radiography and magnetic resonance imaging. Am J Sports Med. 1994;22:204-10.
14. Houseworth SW, Vincent M, Melon B, et al. The intercondylar notch. Am J Sport Med. 1997;15:221-4.
15. Howell SM. Arthroscopic roofplasty: a method for correcting an extension deficit caused by roof impingement of an anterior cruciate ligament graft. Arthroscopy. 1992;8:375-9.
16. Johnson D, Harner CD, Maday MG, et al. Revision anterior cruciate ligament surgery. In: Fu FH, Harner CD, Vince KG (Eds). Knee Surgery. Baltimore: Williams and Wilkins; 1994. pp. 877-95.
17. LaPrade RB, Terry GC, Montgomery RD, et al. The effects of aggressive notchplasty on the normal knee in dogs. Am J Sports Med. 1998;26:193-200.
18. LaPrade RF, Burnett QM 2nd. Femoral intercondylar notch stenosis and correlation to anterior cruciate ligament injuries. A prospective study. Am J Sports Med. 1994;22:198-202.
19. Norwood LA Jr, Cross M. The intercondylar shelf and the anterior cruciate ligament. Am J Sports Med. 1977;5:171-6.
20. Palmer I. On the injuries to the ligaments of the knee joint: a clinical study. Acta Chir Scand. 1938;53:1-28.
21. Souryal TO, Moore HA, Evans JP. Bilaterality in anterior cruciate ligament injuries: associated intercondylar notch stenosis. Am J Sports Med. 1988;16:449-54.
22. Tanzer M, Lenczner E. The relationship of intercondylar notch size and content to notchplasty requirement in anterior cruciate ligament surgery. Arthroscopy. 1990;6:89-93.
23. Trehan RK, Dabbas N, Allwood D, et al. Arthroscopic decompression and notchplasty for long- standing anterior cruciate ligament impingement in a patient with multiple epiphyseal dysplasia: a case report. J Med Case Rep. 2008;2:172.
24. van Eck C, Working Z, Fu F. Current concepts in anatomic single- and double-bundle anterior cruciate ligament reconstruction. Phys Sportsmed. 2011;39:140-8.
25. van Eck CF, Martins CA, Lorenz SG, et al. Assessment of correlation between knee notch width index and the three-dimensional notch volume. Knee Surg Sports Traumatol Arthrosc. 2010;18:1239-44.

CHAPTER

11 Identifying the Femoral Footprint

Freddie H Fu, Soheil Sabzevari, Marcio Albers, Thierry Pauyo

INTRODUCTION

The goal of anterior cruciate ligament (ACL) reconstruction is to restore the native ACL's soft tissue dimensions, collagen fibers and insertion sites.[1] In order to achieve improved long-term clinical outcomes and to prevent early arthritic changes after ACL reconstruction, the surgical technique has changed from the transtibial technique to the anatomical technique in order to restore the native ACL anatomy.[2,3] Therefore, having an adequate visualization of both femoral and tibial footprints is paramount to proper tunnel placement.

Traditionally, two standard portals are used for ACL reconstruction. The anterolateral portal and the anteromedial portal (AMP) are used as viewing portal and working portal, respectively. During ACL reconstruction, the utilization of the AL portal as the viewing portal makes the evaluation of the posterior aspect of the lateral intercondylar notch challenging and further complicates identifying the exact anatomy of the femoral footprint.[4] To overcome this issue, the three-portal technique has been introduced; it consists of a high anterolateral portal (AL), central portal (C), and accessory medial portal (AM) (Fig. 11.1).[5]

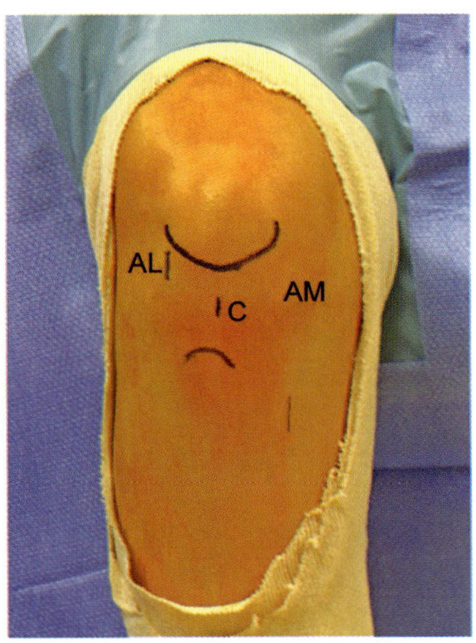

Fig. 11.1: Anterior view of a right knee flexed 90 degrees.
(AL: Anterolateral portal; C: Central portal; AM: Accessory anteromedial portal).

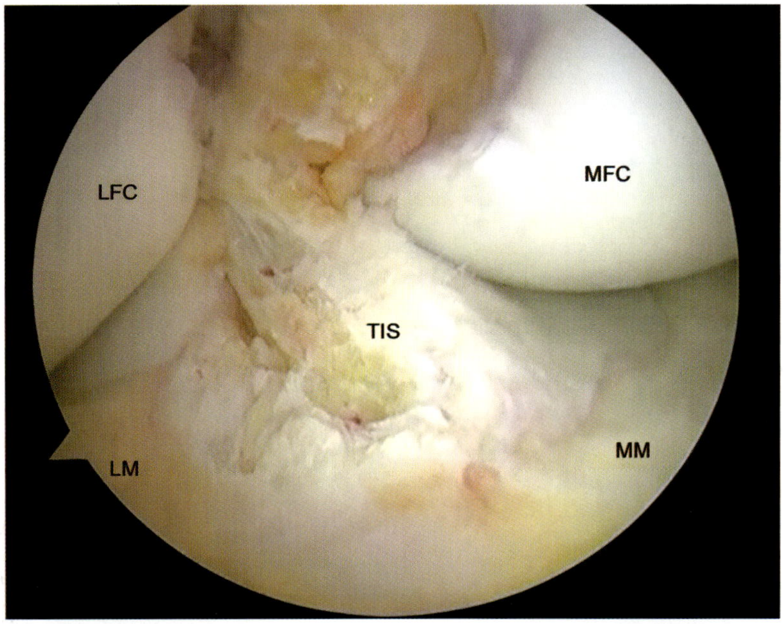

Fig. 11.2: Anterolateral portal view of the anterior cruciate ligament tibial insertion site showing its close relationship with the lateral meniscus (LM). The portal also allows a clear view of the lateral femoral condyle (LFC), medial femoral condyle (MFC) and medial meniscus (MM). (TIS: Tibial insertion site).

"HIGH" ANTEROLATERAL PORTAL

This portal is the first portal created during arthroscopic ACL reconstruction. A number 11 scalpel blade is used to create a "high" anterolateral portal. To avoid cartilage or meniscus damage, the cutting surface of the blade is positioned superiorly. While the knee is flexed to 90°, the portal is created 1 cm lateral to the patellar tendon with the most inferior portion of the portal located at the level of the inferior pole of the patella. The advantage of this portal is to provide a broad overview of the tibial footprint, patellofemoral, medial, and lateral compartments and also avoid penetration into Hoffa's fat pad (Fig. 11.2).

CENTRAL ANTEROMEDIAL PORTAL

The central AMP or "central" portal (CP) plays a critical role for a precise anatomical ACL reconstruction. The advantage of this portal is to provide a direct view of femoral bundles insertion sites that are hardly seen with a standard anterolateral portal. Achieving an adequate view of the lateral intercondylar notch will eliminate the necessity for a notchplasty. Therefore, the native bony anatomy and soft tissue ACL remnants, which are the landmarks for anatomical ACL reconstruction, will be preserved (Fig. 11.3).

While the knee is flexed to 90° and under direct visualization through anterolateral portal, a spinal needle is inserted into the joint through the medial third of the patella tendon just above the joint line. The needle should be in lower third of the intercondylar notch, above the meniscus, and in the central portion of the notch in the coronal plane. After visual confirmation of the location of the portal with the needle, a number 11 scalpel blade is used to make the portal through the patellar tendon. This portal can be used

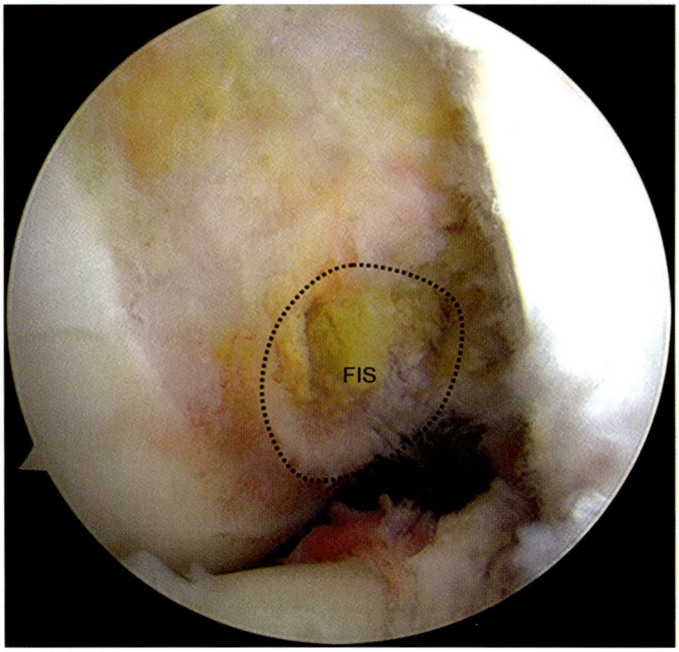

Fig. 11.3: Central portal view of the anterior cruciate ligament's femoral insertion site (FIS).

either as a viewing portal (providing direct visualization of the femoral footprint) and as a working portal (placement of tibial guide during tibial tunnel drilling). The surgeons should be aware not to damage cartilage and meniscus while placing this portal.

ACCESSORY ANTEROMEDIAL PORTAL

The accessory AM or "medial" portal is essentially used as a working portal to create the anteromedial (AM) and posterolateral (PL) femoral tunnels. This portal has been shown to improve the accuracy of femoral tunnel placement while the transtibial technique was less than 50% accurate in creating an anatomical AM bundle in the femoral footprint.[6] The AM portal is placed with the knee positioned at 90° flexion and under direct visualization through central portal. Again, a spinal needle is inserted into the knee joint about 2 cm medial to the medial border of the patella tendon and above the anterior horn of the medial meniscus. The spinal needle should easily reach the anatomical femoral footprint of the ACL on the lateral intercondylar surface. Furthermore, there should be about 2 mm of space between spinal needle and medial femoral condyle to avoid damage to the cartilage surface during drilling the femoral tunnel (Fig. 11.4).

It should be noted that the exact location of the AM will depend on the bony anatomy of each individual and will vary depending on notch width and height. Additionally, the AM can be used as a working portal to place the tibial guide and drill the tibial posterolateral tunnel during ACL double-bundle reconstruction. Finally, this portal is also used as a viewing portal to measure the femoral ACL footprint dimensions with a ruler introduced through the "high" anterolateral portal (Fig. 11.5).

The accessory AM portal enables the evaluation of the femoral tunnel placement and inspection of the integrity of posterior aspect of the lateral femoral condyle after drilling the tunnel.

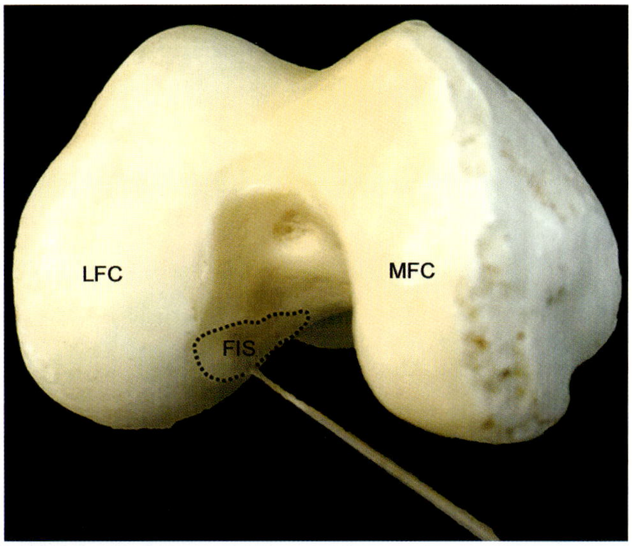

Fig. 11.4: A spinal needle is inserted through the AMP, aiming to the center of the FIS and keeping a minimum distance of 2 mm from the MFC to avoid injuries to the chondral structures.
(AMP: Anteromedial portal; FIS: Femoral insertion site; MFC: Medial femoral condyle; LFC: Lateral femoral condyle).

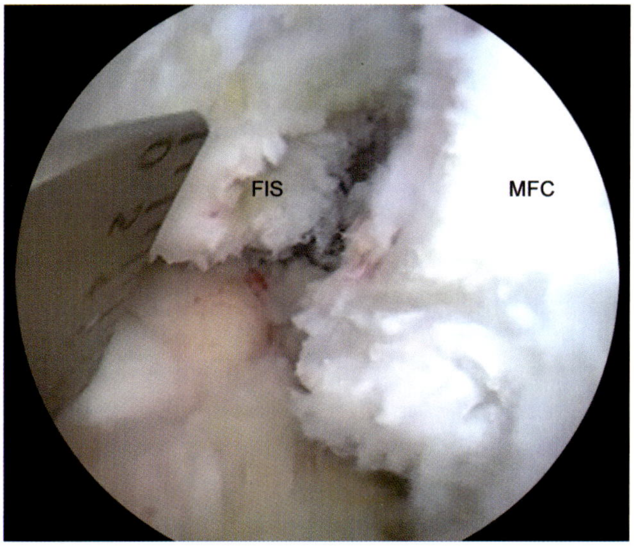

Fig. 11.5: AMP view of the arthroscopic ruler used to measure the FIS of the ACL.
(AMP: Anteromedial portal; MFC: Medial femoral condyle; FIS: Femoral insertion site; ACL: Anterior cruciate ligament).

The most common etiology of failed ACL reconstruction is surgical technical error where tunnel malpositioning is most frequently encountered.[7,8] Among the surgical technical errors, tunnel malpositioning is the most common etiology. Although tunnel malpositioning can be multifactorial, poor visualization of the ACL remnants and bony landmarks contributes in the majority of cases.[9] Therefore, the three-portal technique should be utilized in anatomical ACL reconstruction.

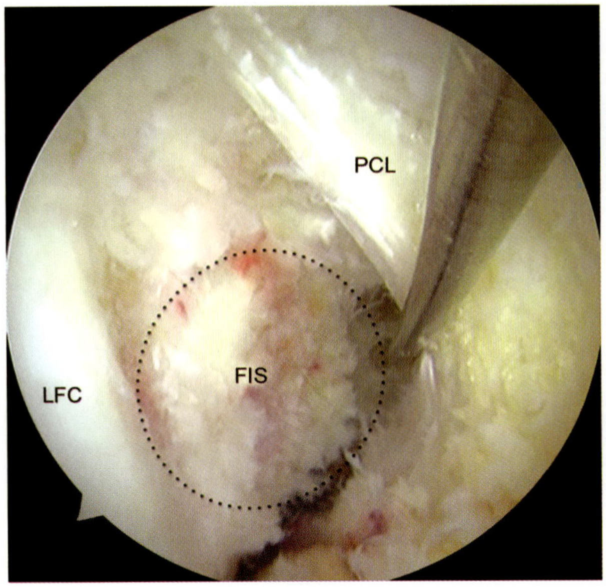

Fig. 11.6: Oval-shaped anterior cruciate ligament FIS.
(LFC: Lateral femoral condyle; FIS: Femoral insertion site; PCL: Posterior cruciate ligament).

FEMORAL ANTERIOR CRUCIATE LIGAMENT FOOTPRINT

The femoral ACL footprint is oval shaped and usually smaller than the tibial footprint (Fig. 11.6).

A previous study by Fujimaki et al.[10] have determined that the femoral footprint actually represents about 70% of the tibial footprint. While the soft tissue remnants of the ruptured ACL and femoral wall bony landmark can be used to correctly identify the femoral ACL footprint, the chronicity of the injury often poses a challenge.

In acute ACL rupture cases, the soft tissue remnant of the ACL provides a clear guide to the exact location of the femoral bundles on the footprint. However, in chronic cases, the ACL remnants on the femoral wall can be attenuated and the bony landmarks on the medial wall of the LFC are the only remaining information to rely on to evaluate the femoral ACL footprint. The two osseous ridges on the medial wall of the LFC define the margins of the femoral ACL footprint.[11] The lateral intercondylar ridge or "resident's ridge" delineates the anterior border of the femoral footprint. This ridge is present in almost all of the knees, starting proximally close to the roof of the intercondylar notch, running distally through the entire ACL insertion to end at the border of the articular cartilage of the femoral condyle.

The lateral bifurcate ridge is another osseous landmark that separates AM and PL bundles. It presents as a change in the slope of the bony surface running perpendicular to the resident's ridge. A study by Ferretti et al.[12] reported this ridge in more than 80% of patients.

In conclusion, the ACL reconstruction with the three-portal technique is an effective method to accurately identify both tibial and femoral ACL footprint in order to recreate native ACL anatomy. The central portal can be especially useful in cases where the anatomy of the patient poses a challenge to identify the femoral footprint precisely. While new efforts are made to individualize anatomic ACL reconstruction with each patient's soft tissue and bony anatomy,[1,13,14] the three-portal technique could prove to be an essential tool to achieve an anatomic ACL reconstruction.

PEARLS AND PITFALLS

- The three-portal technique provides a unique opportunity to optimize the visualization of the femoral footprint.
- The CP is used as a viewing portal to identify the exact location of the femoral footprint. When viewing from the anterolateral portal and when the notch is narrowed, it is often difficult to fully appreciate the ACL femoral footprint on the medial wall of the LFC. In these cases, the CP provides a direct and essential view of the femoral footprint and enables the correct anatomical placement of the femoral tunnel.
- In acute ACL ruptures, the remnant of the torn ACL will help identify the anatomical femoral footprint.
- In chronic cases, the lateral intercondylar ridge (resident ridge) will help determine the anterior border of the femoral footprint, while the lateral bifurcate ridge will help determine the border between AM and PL bundles.

REFERENCES

1. Rahnemai-Azar AA, Sabzevari S, Irarrazaval S, et al. Anatomical individualized ACL reconstruction. Arch Bone Jt Surg. 2016;4(4):291-7.
2. van Eck CF, Schreiber VM, Liu TT, et al. The anatomic approach to primary, revision and augmentation anterior cruciate ligament reconstruction. Knee Surg Sports Traumatol Arthrosc. 2010;18(9):1154-63.
3. Lohmander LS, Ostenberg A, Englund M, et al. High prevalence of knee osteoarthritis, pain, and functional limitations in female soccer players twelve years after anterior cruciate ligament injury. Arthritis Rheum. 2004;50(10):3145-52.
4. Cohen SB, Fu FH. Three-portal technique for anterior cruciate ligament reconstruction: use of a central medial portal. Arthroscopy. 2007;23(3):325 e321-325.
5. Araujo PH, van Eck CF, Macalena JA, et al. Advances in the three-portal technique for anatomical single- or double-bundle ACL reconstruction. Knee Surg Sports Traumatol Arthrosc. 2011;19(8):1239-42.
6. Schreiber VM, van Eck CF, Fu FH. Anatomic double-bundle ACL reconstruction. Sports Med Arthrosc. 2010;18(1):27-32.
7. Bedi A, Altchek DW. The "footprint" anterior cruciate ligament technique: an anatomic approach to anterior cruciate ligament reconstruction. Arthroscopy. 2009;25(10):1128-38.
8. Johnson DL, Swenson TM, Irrgang JJ, et al. Revision anterior cruciate ligament surgery: experience from Pittsburgh. Clin Orthop Relat Res. 1996;(325):100-9.
9. Sommer C, Friederich NF, Muller W. Improperly placed anterior cruciate ligament grafts: correlation between radiological parameters and clinical results. Knee Surg Sports Traumatol Arthrosc. 2000;8(4):207-13.
10. Fujimaki Y, Thorhauer E, Sasaki Y, et al. Quantitative In Situ Analysis of the Anterior Cruciate Ligament: Length, Midsubstance Cross-sectional Area, and Insertion Site Areas. Am J Sports Med. 2016;44(1):118-25.
11. Fu FH, Jordan SS. The lateral intercondylar ridge—a key to anatomic anterior cruciate ligament reconstruction. J Bone Joint Surg Am. 2007;89(10):2103-4.
12. Ferretti M, Ekdahl M, Shen W, et al. Osseous landmarks of the femoral attachment of the anterior cruciate ligament: an anatomic study. Arthroscopy. 2007;23(11):1218-25.
13. Fu FH, van Eck CF, Tashman S, et al. Anatomic anterior cruciate ligament reconstruction: a changing paradigm. Knee Surg Sports Traumatol Arthrosc. 2015;23(3):640-8.
14. Rahnemai-Azar AA, Sabzevari S, Irarrazaval S, et al. Restoring nature through individualized anatomic anterior cruciate ligament reconstruction surgery. Arch Bone Jt Surg. 2016;4(4):289-90.

CHAPTER

12 Creating a Transportal Femoral Tunnel

Freddie H Fu, Soheil Sabzevari, Marcio Albers, Thierry Pauyo

INTRODUCTION

The drive to improve the outcomes of anterior cruciate ligament (ACL) reconstruction has led to tremendous progress during the last two decades. The transtibial drilling technique was used traditionally during ACL reconstruction, and often resulted with the graft being placed outside of the native femoral ACL footprint.[1] The inappropriate placement of tunnels has been shown to decrease range of motion in the knee, increase instability, and alter the physiologic forces applied to the graft leading to potential failure of the reconstruction.[2,3] The efforts to place the ACL in the correct anatomical location has led to the replacement of the transtibial technique. The anatomical ACL reconstruction technique encompasses the following four principles:[1,4]

1. Restoring the anteriormedial (AM) and posteriorlateral (PL) bundles of the ACL
2. Restoring the native ACL footprints by placing the femoral and tibial tunnels in the anatomic location with appropriate graft size
3. Properly tensioning each bundle in the appropriate knee flexion angle
4. Evaluating and considering each patient's individual anatomy to perform individualized-ACL reconstruction.

The reconstruction of the ACL following these principles aims to improve outcomes by reestablishing the characteristics of the native ACL. Previous studies have found that the trans-portal technique was more accurate than the transtibial technique in placing the femoral tunnel in its anatomic footprint (Fig. 12.1).[5]

The transportal technique provides the ability to make the femoral tunnel independently from tibial tunnel. The only disadvantage of this technique is a potentially shorter femoral tunnel compared with transtibial technique.

To achieve anatomical ACL reconstruction, it is critical to have an adequate visualization of the femoral and tibial footprint. In an effort to improve visualization, the standard two-portal arthroscopy technique has been replaced by the three-portal technique. The following is a description of the three-portal technique.

THE THREE-PORTAL TECHNIQUE

1. *"High" anterolateral portal (AL)*: This portal is the first portal placed during ACL reconstruction. With the knee at 90° flexion, the portal is created 1 cm lateral to the patellar tendon and above the joint line. This portal is used as the viewing portal to evaluate the tibial footprint.

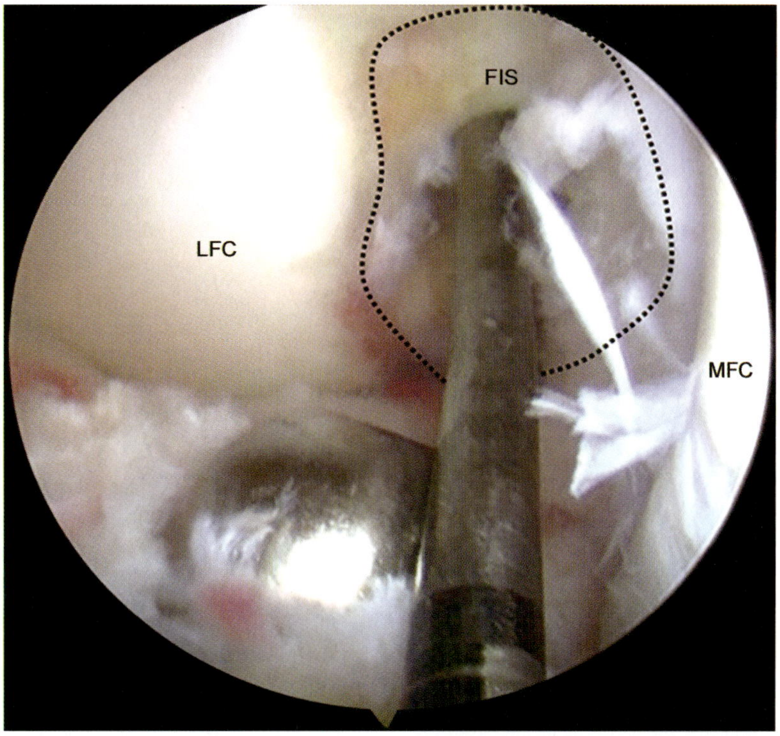

Fig. 12.1: Central portal view of the FIS area. The flexible guide is far enough from the MFC to avoid chondral damage. (FIS: Femoral insertion site; LFC: Lateral femoral condyle; MFC: Medial femoral condyle).

2. *Central anteromedial portal*: The central anteromedial portal or "central" portal (CP) has a key role in anatomical ACL reconstruction. This portal is created under direct visualization from the AL. It is also used as a viewing portal and provides a more central and direct view to the femoral footprint. With the knee at 90° flexion, a spinal needle is entered 1 cm above the joint through the medial third of the patella tendon. As stated above, the main advantage of this portal is to provide a more central and direct visualization of the femoral footprint.
3. *Accessory anteromedial portal*: The accessory medial portal or "medial" portal is used as the working portal to create a transportal femoral tunnel. With the knee at 90° flexion and under direct visualization of the central portal, a spinal needle is inserted above the joint line (care must be taken not to damage the anterior horn of the medial meniscus) and about 2 cm medial to the medial border of the patella tendon. The spinal needle should easily reach the anatomical femoral footprint on the medial wall of the lateral femoral condyle and there should be about 2 mm of space between spinal needle and medial femoral condyle. This space will prevent damage to the articular cartilage of the medial femoral condyle during transportal femoral tunnel drilling. The surgeon should be aware that the exact location of this portal will depend on the patient's distal femoral bone morphology and on other anatomic variables, such as the width of the notch.

SURGICAL TECHNIQUE

Recent studies have aimed at customizing the treatment of ACL reconstruction based on each patient's individual bony and native ligament characteristics. This approach aims to use individualized reconstruction surgery to restore the size and insertion of the native ligament.[4,5] The individualized ACL

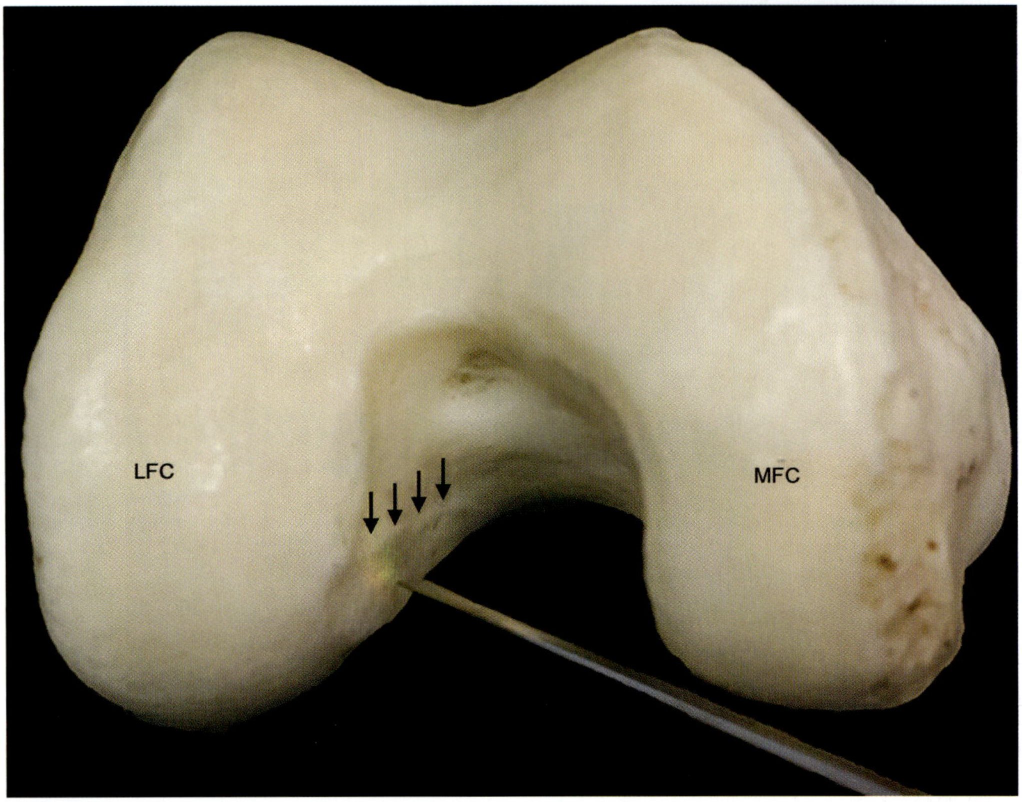

Fig. 12.2: Anterior view of a distal femur model showing the resident's ridge (arrows) and the lateral bifurcate ridge as indicated by the needle.
(LFC: Lateral femoral condyle; MFC: Medial femoral condyle).

reconstruction utilizes three-portal to correctly identify the femoral footprint and uses the transportal drilling technique to place the femoral tunnel.

After creation of the three portals, as mentioned above, a diagnostic arthroscopy is performed and the central portal is used to identify the ACL femoral footprint. In acute cases, the ACL remnant is used to help localize the femoral footprint. In chronic cases, the ACL remaining fiber can be attenuated and the surgeons should use the bony landmarks to correctly identify the femoral footprint. The lateral intercondylar ridge determines the anterior border of the ACL insertion site and the lateral bifurcate ridge determines the border between the AM and PL bundle (Fig. 12.2).[6,7]

During the next step, an arthroscopic ruler is inserted into the joint through the central anteromedial portal to measure the femoral footprint and notch dimensions. As mentioned above, the best approach to ACL reconstruction, regardless of a single- or double-bundle reconstruction, should be determined on an individual basis for each patient. The decision on graft size is made with the preoperative imaging and is corroborated with the intraoperative measurements of the tibial and femoral footprint and intercondylar notch dimensions.[8] The following are the inclusion criteria for double- and single-bundle ACL reconstruction utilizing the anatomic individualized ACL reconstruction. A double-bundle ACL reconstruction should be considered in a patient that meets the following criteria:[8-10]

- Anteroposterior tibial footprint length longer than 14 mm
- Lateral intercondylar notch length and width longer than 14 mm

- Absence of severe bone bruising, concomitant collateral ligament injuries, and severe osteoarthritic changes
- Closed physes.

Single-bundle ACL reconstruction criteria:

- Anteroposterior tibial footprint length less than 14 mm
- Lateral intercondylar notch length and width less than 12 mm
- Multiligamentous injuries
- Severe bone bruising
- Severe osteoarthritic changes
- Open physes.

There is no difference between single- and double-bundle ACL reconstruction regarding restoration of the anteroposterior and rotational stability when patients undergo reconstruction in an anatomic individualized approach.[2]

While performing a double-bundle reconstruction, the AM and PL tunnels should be placed at their respective native insertion sites. There should be a 2-mm bone bridge between two tunnels.

In the terms of single-bundle reconstruction, the femoral tunnel is created at the center of the femoral footprint.

In summary, anatomical individualized ACL reconstructions should be considered while performing ACL reconstruction. This technique is based on a patient's individual bony and native ligament characteristics and aims to recreate the size and insertion of the native ACL. This surgical reconstruction utilizes the three-portal technique in order to appropriately identify the femoral footprint and create the femoral tunnel with transportal drilling. While the central portal provides the best visualization of the native femoral ACL footprint, the medial portal is used to drill the femoral tunnel at the native femoral footprint.

PEARLS AND PITFALLS

- The three-portal technique provides a unique view of the femoral footprint for optimal anatomical placement of the femoral tunnel.
- The accessory anteromedial portal, or medial portal, is used as a working portal to drill the trans-portal femoral tunnel. This is performed while the central portal is used as a viewing portal to optimize the exact placement of an anatomical femoral tunnel.
- There should be at least a 2-mm distance between the femoral guide pin and the medial femoral condyle to avoid articular cartilage damage during femoral tunnel drilling.
- The decision making regarding the diameter of the tunnels (i.e. single/double-bundle reconstruction) should be done on an individual basis and after measurements of the footprints and notch diameter are confirmed.

REFERENCES

1. Rahnemai-Azar AA, Sabzevari S, Irarrázaval S, et al. Anatomical individualized ACL reconstruction. Arch Bone Jt Surg. 2016;4(4):291-7.
2. Hussein M, van Eck CF, Cretnik A, et al. Individualized anterior cruciate ligament surgery: a prospective study comparing anatomic single- and double-bundle reconstruction. Am J Sports Med. 2012;40(8):1781-8.
3. Araujo PH, Asai S, Pinto M, et al. ACL graft position affects in situ graft force following ACL reconstruction. J Bone Joint Surg Am. 2015;97(21):1767-73.

4. Rahnemai-Azar AA, Sabzevari S, Irarrazaval S, et al. Restoring nature through individualized anatomic anterior cruciate ligament reconstruction surgery. Arch Bone Jt Surg. 2016;4(4):289-90.
5. Wolf MR, Murawski CD, van Diek FM, et al. Intercondylar notch dimensions and graft failure after single- and double-bundle anterior cruciate ligament reconstruction. Knee Surg Sports Traumatol Arthrosc. 2015;23(3):680-6.
6. Ferretti M, Ekdahl M, Shen W, et al. Osseous landmarks of the femoral attachment of the anterior cruciate ligament: an anatomic study. Arthroscopy. 2007;23(11):1218-25.
7. Fu FH, Jordan SS. The lateral intercondylar ridge—a key to anatomic anterior cruciate ligament reconstruction. J Bone Joint Surg Am. 2007;89(10):2103-4.
8. van Eck CF, Lesniak BP, Schreiber VM, et al. Anatomic single- and double-bundle anterior cruciate ligament reconstruction flowchart. Arthroscopy. 2010;26(2):258-68.
9. Shen W, Forsythe B, Ingham SM, et al. Application of the anatomic double-bundle reconstruction concept to revision and augmentation anterior cruciate ligament surgeries. J Bone Joint Surg Am. 2008;90(Suppl 4):20-34.
10. Kopf S, Pombo MW, Szczodry M, et al. Size variability of the human anterior cruciate ligament insertion sites. Am J Sports Med. 2011;39(1):108-13.

CHAPTER

13

Creating Transportal Femoral Tunnel Using Flexible Reamers

Anant Joshi, Bhushan Sabnis, Sajeer Usman

INTRODUCTION

The technique of arthroscopic anterior cruciate ligament (ACL) reconstruction has evolved over the past two decades with better understanding of anatomy and development of better instrumentation.

In the 1980s, the focus was on isometric ACL reconstruction. In the past decade, greater emphasis has been placed on anatomical placement of the graft. Anatomical placement implies functional restoration of the ACL to its native dimensions, collagen orientation and insertion sites.

Greater attention has been given to the femoral footprint of the ACL, where even minor variations in tunnel placement may affect the final outcome.[1]

Cain and Clancy initially described the use of flexible reamers in ACL reconstruction surgery.[2]

We now routinely use the flexible reamer system (Stryker VersiTomic™ system) for ACL reconstructions.

BACKGROUND

For anatomic ACL reconstruction, the femoral tunnel is created using the transportal technique, i.e. the femoral tunnel is drilled independent of the tibial tunnel through the standard anteromedial or an accessory medial portal. To get to the desired position of the femoral tunnel, one needs to hyperflex the knee to more than 110° (Fig. 13.1). During this hyperflexion, fat pad usually obscures vision and as a result, necessitates fat pad debridement. Moreover, achieving the desired hyperflexion may not be possible in obese individuals. Thus, compromised knee positioning and obscured vision may lead to a malpositioned femoral tunnel, which ultimately affects the surgical outcome.

Stump preservation has been shown to have significant advantages for the ligamentization process of the ACL graft. In a study on revascularization of the ACL graft analyzed with postoperative MRI comparing standard and minimal debridement of ACL remnant, fat pad and infrapatellar ligament, it was concluded that minimal intra-articular tissue debridement leads to earlier revascularization.[3]

Anatomical accuracy and adequacy of the length of the femoral tunnels using flexible reamers has also been confirmed using CT scan in a cadaveric study.[4]

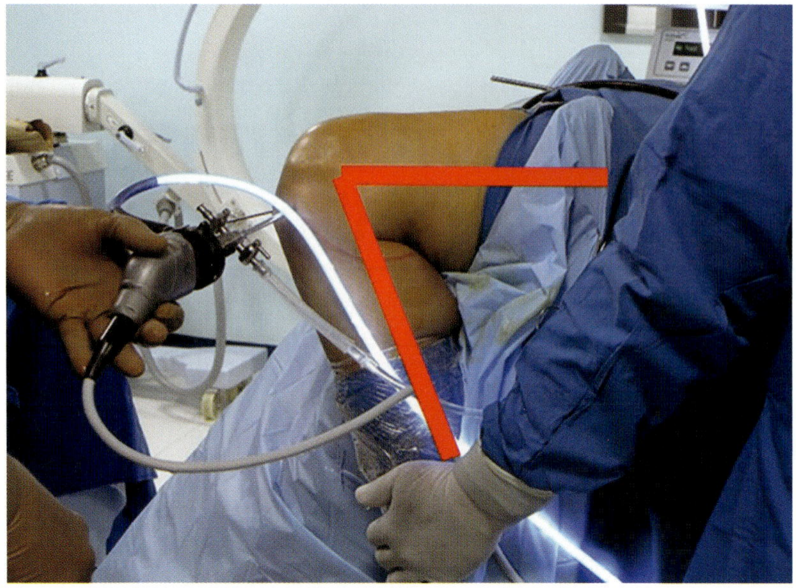

Fig. 13.1: Knee hyperflexion required while transportal drilling of femoral tunnel using rigid reamers.

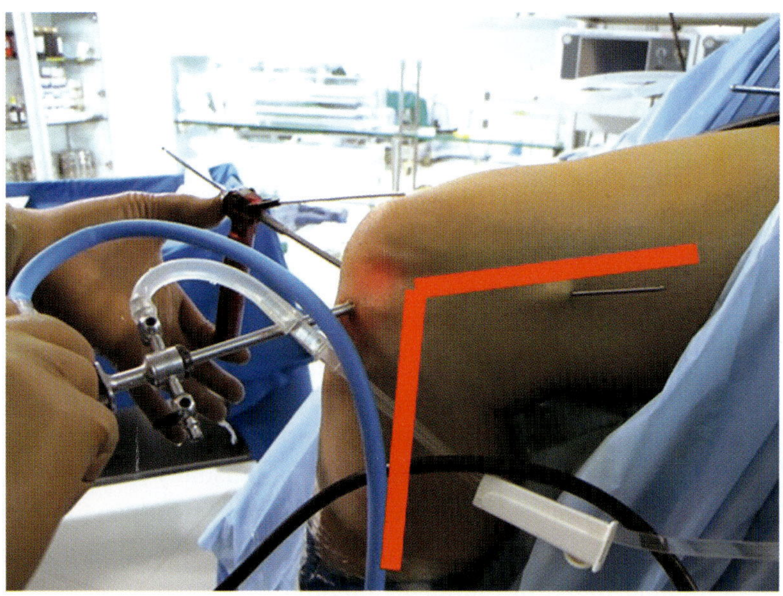

Fig. 13.2: Knee flexion less than 90 degrees during transportal drilling using flexible reamers.

The safety of flexible reamers has also been demonstrated. In a cadaveric study, it was found that with flexible reamers, there is minimal risk to the peroneal nerve and the femoral origin of the lateral collateral ligament (LCL) unless lateral femoral wall blowout occurs.[4,5]

Thus, without hyperflexion of the knee, it has been shown that femoral tunnels of consistent length and obliquity can be drilled safely using flexible reamers (Fig. 13.2).

The authors have used the flexible reamer system for last 2 years and have experience of more than 1,000 cases of anterior cruciate ligament reconstruction (ACLR) using this system.

INSTRUMENTATION

The flexible reamer set consists of an offset jig, shape memory alloy (SMA) flexible guide pins, outside-in depth gauge and flexible reamers (Fig. 13.3A).

The *offset jig* is side specific and color coded. It is curved at 45° at the end which directs the flexible pin in the preferred direction. The jig enables access to the femoral footprint area, transportally, without knee hyperflexion. The offset, which comes in 6 mm, 7 mm and 8 mm sizes, ensures that an adequate posterior cortical wall is preserved.

A flippable *Accupin*-direction guide, attached to this jig, helps the surgeon predict the trajectory of the femoral tunnel and guesstimate the exit point of the flexible pin on the lateral thigh (Fig. 13.3B).

The *SMA guide pin* is a flexible wire and is made up of a SMA whereby it can bend to any shape and yet retain its shape until further manipulation. It has a distinct calibration mark that enables tunnel length measurement using a specific *outside-in depth gauge.*

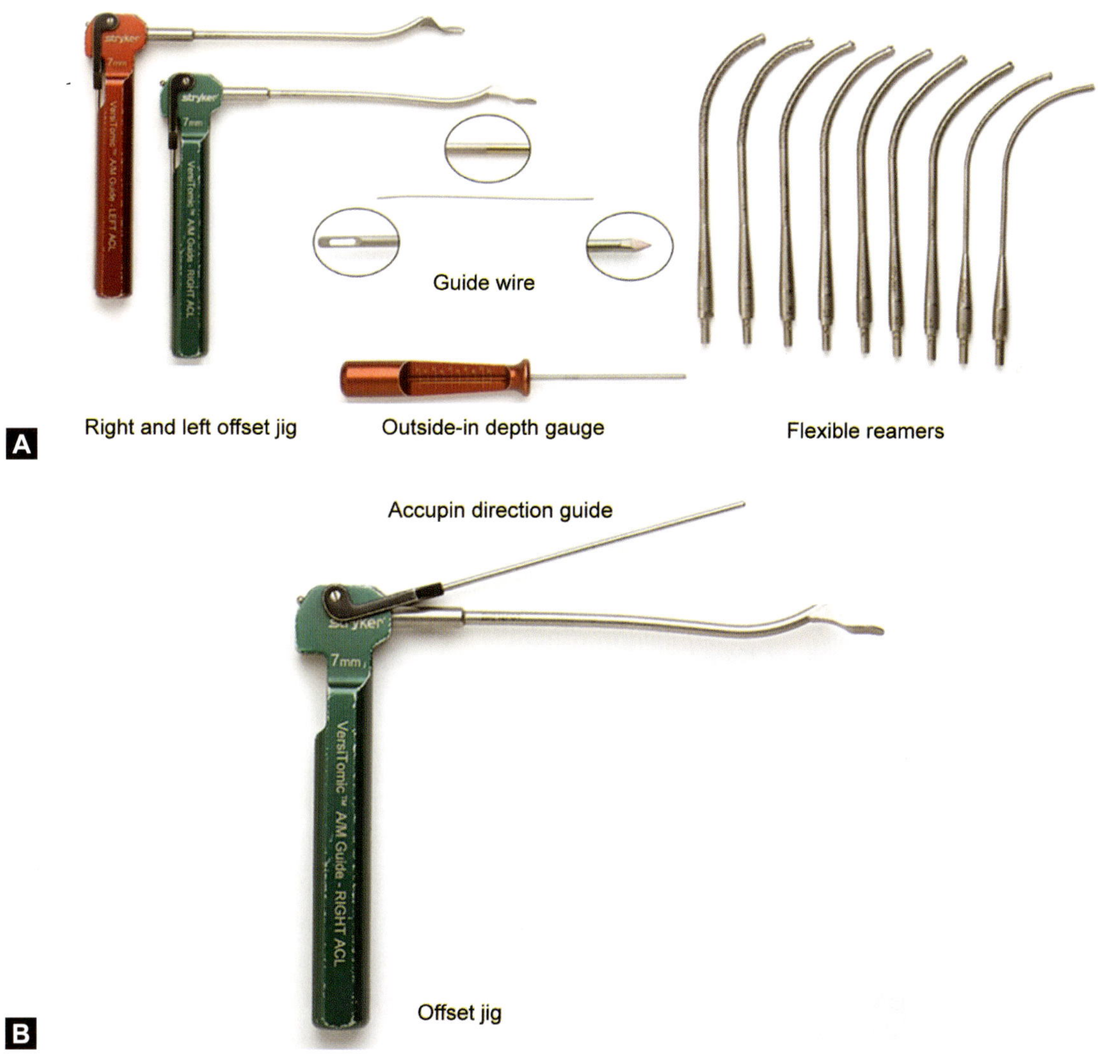

Figs. 13.3A and B: (A) Flexible reamer instrumentation (VersiTomic™ by Stryker). (B) Offset jig with direction guide.

Cannulated flexible reamers come in sizes ranging from 4.5 mm to 12 mm. They have an eccentric cutting flute head with flexible puzzle piece shaft that allows safe intra-articular placement and socket or tunnel creation without damaging the surrounding articular cartilage, bone or soft tissue structures.

SURGICAL TECHNIQUE

Position of Leg: With patient in supine position, the limb to be operated is placed in a leg holder. More than 90° of knee flexion is usually not necessary.

Surgical Steps

Step 1: Portal Creation and Footprint Preparation

Arthroscopy is performed through standard anterolateral and anteromedial portals. The ACL nodule (if present) is debrided sparing the fat pad and the ligamentum mucosum (infrapatellar ligament). After this step, based on the type of ACL lesion, a hamstring graft is harvested and prepared.

Step 2: Placement of Jig (Fig. 13.4A)

Once the site for placement of the offset jig is confirmed, appropriate right or left offset jig is selected. The jig is gently passed around the ligamentum mucosum and placed on the medial wall of the lateral femoral condyle with the guide wire slot on the femoral footprint and the offset hooked on to the posterior wall of the intercondylar notch. This will ensure a sufficient posterior wall margin and avoid a posterior blowout. The knee is at 90° of flexion. The socket height can be adjusted by changing rotation of the jig. The Accupin direction guide is flipped into position to assess the trajectory of the guide pin and the direction of the femoral tunnel.

Step 3: Drilling the Guide Wire and Tunnel Length Measurement (Fig. 13.4B)

The SMA flexible guide pin is drilled across, the tip is retrieved laterally, the offset guide is removed and then the wire is advanced till the calibrated marking is flush with the medial wall of the lateral femoral condyle. A stab incision is made laterally at the guide wire exit for the outside-in depth gauge. The depth gauge is passed until it reaches the lateral femoral cortex. At this position, the tip of the guide wire in the cannulated depth gauge indicates the total femoral tunnel length.

Note: The authors prefer using a fixed length loop device when the tunnel length is more than 30 mm, while an adjustable loop device is used where the measured tunnel length is less than 30 mm.

Step 4: Femoral Socket Preparation (Figs. 13.4C and D)

After confirmation of tunnel length, the femoral socket is prepared. The larger diameter flexible reamer corresponding to the graft size is initially passed over the guide wire on a power drill to the desired length. This is followed by drilling the remaining femur and the lateral cortex with a smaller size flexible reamer (4.5/5 mm), depending upon the choice of fixation implant. Once the tunnel mouth is adequately cleared

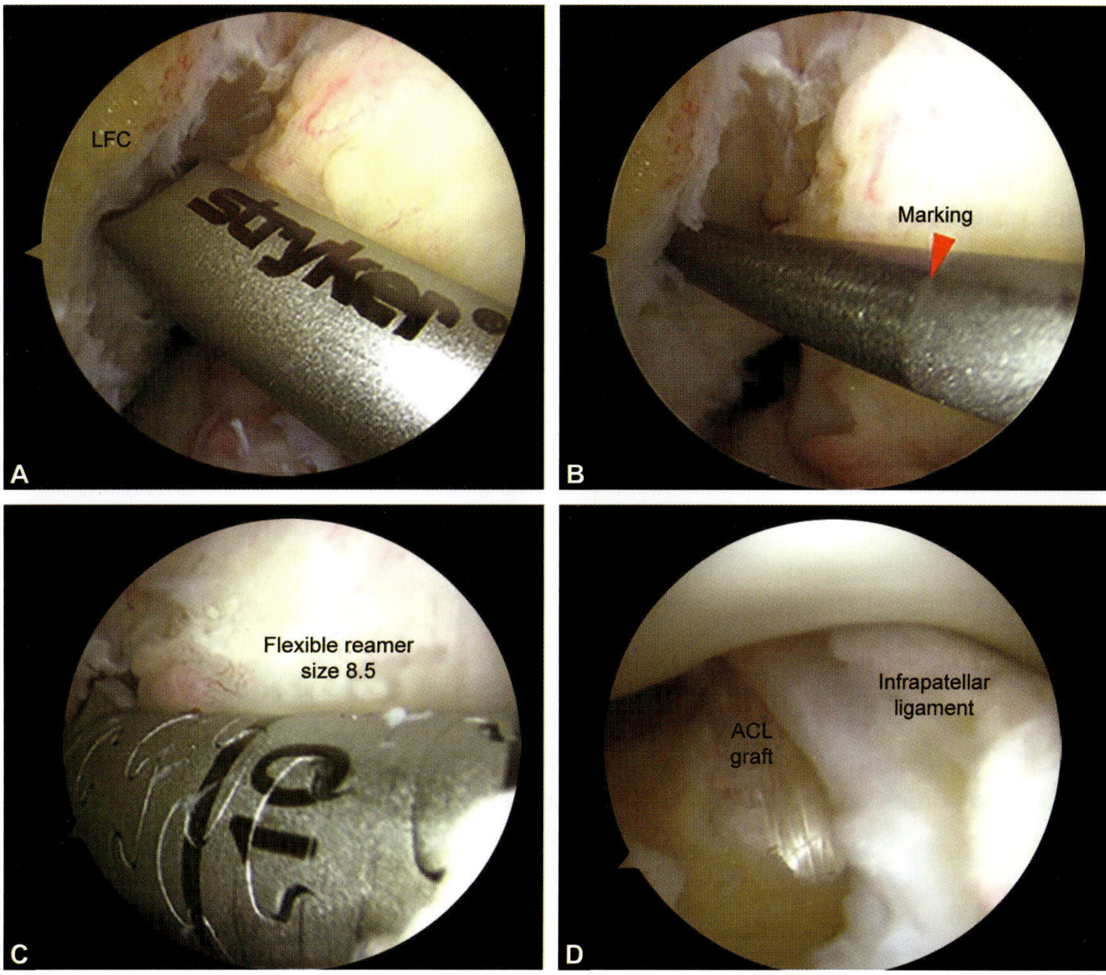

Figs. 13.4A to D: (A) Placement of femoral jig on the ACL femoral footprint; (B) Drilling of flexible guide wire depicting the marking up to which the drilling has to be done; (C) Drilling the femoral socket with the desired size flexible reamer; (D) ACL graft following a biological ACL reconstruction with intact infrapatellar ligament.
(ACL: Anterior cruciate ligament; LFC: Lateral femoral condyle).

with a debrider, a passing suture loop is passed through the guide wire eyelet. After a standard tibial tunnel preparation, the loop is retrieved through the tibial tunnel and the graft is passed.

ESSENTIAL TIPS AND TRICKS

- For a precise placement of the offset femoral jig, one must ensure proper creation of an anteromedial or an accessory anteromedial portal.
- Using the flexible reamers and with the knee not in hyperflexion, the fat pad and the infrapatellar ligament can be conserved. ACL stump is usually preserved to perform a true biological ACL reconstruction. Adequate joint distention improves visualization and prevents iatrogenic chondral injury.
- The femoral tunnel mouth needs to be cleared prior to passing the suture loop.

POSTOPERATIVE MANAGEMENT

There is no difference in the postoperative management and rehabilitation.

COMPLICATIONS

The authors have performed more than 1,000 cases of ACL reconstruction using flexible reamer system over the past 2 years. There were two cases of broken guide wires which could be retrieved easily. One flexible reamer had to be replaced due to break in one of the links after 1 year of use.

One direct fixation device (Endobutton® Direct by Smith & Nephew, Andover, MA) got impacted in the femoral socket, could not be retrieved and was left in situ without any complications. We have not had any incidence of peroneal nerve or LCL injury. The average surgical time for a standard ACLR has also reduced when using the flexible reamers.

AUTHORS' EXPERIENCE

The authors emphasize attention to the *a*natomical placement, preservation of *b*iology and a strong *c*onstruct of the ACL (ABC approach to ACLR). Flexible reamers help in fulfilling all of these.

Use of flexible reamers allows preservation of fat pad and ligament mucosum, thus preserving biology without compromising the femoral tunnel position. A consistent femoral tunnel length can be achieved using this technique. In our series, the average length was 40 mm +/-5 mm.

We believe the flexible reamer system has following distinct advantages:

- The flexible reamer system simplifies the technique of femoral tunnel drilling as compared to rigid reamers.
- Flexible reamers permit superior visualization without hyperflexion during creation of the femoral socket.
- The flexible system allows creation of tunnel in a new direction which is beneficial in revision cases.

CONCLUSION

The flexible reamers facilitate less invasive and anatomic remnant preserving ACL reconstruction. Consistent and adequate femoral tunnels can be safely created using this system. The instrumentation is technically easy to use and is the author's preferred method for primary and revision ACLR using a hamstring graft.

PEARLS AND PITFALLS

- In obese individuals and in cases where the iliotibial band (ITB) is strong and thick, retrieving the wire laterally may be difficult, as the wire tends to skive off the inner aspect of ITB.
- The guide wire, if broken, is difficult to retrieve due to its curved nature.

Contd...

Contd...

- The guide wire or loop once withdrawn or lost from the femoral socket is difficult to re-loop in the same tunnel due to the curved nature of the sockets created.
- In case of a lateral cortex blowout or to use a direct fixation device primarily, passage is difficult due to curved nature of the socket and such a device may get impacted in the tunnel. This is a limitation of this technique.
- Another limitation is its incompatibility with a bone-tendon-bone graft as negotiating the bone plug through a curved tunnel can be challenging.
- In the authors' series, there has been no significant difference in tunnel length created using flexible reamer system compared to rigid reamers, contrary to some of the studies.

REFERENCES

1. Morgan J, Dahm D, Levy B, et al. Femoral tunnel malposition in acl revision reconstruction. J Knee Surg. 2012;25(05): 361-8.
2. Cain EL, Clancy WG. Anatomic endoscopic anterior cruciate ligament reconstruction with patella tendon autograft. Orthop Clin North Am. 2002;33(4):717-25.
3. Russell R, Dumont G, Robertson W. Flexible reamers provide similar length and safer ACL tunnels without the need for knee hyperflexion: A Cadaveric assessment of flexible and rigid reamers. *Texas Orthopaedic Journal.* 2015;1(1):19-84.
4. Silver AG, Kaar SG, Grisell MK, et al. Comparison between rigid and flexible systems for drilling the femoral tunnel through an anteromedial portal in anterior cruciate ligament reconstruction. Arthroscopy. 2010;26(6):790-5.
5. Steiner ME, Smart LR. Flexible instruments outperform rigid instruments to place anatomic anterior cruciate ligament femoral tunnels without hyperflexion. Arthroscopy. 2012;28(6):835-43.

CHAPTER

14

Creating an Outside-in Femoral Tunnel

Raju Easwaran

INTRODUCTION

In the field of anterior cruciate ligament (ACL) surgery, some recent new developments just represent a refinement of what was being practiced previously. A perfect case in point is "outside-in" drilling for the femoral tunnel, a practice that was in vogue in the 1980s[1,2] and that has now found a new role in the modern ACL surgeon's toolkit for performing an anatomic ACL reconstruction, especially in a revision scenario. In the initial years of the outside-in drilling method, the technique suffered from problems with cumbersome jigs and inadequate visualization of the femoral stump resulting in the placement of a nonanatomic graft.[3] The need for an additional lateral incision was also perceived as a disadvantage especially from the cosmesis point of view and all thrust was on the development of an all-endoscopic transtibial technique[3] with the outside-in technique getting relegated to the history textbooks. With renewed interest in the femoral footprint and anatomic drilling, newer and sleeker jig designs have allowed us to revisit this technique for femoral tunnel drilling.

WHY OUTSIDE-IN?

1. Easy visualization of the femoral stump with the knee at or even below 90° flexion, without having to remove any patellar fat pad or hyper-flexing the knee.
2. Predictability of getting a consistent tunnel length, with the option to know the length of the tunnel even before drilling and to have the luxury of adjusting it to suit one's requirements. Less likely to get tunnels shorter than 30 mm.[4]
3. Safe drilling, avoiding potential damage to the medial femoral cartilage resulting from inside-out drilling with an excessively medial trajectory.
4. Multiple options with drill angles and trajectories available for revision surgeries where a good femoral tunnel is already in place and cannot be reused.
5. Cylindrical tunnel inlet versus the elliptical tunnel created by standard anteromedial (AM) portal drilling.
6. Adaptability to suit all grafts used for ACL reconstruction.
7. Elimination of divergence while putting in an interference screw for femoral fixation, especially with the bone-tendon-bone (BTB) graft.
8. Versatility of creating a custom tunnel trajectory to avoid tunnel collision in multiligament reconstruction, especially with anatomic lateral-sided reconstructions.

The main reasons for inertia amongst ACL surgeons to adopt this method are the need for an additional lateral incision and the initial learning curve associated with this technique. Another concern is the potential injury to the lateral collateral ligament (LCL) with a very low tunnel.[4] One may need to change usual fixation methods and use interference screws with this type of tunnel drilling especially if through and through drilling is done, as standard button devices will not find purchase on the lateral cortex of the femur. Endobutton® Direct (Smith & Nephew, Andover, MA) may still be used. Difficulties with graft passage may also be encountered as the trajectories of the tibial and femoral tunnel are totally different and a simple pulling action is at times insufficient to coax the graft to enter both tunnels. One also needs a skilled assistant to help with good sleeve placement and drilling of the tunnel.

ESSENTIAL HARDWARE

- Outside-in jig for ACL, with its sleeve and guide wire (Fig. 14.1)
- Standard ACL tibial reamers can be used for through and through drilling of the femoral tunnel.
- Specialized flip-cutting devices can be used (expensive) if drilling of a socket is desired while using a hamstring graft with a button device for fixation (Fig. 14.2).

SURGICAL TECHNIQUE

1. Viewing the femoral footprint from the AM portal is required as an essential step. AM portal gives a direct view of the femoral footprint (Fig. 14.3) compared to the tangential view afforded by the conventional anterolateral (AL) viewing portal (Fig. 14.4).
2. The jig (Fig. 14.1) is introduced from the AL portal. It is useful to enlarge this portal both externally (with a No. 11 blade) and internally (using a soft tissue shaver) to facilitate its smooth introduction. The surgeon should be holding the scope in one hand and the jig in the other, whereas the assistant should be responsible for inserting the sleeve and drilling the guide wire.

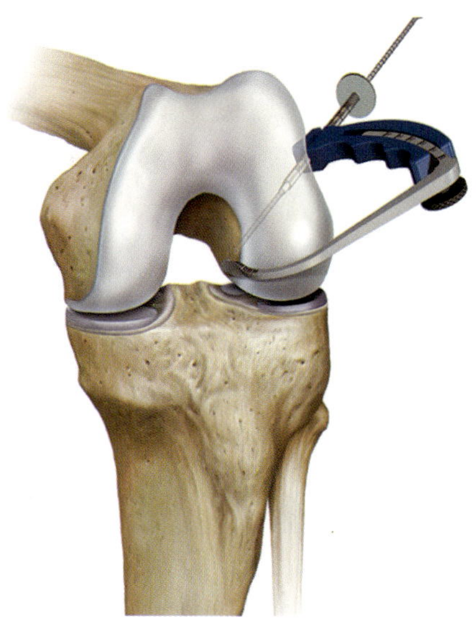

Fig. 14.1: Outside-in jig for anterior cruciate ligament, with its sleeve and guide wire.

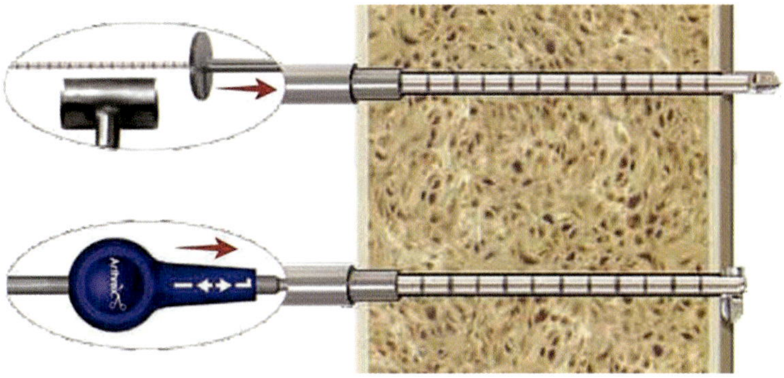

Fig. 14.2: FlipCutter® (Arthrex, Naples, FL).

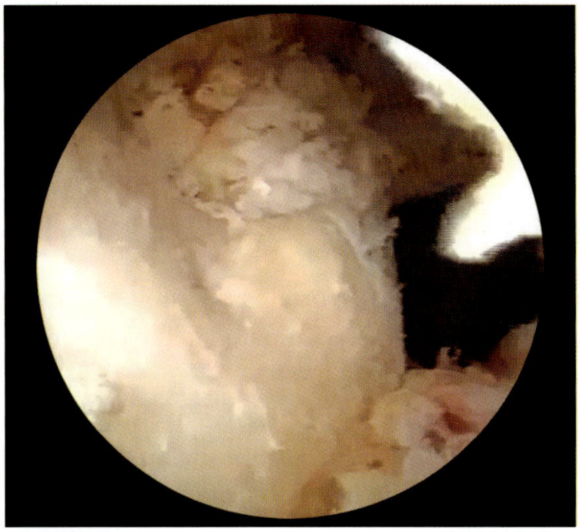

Fig. 14.3: Direct visualization of the femoral footprint from the anteromedial portal.

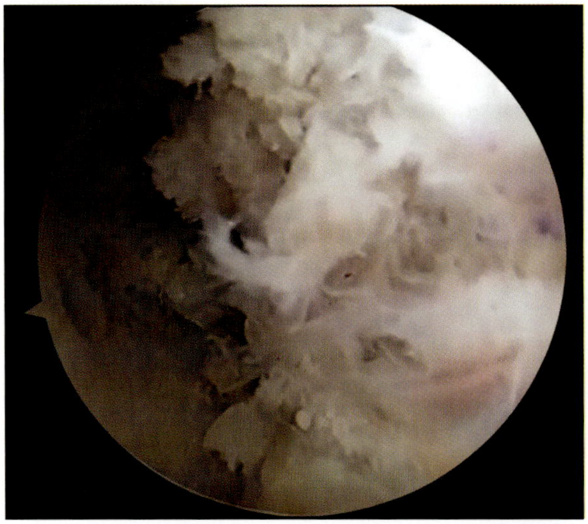

Fig. 14.4: Tangential view of the femoral footprint usually seen from the anterolateral portal.

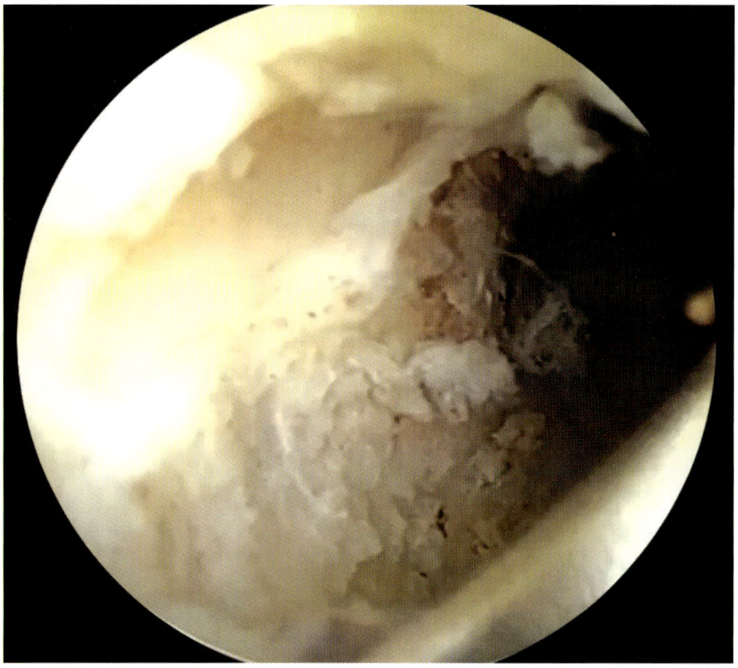

Fig. 14.5: Placement of the aiming tip of the jig in the femoral footprint of the anterior cruciate ligament.

3. Insert the aiming tip of the jig into the center of the femoral footprint (Fig. 14.5). Some jigs have an oval that can encompass the entire footprint, with the guide wire emanating from the center of the oval. The sagittal angle on the jig can be set at any convenient angle that allows a good femoral tunnel placement. Some jigs have their angle fixed and nothing much can be done apart from rotating the jig in the coronal plane to get the correct trajectory.
4. Once you are satisfied with the placement of the aiming tip or oval on the femoral footprint, rotate the jig in the coronal plane to get the appropriate placement for the sleeve on the lateral aspect of the distal thigh. The assistant inserts the sleeve in the appropriate slot and pushes it onto the skin to create a marking dimple. A skin incision is made and tissues are sharply dissected till the bone, to approach the lateral cortex of the femur (Fig. 14.6). The sleeve is advanced till it hits the bone and one can directly read the length of the tunnel off the markings on the sleeve (Fig. 14.7). If one needs more length, minor adjustments are still possible by altering the coronal inclination of the jig.
5. Aim to place the tip of the sleeve on the flat surface of the lateral distal femur, 10 mm proximal and anterior to the lateral epicondyle (Fig. 14.8) to get the best surface for the tunnel, avoiding injury to the LCL.[4]
6. The assistant then drills the guide wire, through both cortices of the femur, till it becomes visible to the chief surgeon, arthroscopically from the medial viewing portal (Fig. 14.9).
7. The jig is then removed and the position of the guide wire is rechecked. Further steps depend on the femoral fixation method desired. If a standard interference screw fixation is desired, through and through drilling is done using a standard tibial reamer of the appropriate diameter. It is useful to prevent the forward migration of the guide wire with a scoop curette introduced through the AL portal (Fig. 14.10) while the assistant is reaming the tunnel. Absolute parallelism can be achieved with this technique, especially with the BTB graft (Fig. 14.11).

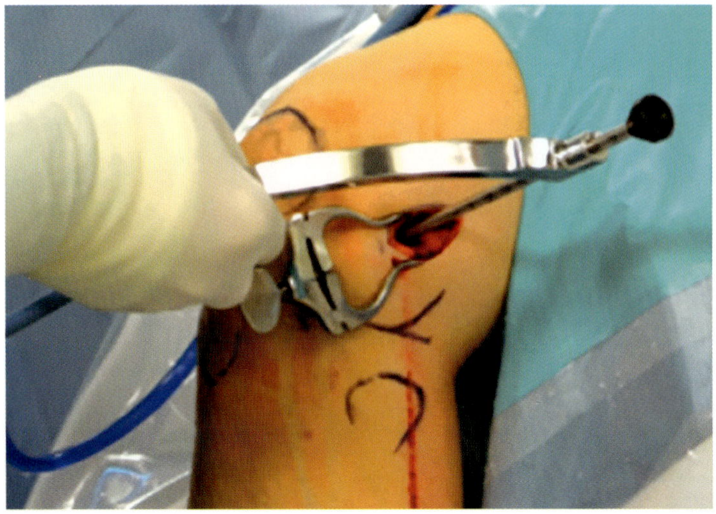

Fig. 14.6: External dissection required to place the aiming bullet of the jig.

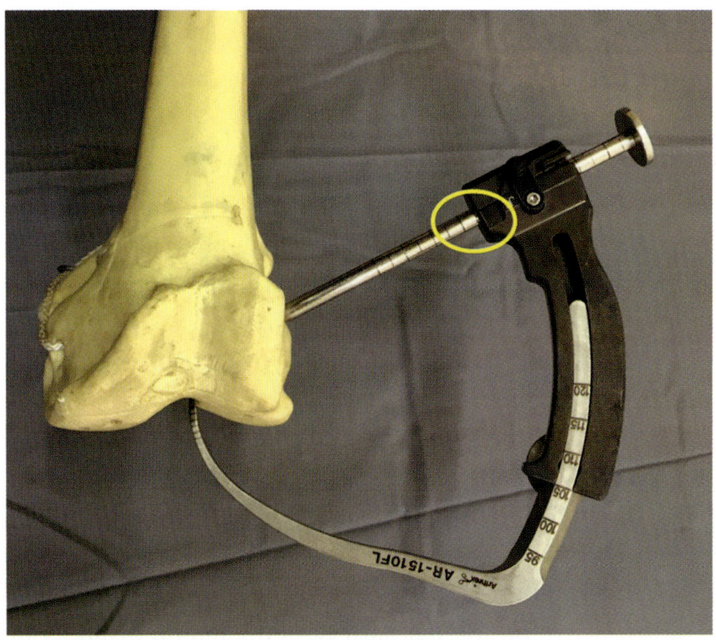

Fig. 14.7: Direct measurement of the femoral tunnel length from the jig sleeve.

8. If a button fixation is desired for a looped soft tissue graft like the hamstring, then a special device known as the FlipCutter® (Arthrex, Naples, FL) needs to be used for creating a socket in the femur *(discussed in Chapter 22).*
9. Once the tunnel is in place, a suture shuttle is passed from the femoral to the tibial tunnels and fixation is completed after graft passage. Due to the different trajectories of the tunnels, sometimes pulling the graft into the tunnels may be a bit difficult, especially with the BTB graft. It may be easier to push the graft into the femoral tunnels with the assistance of a probe/Wissinger rod's blunt cylindrical end/standard 4.5-mm screwdriver, introduced from the AM portal while viewing from the AL portal.

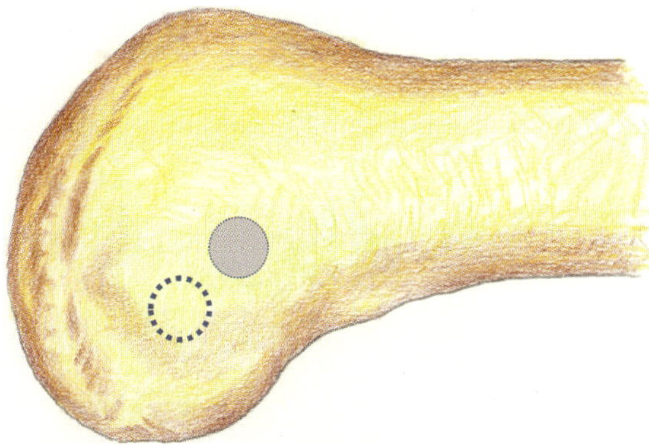

Fig. 14.8: The ideal flat surface for seating the tip of the bullet in the femoral aimer.

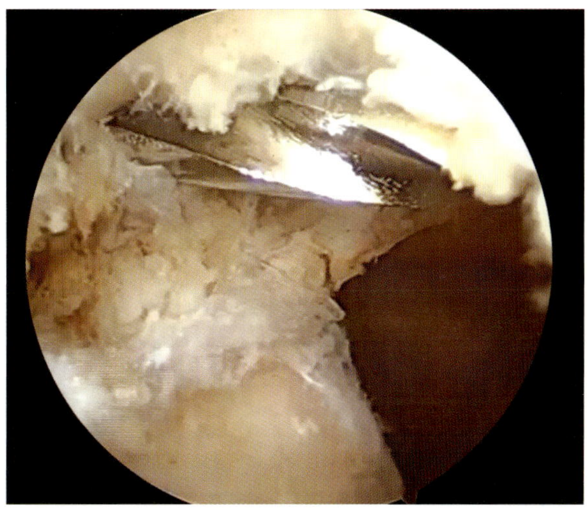

Fig. 14.9: Seeing the guide wire from the anteromedial portal.

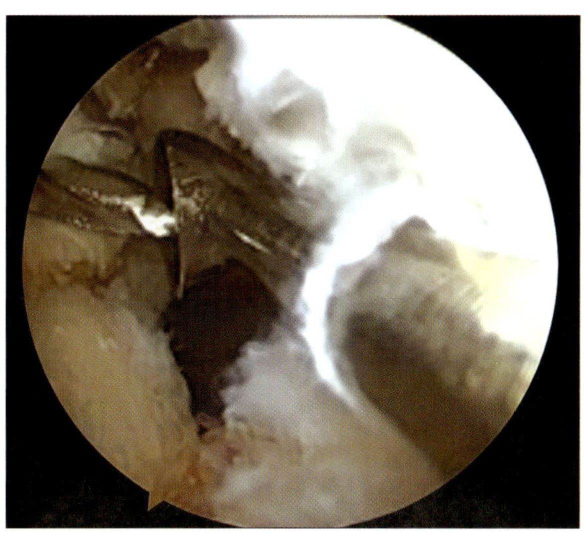

Fig. 14.10: Protecting the tip of the guide wire with a curette to prevent forward migration while reaming.

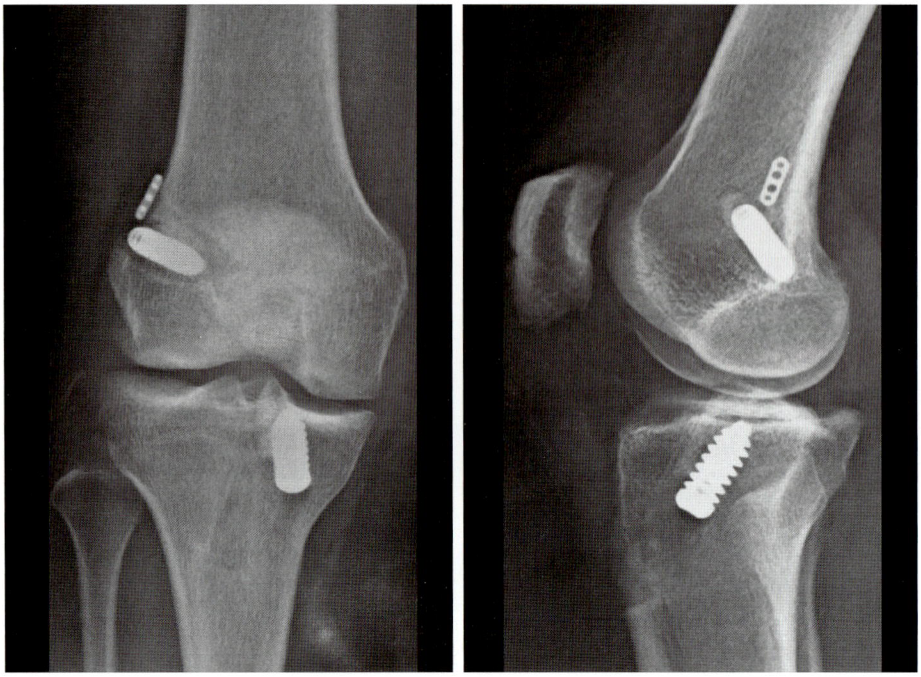

Fig. 14.11: Check X-ray showing no screw divergence (bone-tendon-bone graft).

PEARLS AND PITFALLS

- *Jig does not go in smoothly from the AL portal*: Solution is to enlarge the portal both externally, by increasing the skin incision, and internally, by shaving off the periportal fat pad.
- *Jig goes in but does not sit over the femoral footprint*: This may be due to a high AL portal being used, especially in very tall people or ones with patella alta. It is worthwhile to create a low AL portal to ensure a straighter trajectory for the jig's aiming arm to reach the footprint.
- *A good view of the footprint is not obtained*: This is usually due to a far medial portal being created. Always check the trajectory of the medial portal with a spinal needle to ensure a direct trajectory to the femoral footprint. Creation of a horizontal portal gives the freedom to extend it laterally (towards the patellar tendon) if the view is less elaborate than what is desired.
- *The guide sleeve does not sit in the proper place in the lateral aspect of the thigh*: This can be easily solved by altering the sagittal and coronal inclination of the jig, to seat it at a spot approximately 10 mm proximal and anterior to the lateral epicondyle.
- *Too short a tunnel marking* (<30 mm) *is read off the sleeve*: This is a rare occurrence with the outside-in technique, but if this happens, altering the jig trajectory (even at the expense of an additional incision) should be tried.
- *The graft does not go in despite matching with the tunnel diameter*: One must remember that this technique relies more on pushing the graft (BTB) or levering it into the femoral tunnel with a Wissinger rod acting as a pulley (hamstring graft) rather than pulling.

KEY TECHNIQUE TIP

It is useful to remember that sometimes the jig may not seat perfectly on the femoral footprint in the same way that the ACL tibial jig sits on the tibial footprint. One should try to apply appropriate pressure (in the outward direction) to ensure good seating of the aiming tip or oval on the femoral footprint. The rest of the steps usually follow smoothly thereafter.

REFERENCES

1. Clancy WG Jr, Narechania RG, Rosenberg TD, et al. Anterior and posterior cruciate ligament reconstruction in rhesus monkeys-A histological, microangiographic, and biomechanical analysis. J Bone Joint Surg Am. 1981;63(8):1270-84.
2. Noyes FR, Matthews DS, Mooar PA, et al. The symptomatic anterior cruciate-deficient knee. Part II. The results of rehabilitation, activity modification, and counseling on functional disability. J Bone Joint Surg Am. 1983;65(2):163-74.
3. Getgood A, Spalding T. The Evolution of Anatomic Anterior Cruciate Ligament Reconstruction. Open Orthop J. 2012;6:287-94. doi:10.2174/1874325001206010287.
4. Chang MJ, Chang CB, Won HH, et al. Anteromedial portal versus outside-in technique for creating femoral tunnels in anatomic anterior cruciate ligament reconstructions. Arthroscopy. 2013;29(9):1533-9.

CHAPTER

15 Creating a Transtibial Femoral Tunnel

Arumugam S, B Bhupesh Karthik, Sadem Amer

INTRODUCTION

Tunnel placement is the most important surgical step determining the successful outcome of anterior cruciate ligament (ACL) reconstruction. But we still do not have consensus on ideal method of tunnel placement.

Transtibial tunnel drilling was commonly used in the era when "clock position" was used to identify the femoral tunnel position. With better understanding of the anatomy of ACL, this high position of femoral tunnel has become obsolete. The new concept of transportal technique has pushed the concept of transtibial technique out of fashion. Main criticism of the transtibial tunnel placement is that it results in nonanatomic femoral tunnel placement and leads to rotatory instability.

This chapter describes the author's technique of creating anatomic tunnels through transtibial method by optimizing the technique.

COMMON WAY OF DOING THE SURGICAL STEP

Conventional transtibial drilling involved drilling the tibial tunnel with ACL jigs and "clock position" was used to identify the femoral tunnel placement.

The entry point for tibial tunnel was 1 cm medial to tibial tuberosity. The femoral aimer was introduced through the tibial tunnel and the aimer was placed abutting the posterior wall of the femoral notch. The femoral tunnel was aimed at either 1 o'clock or 11 o'clock position.

This position was usually high in the notch and in continuity with the tibial tunnel. The guide wire was passed through the femoral aimer and was exited from the anterior thigh. Sequential remaining of the femoral tunnel was done by introducing the reamers through the tibial tunnel.

This technique usually led to a tunnel which was placed high and missed the anatomical footprint of ACL and failed to reproduce the biomechanical functions of a normal ACL.

Many reports in literature have shown that it is not possible to have anatomic femoral tunnels by transtibial technique.[1,2] But, all these studies have used only hamstring tendon graft. Transtibial technique with hamstring grafts, which usually had tibial tunnels less than 9 mm in diameter, will always lead to nonanatomic, superiorly placed femoral tunnels.[3]

The optimized transtibial technique can be used to achieve anatomical femoral tunnel placement in ACL reconstructions with bone-patellar tendon-bone grafts which has a tibial tunnel diameter of 11 mm.

The Way I Do It

The transtibial technique can be optimized to get an anatomical femur tunnel placement. There are 3 steps of optimization:

1. *Graft*: Bone-tendon-bone (BTB) graft which has an 11-mm tibial bone plug with a tibial tongue and a 10-mm patellar bone plug is harvested (*technique described in Chapter 2*).
2. *Femoral Tunnel Entry*: Femoral tunnel position is marked at an equidistant point on the medial surface of the lateral condyle.[4] This point is marked through the medial portal. This equidistant point is chosen because high position is proven to be nonanatomic. On the other hand, very low positions should also be avoided since long-term follow up of double-bundle ACL reconstructions show failure of posterolateral bundle.[5]
3. *Tibial Tunnel Entry*: It is about 2.5 cm away from tuberosity (midway between tibial tuberosity and posteromedial border of tibia) as described by Chhabra et al.[6] This gives better trajectory in the coronal plane and helps to reach the femoral entry point marked through medial portal by transtibial technique (Fig. 15.1).

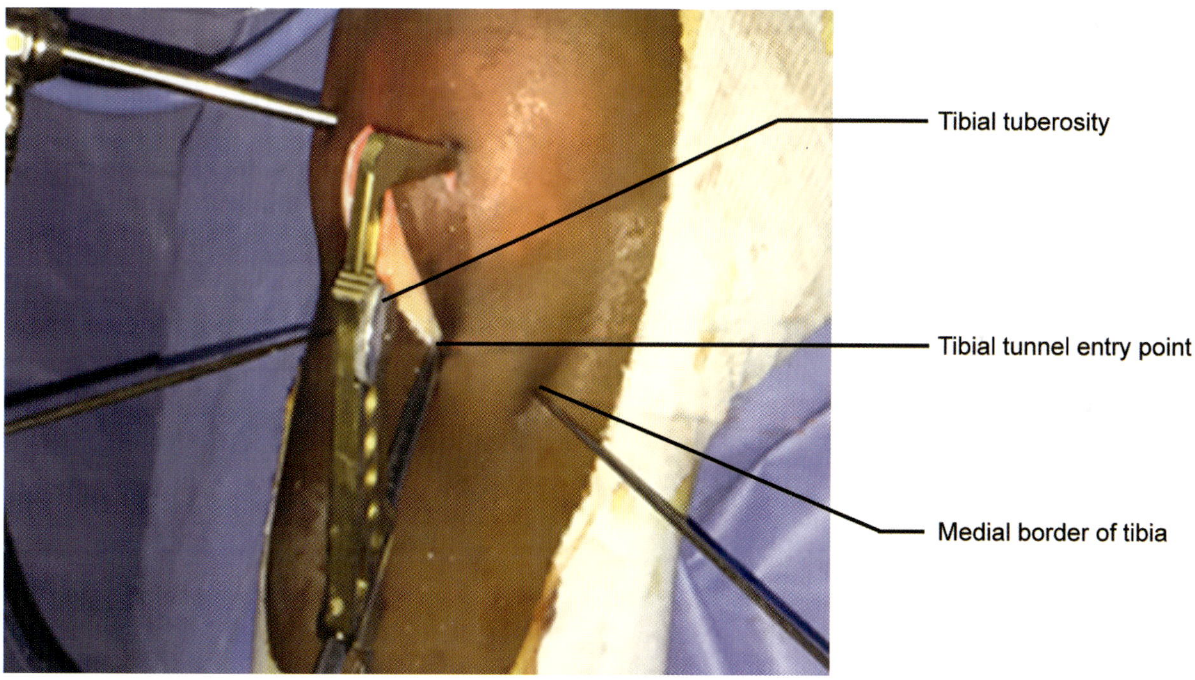

Fig. 15.1: Tibial entry point midway between tibial tuberosity and medial border of tibia.

Once diagnostic arthroscopy is done and ACL tear is confirmed, the BTB graft is harvested and prepared. The graft is sized to an 11-mm tibial bone plug and a 10-mm femoral bone plug. The advantage of larger bone plugs is that they will cover more of the native ACL insertion at femoral and tibial ends.

First, the femoral tunnel entry point is marked through the medial portal as described above (Fig. 15.2). The standard ACL tibial jig is set at 50° and is placed at the anatomical footprint of ACL. The tibial entry point is made midway between the tibial shin and the posteromedial border of the tibia. With knee in 90° of flexion, the tibial tunnel is drilled to the center of the native ACL. Sequential reaming is done and the tunnel is reamed up to 11 mm.

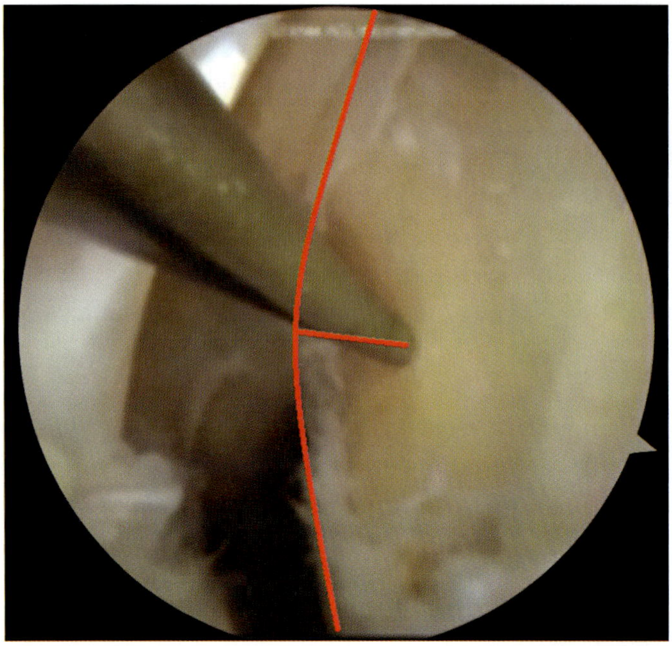

Fig. 15.2: Osseous landmarks of anterior cruciate ligament femoral attachment and the equidistant point for femoral tunnel placement.

If the tibial jig is set at an angle over 50°, the resulting tibial tunnel will become more vertical. In transtibial technique, the femoral tunnel placement is dependent on the tibial tunnel angle. Vertically placed tibial tunnel will place the resulting femoral tunnel more anterior and superior. Hence, an optimum angle of 50° is chosen.

The 11-mm tibial tunnel that is made allows the surgeon to play with the femoral aimer and reach the desired anatomical spot. This is not possible in reconstructions where the tibial tunnel is less than 9 mm in diameter.

A femoral aimer with a 7-mm offset is used for a graft with 10-mm femoral bone plug. The surgeon must be aware of the different types of femoral aimers that are commercially available. The transtibial aimer will have the offset at right angles to the shaft of the aimer. In a transportal aimer, the offset is at 30° to the shaft of the aimer (Fig. 15.3).

With the knee in 90° of flexion using the 7-mm transtibial aimer, the back of the lateral femoral condyle is hooked. This position is usually superior to the center of native ACL. Now the aimer is internally rotated to bring the femoral guide pin more inferior. Internally rotating the aimer effectively brings down the femoral offset by 1 mm. Hence, for a 10-mm femoral tunnel, it is mandatory to use a 7-mm offset to prevent posterior blowout.

The exit point of the femoral guide pin in the lateral aspect of distal thigh also gives a rough idea on the position of the tunnel. A superiorly placed nonanatomic femoral tunnel will have the guide pin exiting more anterior than lateral. An anatomically placed femoral tunnel will result in the guide pin exiting more lateral than anterior (Figs. 15.4A and B).

Once the tunnels are reamed at the anatomical footprints of ACL, the BTB graft is passed through the tunnels. The graft is secured with interference screw on femoral end with knee in 120° of flexion and at tibial end with knee in near-full extension.

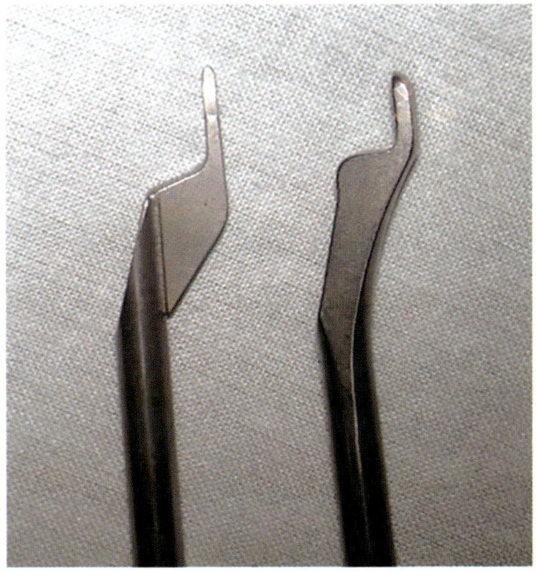

Fig. 15.3: Both are 7-mm offset femoral aimers. Left: Transportal aimer. Right: Transtibial aimer.

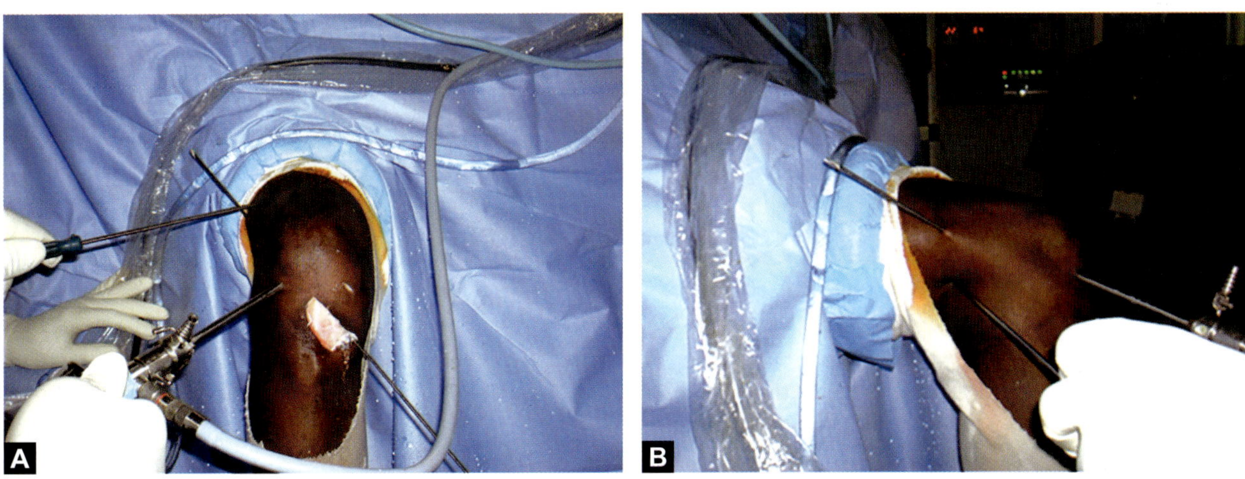

Figs. 15.4A and B: The femoral guide pin exiting at a much lower level than in the traditional transtibial technique.

ADVANTAGES

- Transtibial technique is easy to perform since the orientation of anatomy is familiar.
- This technique avoids the potential problems of transportal technique such as obscured field due to fat pad obstruction in hyperflexion, risk of neurovascular injury and scuffing of medial femoral condyle during reaming.

CONCLUSION

One should remember that this technique is described for BTB graft where we have a tibial tunnel of size 11 mm. This technique cannot be implemented in reconstructions where the tibial tunnel is smaller than 10 mm. This technique of creating a transtibial femoral tunnel is reproducible and produces anatomical femoral tunnels.

PEARLS AND PITFALLS

- Sometimes it may be difficult to pass the reamer over the guide wire from tibia to femur. In these occasions, the guide wire can be advanced into intra-articular position by reversing it from the femoral side, and the flower tip reamer can be inserted free hand through tibial tunnel and rail road over the guide wire (Figs. 15.5 to 15.10).

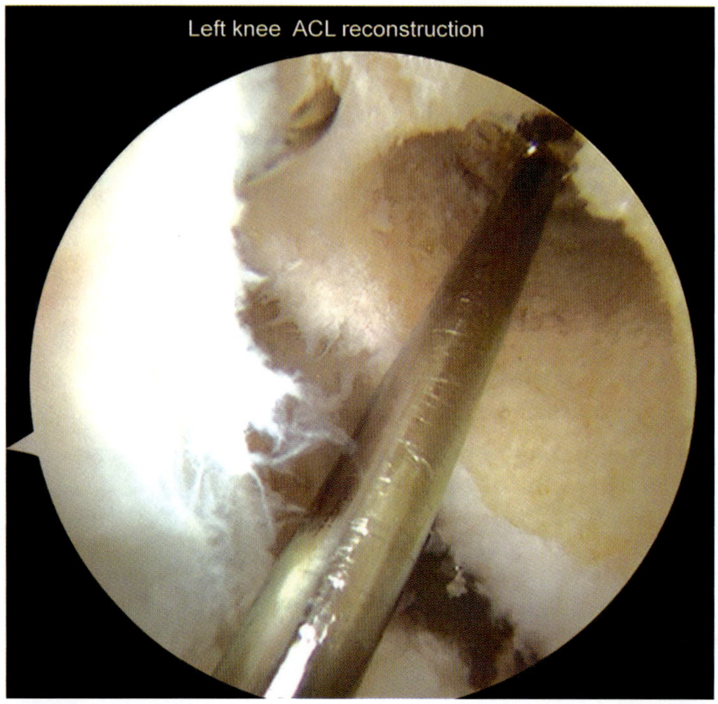

Fig. 15.5: A 10-mm low-posterior femoral tunnel, covering most of the native anterior cruciate ligament footprint.

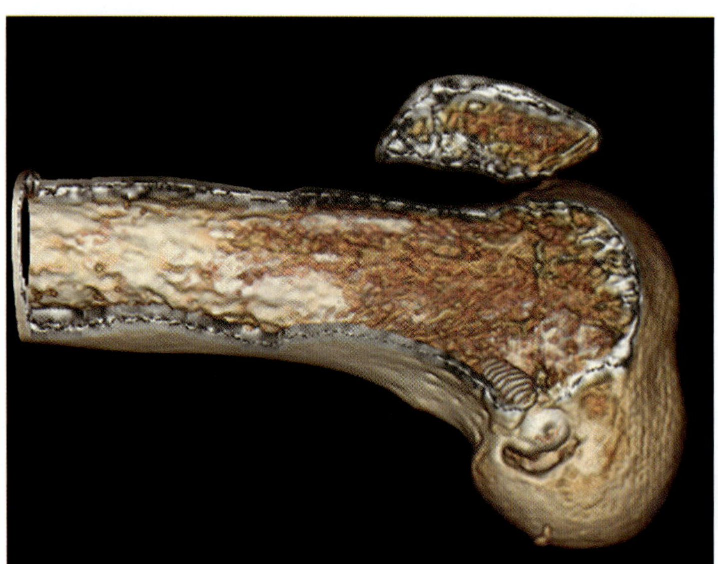

Fig. 15.6: A postoperative, three-dimensional computed tomography showing anatomically placed femoral tunnel optimized by transtibial technique.

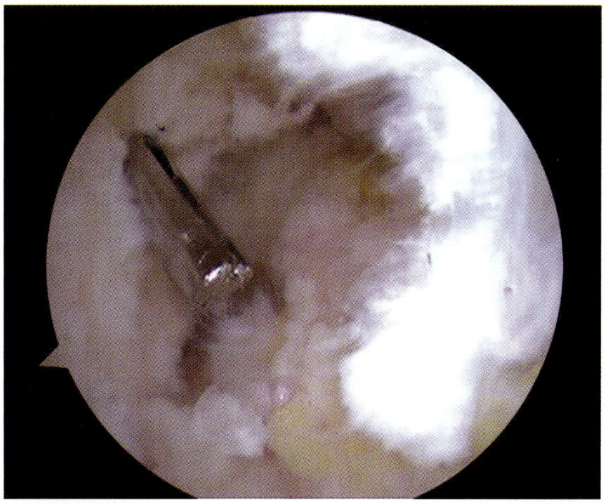

Fig. 15.7: Femoral guide pin advanced into intra-articular space.

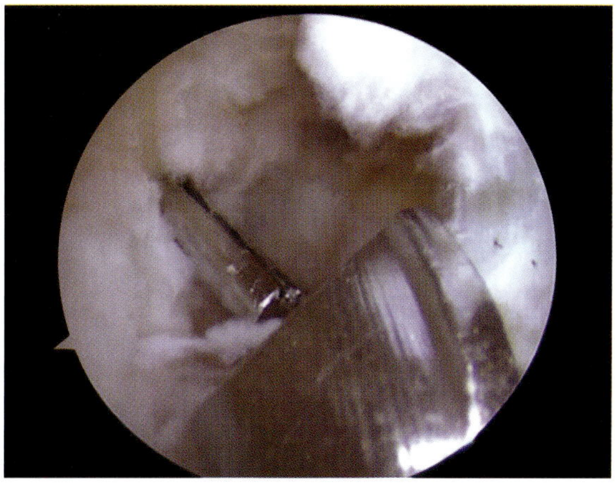

Fig. 15.8: Reamer railroaded into the guide pin through tibial tunnel.

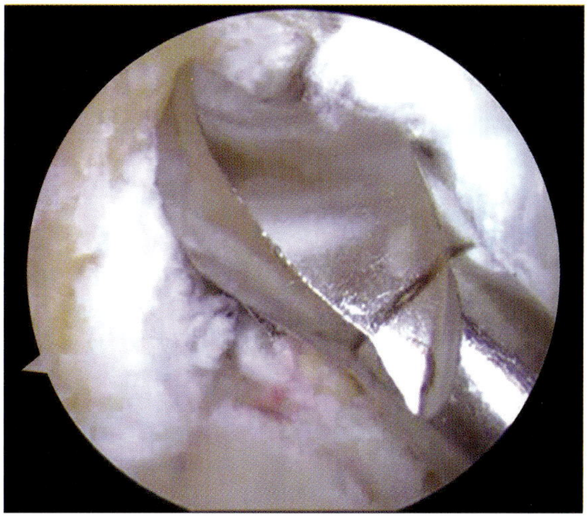

Fig. 15.9: Reamer in position for drilling the femoral tunnel.

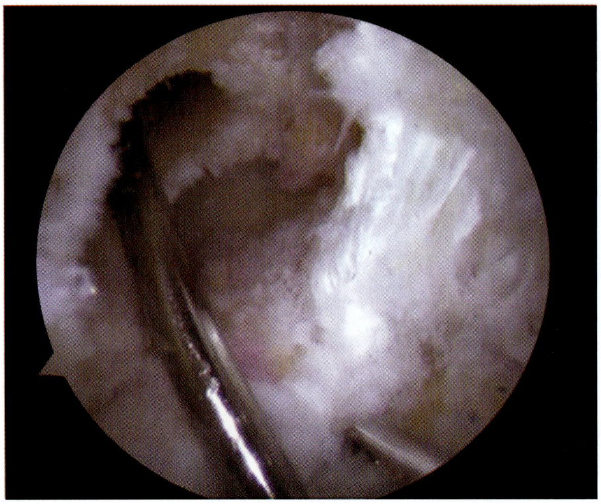

Fig. 15.10: Final anatomical femoral tunnel, made by transtibial rail-road technique.

REFERENCES

1. Shin YS, Ro KH, Lee JH, et al. Location of the femoral tunnel aperture in single-bundle anterior cruciate ligament reconstruction comparison of the transtibial, anteromedial portal, and outside-in techniques. Am J Sports Med. 2013;41(11):2533-9.
2. Pearle AD, Shannon FJ, Granchi C, et al. Comparison of 3-dimensional obliquity and anisometric characteristics of anterior cruciate ligament graft positions using surgical navigation. Am J Sports Med. 2008;36(8):1534-41.
3. Strauss EJ, Barker JU, McGill K, et al. Can anatomic femoral tunnel placement be achieved using a transtibial technique for hamstring anterior cruciate ligament reconstruction? Am J Sports Med. 2011;39(6):1263-9.
4. Howell SM, Gittins ME, Gottlieb JE, et al. The relationship between the angle of the tibial tunnel in the coronal plane and loss of flexion and anterior laxity after anterior cruciate ligament reconstruction. Am J Sports Med. 2001;29:567-74.
5. Rahr-Wagner L, Thillemann TM, Pedersen AB, et al. Increased risk of revision after anteromedial compared with transtibial drilling of femoral tunnel during primary ACL reconstruction. Results from Danish Knee Ligament Registry. Arthroscopy. 2013;29:98-105.
6. Chhabra A, Diduch DR, Blessey PB, et al. Recreating an acceptable angle of the tibial tunnel in the coronal plane in anterior cruciate ligament reconstruction using external landmarks. Arthroscopy. 2004;20:328-30.

CHAPTER

16

Identifying the Tibial Footprint

Mao Weijia David, Lee Yee Han Dave

FETAL AND ADULT ANTERIOR CRUCIATE LIGAMENT ANATOMY

The anterior cruciate ligament (ACL) starts to form in the 8th week of gestation.[1] Ferretti and Fu identified two differentiated anteromedial (AM) and posterolateral (PL) bundles in their fetal anatomy study.[2] The AM and PL bundles become apparent by week 16 of gestation.[3] The fetal ACL is similar to the adult ligament except that the bundles are more parallel and have a higher amount of cellularity and vascularity.[3] In the adult, the ACL is described as being composed of two bundles, separated by a vascular septum containing a branch of the medial geniculate artery, with innervation from the tibial nerve.[1,4]

MACROSCOPIC AND MICROSCOPIC ANATOMY

The ACL originates from the medial surface of the lateral femoral condyle, and runs obliquely from PL to AM, inserting into the broad base of the central tibial plateau.[5] Many ligamentous fibers make up the ACL, each attaching a specific point from the femur to the tibia. These fibers undergo a cascade of tightening and loosening as the knee moves through flexion and extension.[4] Tampere et al. demonstrated with a three-dimensional (3D) computed tomography (CT) model the recruitment pattern behavior of the ACL, where PL fibers are recruited in extension and AM fibers in flexion.[6]

The intra-articular course is approximately 2.0–2.5 cm and ends in a triangular footprint insertion in the anterior intercondylar area, from a fossa in front of and lateral to the anterior spine.[4,7] Two consistent bony landmarks are the medial tibial intercondylar ridge as the medial border of the ACL, and the anterior intertubercular ridge of the tibial spine acting as the posterior border.[8] The mean footprint measures 11 mm mediolateral and 17 mm anteroposterior.[4,9-11]

Furumatsu investigated histology to identify an ACL tibial insertion—lateral meniscus anterior insertion complex, composed of a connection of disorganized bridging Type I collagen fibers in the transition zone, which may play a role in stabilizing these tibial attachments. Dense anterior fiber connections on the tibial surface were also found in the study.[12]

EVOLUTION AND NEW INSIGHTS ON ANTERIOR CRUCIATE LIGAMENT TIBIAL FOOTPRINT

The understanding of the anatomy of the ACL has evolved over time. We learnt the two bundle nature of the ACL, with a later shift to a flat ribbon-shaped ligament concept. More recently, studies have looked at the tibial footprint being more of a C-shaped insertion.[13-15]

The double-bundle concept was first described in 1938. Anatomical and biomechanical studies subsequently guided our understanding of this important anatomic and functional difference. Double-bundle ACL reconstruction can improve subjective outcome scores and manual joint laxity tests.[16] The ACL has been described as having an AM and PL bundle, with each bundle having a distinct origin and insertion on the femur and tibia. The AM bundle controls more of the anterior movement while the PL bundle controls more of tibiofemoral rotation.[4,5] Double-bundle reconstruction techniques were developed to provide more anatomic reconstruction and restore knee rotational stability.[5]

The tibial footprint has been described to be oval shaped with the AM bundle inserting into the AM aspect of the footprint in direct relationship with the medial tibial spine, while the PL bundle inserts into the PL aspect close to the lateral tibial spine, in front of the posterior root of the lateral meniscus.[9,17-19] The ACL footprint area was reported as being 136 ± 33 mm^2 with the AM footprint between 35 mm^2 and 77 mm^2 and the PL footprint between 32 mm^2 and 64 mm^2.[9,18]

The concept of a two bundle ACL is still somewhat controversial, as ACL fibres can often be difficult to separate macroscopically. The ACL has a twisted, ribbon-like appearance, with differing fiber alignments at varying knee flexion.[1,9] Several authors describe no histological evidence for two separate bundles, while others described between 2 and even 3 histological bundles.[9-11,20-22]

C-SHAPED INSERTION

The fascicles of the anterior ACL may blend with the anterior horn of the lateral meniscus as some posterior fibers may blend with its posterior horn.[9,10] Many previous authors described the ACL insertion to have footprints of the AM and PL bundles.[18,19,21] However, Guenther and Fu[23] found the tibial insertion shape to be either elliptical (51%), triangular (33%) or C-shaped (16%) (Fig. 16.1).

Smigielski has also described the ACL to be a ribbon and the tibial ACL insertion to be C-shaped.[9,24] In both Smigielski's and Siebold's studies, a key step was careful dissection under magnification of the synovial tissue surrounding the collagen fibers.[9,24,25] At 5 mm from the tibial insertion, the midsubstance was ribbon-like, with mean measurements of diameter of 12.2 mm × 3.5 mm.

The footprint was found to be a C-shaped bony insertion along the medial tibial spine to the anterior aspect of the anterior root of the lateral meniscus. Smigielski reported no PL fibers, but rather, the posterior fibers inserted medially along the tibial spine and were named posteromedial fibers. Anterior and posterior horn fibers from the lateral meniscus blended in with the C-shaped insertion of the ACL. The average length and width were measured to be 13.7 mm × 3.3 mm. The anterior part was 8.7 mm in length mediolaterally. The medial part was 10.8 mm anteroposteriorly on average, which was the same as the width of the anterior horn of the lateral meniscus. The most posterior fibers were on average 2.8 mm anterior to the medial intercondylar tubercle.

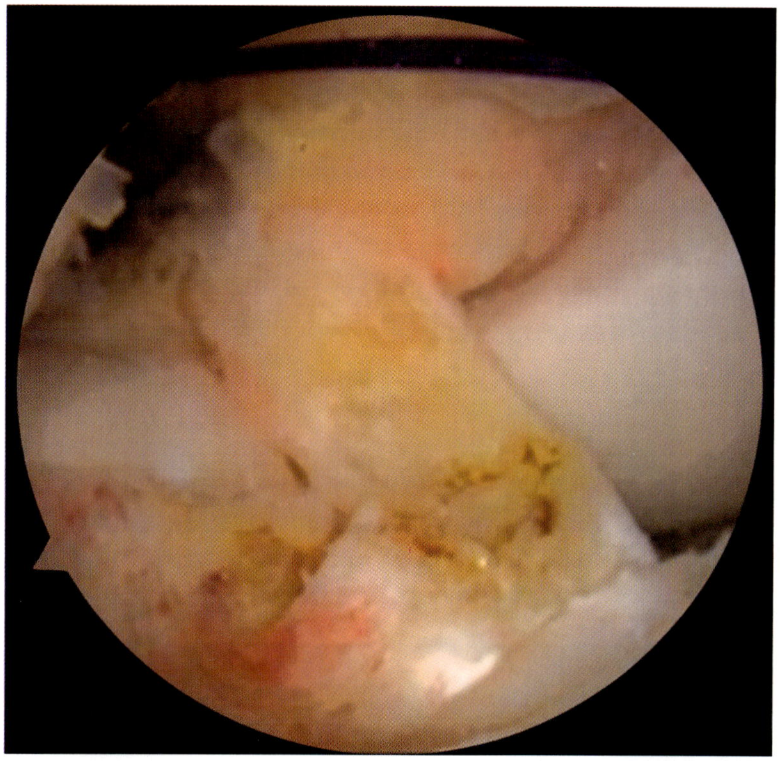

Fig. 16.1: C-shaped tibial insertion.

There were no ACL fibers inserting into the center of the C-shaped footprint and no PL tibial ACL insertion. The center of the "C" was the bony insertion of the anterior root of the lateral meniscus. The root was covered by fat and was overpassed by the flat ACL anteriorly. There was a direct insertion which was the C-shaped insertion of the midsubstance fibers and an indirect insertion which consisted of the anterior and broader attachment of the fan-like extension of fibers. Both parts together formed a duckfoot-like bony footprint.[9]

Smigielski described three types of C-shaped insertions: (1) C-type, (2) J-type and (3) Cc-type.[24] Oka also found the tibial ACL insertion to be duckfoot-like in a C-shaped configuration. There were no PL fibers, nor ACL bundles found histologically.[26] Janovsky found the insertions to be C-shaped and histological findings revealed that the ligament (vertical parallel collagen fibers) occupied only 30.8% of the complete insertion. The remaining area was filled with synovial tissue.[27]

The difference in findings may be due to difference in dissection methods amongst the authors. Similar to Smigielski, Siebold was not able to clearly separate the collagen fibers into bundles.[9]

ARTHROSCOPIC LANDMARKS AND GUIDE POINTS, HOW TO FIND IT

Arthroscopic orientation is essential for anatomical placement of bone tunnels. The best individual landmark for orientation is the ACL stump[28] (Fig. 16.2). Other important landmarks are the anterior horn of the lateral meniscus, transverse intermeniscal ligament (Fig. 16.3), the medial and lateral tibial spine (Fig. 16.4)

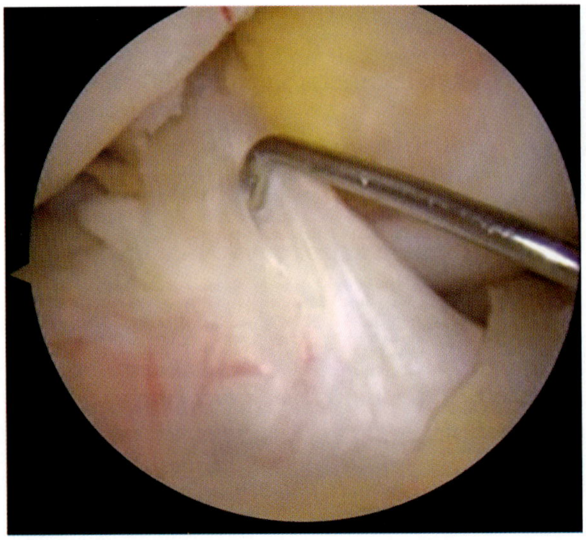

Fig. 16.2: Anterior cruciate ligament (ACL) stump midpoint.

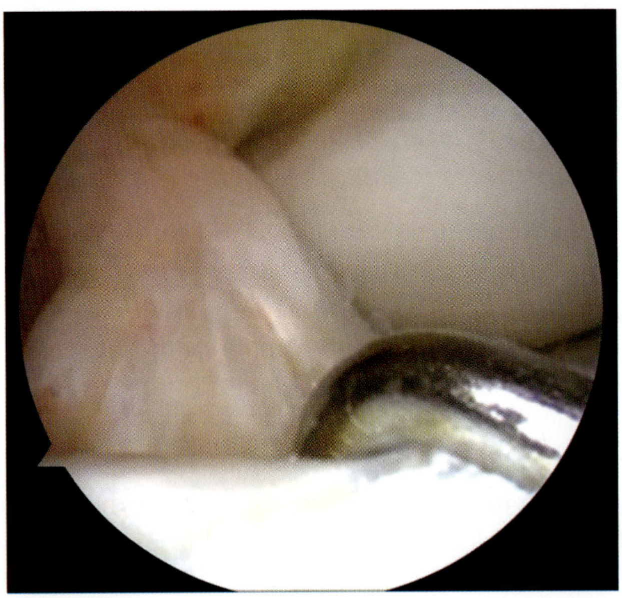

Fig. 16.3: Transverse intermeniscal ligament.

and posterior horn of the lateral meniscus (Fig. 16.5). These become especially important when ACL remnants are lacking such as in revision surgery. Other suggested key arthroscopic landmarks were the anterior border of the AM bundle (Fig. 16.6), posterior border of the PL bundle as well as the AM rim, anterolateral rim and the eminentia intercondylaris.[19] Kassam suggested the posterior border of the anterior horn of the lateral meniscus as a reproducible and anatomical marker for the midpoint of the ACL footprint.[29] Though Werner found the anterior horn of the lateral meniscus to yield an inconsistent tunnel location.[30] Jackson identified the ACL footprint to be 7 mm anterior to the anterior border of the posterior cruciate ligament (PCL).[31]

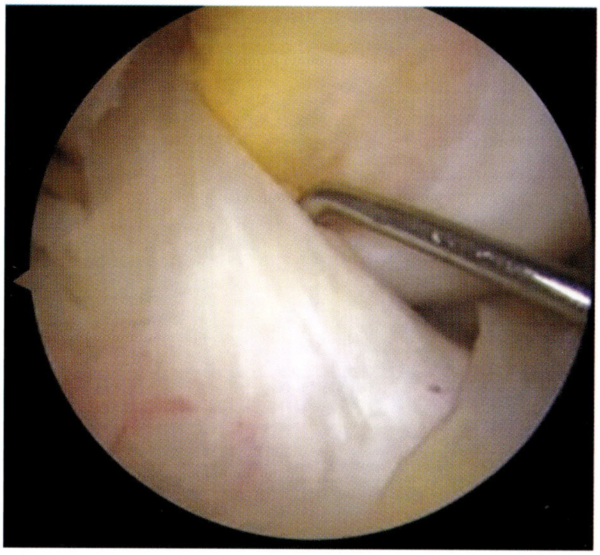

Fig. 16.4: Medial tibial spine.

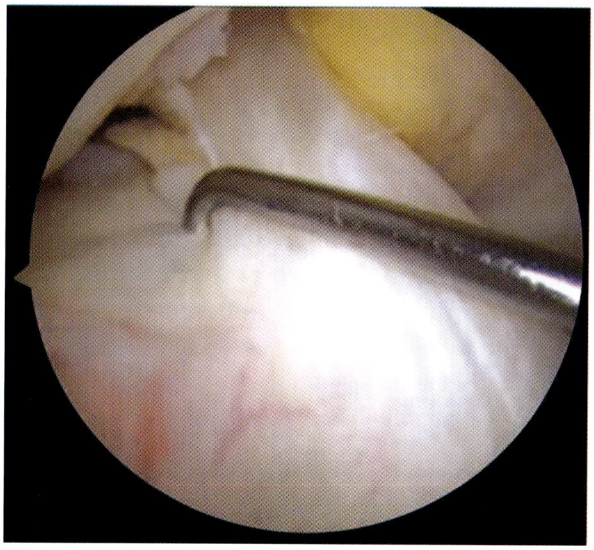

Fig. 16.5: Posterior horn of the lateral meniscus.

Key landmarks can be found on the tibial eminence, which features two tubercles, the lateral tibial eminence and the medial tibial eminence, separated by an intertubercular ridge. The medial condylar ridge extends anterior from the medial tubercle. The insertion of the ACL is from the fovea at the base of the intertubercular ridge to the posterior border of the lateral meniscus. Fibers may extend up to the intertubercular ridge and the medial condylar ridge.[32] A retroeminence or "over the back" ridge has also been described that provides a consistent landmark that is 17.0–17.5 mm (±1.7–2.0 mm) from the center of the AM bundle.[17,33] Ziegler described the tibial ACL attachment center to be 7.5 mm medial the anterior horn of the lateral meniscus, 13 mm anterior to the retro eminence ridge and 10.5 mm posterior to the ACL ridge.[34]

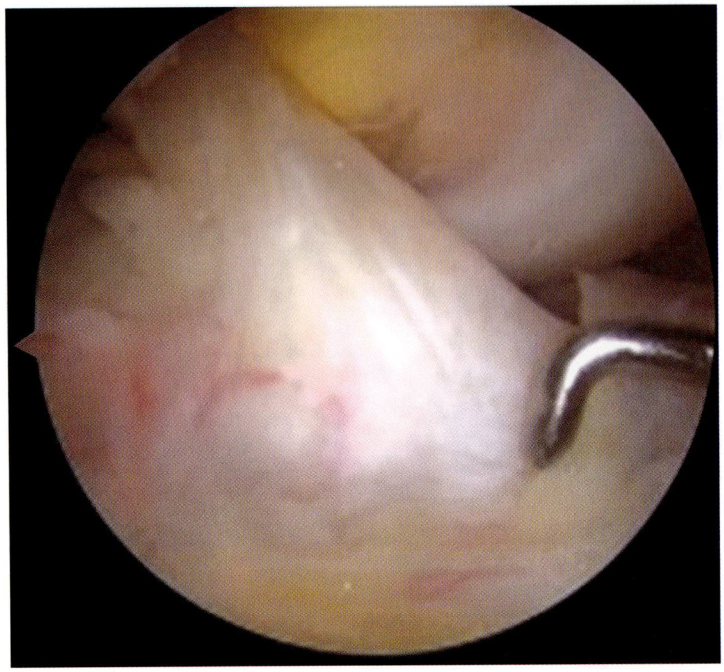

Fig. 16.6: Anterior limit of the anterior cruciate ligament (ACL) footprint.

TUNNEL ANGLE AFFECTING THE RECONSTRUCTED FOOTPRINT

When planning the tibial tunnel for ACL reconstruction, there must be consideration for how the tunnel angle affects the final footprint. It should be noted that the tibial tunnel drilled at an angle will create an oblong hole.[8] A 10 mm reamer drilled at 40° will create a 15.5 mm long footprint. More than 95% of the footprint surface area can be restored by applying different approaches to graft diameters and drill angles.[35] In larger footprints, double bundle can replicate up to 63% more area and 27% more length than a single bundle ACL reconstruction.[36]

COMPLICATIONS OF INCORRECT POSITION

Anterior placement of the tibial tunnel can cause notch impingement, while posterior placement will cause the graft to impinge with the PCL.[37] Reconstructing the tibial footprint should more closely restore the natural function of the ACL.[4] Siebold recommended to avoid a central or PL tibial bone tunnel placement as it is nonanatomical and may compromise biomechanics and may damage the anterior root of the lateral meniscus.[9] Kodama also found this to be true, with a more PL positioning of the tibial tunnel aperture inducing lateral meniscal extrusion after ACL reconstruction.[38]

REFERENCES

1. Sonnery-Cottet B. Single or double bundle. In: Dunbar M, Sripada S, Kjar R (Eds). The Knee Joint: Surgical Techniques and Strategies. Paris, France: Springer-Verlag; 2012. pp. 227-34.
2. Ferretti M, Levicoff EA, Macpherson TA, et al. The fetal anterior cruciate ligament: an anatomic and histologic study. Arthroscopy. 2007;23(3):278-83.

3. Irarrázaval S, Albers M, Chao T, et al. Gross, arthroscopic, and radiographic anatomies of the anterior cruciate ligament: Foundations for anterior cruciate ligament surgery. Clin Sports Med. 2017;36(1):9-23.
4. Shelton W. Anterior cruciate ligament repair. In: Hunter RE, Sgaglione NA (Eds). AANA Advanced Arthroscopy: The Knee, 1st edition. Philadelphia, PA: Saunders-Elsevier; 2010. pp. 178-83.
5. Andrews JR, Meisterling SW. Anterior cruciate ligament reconstruction: Overview of anatomy, biomechanics, and indications for surgery. In: Lieberman JR, Berry DJ, Azar FM (Eds). Advance Reconstruction: Knee. Rosemont, IL, USA: American Academy of Orthopaedic Surgeons; 2011. pp. 551-4.
6. Tampere T, Van Hoof T, Cromheecke M, et al. The anterior cruciate ligament: a study on its bony and soft tissue anatomy using novel 3D CT technology. Knee Surg Sports Traumatol Arthrosc. 2017;25(1):236-44.
7. Strobel MJ. Anterior cruciate ligament. In: Manual of Arthroscopic Surgery, 1st edition. Heidelberg, Germany: Springer-Verlag; 2012. p. 367.
8. Purnell ML, Larson AI. Mini-incision patellar tendon harvest and anterior cruciate ligament reconstruction using critical bony landmarks. Sports Med Arthrosc. 2009;17(4):234-41.
9. Siebold R, Schuhmacher P, Brehmer A, et al. Tibial C-shaped insertion of the anterior cruciate ligament without posterolateral bundle. In: Siebold R, Dejour D, Zaffagnini S (Eds). Anterior Cruciate Ligament Reconstruction: A Practical Surgical Guide. Heidelberg, Germany: Springer-Verlag. 2014. pp. 19-27.
10. Arnoczky SP. Anatomy of the anterior cruciate ligament. Clin Orthop Relat Res. 1983;(172):19-25.
11. Girgis FG, Marshall JL, Monajem A. The cruciate ligaments of the knee joint. Anatomical, functional and experimental analysis. Clin Orthop Relat Res. 1975;(106):216-31.
12. Furumatsu T, Kodama Y, Maehara A, et al. The anterior cruciate ligament-lateral meniscus complex: A histological study. Connect Tissue Res. 2016;57(2):91-8.
13. Siebold R. Flat ACL anatomy: fact no fiction. Knee Surg Sports Traumatol Arthrosc. 2015;23(11):3133-5.
14. Śmigielski R, Zdanowicz U, Drwięga M, et al. Ribbon like appearance of the midsubstance fibres of the anterior cruciate ligament close to its femoral insertion site: a cadaveric study including 111 knees. Knee Surg Sports Traumatol Arthrosc. 2015;23(11):3143-50.
15. Śmigielski R, Zdanowicz U, Drwięga M, et al. The anatomy of the anterior cruciate ligament and its relevance to the technique of reconstruction. Bone Joint J. 2016;98-B(8):1020-6.
16. Siebold R, Branch TP, Freedberg HI, et al. A matched pairs comparison of single- versus double-bundle anterior cruciate ligament reconstructions, clinical results and manual laxity testing. Knee Surg Sports Traumatol Arthrosc. 2011;19(Suppl 1):S4-11.
17. Colombet P, Robinson J, Christel P, et al. Morphology of anterior cruciate ligament attachments for anatomic reconstruction: a cadaveric dissection and radiographic study. Arthroscopy. 2006;22(9):984-92.
18. Harner CD, Baek GH, Vogrin TM, et al. Quantitative analysis of human cruciate ligament insertions. Arthroscopy. 1999;15(7):741-9.
19. Siebold R, Ellert T, Metz S, et al. Tibial insertions of the anteromedial and posterolateral bundles of the anterior cruciate ligament: morphometry, arthroscopic landmarks, and orientation model for bone tunnel placement. Arthroscopy. 2008;24(2):154-61.
20. Dargel J, Pohl P, Tzikaras P, et al. Morphometric side-to-side differences in human cruciate ligament insertions. Surg Radiol Anat. 2006;28(4):398-402.
21. Duthon VB, Barea C, Abrassart S, et al. Anatomy of the anterior cruciate ligament. Knee Surg Sports Traumatol Arthrosc. 2006;14(3):204-13.
22. Otsubo H, Shino K, Suzuki D, et al. The arrangement and the attachment areas of three ACL bundles. Knee Surg Sports Traumatol Arthrosc. 2012;20(1):127-34.
23. Guenther D, Irarrázaval S, Nishizawa Y, et al. Variation in the shape of the tibial insertion site of the anterior cruciate ligament: classification is required. Knee Surg Sports Traumatol Arthrosc. 2015 Dec 12. [Epub ahead of print].
24. Smigielski R, Zdanowicz U, Drwiega, et al. Variations of the tibial insertion of the anterior cruciate ligament: An anatomical study. In: Siebold R, Dejour D, Zaffagnini S (Eds). Anterior Cruciate Ligament Reconstruction: A Practical Surgical Guide. Heidelberg, Germany: Springer-Verlag; 2014. pp. 29-32.
25. Siebold R, Schuhmacher P, Fernandez F, et al. Flat midsubstance of the anterior cruciate ligament with tibial "C"-shaped insertion site. Knee Surg Sports Traumatol Arthrosc. 2015;23(11):3136-42. [Erratum in: Knee Surg Sports Traumatol Arthrosc. 2016;24(9):3046. Knee Surg Sports Traumatol Arthrosc. 2016;24(9):3046].
26. Oka S, Schuhmacher P, Brehmer A, et al. Histological analysis of the tibial anterior cruciate ligament insertion. Knee Surg Sports Traumatol Arthrosc. 2016;24(3):747-53.

27. Janovsky C, Kaleka CC, Alves MT, et al. Synovial C-shaped tibial footprint of the anterior cruciate ligament. Orthop J Sports Med. 2016;4(11):2325967116671300.
28. Siebold R, Smigielski R. Arthroscopic appearance of the "C"-shaped insertion of the anterior cruciate ligament. In: Siebold R, Dejour D, Zaffagnini S (Eds). Anterior Cruciate Ligament Reconstruction: A Practical Surgical Guide. Heidelberg, Germany: Springer-Verlag; 2014. pp. 33-38.
29. Kassam AM, Tillotson L, Schranz PJ, et al. The lateral meniscus as a guide to anatomical tibial tunnel placement during anterior cruciate ligament reconstruction. Open Orthop J. 2015;9:542-7.
30. Werner BC, Burrus MT, Gwathmey FW, et al. A prospective evaluation of the anterior horn of the lateral meniscus as a landmark for tibial tunnel placement in anterior cruciate ligament (ACL) reconstruction. Knee. 2016;23(3):478-81.
31. Jackson DW, Gasser SI. Tibial tunnel placement in ACL reconstruction. Arthroscopy. 1994;10(2): 124-31.
32. Carmont MR, Scheffler S, Spalding T, et al. Anatomical single bundle anterior cruciate ligament reconstruction. Curr Rev Musculoskelet Med. 2011;4(2):65-72.
33. Edwards A, Bull AM, Amis AA. The attachments of the anteromedial and posterolateral fibre bundles of the anterior cruciate ligament: Part 1: tibial attachment. Knee Surg Sports Traumatol Arthrosc. 2007;15(12):1414-21.
34. Ziegler CG, Pietrini SD, Westerhaus BD, et al. Arthroscopically pertinent landmarks for tunnel positioning in single-bundle and double-bundle anterior cruciate ligament reconstructions. Am J Sports Med. 2011;39(4):743-52.
35. Siebold R. The concept of complete footprint restoration with guidelines for single- and double-bundle ACL reconstruction. Knee Surg Sports Traumatol Arthrosc. 2011;19(5):699-706.
36. Siebold R, Schuhmacher P. Restoration of the tibial ACL footprint area and geometry using the Modified Insertion Site Table. Knee Surg Sports Traumatol Arthrosc. 2012;20(9):1845-9.
37. Howell SM, Clark JA. Tibial tunnel placement in anterior cruciate ligament reconstructions and graft impingement. Clin Orthop Relat Res. 1992;(283):187-95.
38. Kodama Y, Furumatsu T, Miyazawa S, et al. Location of the tibial tunnel aperture affects extrusion of the lateral meniscus following reconstruction of the anterior cruciate ligament. J Orthop Res. 2016 Sep 27. [Epub ahead of print].

CHAPTER

17

Creating a Tibial Tunnel

Lim Wei-an Joel, Lee Yee Han Dave

INTRODUCTION

Incorrect tunnel position is the most common surgical technique error in anterior cruciate ligament (ACL) surgery.[1] An incorrect tibial tunnel position has a significant effect on clinical outcomes.[2] Accurate anatomic placement of the tibial tunnel has been shown to resist anterior tibia translation and rotational instability and the failure to do so results in increased graft stress and early failure.[3-6]

There is a risk of intercondylar roof and posterior cruciate ligament (PCL) impingement when the tunnel is drilled too anterior or posterior, respectively. Howell has demonstrated that a tibial tunnel that is placed too anterior results in graft impingement by the intercondylar notch which can result in a fixed flexion deformity of the knee and graft failure due to attritional damage from impingement.[7,8] Traditionally, many surgeons have performed a notchplasty during ACL reconstruction to reduce the risk of notch impingement.[2,8-14] However, with recent trends favoring anatomic ACL reconstructions, the practice of routine notchplasty has fallen out of favor.[15]

Magnetic resonance imaging (MRI) studies have shown that a tibial tunnel placed in the anterior part of the tibial ACL footprint requires a 5–6-mm notchplasty to prevent impingement.[13] Howell, therefore, recommended a posteriorly placed tibial tunnel to avoid femoral roof impingement as it has been shown that a tibial tunnel placed 3 mm posterior to the native ACL insertion does not require a notchplasty.[2,13] On the contrary, there are problems with a posteriorly placed tibial tunnel as Silva et al. demonstrated recurrent high-grade pivot shift and inferior outcomes when a tibial tunnel was placed too posterior.[5] Based on the Amis-Jakob line on intraoperative radiographs, Kasten described the ideal tibia ACL insertion to be 41% (SD 4.4%, range 37–52%) of the anteroposterior (AP) direction.[16] In cadaveric studies, Colombet established that the centers of the anteromedial (AM) and posterolateral (PL) bundles to be at 36% and 52% of the Amis-Jakob line, respectively, while Zantop found that the centers of the AM and PL bundles to be at 30% and 44%.[17,18]

There has been much debate on the ACL footprint and optimal position of the tibial tunnel. Kato et al. reported in their biomechanical study that using the midpoint insertions between the AM and PL bundles on both the femoral and tibia had the best stability in anterior translation and rotational stability.[19] Karlsson et al. recommended individualizing ACL reconstruction with the goals of restoring the native insertion site of the ACL, achieving two functional bundles and applying appropriate graft tension.[20]

ANTERIOR CRUCIATE LIGAMENT TIBIA FOOTPRINT

The understanding of the dimensions and position of the native ACL is essential to guide accurate tibial tunnel placement. The native ACL inserts into the footprint between the tibial spines at the posterior edge of the anterior horn of the lateral meniscus. Morgan has recommended choosing a point 7 mm anterior to the anterior border of the PCL in 120° of knee flexion while Jackson and Gasser have recommended a point halfway between the line connecting the attachment of the anterior horn of the lateral meniscus and the medial tibial spine (Figs. 17.1A to C).[21-23]

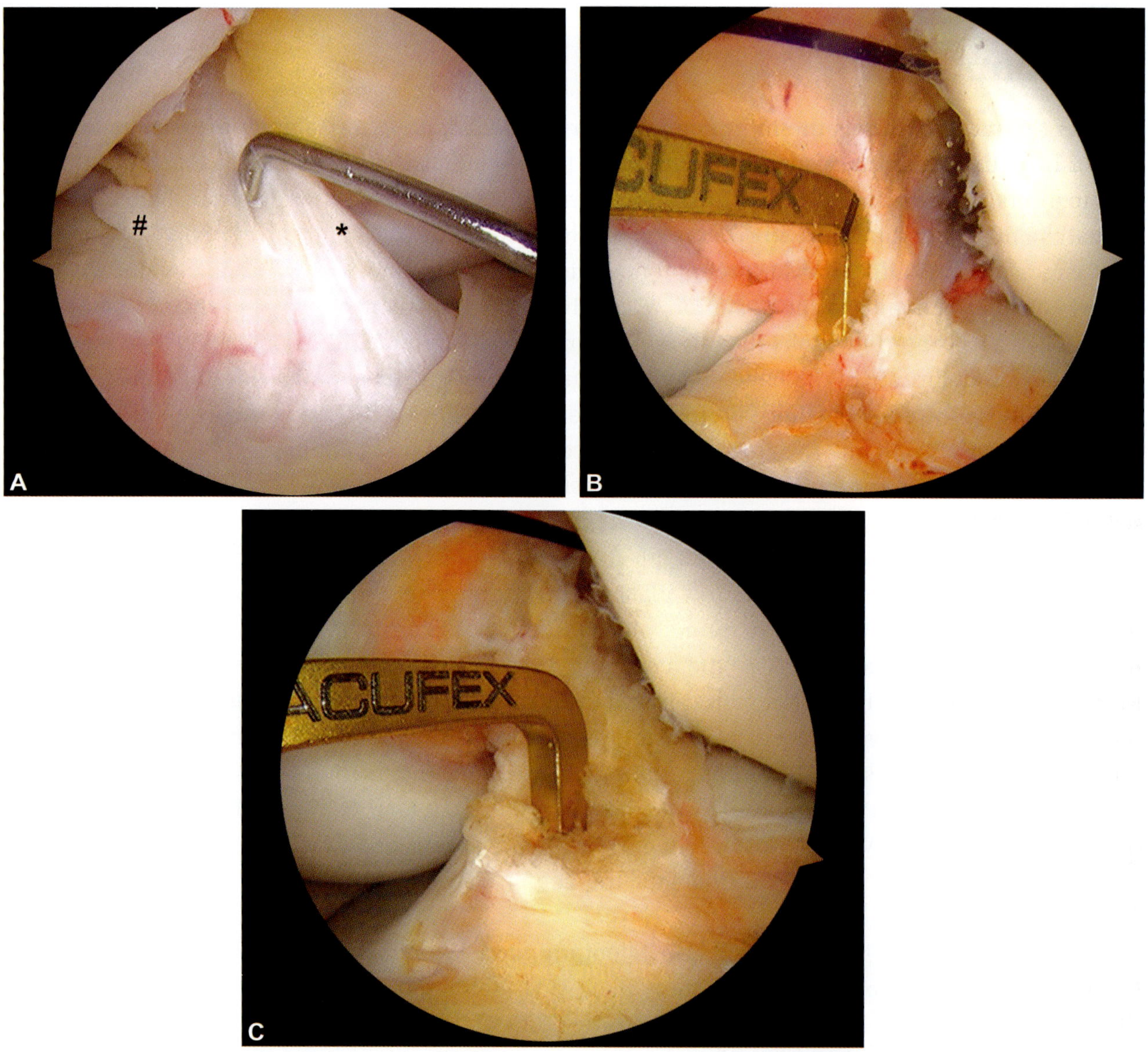

Figs. 17.1A to C: (A) Anterior cruciate ligament (ACL) footprint midpoint between medial tibia spine (*) and anterior horn of lateral meniscus (#) as described by Jackson and Gasser.[23] ACL footprint 7 mm in front of the posterior cruciate ligament (PCL) as described by Morgan et al.[22] (B) with elbow aimer and (C) with tip aimer.

TUNNEL LENGTH

The tibial tunnel length should be varied according to the graft length to prevent an excessively protruding graft or a disappearing graft. Tunnel length is especially important for bone-patella tendon-bone grafts, where a common intraoperative complication during ACL reconstruction is graft tunnel length mismatch.[23-29]

The adjustment of the tibial tunnel length is recommended to manage this mismatch. There are multiple studies that have proposed achieving the optimal tibial tunnel length according to the graft length. Miller and Hinkin proposed drilling the tibial length 'N + 7,' where N is the patella tendon length, in order to achieve an adequate tibial tunnel length.[30] Kenna et al. calculated the tibial tunnel length by subtracting 50 mm off the total graft length while Olszewski recommened the 'N + 2' rule.[31,32] A study by Wallace et al. showed that varying the drill angle at 45°, 50°, and 55° had no significant change in tibial tunnel length.[33] Therefore it is, recommended to set the drill guide for the tibia cortex entry at an angle between 40° and 60° to the horizontal.

For hamstring graft fixation, the tibial tunnel length is more forgiving, however, attention must be paid to avoid protrusion of the interference screw intra-articular.[34,35] It has been suggested by Herrera et al. that the minimum tibial tunnel length should be 28 mm for adequate fixation of the soft tissue graft by interference screws as the 28-mm screw fixation fails at loads above 500 N, which can occur during aggressive rehabilitation.

A short tibial tunnel has been discouraged as short interference screws (<23 mm) have been shown not to achieve optimal fixation strength.[36] Selby et al. have also demonstrated that using 35-mm interference screws has significantly higher load to failure than 28-mm interference screws, which provides secure graft fixation during graft incorporation.[37] Figueroa has shown that when the tibia drill guide is set at 55°, the average tibial tunnel length was 43 mm, allowing consistent use of a 35-mm interference screw fixation.[27]

With the advent of newer fixation devices, there has been recent hype on short grafts for ACL reconstruction as a new concept. It involves a rethink of the biomechanical and biological concepts in ACL reconstruction from graft selection to tunnel lengths. The creation of long tibia tunnels may not be necessary as it has been suggested that intratunnel healing only has a temporary role.[38] More recent evidence has proven that there is no statistical difference in pull out strength and biological remodeling of 5-mm and 15-mm tibia sided grafts—this has been validated by various authors.[39,40]

TUNNEL START POINT

Morgan described that the ideal extra-articular tibial starting point is 1 cm above the pes anserinus and 1.5 cm medial to the tibial tuberosity.[22] If the tibial tunnel starting point is too medial, the medial collateral ligament is at risk of being damaged. If the tunnel is too shallow, there is a risk of breaching the medial tibial joint surface causing chondral damage. Miller et al. have recommended using the midpoint between the tibial tubercle and posteromedial tibia border as an easily identifiable landmark, which can reliably reproduce tibial tunnel drilling without the need for intraoperative radiographs (Fig. 17.2).[41]

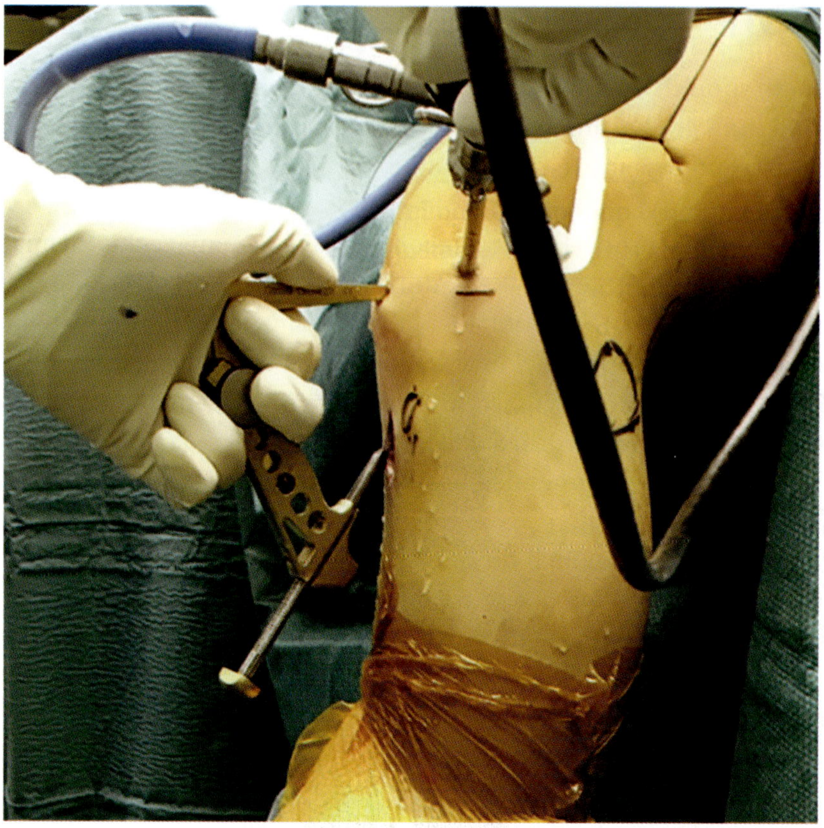

Fig. 17.2: Tibial cortex starting point midway between the tibia tubercle and posteromedial tibia cortex.

TUNNEL ANGLE AND APERTURE

The tibial tunnel angle must be considered to prevent risk of tunnel enlargement. Kopf et al. demonstrated that the angle between the tibia plateau and tibia tunnel influences the shape and size of the tibial tunnel aperture.[42] A shallow tibial tunnel will produce a tunnel outlet that is elliptical rather than circular. If the tunnel is too elliptical, the graft cannot stay in full contact with the walls during range of motion resulting in an inflexion point within the tunnel, leading to graft tunnel aperture motion, potentially causing tibial tunnel enlargement.[43]

Howell showed that a tibial tunnel angle greater than 75° in the coronal plane is associated with greater tension in the ACL graft during flexion, loss of knee flexion, and increased anterior laxity.[44]

Oversizing of the tibial tunnel aperture can also result in graft overhang with potential PCL impingement and intra-articular injury to the anterior horn of the lateral meniscus.[23,45] 20% of patients had definite notch impingement with an additional 45% of patients at risk of notch impingement when a 10 mm diameter tunnel is drilled at 45°.[46]

TIBIAL TUNNEL PREPARATION

There are four techniques of creating a tibial tunnel, sequential drilling, sequential dilation, cancellous bone plug harvesting, and retrodrilling.

Sequential drilling is a quick and efficient surgical technique used by most surgeons. In sequential drilling, a K wire is drilled through the upper tibia to determine the intra-articular insertion site of the ACL graft. The K wire is subsequently overdrilled to the desired graft diameter. The surgeon is able to make minute adjustments to tibial tunnel placement by pressing the K wire against the walls during drilling. The disadvantage of sequential drilling is the excavation of soft cancellous bone with more bone removed than desired; and uncontrolled plunging into the joint with inadvertent chondral damage.

Serial tibia tunnel dilation is an alternative technique. Due to the presence of soft cancellous bone in the upper tibia, this technique has been shown to increase pullout strength and bone strength for better support of interference screws.[47,48] This method is especially recommended for revision procedures as drilling preexisting tunnels might remove more tissue than desired. The last technique involves harvesting a cancellous bone plug while creating the tibial tunnel, allowing the surgeon to use the plug to augment graft fixation.[49] This is especially useful in implant-free ACL graft fixation surgical techniques.

Standard drilling techniques can result in fragmentation of the bone tunnels. Retrograde drilling of the tibial tunnel is not only essential in short graft ACL reconstruction but has been shown to be less aggressive, resulting in less fragmentation, fewer microfractures, less postoperative pain, and produce a smooth consistent tunnel wall.[50] The recently introduced FlipCutter® (Arthrex, Naples, FL) is an all-in-one guide pin and drill that allows for minimally invasive retrodrilling of the tunnel sockets. This results in an intact cortical rim which provides a better graft-tunnel interface and consequently superior graft fixation and decreased tunnel widening.[51]

THE WAY I DO IT

When drilling the tibial tunnel, I usually keep the lower extremity free and flexed at the knee. I would utilize a high lateral portal for visualization of the ACL footprint and a medial portal to visualize the medial wall of the lateral femoral condyle. After performing complete evaluation of the knee arthroscopically, I would define the landmarks of the ACL footprint. I prefer to leave any remnant ACL fibers and an ACL stump of at least 5 mm as it not only guides placement of the tibia drill guide but also provides early postoperative mechanical strength, blood supply preservation, and proprioception (Fig. 17.3).[52]

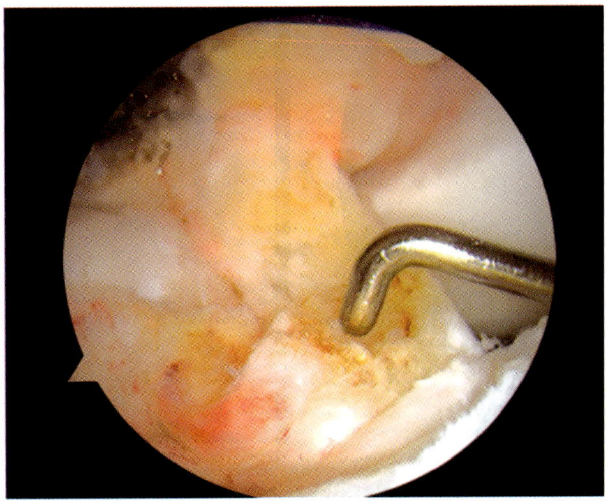

Fig. 17.3: Prepared anterior cruciate ligament (ACL) footprint with preserved remnant ACL.

I usually use a tip aimer guide set at 50° to the horizontal. Setting the drill angle 50° to the horizontal consistently yields sufficient tibial tunnel length of approximately 35 cm. Placing the guide through the medial portal, I aim for the midpoint of the ACL footprint and set the elbow of the guide against the PCL, which results in a tibia intra-articular insertion point 7 mm anterior to the PCL. Careful attention must be paid to the anterior horn of the lateral meniscus, PCL, intercondylar femoral roof before drilling as malpositioning of the tibia tunnel can lead to iatrogenic damage of the lateral meniscus, graft impingement, and failure. The guidewire is next inserted through the medial tibia cortex at a point midway between the tibial tubercle and the posteromedial edge of the tibia.

The guidewire is advanced into the joint leaving 2 cm of the wire projecting inside the joint. It is important to note that the guidewire's exit is a poor way to define the insertion point because of the remnant ACL stump and an oblique drill angle which may result in a more medially placed insertion point than observed. Proper placement is indicated when the guidewire bisects the tibial spines and enters the notch lateral to the PCL. Potential graft impingement is assessed using the guidewire with the knee in extension. Appropriate notchplasty should be performed until the tip of the guidewire passes freely towards the lateral femoral condyle. Guidewire malpositioning must be addressed at this point and upon confirming the desired tibial tunnel position.

I sequentially overdrill the guidewire to the desired tibial tunnel diameter. A closed curette is placed over the guidewire (Fig. 17.4) during drilling to prevent inadvertent pin migration and meticulous

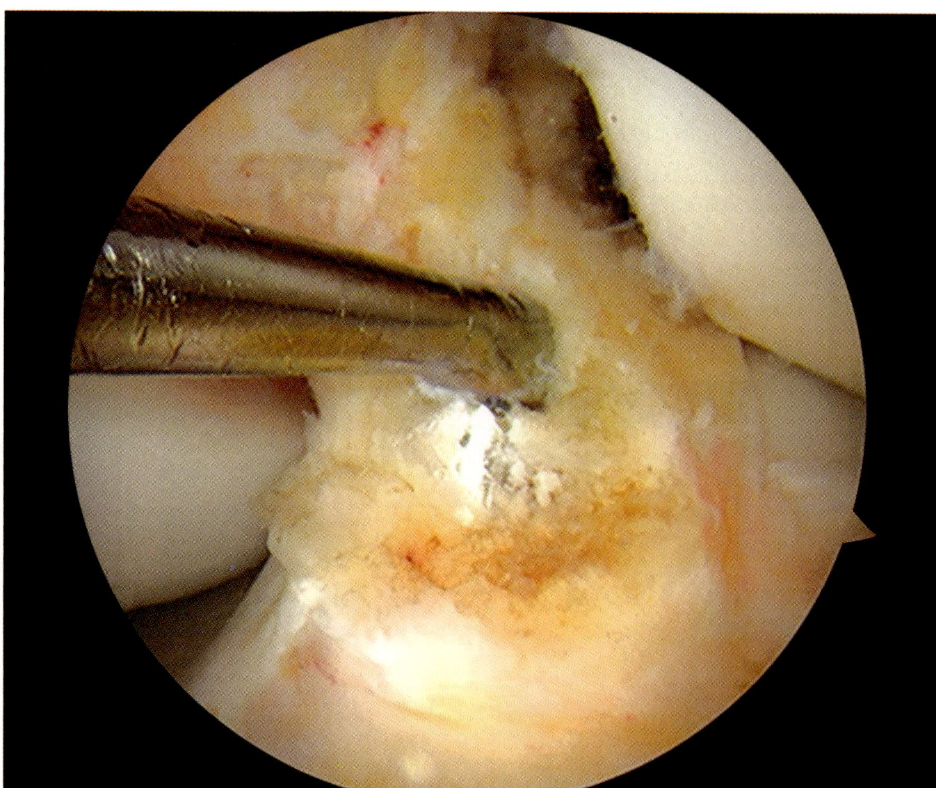

Fig. 17.4: Guide pin placed and protected with a curette during reaming.

care is taken not to disrupt the anterior horn of the lateral meniscus and the intermeniscal ligament. After completion of tibia tunnel drilling, the intra-articular edge of the tibia tunnel and debris are cleared with a radiofrequency probe and shaver.

COMPLICATIONS AND PEARLS

Placement of a correct tibial tunnel is relevant to achieve good knee kinematics.[3] There are numerous occasions during tibial tunnel drilling that malposition can occur and the surgeon should be aware of the potential pitfalls. Occasionally, unfavorable placement of the AM portal can deflect the drill guide and prevent its accurate placement - this can be bypassed by making another portal. Next, identifying the appropriate ACL footprint is important to prevent malpositioning of the tibial intra-articular insertion point.

The tibia insertion point, drill size, and drill angle point influence tibial tunnel positioning, aperture size, and shape, respectively. If the tibia insertion point is too anterior, it can cause graft impingement with the intercondylar notch and also potential iatrogenic damage to the anterior horn of the lateral meniscus and intermeniscal ligament.[53] If the tibial tunnel is placed too posteriorly, there is a risk of PCL impingement.[54] If the surgeon discovers that the tibial tunnel is too anterior or posterior, the guidewire must be repositioned by eccentric drilling with a 4.5 mm drill bit.

The ideal tibial tunnel length is 3.5–4 cm for adequate fixation strength of the graft by interference screw. A horizontal drill angle can also result in damage to the medial tibia condyle with a very elliptical aperture. A more vertical drill angle will conversely result in a more circular aperture, which results in less movement of the graft and less synovial fluid leakage into the tunnel that can interfere with graft bone healing.[55]

During guidewire insertion and after tibial tunnel drilling, potential graft impingement must be reassessed repeatedly to prevent early graft failure and fixed flexion deformity postoperatively. Appropriate notchplasty should be performed if intercondylar notch impingement is present.

REFERENCES

1. Yasuda K, van Eck CF, Hoshino Y, et al. Anatomic single- and double-bundle anterior cruciate ligament reconstruction. Part 1: Basic science. Am J Sports Med. 2011;39(8):1789-99.
2. Howell SM, Clark JA. Tibial tunnel placement in anterior cruciate ligament reconstructions and graft impingement. Clin Orthop Relat Res. 1992;(283):187-95.
3. Zantop T, Diermann N, Schumacher T, et al. Anatomical and nonanatomical double-bundle anterior cruciate ligament reconstruction: importance of femoral tunnel location on knee kinematics. Am J Sports Med. 2008;36(4):678-85.
4. Pinczewski LA, Salmon LJ, Jackson WF, et al. Radiological landmarks for placement of the tunnels in single-bundle reconstruction of the anterior cruciate ligament. J Bone Joint Surg Br. 2008;90(2):172-9.
5. Silva A, Sampaio R, Pinto E. ACL reconstruction: comparison between transtibial and anteromedial portal techniques. Knee Surg Sports Traumatol Arthrosc. 2012;20(5):896-903.
6. Clancy WG, Nelson DA, Reider B, et al. Anterior cruciate ligament reconstruction using one-third of the patellar ligament augmented by extra-articular tendon transfers. J Bone Joint Surg Am. 1982;64(3):352-9.

7. Howell SM. Principles for placing the tibial tunnel and avoiding roof impingement during reconstruction of a torn anterior cruciate ligament. Knee Surg Sports Traumatol Arthrosc. 1998;6 Suppl 1:S49-55.
8. Jackson DW, Schaefer RK. Cyclops syndrome: Loss of extension following intra-articular anterior cruciate ligament reconstruction. Arthroscopy. 1990;6(3):171-8.
9. Howell SM. Arthroscopic roofplasty: A method for correcting an extension deficit caused by roof impingement of an anterior cruciate ligament graft. Arthroscopy. 1992;8(3):375-9.
10. Howell SM, Berns GS, Farley TE. Unimpinged and impinged anterior cruciate ligament grafts: MR signal intensity measurements. Radiology. 1991;179(3):639-43.
11. Howell SM, Clark JA, Blasier RD. Serial magnetic resonance imaging of hamstring anterior cruciate ligament autografts during the first year of implantation: A preliminary study. Am J Sports Med. 1991;19(1):42-7.
12. Howell SM, Clark JA, Farley TE. Serial magnetic resonance study assessing the effects of impingement on the MR image of the patellar tendon graft. Arthroscopy. 1992;8(3):350-8.
13. Howell SM, Clark JA, Farley TE. A rationale for predicting anterior cruciate graft impingement by the intercondylar roof: A magnetic resonance imaging study. Am J Sports Med. 1991;19(3):276-82.
14. Howell SM, Taylor MA. Failure of reconstruction of the anterior cruciate ligament due to impingement by the intercondylar roof. J Bone Joint Surg. 1993;75(7):1044-55.
15. Keklikci K, Yapici C, Kim D, et al. The effect of notchplasty in anterior cruciate ligament reconstruction: a biomechanical study in the porcine knee. Knee Surg Sports Traumatol Arthrosc. 2013;21(8):1915-21.
16. Kasten P, Szczodry M, Irrgang J, et al. What is the role of intra-operative fluoroscopic measurements to determine tibial tunnel placement in anatomical anterior cruciate ligament reconstruction? Knee Surg Sports Traumatol Arthrosc. 2010;18(9):1169-75.
17. Colombet P, Robinson J, Christel P, et al. Morphology of anterior cruciate ligament attachments for anatomic reconstruction: a cadaveric dissection and radiographic study. Arthroscopy. 2006;22(9):984-92.
18. Zantop T, Wellmann M, Fu FH, et al. Tunnel positioning of anteromedial and posterolateral bundles in anatomic anterior cruciate ligament reconstruction: anatomic and radiographic findings. Am J Sports Med. 2008;36(1): 65-72.
19. Kato Y, Ingham SJ, Kramer S, et al. Effect of tunnel position for anatomic single-bundle ACL reconstruction on knee biomechanics in a porcine model. Knee Surg Sports Traumatol Arthrosc. 2010;18(1):2-10.
20. Karlsson J, Hirschmann MT, Becker R, et al. Individualized ACL surgery. Knee Surg Sports Traumatol Arthrosc. 2015;23(8):2143-4.
21. Miller MD, Harner CD. Revision anterior cruciate ligament surgery. In: Chow JC (Ed). Advanced Arthroscopy. New York: Springer-Verlag; 2001. pp. 471-88.
22. Morgan CD, Kalman VR, Grawl DM. Definitive landmarks for reproducible tibial tunnel placement in anterior cruciate ligament reconstruction. Arthroscopy. 1995;11(3):275-88.
23. Jackson DW, Gasser SI. Tibial tunnel placement in ACL reconstruction. Arthroscopy. 1994;10(2):124-31.
24. Kohn D, Busche T, Carls J. Drill hole position in endoscopic anterior cruciate ligament reconstruction. Results of an advanced arthroscopy course. Knee Surg Sports Traumatol Arthrosc. 1998;6 Suppl 1:S13-5.
25. Sommer C, Friederich NF, Muller W. Improperly placed anterior cruciate ligament grafts: Correlation between radiological parameters and clinical results. Knee Surg Sports Traumatol Arthrosc. 2000;8(4):207-13.
26. Prodromos CC, Fu FH, Howell SM, et al. Controversies in soft-tissue anterior cruciate ligament reconstruction: Grafts, bundles, tunnels, fixation, and harvest. J Am Acad Orthop Surg. 2008; 16(7):376-84.
27. Figueroa D, Calvo R, Vaisman A. Variation in the length of the tibial tunnel in anterior cruciate ligament reconstruction: Is it safe to use a 35-mm screw? Arthroscopy. 2006;22(5):e1-3.
28. Shaffer B, Gow W, Tibone JE. Graft-tunnel mismatch in endoscopic anterior cruciate ligament reconstruction: A new technique of intraarticular measurement and modified graft harvesting. Arthroscopy. 1993;9(6):633-46.
29. Hartman GP, Sisto DJ. Avoiding graft-tunnel mismatch in endoscopic anterior cruciate ligament reconstruction: A new technique. Arthroscopy. 1999;15(3):338-40.

30. Miller MD, Hinkin DT. The "N + 7 rule" for tibial tunnel placement in endoscopic anterior cruciate ligament reconstruction. Arthroscopy. 1996;12(1):124-6.
31. Kenna B, Simon TM, Jackson DW, et al. Endoscopic ACL reconstruction: A technical note on tunnel length for interference fixation. Arthroscopy. 1993;9(2):228-30.
32. Olszewski AD, Miller MD, Ritchie JR. Ideal tibial tunnel length for endoscopic anterior cruciate ligament reconstruction. Arthroscopy. 1998;14(1):9-14.
33. Wallace M, Bedi A, Lesniak BP, et al. What effect does anterior cruciate ligament tibial guide orientation have on tibial tunnel length? Arthroscopy. 2011;27(6):803-8.
34. Hall MP, Hergan DM, Sherman OH. Early fracture of a Bioabsorbable Tibial Interference Screw after ACL reconstruction with subsequent chondral injury. Orthopedics. 2009;32(3):208.
35. Appelt A, Baier M. Recurrent locking of knee joint caused by intraarticular migration of bioabsorbable tibial interference screw after arthroscopic ACL reconstruction. Knee Surg Sports Traumatol Arthosc. 2007;15(4): 378-80.
36. Herrera A, Martínez F, Iglesias D, et al. Fixation strength of biocomposite wedge interference screw in ACL reconstruction: effect of screw length and tunnel/screw ratio. A controlled laboratory study. BMC Musculoskelet Disord. 2010;11:139.
37. Selby JB, Johnson DL, Hester P, et al. Effect of screw length on bioabsorbable interference screw fixation in a tibial bone tunnel. Am J Sports Med. 2001;29(5):614-9.
38. Weiler A, Hoffmann RFG, Bail HJ, et al. Tendon healing in a bone tunnel. Part II. Histologic analysis after biodegradable interference fit fixation in a model of anterior cruciate ligament reconstruction in sheep. Arthroscopy. 2002;18: 124-35.
39. Yamazaki S, Yasuda K, Tomita F, et al. The effect of intraosseous graft length on tendon bone healing in anterior cruciate ligament reconstruction using flexor tendon. Knee Surg Sports Traumatol Arthrosc. 2006;14: 1086-93.
40. Zantop T, Ferretti M, Bell KM, et al. Effect of tunnel-graft length on the biomechanics of anterior cruciate ligament–reconstructed knees intra-articular study in a goat model. Am J Sports Med. 2008;36(11):2158-66.
41. Chhabra A, Diduch DR, Blessey PB, et al. Recreating an acceptable angle of the tibial tunnel in the coronal plane in anterior cruciate ligament reconstruction using external landmarks. Arthroscopy. 2004;20(3):328-30.
42. Kopf S, Martin DE, Tashman S, et al. Effect of tibial drill angles on bone tunnel aperture during anterior cruciate ligament reconstruction. J Bone Joint Surg Am. 2010;92(4):871-81.
43. Jagodzinski M, Foerstemann T, Mall G, et al. Analysis of forces of ACL reconstructions at the tunnel entrance: is tunnel enlargement a biomechanical problem? J Biomech. 2005;38(1):23-31.
44. Howell SM, Gittins ME, Gottlieb JE, et al. The relationship between the angle of the tibial tunnel in the coronal plane and loss of flexion and anterior laxity after anterior cruciate ligament reconstruction. Am J Sports Med. 2001;29(5):567-74.
45. Purnell ML, Larson AI, Clancy W. Anterior cruciate ligament insertions on the tibia and femur and their relationships to critical bony landmarks using high resolution volume-rendering computed tomography. Am J Sports Med. 2008;36(11):2083-90.
46. Van der Bracht H, Verhelst L, Stuyts B, et al. Anatomic single-bundle ACL surgery: consequences of tibial tunnel diameter and drill-guide angle on tibial footprint coverage. Knee Surg Sports Traumatol Arthrosc. 2014;22(5): 1030-9.
47. Fu FH, Bennett CH, Ma CB, et al. Current trends in anterior cruciate ligament reconstruction. Part II: operative procedures and clinical correlations. Am J Sports Med. 2000;28(1):124-30.
48. Johnson LL. Bone compaction techniques in knee ligament reconstruction. Tech Orthop. 1998;13:341-52.
49. Fowler BL, DiStefano VJ. Tibial tunnel bone grafting: a new technique for dealing with graft- tunnel mismatch in endoscopic anterior cruciate ligament reconstruction. Arthroscopy. 1998;14(2):224-8.

50. Lopes R, Klouche S, Odri G, et al. Does retrograde tibial tunnel drilling decrease subchondral bone lesions during ACL reconstruction? A prospective trial comparing retrograde to antegrade technique. Knee. 2016;23(1): 111-5.
51. McAdams TR, Biswal S, Stevens KJ, et al. Tibial aperture bone disruption after retrograde versus antegrade tibial tunnel drilling: a cadaveric study. Knee Surg Sports Traumatol Arthrosc. 2008;16(9):818-22.
52. Bak K, Scavenius M, Hansen S, et al. Isolated partial rupture of the anterior cruciate ligament. Long-term follow-up of 56 cases. Knee Surg Sports Traumatol Arthrosc. 1997;5(2):66-71.
53. Karakasli A, Acar N, Basci O, et al. Iatrogenic lateral meniscus anterior horn injury in different tibial tunnel placement techniques in ACL reconstruction surgery—A cadaveric study. Acta Orthop Traumatol Turc. 2016;50(5): 514-8.
54. Matsumoto A, Howell SM. Avoiding posterior cruciate ligament and roof impingement with transtibial anterior cruciate ligament reconstruction: keys to correct tunnel placement. Tech Orthop. 2005;20:211-7.
55. Bonnin M, Amendola NA, Bellemans J, MacDonald SJ, Menetrey J. The Knee Joint: Surgical Techniques and Strategies. Philadelphia: Springer; 2013. pp. 187-8.

CHAPTER

18

Suspensory Femoral Fixation Using a Fixed Loop Device

Raju Easwaran

INTRODUCTION

Suspensory fixation using a fixed loop device is arguably the most popular method of femoral fixation of looped soft tissue grafts like the hamstrings. This popularity stems from the ease of execution of the fixation coupled with the extreme versatility that it offers in terms of double looping the grafts, tripling the semitendinosus, making a 5 stand graft, 6 strand graft, double bundle reconstruction and so on. The fixation relies upon the strength of the lateral cortex of the femur and allows the graft to osteointegrate with the tunnel along its entire length and aperture. In the hands of the average surgeon, this fixation is fast, reproducible, secure and there is very little that can go wrong with this type of fixation. Recent biomechanical studies show minimal elongation of the loop with cyclic loading (1.05–1.09 mm across two of the most popular devices) compared to a significantly more elongation (2.2 mm) for the adjustable loop ones.[1]

MINIMUM REQUIREMENTS

- Soft tissue graft like the hamstrings that can be looped over [these devices are also available for the Bone-patella tendon-bone (BTB) graft and can be used with the quadriceps tendon].
- Intact lateral cortex of the distal femur (can still be used with posterior wall blow-out).
- Loop lengths of all sizes ranging from 10 mm to 40 mm (most common used sizes are 15 mm and 20 mm).
- One should strive to put at least 15 mm of the graft inside the tunnel.

MUST KNOW THINGS

- Every button has a parameter called the *flipping distance* that must be accounted for while preparing the femoral socket. This is the minimum distance required to successfully flip the button over the femoral cortex, over and above the length reamed for the graft. It is usually 6 mm. It means that the socket must at least be over-reamed by 6 mm to allow the button to pass through the lateral cortex so that it may be flipped. Ground reality however requires us to over-ream by 10 mm to easily flip the button (Fig. 18.1). Over-reaming may cause the button to flip over the soft tissues of the lateral extensor mechanism. This makes the fixation less secure and results in pain over the lateral thigh.

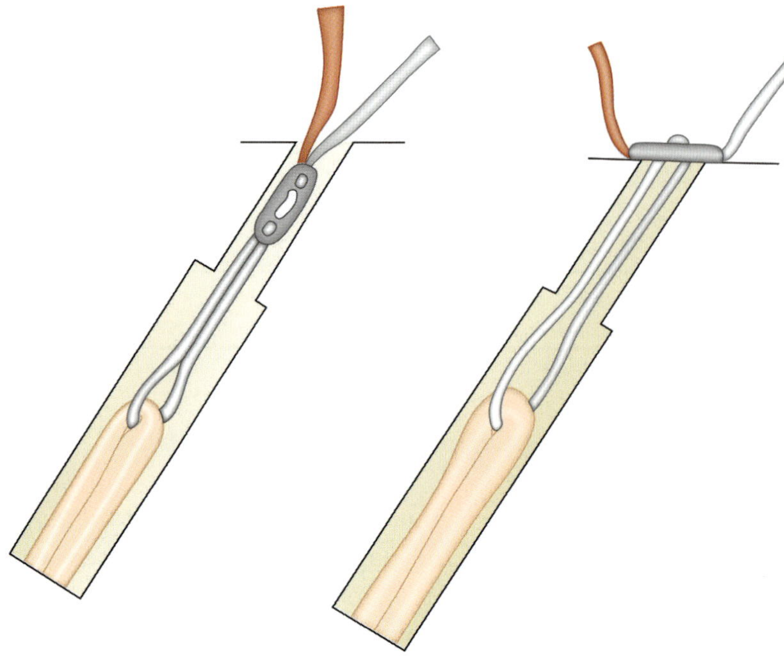

Fig. 18.1: Flipping the button over the lateral cortex requires over-reaming.

- For very small fixed loop lengths like 10 mm, there is an upper limit of the graft diameter that can be used. It is not recommended to use a graft greater than 9 mm diameter with a 10 mm loop because the portion of the loop that is left behind after the graft is looped over, is insufficient for the construct to flip over the lateral cortex of the femur. The bulk of the graft prevents the button from orienting itself parallel to the loop to allow it to flip (Fig. 18.2)!

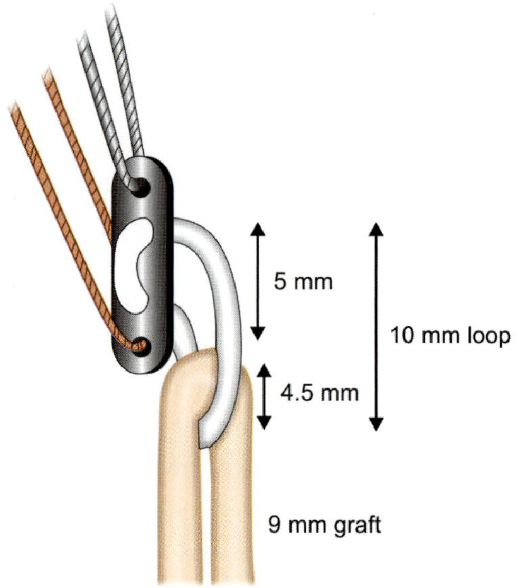

Fig. 18.2: Using a critical upper graft size with the 10 mm loop is important.

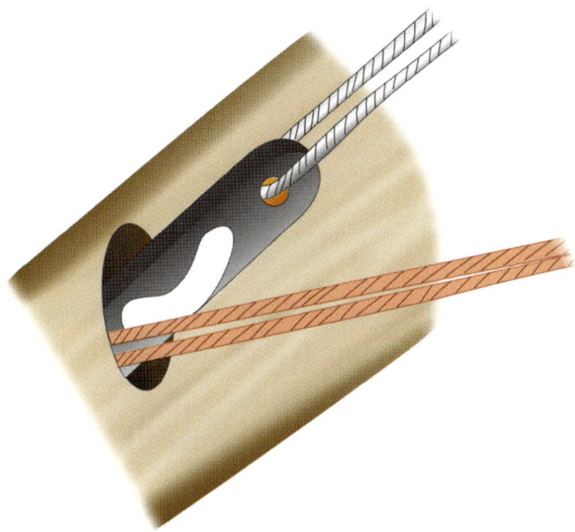

Fig. 18.3: Close-up of the exit point of the femoral tunnel showing a small discrepancy in the anterior and posterior length measurements due to the obliquity of the cylinder.

- It is useful to keep the leading suture oriented posteriorly for easier flipping of the button. The femoral tunnel due to its obliquity is a few millimeters shorter anteriorly, thereby allowing the button to flip easily (Fig. 18.3).
- All available fixed loop buttons allow tactile feedback of the flipping by toggling the 2 sets of sutures attached to the button, as a haptic confirmation of button flipping. If this feedback is not appreciated, it is desirable to check the flipping of the button on the C arm. Sometimes the button flips over the iliotibial band (over-reaming the socket) and the tactile feedback is either not appreciated fully or is felt as being a bit muffled. If the calculations are not in order (meaning the socket is under-reamed), the button will not flip at all as it has not been given the requisite distance to exit the femoral cortex fully (Fig. 18.4). Very rarely despite accurate calculations, the button gets jammed in the femoral tunnel

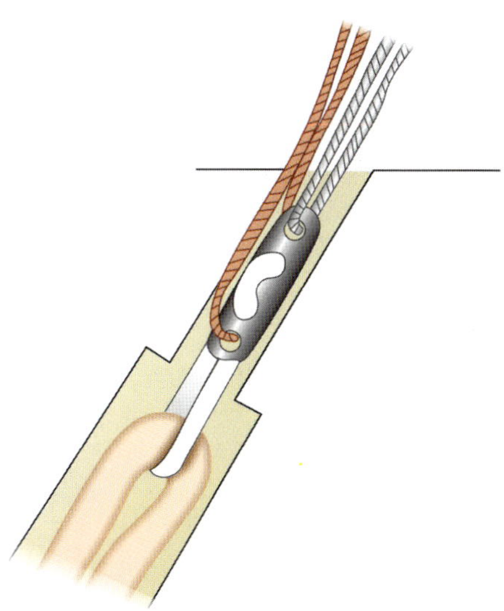

Fig. 18.4: Under-reaming the femoral socket makes it impossible to flip the button.

and does not come out of the lateral cortex. This is confirmed by intraoperative C arm imaging. In such circumstances it is recommended to use an additional fixation like an interference screw in the femoral tunnel. There are case reports of leaving a jammed button in situ as in most instances it gives sufficient fixation stability by acting as a femoral anchor, to allow optimal graft healing.[2,3]

MATHS

As mentioned earlier, a minimum amount of reaming needs to be done over and above the desired graft length inside the tunnel to allow the button to flip. It is very easy to calculate this and can be done in one of several ways.

- Subtract the loop length (l) from the tunnel length (L) and add 10 mm, to know the amount of reaming (S) to be done.
  $S = L - l + 10$. (Not recommended with the 10 mm fixed loop)
- Instead of adding 10 mm, simply add 6 mm as the minimum flipping distance to the above equation.
  $S = L - l + 6$. (Recommended especially for the 10 mm fixed loop)
- Ream 5 mm less than the total tunnel length and use a loop of any size (from 15 mm loop size onwards).
  $S = L - 5$

If any of these calculations yields a graft inside the tunnel shorter than 15 mm, then a 5 mm shorter loop needs to be used. If that is not possible, then the fixation technique should be changed to allow more graft to fill the tunnel. Intraoperative comfort and convenience should not be at the expense of putting in less graft inside the femoral tunnel.

COMMON SENSE POINTS

- The bigger the loop, the lesser the amount of graft sitting inside the tunnel. In these days of anatomic anterior cruciate ligament (ACL) reconstruction, loop lengths exceeding 20 mm are rarely used. At least 15 mm of the graft should be inside the tunnel.
- The smaller the loop, the greater the chances of blowing out the lateral cortex of the femur with reckless drilling. It is preferable to hand ream/use a very low rotation speed while reaming the last 10 mm of the femur.
- The bigger the loop, the greater the chances of bungee jumping and windshield wiper effects. The bungee jumping effect refers to the longitudinal pistoning of the graft within the tunnel. The windshield wiper effect refers to movement of the graft in a perpendicular plane to the tunnel at the aperture. Both movements are detrimental to the long-term health of the graft within the joint and contribute to the tunnel widening seen on postoperative radiographs. The smaller the loop, the greater chances of a difficult flipping.

TECHNIQUE

- Prepare the femoral tunnel as per standard methods. Use the manufacturer recommended drill bit (generally 4.5 mm) to drill over the drill tip passing pin inserted for the femoral tunnel. Drill through the lateral femoral cortex with this bit (Fig. 18.5). Measure the length of the entire femoral tunnel (L) with the

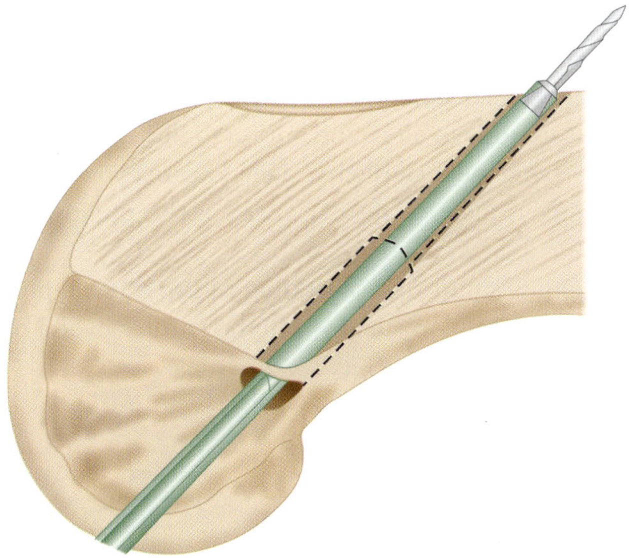

Fig. 18.5: Drilling of the lateral femoral cortex using the design-specific drill bit over the drill tip passing pin.

depth gauge. Use the minimum loop size (*l*) (typically 15 mm) to calculate the amount of reaming (*S*) to be done for the desired socket length.

- Once the tunnel has been reamed to the desired length, use the drill tip passing pin to shuttle a looped suture (usually No. 5 Ethibond) through the femoral tunnel. Pullout the loop through the anteromedial portal and the free ends through the lateral aspect of the thigh. Secure the threads with a hemostat at either ends.
- Pull the loop out of the tibial tunnel. The graft is now ready to be pulled into the joint for femoral fixation.
- Load the graft onto the button with the loop of the desired length and mark it circumferentially at a distance equal to the amount of reaming done (*S*) from the tip of the loop (Fig. 18.6).
- Loop the tails of the leading and flipping sutures of the button into the suture loop coming out of the tibial tunnel. Pull them out of the lateral aspect of the thigh. Designate one suture as the pulling and the

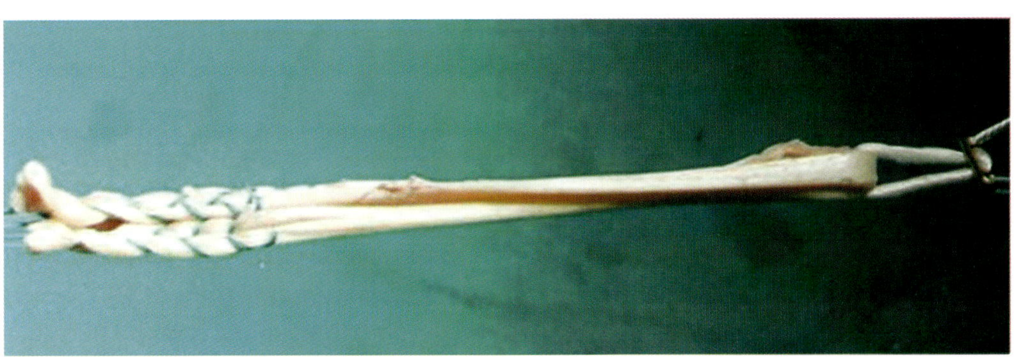

Fig. 18.6: Marking the graft correctly ensures visual feedback and confirmation of button flipping when viewing arthroscopically.

other as the flipping suture. Generally any suture can be used as the pulling or the flipping sutures but follow the manufacturer's recommendations. Attach a hemostat to the end of the flipping suture and cross this over to the medial aspect of the thigh for convenience and avoiding entanglement.

- Orient the leading suture posteriorly to allow the button to flip against the slightly short anterior wall of the tunnel. Use a folded sponge or a sterile bandage to assist you with the grip on the suture. This avoids lacerations on your fingers that may result from excessive pulling on these high strength sutures with the gloved hand.
- Remove the slack on the flipping suture, as the leading suture is being pulled. Maintain a steady pull, avoiding jerky movements. It is useful to steadily roll the sutures over a bandage, thereby allowing a more controlled pull with a short lever arm (Fig. 18.7).

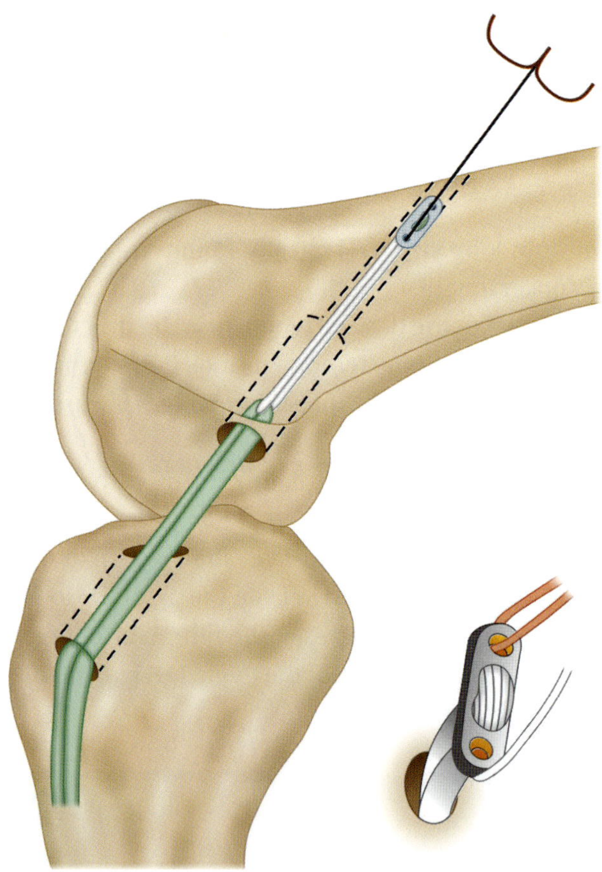

Fig. 18.7: Controlled pulling on the button sutures.

- Observe the entire process with the arthroscope in the anterolateral portal. Stop pulling when the mark on the graft reaches the mouth of the tunnel. Continuous observation of the process prevents pulling the graft too much into the tunnel that may result from over-reaming and cause the button to flip over the iliotibial band. It also prevents the premature urge to tug on the flipping suture before the graft has passed adequately inside the tunnel, risking breakage of the flipping suture.

- Once the desired length of the graft has traversed the femoral tunnel, pull on the flipping suture and toggle pull between the pulling and flipping sutures to get a tactile feedback of the entire flipping process, as the button rocks over the lateral femoral cortex.
- Check the strength of the fixation by pulling on the tibial end of the graft. Normally one is able to rock the patient on the operating table by pulling on the tibial end.
- Pull on the tibial end of the graft and complete the tibial fixation after cycling the knee. Remove the pulling and flipping sutures by pulling at one end of each of the sutures.

PEARLS AND PITFALLS

Graft Does Not Go in at All!
Recheck the graft diameter. If it is too tight, remove everything and over-ream by 0.5 mm over guide wire. Remove soft tissues circumferentially at the mouth of the tibial tunnel. It is useful not to soak the graft in saline and to keep it dry while on the back table. It causes a slight shrinkage of the graft and facilitates its passage through the tunnels. Avoid soaking the graft in saline as it causes the graft to swell up.

Graft Goes Inside the Tibia But Gets Stuck at the Femur
The most common cause of this is wrong sequence pulling on the leading/flipping sutures that causes the button to orient itself perpendicular to the femoral aperture, instead of being parallel to it. Withdraw the graft slightly, pull on the leading suture to reorient the button parallel to the femoral tunnel and advance the construct. Direct visualization of the entire process prevents this from happening and if required the button may be reoriented with the help of a probe inserted into the joint.

The Button Does Not Flip
Something is wrong with the measurements. See the process with the arthroscope. If the mark on the graft has not reached the femoral aperture, the graft needs to be pulled further into the socket. If the button still does not flip even after pulling all the graft into the socket, there could be under-reaming of the socket. Remove the entire construct and over-ream by the desired length (usually 5 mm). If the mark on the graft is not visible, or just barely visible, there may be over-reaming of the socket. In this case the button has exited the lateral femoral cortex and flipped over the IT band. Pull at the tibial end of the graft to confirm flipping and reconfirm it with the image intensifier.

Graft Has Traveled the Distance, the Button Has a Muffled Flip But on Pulling the Tibial End, the Graft Comes Out
The only cause of this phenomenon is blow-out of the lateral femoral cortex. Remove the entire construct and confirm the blow-out by direct visualization of the femoral tunnel from the anteromedial portal. Use a button extender (Figs. 18.8 and 18.9) or a direct button to complete the femoral fixation. Alternatively, an interference screw may be used in the femur.

The Button Does Not Flip, But the Graft Also Does Not Come Out on Pulling at the Tibial End
The button is now jammed inside the femoral tunnel beyond the socket. Confirm this with the image intensifier. There are two case reports[2,3] in literature of this occurrence being managed successfully by going ahead with the tibial fixation and going a bit slow on the rehab in the initial phases. The button here acts like an anchor in the femur during the initial healing process.

One of the Sutures (Usually Flipping Suture) Breaks
The entire construct can still be pulled out of the tibia. A new suture can be threaded into the hole and the process can be repeated.

Both Sutures Break
This is a rare occurrence especially considering the high strength sutures used nowadays. There is a risk of the button being jammed if the construct is pulled out from the tibia.

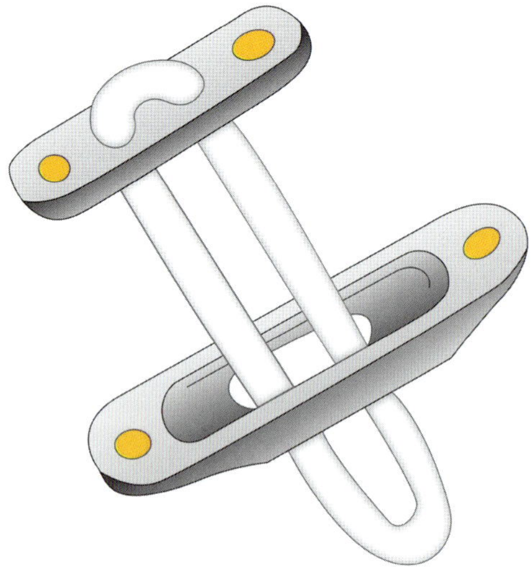

Fig. 18.8: Fixed loop button being assembled over a button extender.

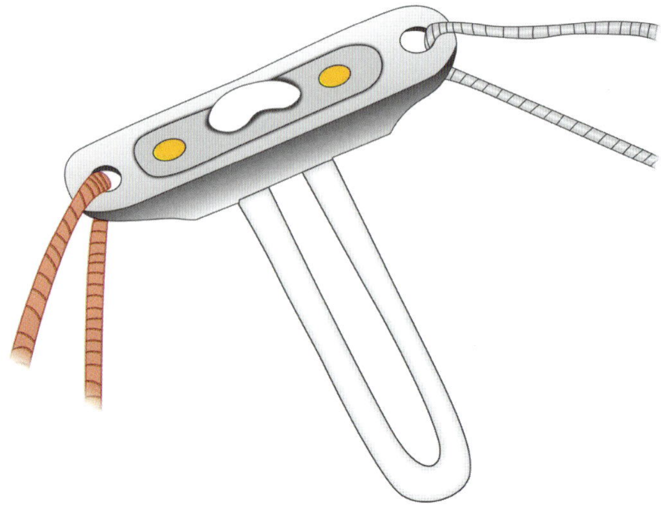

Fig. 18.9: The final assembled construct with a button extender.

TAKE HOME MESSAGE

If one needs to apply excessive force to deploy the button, something is wrong somewhere. At this stage of the surgery, it is better to pause, reassess and recheck measurements. Meticulous calculation of femoral tunnel lengths while drilling the guide pin, reaming with the button reamer and direct measurement with the depth gauge is the key to success. Extra time spent on these seemingly small steps will pay rich dividends in reducing intraoperative time and stress.

REFERENCES

1. Johnson JS, Smith SD, LaPrade CM, et al. A biomechanical comparison of femoral cortical suspension devices for soft tissue anterior cruciate ligament reconstruction under high loads. Am J Sports Med. 2015;43:154-60.
2. Karaoglu S, Halici M, Baktir A. An unidentified pitfall of EndoButton use: Case report. Knee Surg Sports Traumatol Arthrosc. 2002;10:247-9.
3. Vega R, Irribarra L, Filippi J. Simple solution for failure of trailing sutures when using the EndoButton in anterior cruciate ligament reconstruction: the "rescue rein." Arthroscopy. 2005;21:1013.

CHAPTER

19 Adjustable-Loop Suspensory Fixation Device

SR Sundararajan, Balaji Sambandam, Amit Kumar Jha, S Rajasekaran

INTRODUCTION

Various fixation devices are used for arthroscopic anterior cruciate ligament reconstruction. Fixation device plays a major role in this surgery particularly during the graft healing period. It varies from 12 weeks to 26 weeks for bone-to-bone healing, 38 weeks for tendon-to-bone healing[1] and it is more for the allografts.[2,3] Further, because of the early rehabilitation the graft is subjected to higher stress particularly at the fixation site. An ideal fixation device must be strong, biocompatible, and easily usable with minimal complications.

These fixation devices can be divided into three types, based on the mechanism in which they work:

1. Aperture/Compression fixation devices (Interference screw)
2. Expansion fixation devices (Cross pin)
3. Suspensory fixation devices: Suspensory fixation devices consist of a loop for holding the graft, which is fixed to a titanium button. This button suspends the entire set up over the bony cortex. There are sutures attached to these buttons for negotiating them through the tunnel and then flipping them out of the tunnel. These suspensory fixation devices offer several advantages over the traditional aperture fixation devices and expansion devices. They have a high pull out strength, perforation of the posterior femoral cortex while drilling will not compromise fixation, provides a 360° bone graft contact, avoids complications like graft cut through, screw divergence, and finally, revision is easier as these implants are extraosseous and can be removed easily.[4-6]

Initial suspensory fixation devices had a loop whose length was constant. These are called the fixed-loop suspensory fixation devices (for example Endobutton CL Ultra®, Smith & Nephew, Andover, MA; Ret-robutton®, Arthrex, Naples, FL, etc.). In these implants the loop length cannot be adjusted and remains constant. Instead, these are available in varying sizes viz 15 mm, 20 mm, and 25 mm. Depending on the graft length, total tunnel length, and desired socket length, a particular implant size is selected. In these devices we need to drill an extra 6 mm more than that of the length of the graft desired in the socket. This enables the button to flip outside the outer cortex and is called the turning space. The extra 6 mm theoretically provides a space for the loop micromotion during rehabilitation and eventually leads to micromotion at the loop graft interface. Consequently, this hinders healing and can cause tunnel widening. To obviate these problems, adjustable-loop suspensory fixation devices were developed. Advantages of adjustable loop are:

- It allows a complete fill of the graft in the tunnel with no empty space
- Single implant fits different tunnel lengths and graft dimensions
- This implant is particularly useful when the total tunnel length is less where we may not be able to give an adequate turning space for the fixed-loop button to flip while ensuring enough collagen within the femoral socket.

TightropeRT® (Arthrex Inc, Naples, FL) and ToggleLoc with ZipLoop® (Biomet Inc, Warsaw, IN) are the commercially available suspensory devices with adjustable loop. In this chapter we discuss the technical aspects and usage of TightropeRT®. Similar to the fixed-loop devices, it has a loop and a titanium button with two different colored sutures attached to it. One is blue colored, which is the guiding suture and is used to pull the button out of the tunnel. The other one is white colored and is in direct continuation with the loop (Figs. 19.1 and 19.2). It uses a friction locking mechanism similar to the "Chinese finger trap"

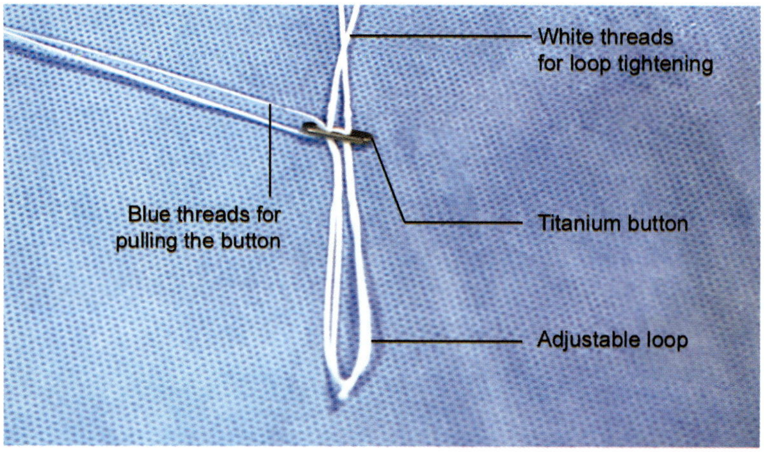

Fig. 19.1: Tightrope® (Arthrex) showing titanium button, adjustable loop, and the two types of suture threads.

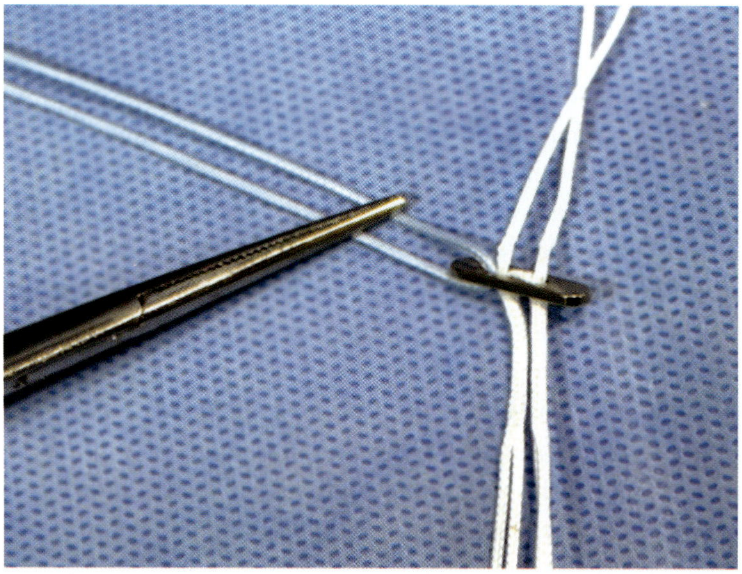

Fig. 19.2: A closer look at the button with the loop. Note that the white suture is in continuation with the loop.

to shorten the loop.[7] Once the loop is shortened by pulling the white sutures it is a one-way journey, it cannot be reversed back. The adjustable loop has a four-point, knotless locking mechanism that depends on multiple points of friction to create resistance to cyclic displacement and slippage under tension.[8]

TECHNIQUE

The anatomical femoral footprint is identified through standard anterolateral and far anteromedial portals. With the help of a femoral anterior cruciate ligament (ACL) jig/aimer a spade guide pin (ACL Tightrope drill pin, open eyelet 4 mm) is drilled inside out at the center of femoral footprint. Tip of this guide pin is spade shaped which is 4 mm wide (Fig. 19.3A). Advantage of using the spade guide pin is it avoids multiple steps which have to be followed when a standard guide pin is used and saves operative time. First, it avoids reaming with an additional 4 mm reamer over the standard guide pin which is required for the button to pass through the tunnel, because the tip of the spade guide pin is itself 4 mm wide. Second, it has markings on its shaft to measure the total tunnel length or aperture-cortex distance (Fig. 19.3B), thereby eliminating the additional step where a depth gauge has to be used to measure this length.

Using a flower tip reamer, a femoral socket of the desired diameter and length is drilled over the spade guide pin. After loading the graft on the adjustable-loop suspensory device, two marks are made on the loop and graft. Using a measuring ruler, the first mark is made on the loop measured from the distal tip of the button and is the aperture-cortex distance as measured using the spade guide pin (Figs. 19.4A and B). The second mark is made on the graft measured from the proximal end and is equal to the socket length (Figs. 19.5A and B). The graft with the fixation device is then passed through the tunnel over a loop. Pulling the TightropeRT® loaded with graft can be done in two ways. First, the blue sutures alone can be used to pull the button out of the tunnel. In this method there is a possibility of the white sutures getting entangled inside the joint or the tunnel, thereby shortening the loop length. To

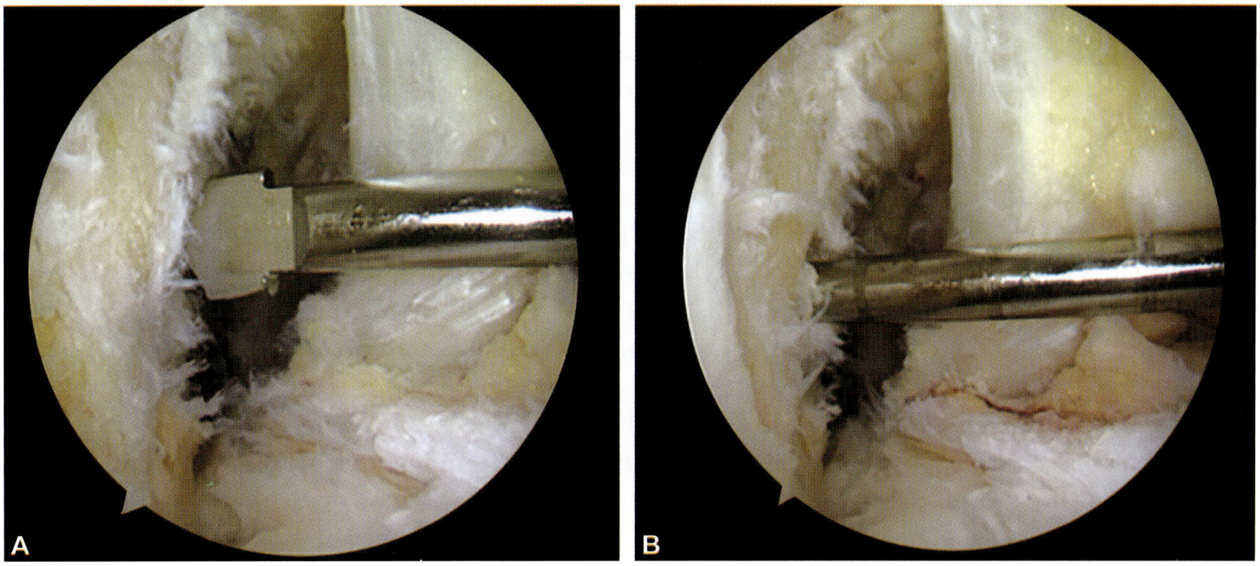

Figs. 19.3A and B: (A) Spade guide pin with 4 mm tip. (B) Shaft with markings for calculating the aperture to cortex distance.

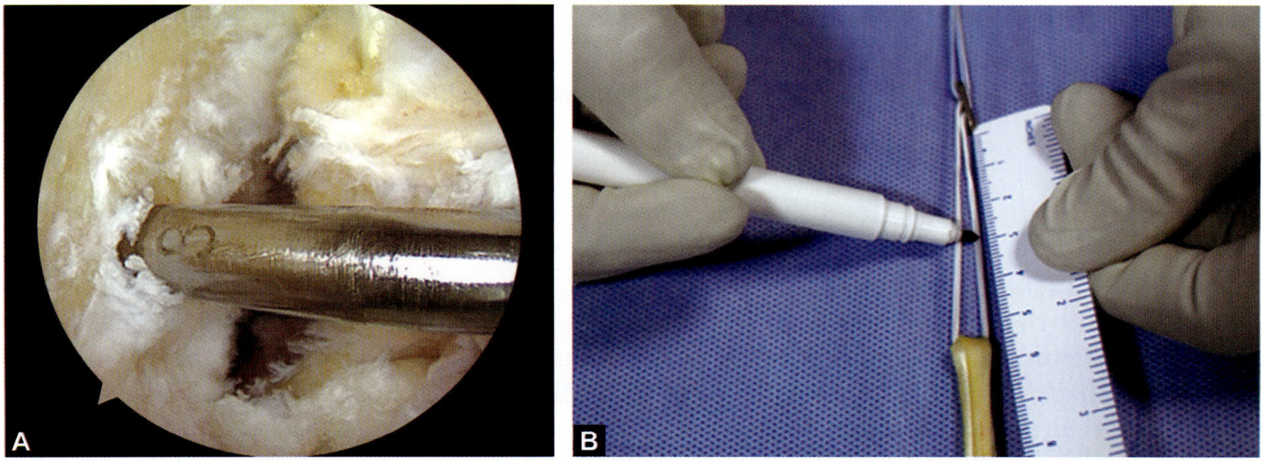

Figs. 19.4A and B: (A) Aperture-cortex distance as measured from the spade guide pin (30 mm). (B) Marking on the loop equal to the aperture-cortex distance (30 mm). Note that the button is held longitudinally.

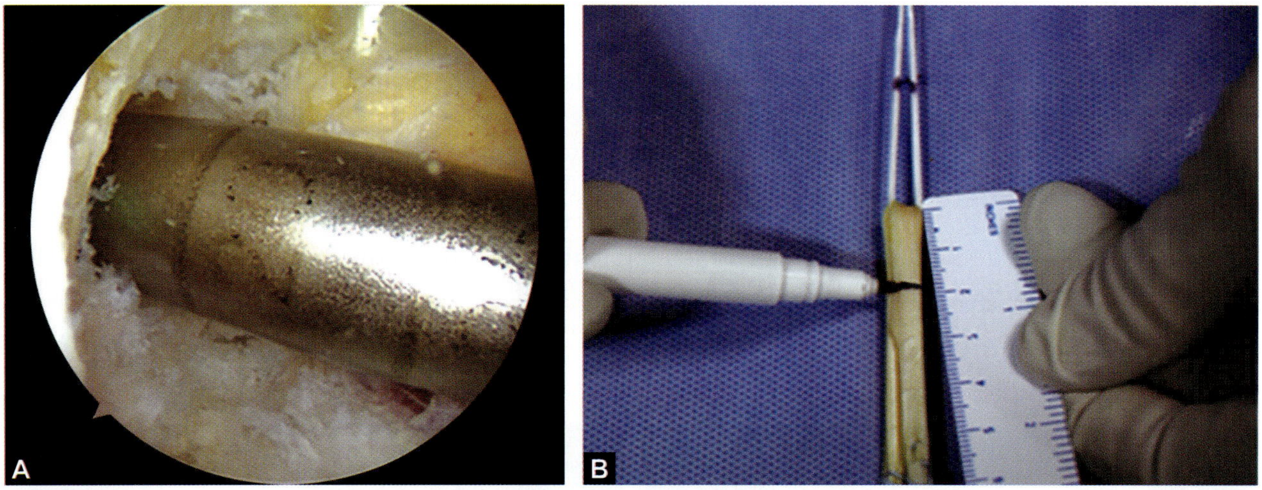

Figs. 19.5A and B: Socket length as measured from the reamer (18 mm). (B) Marking on the graft equal to the socket length (18 mm).

avoid this and to get a better grip, the other technique of holding and pulling both the blue and white sutures together is better. One has to pull till the first mark on the loop reaches the entry of the femoral socket (Fig. 19.6). At this point, the button will be out of the tunnel and would have flipped over the outer cortex which can be confirmed by three ways. First, by observing through the far anteromedial portal when the mark will be at the level of the entry of the socket and the button will not be visible inside the socket (Fig. 19.7). Second, by pulling the graft firmly on the tibial side. A flipped button will not allow the graft to slide back. Third, we can also confirm the button flipping arthroscopically by reaching the lateral gutter. After this, the loop can be shortened by alternatively pulling the white sutures which will pull the graft into the socket. Once the mark on the graft comes to the level of the socket entry it means that the loop is adequately tightened and graft is completely within the socket (Fig. 19.8). Subsequently, one can perform cyclical loading and fixation at the tibial side.

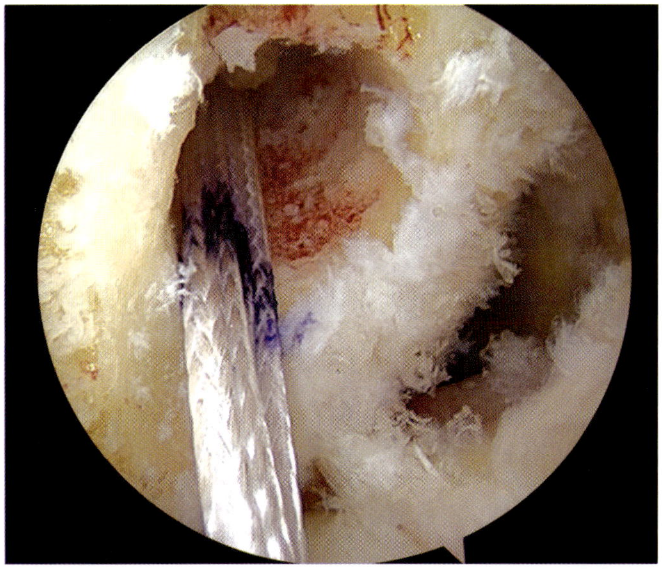

Fig. 19.6: Point when the mark on the loop reaches the entry of the socket, indicating the button is outside the outer cortex.

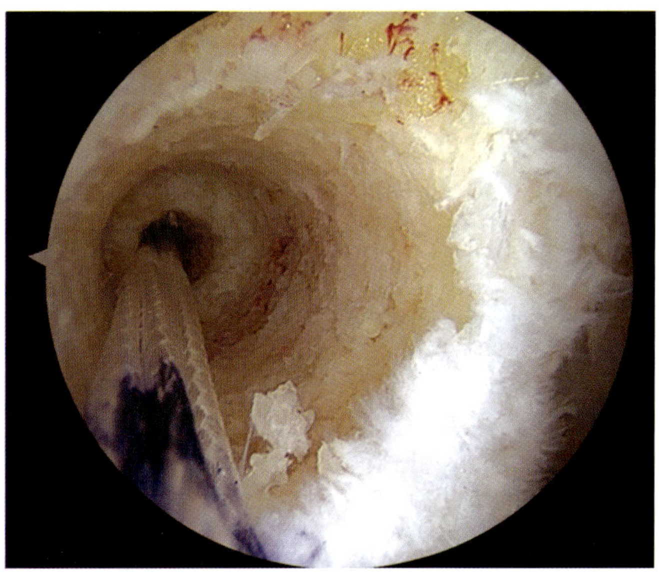

Fig. 19.7: Femoral socket as observed from far anteromedial portal. Titanium button is not within the socket indicating it has flipped over the outer cortex.

TECHNICAL PEARLS

- The button needs to be flipped over the femoral cortex before tightening the adjustable loop. However, when the sutures are pulled with excessive force there is a possibility that the button will pass through the soft tissues and flip over the fascia lata or sometimes on the skin. In such a situation, one should be careful not to tighten the loop by pulling the white sutures. If it flips outside the skin then it will be obvious (Fig. 19.9). If it gets flipped over the fascia lata, there is a chance one can miss it.

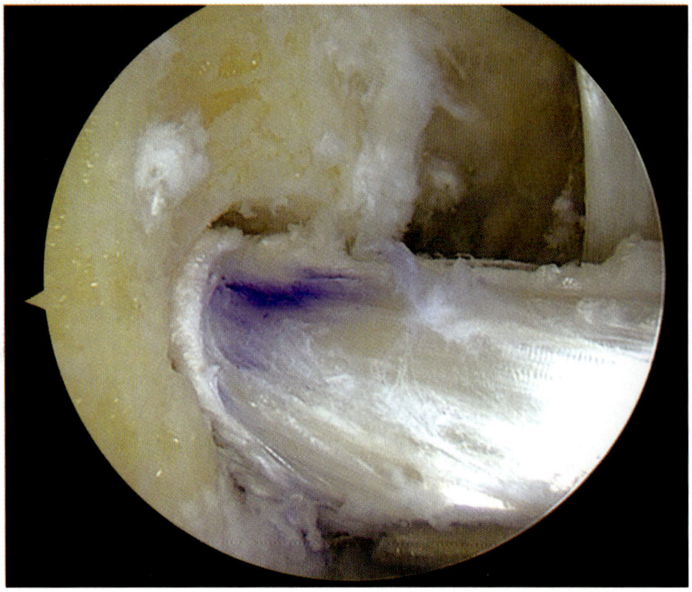

Fig. 19.8: Marking on the graft at the entry of femoral socket indicating that the loop has been tightened adequately and the tip of the graft has reached the far end of the socket.

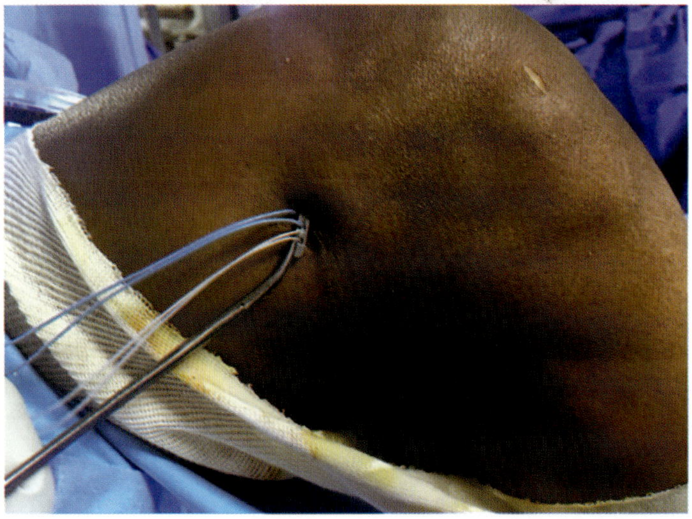

Fig. 19.9: Button flipped outside the skin due to excessive force applied while pulling the graft.

This situation can be identified by observing the mark on the loop. If the mark is inside the tunnel (Fig. 19.10) instead of at the level of the femoral socket entry, it suggests that the button has traveled beyond the outer cortex. Further, one can feel a bungee-like movement when the graft is pulled on the tibial side. In such situations, the button should be carefully repositioned on the bone by gradually dissecting the tissues. Making a small incision on the lateral thigh, the button can be guided to the outer cortex using an artery forceps. This can be confirmed by checking the mark on the loop which has to reach the level of the socket entry and not inside the socket. Once it is repositioned on the bony cortex,

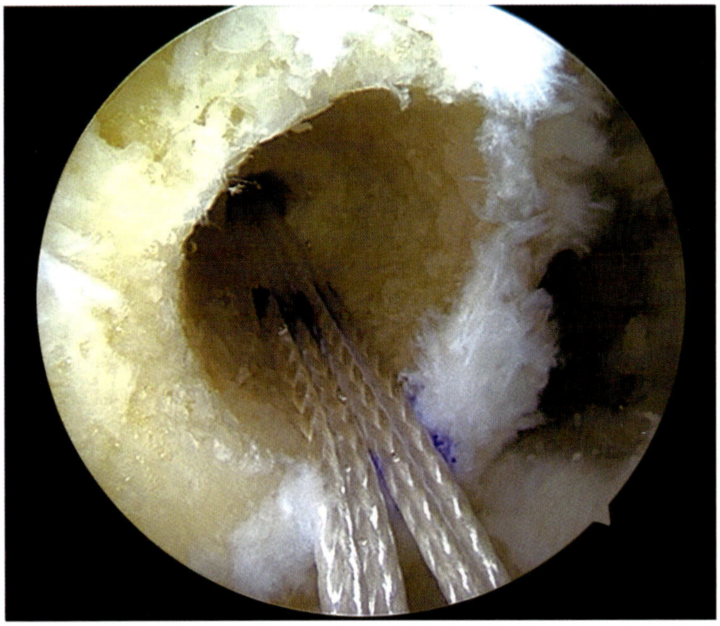

Fig. 19.10: Marking on the loop inside the socket indicating that the button has traveled away from the bony cortex and flipped over fascia lata or skin.

the loop can be tightened. If one fails to identify this situation then the graft will get loose at a later date leading to failure of the surgery. Also, the patient will have persistent pain on lateral aspect of knee during knee movement due to abutment of button on fascia lata. To avoid this complication, excessive force should not be applied while pulling the sutures. While the sutures are being pulled, some amount of counter pull has to be given in the opposite direction so that the button does not travel beyond the desired location on the outer cortex.

- When the white sutures are pulled before the button flips over the outer cortex, it can cause premature tightening of the loop. If it gets shorter than the transosseous length, the button will never come out of the bone. In such a case either a new implant has to be taken or the socket length should be increased. To avoid this situation it is always advised to be very careful while pulling the graft and the white sutures should be pulled only after confirming that the button has flipped.
- Sometimes due to accidental excessive reaming, the femoral socket length will be more than what is intended. If the entire socket is filled with the graft then there can be inadequate graft to fill the tibial socket. In such cases, we should make a mark on the graft up to which we want to fill the femoral socket. While pulling the graft inside, one has to stop once the mark on the graft reaches the entry of the femoral socket. At this point the graft should be held tightly and then the loop should be tightened. Tibial fixation can then be performed.

There are few concerns with the use of adjustable-loop suspensory fixation devices. Theoretically, the loop once tightened will not get loose. But there can be some amount of loosening with overloading. If the loop gets loosened it will increase the laxity of the graft. There is mixed evidence in literature about this phenomenon[9,10] but the amount of loosening is not clinically relevant. One way of preventing this is retightening after cyclic loading and tying a knot.[11] Strength of the loop is also a cause of concern when compared to fixed-loop devices. Biomechanical studies showed lesser strength than the fixed-loop device but the clinical significance of this is not proven.[7,12] At present, there is no clinical study to prove that adjustable-loop devices have lesser strength than fixed-loop devices. Also, there is no study to prove that adjustable loop had increased failure due to insufficient strength when compared to a fixed-loop device.

A special adjustable-loop fixation device (Tightrope BTB®, Arthrex) that can be used for bone-patellar tendon-bone grafts is also available. This allows fixation of the graft into anatomical femoral socket that can be difficult to reach while using an interference screw. Another recent advance in this implant is the button extender (Tightrope Button Extender®, Arthrex) which can be attached to TightropeRT® button to increase the cortical contact area. This is particularly useful whenever there is an accidental lateral cortical blowout, revision surgery, and in cases where full tunnel is used for graft incorporation. Adjustable-loop suspensory devices can be used in all-inside ACL reconstruction where the graft is fixed with adjustable-loop devices on both tibial and femoral sides.

REFERENCES

1. Deehan DJ, Cawston TE. The biology of integration of the anterior cruciate ligament. J Bone Joint Surg Br. 2005;87(7):889-95.
2. Malinin TI, Levitt RL, Bashore C, et al. A study of retrieved allografts used to replace anterior cruciate ligaments. Arthroscopy. 2002;18(2):163-70.
3. Hortsman JK, Ahmadu-Suka F, Norrdin RW. Anterior cruciate ligament fascia lata allograft reconstruction: progressive histological changes towards maturity. Arthroscopy. 1993;9(5):509-18.
4. Milano G, Mulas PD, Ziranu F. Comparison between different femoral fixation devices for ACL reconstruction with doubled hamstring tendon graft: a biomechanical analysis. Arthroscopy. 2006;22(6):660-8.
5. Lubowitz JH, Schwartzberg R, Smith P. Cortical Suspensory Button Versus Aperture Interference Screw Fixation for Knee Anterior Cruciate Ligament Soft-Tissue Allograft: A Prospective, Randomized Controlled Trial. Arthroscopy. 2015;31(9):1733-9.
6. Aydin D, Ozcan M. Evaluation and comparison of clinical results of femoral fixation devices in arthroscopic anterior cruciate ligament reconstruction. Knee. 2016;23(2):227-32.
7. Eguchi A, Ochi M, Adachi N, et al. Mechanical properties of suspensory fixation devices for anterior cruciate ligament reconstruction: comparison of the fixed-length loop device versus the adjustable-length loop device. Knee. 2014;21(3):743-8.
8. Lanzetti RM, Monacoa E, De Carli A, et al. Can an adjustable-loop length suspensory fixation device reduce femoral tunnel enlargement in anterior cruciate ligament reconstruction? A prospective computer tomography study. Knee. 2016;23(5):837-41.
9. Barrow AE, Pilia M, Guda T, et al. Femoral suspension devices for anterior cruciate ligament reconstruction: do adjustable loops lengthen? Am J Sports Med. 2014;42(2):343-9.
10. Boyle MJ, Vovos TJ, Walker CG, et al. Does adjustable-loop femoral cortical suspension loosen after anterior cruciate ligament reconstruction? A retrospective comparative study. Knee. 2015;22(4): 304-8.
11. Noonan BC, Dines JS, Allen AA, et al. Biomechanical Evaluation of an Adjustable Loop Suspensory Anterior Cruciate Ligament Reconstruction Fixation Device: The Value of Retensioning and Knot Tying. Arthroscopy. 2016;32(10): 2050-9.
12. Johnson JS, Smith SD, LaPrade CM, et al. A biomechanical comparison of femoral cortical suspension devices for soft tissue anterior cruciate ligament reconstruction under high loads. Am J Sports Med. 2014;43(1):154-60.

CHAPTER

20 Tibial Fixation

Sagar Kakatkar, Jonathan Herald

INTRODUCTION

Tibial fixation in anterior cruciate ligament (ACL) reconstruction is the Achilles heel for the whole construct.[1] Tibial fixation is the most stressed segment of the reconstructed ACL. Published literature also suggests that failure of the ACL graft is more commonly seen on the tibial side of the graft, and there are various reasons for the same.[2-7] For instance, cancellous bone morphology in the metaphyseal region of the proximal tibia makes it anatomically weaker to act as a holding ground for the reconstructed ACL.[8-10] Also, the tail end of the soft tissue grafts is difficult to secure.[11] Finally, the forces acting on the ACL tibial graft are parallel to the tibial tunnel which makes it prone for slippage.[3-6]

Most of the studies done for tendon to bone healing on the tibial side have been primarily animal studies and the results have been extrapolated to humans.[11] Hence it is difficult to make conclusive comments about ideal tibial fixation method which will have adequate pullout strength, least tunnel widening and which can enhance the graft to tunnel healing.

WAYS TO DO THE TIBIAL FIXATION AND REVIEW OF LITERATURE

There are various aspects of the tibial fixation which should be considered before selecting a tibial fixation method (Flowchart 20.1).

Flowchart 20.1: Tibial fixation aspects.

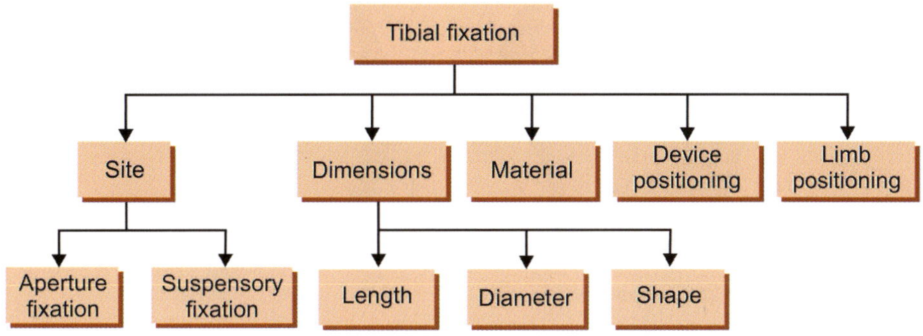

Site

Based on the site of tibial fixation, it can be either an "aperture fixation" or "suspensory fixation".

Aperture Fixation

- In aperture fixation, such as with interference screw fixation the graft is fixed closer to the tibial joint line. This decreases the micromotion of the graft by decreasing the length of the intratunnel mobile segment of the graft. Shorter mobile segments have an advantage that they cause less tunnel dilatation.[12-21]
- Since aperture fixation is based on the principle of compressing the graft on metaphyseal tibial bone in the tunnel, its strength vastly depends on the quality of tibial metaphyseal bone. Being a cancellous weak bone, tibial fixation is the weak link leading to graft pullout or slippage especially, if patient is started on aggressive physiotherapy in early postoperative period.[22-27]

Suspensory Fixation

- Suspensory fixation is the other type of tibial fixation in which fixation is done outside the tibial tunnel on the tibial cortex. Since the cortical bone is stronger, it gives better pullout strength to the construct.[22-27]
- But the mobile segment of the graft in the tunnel with suspensory fixation is longer which increases the working length. When subjected to early and aggressive rehabilitation, there are high chances of tunnel widening because of "wind-shield wiper effect" (Figs. 20.1A and B).[28-33]
- Also, excessive micromotion at the graft tunnel interface interferes with the incorporation of the graft.[29-32]

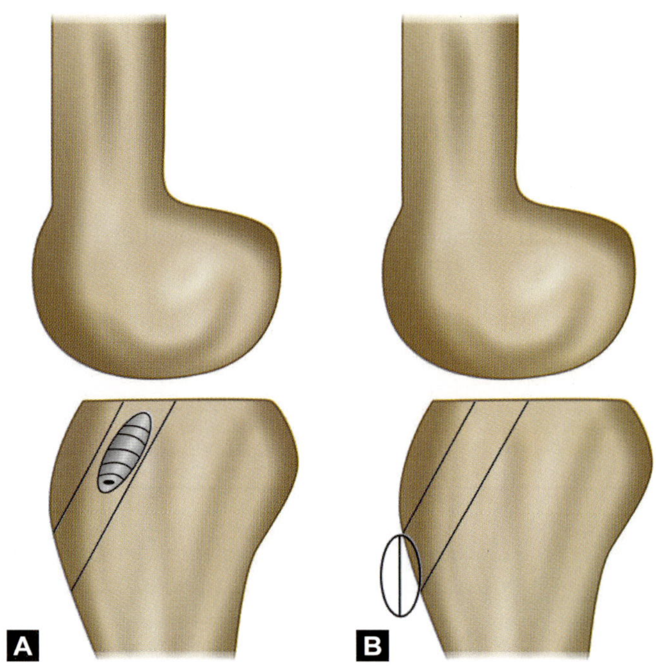

Figs. 20.1A and B: Aperture fixation and suspensory fixation.

Dimensions of the Fixation Device

Dimensions of the fixation device are vital in aperture fixation, since these devices are in contact with the graft and their structural properties affect the biomechanics of the construct.

- *Length*: Shorter interference screws, i.e. less than 23 mm cannot resist loads on a greater scale and have poor pullout strength. While screws which are longer in length and which engage in both proximal and distal cortices prevent graft slippage.[20,34-36]
- *Diameter*: Apart from few studies such as by Morris et al.[46] which showed that wider screws can lead to serious structural damage to the graft; most of the literature supports use of wider screws. Interference screw diameter which is at least 1 mm wider than the tunnel diameter gives better strength to the construct and increases pullout strength.[20,34-36]
- *Shape*: Tapered screws are shown to reduce the damage to the graft during the screw insertion. But these screws reduce the advantages of having better graft compression closer to the joint line since the distal part of the screw being tapered cannot compress the graft to the tunnel.[34,35]

Material

- Bioabsorbable screws have similar or better fixation strength compared to the metallic screws and they cause less damage to the graft during the insertion compared to metallic screws.[37-40]
- These bioabsorbable screws do not interfere with tunnel to graft incorporation.[40,41]

Device Positioning

Positioning of interference screws is a topic of debate when bone patellar tendon bone graft is used. Screws when put on the cancellous side of the bone plug compress the cortical side of the bone plug to the wall of the tunnel which can hamper graft incorporation. Hence most studies recommend putting the screws on the cortical side of the bone plug. But there are also chances of suture cut outs while putting the interference screws on the cortical side of the bone plug. These sutures which hold the bone plug and allow traction to be applied on the graft during fixation if cut, can lead to graft slippage.[42]

Limb Positioning

- Conventional technique of doing ACL tibial side fixation with knee in flexion led to decreased knee extension in patients who had physiological hyperextension.
- Hence Pinczewski et al. recommended fixing the ACL tibial side with knee in extension or hyperextension. But literature regarding the same does not show much difference in long-term outcome following ACL tibial fixation by hyperextension method and by conventional method.[15]
- Hybrid tibial fixation using two modalities of tibial fixation has been found to be biomechanically more stable. With such fixations, aggressive rehabilitation strategies can be followed.
- The hybrid fixations can also be used when the tibial metaphyseal bone quality is very poor or in revision cases.[43-45]

ACT OF BALANCING: THE WAY WE DO IT

- We have always used the aperture fixation with interference screws for the ACL tibial side fixation and bioabsorbable screws are our implants of choice (Fig. 20.2).
- We always use tibial screws longer than 25 mm length which tend to compress the graft at both proximal and distal ends of the tibial tunnel.

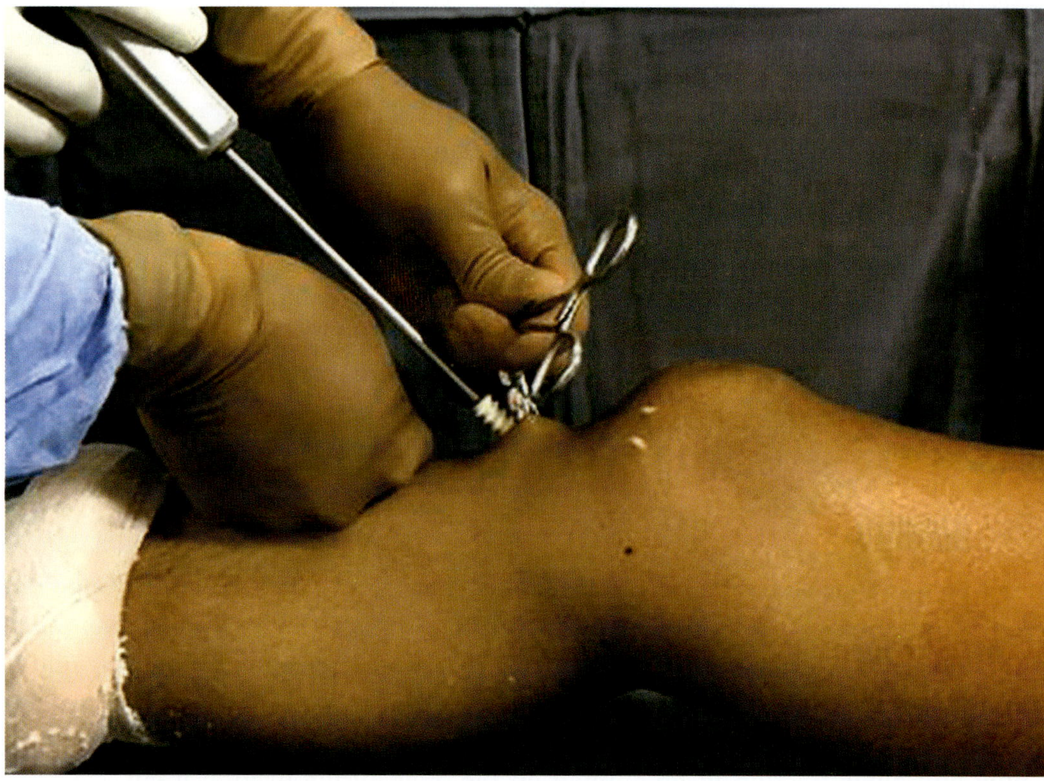

Fig. 20.2: Tibial fixation of the graft being done using a bioabsorbable screw. Note that while traction is applied to the graft, an assistant exerts a posterior drawer force to the proximal tibia and knee is maintained in 30 degrees flexion.

- For the bone-patellar tendon-bone (BPTB) graft, we put the screws on the cortical side of the bone plug so that the cancellous side is compressed against the bone tunnel which promotes healing. We often use stronger suture material such as No 2 FiberWire® (Arthrex, Naples, FL) passed through the bone plug which does not get damaged during interference screw insertion next to the bone plug.
- In our patients with hyperextension of the knee on the unaffected side, we perform tibial fixation with the knee in full extension.
- We choose a screw diameter 1–2 mm larger than the size of the tunnel for soft tissue ACL grafts but whenever we have to use a metallic interference screw, we use a screw of the same diameter as that of the tunnel to avoid excessive soft tissue graft damage by the screw.

- We do not usually perform double fixation routinely unless the tibial bone quality is poor. In this situation, we first use a screw 2 mm larger and if too loose (e.g. revision situation) use cortical fixation with a Suture Washer® (Smith and Nephew, Andover, MA) or bicortical screw post with washer or staple.

PITFALLS IN TIBIAL FIXATION

- Using interference screw shorter than 23 mm is associated with low pullout strength.
- When using interference screws which are not extending up to the tibial joint line, aggressive postoperative mobilization should be avoided.

REFERENCES

1. Chizari M, Wang B, Snow M, et al. Experimental and numerical analysis of screw fixation in anterior cruciate ligament reconstruction. AIP Conf Proc. 2008;1045:61-70.
2. Burks R, Daniel D, Losse G, et al. The effect of continuous passive motion on anterior cruciate ligament reconstruction stability. Am J Sports Med. 1984;12:323-7.
3. Ishibashi Y, Rudy TW, Livesay GA, et al. The effect of anterior cruciate ligament graft fixation site at the tibia on knee stability: evaluation using a robotic testing system. Arthroscopy. 1997;13:177-82.
4. Kousa P, Jarvinen TL, Vihavainen M, et al. The fixation strength of six hamstring tendon graft fixation devices in anterior cruciate ligament reconstruction: part II. Tibial site. Am J Sports Med. 2003;31:182-8.
5. Martin SD, Martin TL, Brown CH. Anterior cruciate ligament graft fixation. Orthop Clin North Am. 2002;33:685-96.
6. Robbe R, Paletta GA Jr. Soft-tissue graft fixation in anterior cruciate ligament reconstruction. Oper Tech Sports Med. 2004;12:188-94.
7. Scheffler SU, Sudkamp NP, Gockenjan A, et al. Biomechanical comparison of hamstring and patellar tendon graft anterior cruciate ligament reconstruction techniques: the impact of fixation level and fixation method under cyclic loading. Arthroscopy. 2002;18:304-15.
8. Brand JJ, Pienkowski D, Steenlage E, et al. Interference screw fixation strength of a quadrupled hamstring tendon graft is directly related to bone mineral density and insertion torque. Am J Sports Med. 2000;28:705-10.
9. Vuori I, Heinonen A, Sievanen H, et al. Effects of unilateral strength training and detraining on bone mineral density and content in young women: a study of mechanical loading and deloading on human bones. Calcif Tissue Int. 1994;55:59-67.
10. Shatzmann L, Brunner P, Staubli HU. Effect of cyclic preconditioning on the tensile properties of human quadriceps. Knee Surg Sports Traumatol Arthrosc. 1998;6:S56-S61.
11. Chizari M, Snow M, Wang B. Post-operative analysis of ACL tibial fixation. Knee Surg Sports Traumatol Arthrosc. 2009;17:730-6
12. Berg EE, Pollard ME, Kang Q. Interarticular bone tunnel healing. Arthroscopy. 2001;17:189-95.
13. Eriksson K, Kindblom LG, Wredmark T. Semitendinosus tendon graft ingrowth in tibial tunnel following ACL reconstruction. A histological study of 2 patients with different types of graft failure. Acta Orthop Scand. 2000; 71:275-9.
14. Nebelung W, Becker R, Urbach D, et al. Histological findings of tendon-bone-healing following anterior cruciate ligament reconstruction with hamstring grafts. Arch Orthop Trauma Surg. 2003;123:158-63.
15. Pinczewski LA, Clingeleffer AJ, Otto DD, et al. Integration of hamstring tendon graft with bone in reconstruction of the anterior cruciate ligament. Arthroscopy. 1997;13:641-3.
16. Yamazaki S, Yasuda K, Tomita F, et al. The effect of graft tunnel diameter disparity on intraosseous healing of the flexor tendon graft in anterior cruciate ligament reconstruction. Am J Sports Med. 2002;30:404-98.
17. Choi NH, Lee JH, Son KM, et al. Tibial tunnel widening after anterior cruciate ligament reconstructions with hamstring tendons using Rigidfix femoral fixation and Intrafix tibial fixation. Knee Surg Sports Traumatol Arthrosc. 2010; 18:92-7.

18. Tsuda E, Fukuda Y, Loh JC, et al. The effect of soft-tissue graft fixation in anterior cruciate ligament reconstruction on graft-tunnel motion under anterior tibial loading. Arthroscopy. 2002;18:960-7.
19. Buelow JU, Siebold R, Ellermann A. A prospective evaluation of tunnel enlargement in anterior cruciate ligament reconstruction with hamstrings: extracortical versus anatomical fixation. Knee Surg Sports Traumatol Arthrosc. 2002;10:80-5.
20. Herrera A, Martínez F, Iglesias D, et al.: Fixation strength of biocomposite wedge interference screw in ACL reconstruction: effect of screw length and tunnel/screw ratio. A controlled laboratory study. BMC Musculoskeletal Disord. 2010;11:139.
21. Shelbourne KD, Klotz C. What I have learned about ACL: utilizing a progressive rehabilitation scheme to achieve total knee symmetry after anterior cruciate ligament reconstruction. J Orthop Science. 2006,11:318-25.
22. Beynnon BD, Amis AA. In vitro testing protocols for the cruciate ligaments and ligament reconstructions. Knee Surg Sports Traumatol Arthrosc. 1998;6:S70-S76
23. Papageorgiou CD, Ma CB, Abramowitch SD, et al. A multidisciplinary study of the healing of an intraarticular anterior cruciate ligament graft in a goat model. Am J Sports Med. 2001;29:620-6.
24. Park MJ, Lee MC, Seong SC. A comparative study of the healing of tendon autograft and tendon-bone autograft using patellar tendon in rabbits. Int Orthop. 2001;25:35-9.
25. Singhatat W, Lawhorn KW, Howell SM, et al. How four weeks of implantation affect the strength and stiffness of a tendon graft in a bone tunnel: a study of two fixation devices in an extraarticular model in ovine. Am J Sports Med. 2002;30:506-13.
26. Zantop T, Weimann A, Wolle K, et al. Initial and 6 weeks' postoperative structural properties of soft tissue anterior cruciate ligament reconstructions with cross-pin or interference screw fixation: an in vivo study in sheep. Arthroscopy. 2007;23:14-20.
27. Jagodzinski M, Scheunemann K, Knobloch K, et al. Tibial press-fit fixation of the hamstring tendons for ACL-reconstruction. Knee Surg Sports Traumatol Arthrosc. 2006;14:1281-7.
28. Becker R, Schroder M, Ropke M, et al. Structural properties of sutures used in anchoring multi-stranded hamstrings in anterior cruciate ligament reconstruction: a biomechanical study. Arthroscopy. 1999;15:297-300.
29. Brand J Jr, Hamilton D, Selby J, et al. Biomechanical comparison of quadriceps tendon fixation with patellar tendon bone plug interference fixation in cruciate ligament reconstruction. Arthroscopy. 2000;16:805-12.
30. Fink C, Zapp M, Benedetto KP, et al. Tibial tunnel enlargement following anterior cruciate ligament reconstruction with patellar tendon autograft. Arthroscopy. 2001;17:138-43.
31. L'Insalata JC, Klatt B, Fu FH, et al. Tunnel expansion following anterior cruciate ligament reconstruction: a comparison of hamstring and patellar tendon autografts. Knee Surg Sports Traumatol Arthrosc. 1997;5:234-8.
32. Jansson KA, Harilainen A, Sandelin J, et al. Bone tunnel enlargement after anterior cruciate ligament reconstruction with the hamstring autograft and endobutton fixation technique: a clinical, radiographic and magnetic resonance imaging study with 2 years' follow-up. Knee Surg Sports Traumatol Arthrosc.1999;7:290-5.
33. Hoher J, Moller HD, Fu FH. Bone tunnel enlargement after anterior cruciate ligament reconstruction: fact or fiction? Knee Surg Sports Traumatol Arthrosc. 1998;6:231-40.
34. Selby JB, Johnson DL, Hester P, et al. Effect of screw length on bioabsorbable interference screw fixation in a tibial bone tunnel. Am J Sports Med. 2001;29:614-9.
35. Harvey AR, Thomas NP, Amis AA. The effect of screw length and position of fixation of four-stranded hamstring grafts for anterior cruciate ligament reconstruction. Knee. 2003;10:97-102.
36. Brown GA, Pena F, Grontvedt T, et al. Fixation strength of interference screw fixation in bovine, young human, and elderly human cadaver knees: influence of insertion torque, tunnel bone block gap, and interference. Knee Surg Sports Traumatol Arthrosc. 1996;3:238-44.
37. Caborn DN, Cohen M, Neef R, et al. Quadrupled semitendinosus-gracilis autograft fixation in the femoral tunnel: a comparison between a metal and a bioabsorbable interference screw. Arthroscopy. 1998;14:241-5.
38. Kousa P, Järvinen TLN, Pohjonen T, et al. Fixation strength of a biodegradable screw in anterior cruciate ligament reconstruction. J Bone J Surg Br. 1995;77:901-5.
39. Walton M. Absorbable and metal interference screws: comparison of graft security during healing. Arthroscopy. 1999;15:818-26.

40. Woo SL, Wu C, Dede O, et al. Biomechanics and anterior cruciate ligament reconstruction. J Orthop Surg Res. 2006;25:2-11.
41. Shapiro JD, Jackson DW, Aberman HM, et al. Comparison of pullout strength for seven- and nine-millimetre diameter interference screw size as used in anterior cruciate ligament reconstruction arthroscopy. Arthroscopy. 1995;11: 596-9.
42. Danial Cooper, Tad Wilson, et al. Clinical failure of tibial interference screw fixation after anterior cruciate ligament reconstruction: a report of two cases. Am J Sports Med. 1996;24(5).
43. Smith KE, Garcia M, McAnuff K, et al. Anterior cruciate ligament fixation: Is radial force a predictor of the pullout strength of soft-tissue interference devices? Knee. 2012;19:786-92.
44. Stadelmaier DM, Lowe WR, Ilahi OA, et al. Cyclic pull-out strength of hamstring tendon graft fixation with soft tissue interference screws: influence of screw length. Am J Sports Med. 1999;27:778-83.
45. Balazs GC, Brelin AM, Grimm PD, et al. Hybrid Tibia Fixation of Soft Tissue Grafts in Anterior Cruciate Ligament Reconstruction: a Systematic Review. Am J Sports Med. 2016;44:2724-32.
46. Morris MW, Williams JL, Thake AJ, et al. Optimal screw diameter for interference fixation in a bone tunnel: a porcine model. Knee Surg Sports Traumatol Arthrosc. 2004;12(5):486-9.

CHAPTER

21 Graft Tensioning and Conditioning

Miten Sheth, Sachin Tapasvi

INTRODUCTION

The goal of anterior cruciate ligament (ACL) reconstruction is to restore normal knee mechanics in terms of stability and mobility. Graft tension along with graft type, size, position and fixation are important factors implicated in the success and failure of ACL surgery. Assuming that an ideal graft has been selected and tunnels positioned optimally, ensuring optimal tension of the graft is thought to contribute to the restoration of knee joint biomechanics.[1] It is generally acknowledged, first mentioned by Jones in 1963 that tension applied to ACL graft at the time of surgery should be sufficient to eliminate an anterior drawer sign and yet allow full range of motion.[2]

There is a wide variation in methods and amount of graft tensioning reported in literature and a genuine lack of information on the adequate tension required in various surgical scenarios. The aim of this chapter is to discuss the rationale for an acceptable ACL tensioning and conditioning technique.

First and foremost, it is essential to understand the meaning of these terms. "Initial Tension" refers to tension in graft at the time of final fixation during ACL reconstruction. To achieve this initial tension, there are a few described techniques that can be used sequentially during ACL surgery. "Pretensioning" or "isometric preconditioning" refers to loading of ACL graft that is performed before it is pulled into the knee. "Conditioning" or "cyclic preconditioning" refers to cyclic loading of ACL graft that is performed after fixation within one bone tunnel and immediately before final graft fixation at the other bone tunnel. "Tensioning" refers to isometric loading of ACL graft that is performed at a selected angle of knee flexion just before final fixation.[3]

No graft in use matches the complex anatomy of the native ACL. To understand and recreate normal knee biomechanics it is essential to review literature concerning the native ACL.

NATIVE ACL

Biomechanical properties of the ACL are determined by the relationship between ligament length and ligament tension.[4-6] These can be measured by simultaneously measuring load and corresponding elongation during experimental tensile testing. The resultant load-elongation curve of the native ACL can be divided into four phases.[7] The first nonlinear phase is due to crimped collagen fibers which easily extend under low axial forces. In the second linear phase, fibers progressively elongate (reversibly deform)

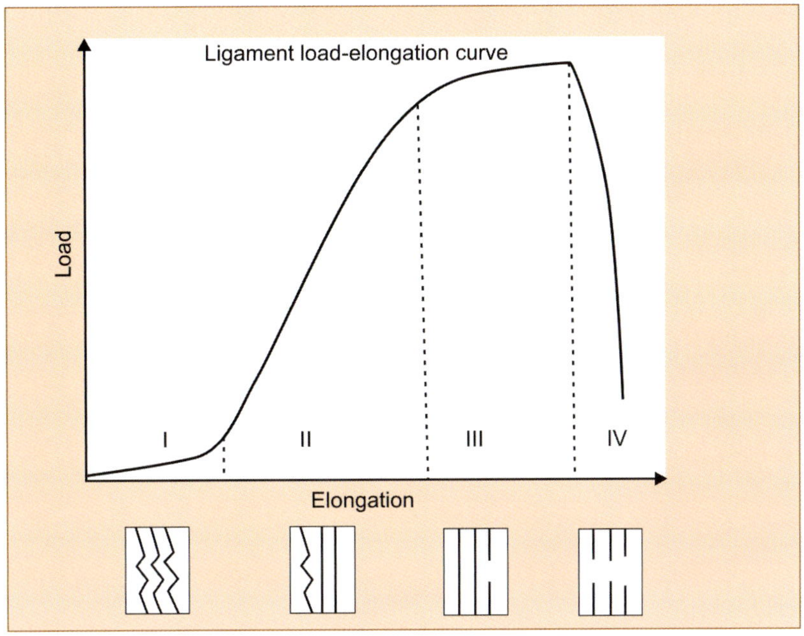

Fig. 21.1: Properties of ligament substance: Load-elongation curve. Demonstration of crimped collagen fibers–reversible elongation–plastic deformation–failure at yield point.
Source: Modified from Takeda et al.[15]

and the ligament structure becomes increasingly stiff. The slope of the linear region allows for reproducible determination of ligament stiffness and corresponds to loads acting on the ACL. In the intact knee, first two phases of the ACL loading curve represent the clinical situation where the tibia translates anteriorly for several millimeters during knee motion. With additional loading, slope of the load-elongation curve decreases as plastic deformation of collagen fibers occurs. Finally, the curve reaches ultimate load point (failure of the bone-ligament-bone complex) (Fig. 21.1). In summary, applying high loads (within yield limit) to the ACL will increase stiffness and may therefore sufficiently restrict excessive joint motion. Varying degrees of ligament stiffness are necessary for various loads and various ranges of joint motion.

Ligaments are capable of both "creep" and "relaxation" activity and exhibit these behaviors in an attempt to prevent overstretching and disruption. Creep is defined as deformation or elongation of a ligament over time under a constant load or stress. Relaxation refers to a decrease in stress of tissue over time when the ligament is subjected to a constant elongation. In vivo, cyclic loading of any ligament will cause gradual creep and relaxation, which results in increased knee laxity after physical activity. However, it will return to the original stiffness after a period of rest.[6,8]

ACL loads of 169 N may be expected during normal level walking, while descending stairs generates 445 N of in situ force due to the activation of the knee extensor apparatus. In contrast, ascending stairs generated in situ forces below 100 N.[9,10] Tensile testing of the ACL has revealed the mean ligament stiffness to be 242 ± 28 N/mm and ultimate failure load as 2160 ± 157 N in younger cadaveric specimens.[11] The ultimate load to failure for younger humans is on average 2.4 times higher than in older humans.[12] In the native ACL, there is no true isometry due to complex geometry and different kinematic properties of individual fibers and bundles.[13-15] In the normal knee, ACL tension decreases with knee flexion from the maximum value at full extension to the minimum value between 20 degrees and 40 degrees and then marginally increases with extreme flexion. This relationship between ACL tension and knee flexion angle is known as the tension-flexion curve.[16-18] Passive extension of the knee generates forces only during the last 10 degrees of extension, with greatest forces in hyperextension.[19] Active knee extension also increases forces in the native ACL especially from 40 degrees of flexion to full extension.[20]

ACL Graft

No graft material commonly used has stiffness or ultimate failure strength comparable to the native ACL. Although ultimate failure loads of a native bone-patellar tendon-bone complex, a quadrupled hamstring tendon complex, or a quadriceps tendon-bone complex average 2977, 4140 and 2353 N, respectively (exceed values for the native ACL), graft harvest and artificial graft fixation into bone significantly decrease both linear stiffness and ultimate strength.[21-24] Load-elongation curve of these grafts is similar to the load-elongation curve of the native ACL. The extent of preload of the ACL graft has no influence on the load elongation curve. However, by enhancing the preload, maximal force in the ACL graft increases significantly.[24]

Isometric bone tunnel placement during ACL reconstruction is not supported by literature. In fact, it has been proved that anatomic graft placement results in kinematics closer to the normal knee than isometric graft placement.[25,26] Considering that ACL reconstruction has now moved toward anatomic tunnel placements, the ACL graft tension-flexion curve is very similar to the native ACL[24,27-29] (Fig. 21.2).

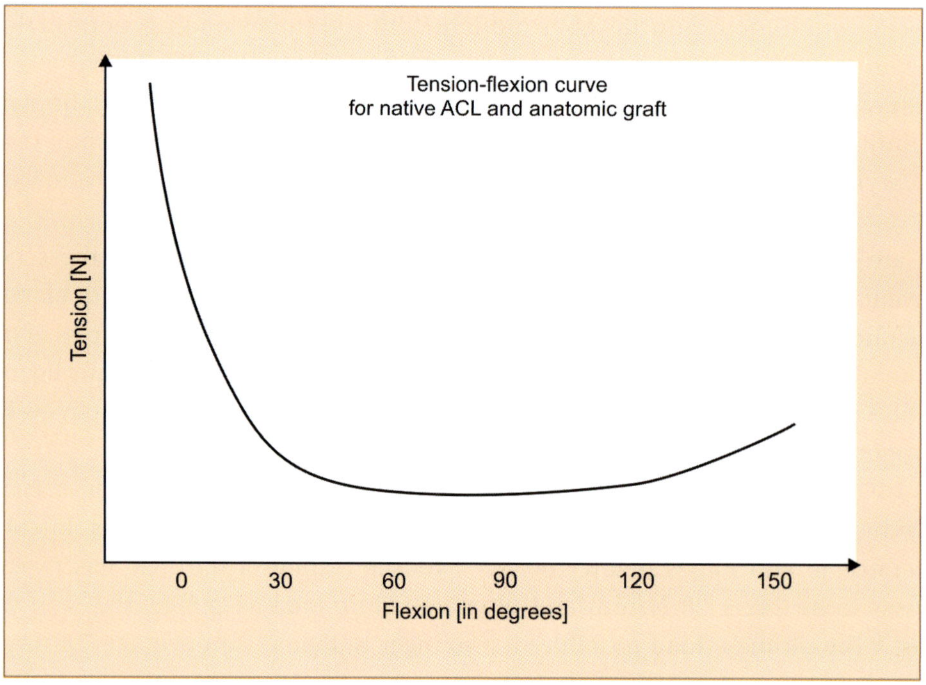

Fig. 21.2: Graphic representation of the tension-flexion curve for native ACL and graft with anatomically placed bone tunnels. *Source*: Modified from Schmitt-Sody et al.[24]

Having reviewed biomechanics of the native ACL and ACL graft, we can now focus on the subject of tensioning and conditioning. Several questions arise when discussing about initial tension in ACL reconstruction.

- Why is the concept of initial tension important?
- How much initial tension is sufficient?
- What are the surgical steps vital to ideal ACL tensioning and conditioning?

Though literature and evidence have a majority of answers, it is personal experience that influences surgeons' techniques maximally. There may be myriad ways of tensioning and conditioning ACL grafts. We will discuss the rationale behind the commonest (which happens to be our way as well) method of achieving ideal initial graft tension.

Why is the Concept of Initial Tension Important?

Initial tension in the graft at the time of fixation can decide the clinical outcome after ACL reconstruction in terms of stability and range of motion. An increase of ACL tension decreases degree of anterior translation of the tibia to the femur.[30-32] In case initial tension of the graft is lower compared to the native ACL, knee stability is decreased. On the other hand, if the graft tension is excessive, nonphysiological movements result putting the knee joint at risk for reduced range of motion. Hence, the goal must be to apply physiologic forces to the ACL graft, enough to stabilize the knee compared to the contralateral knee.

All Grafts Lose Tension after Surgery

Graft relaxation (creep elongation) and/or transposition of the graft in bone tunnel occurs with repetitive submaximal cyclic loading in a relatively early phase after surgery and has the potential to cause "loosening" of the graft over time. Hence, insufficient tension applied on the graft during fixation may result in a slack reconstructed ligament. Rate and degree of graft relaxation depends on the combination of graft type and material used for fixation.[33-37]

Excessively High Initial Tension in Grafts is Dangerous

Excessive tension in the ACL graft can lead to posterior, lateral, and external tibial subluxation. Graft tension-related posterior tibial subluxation can result in an increase in quadriceps force needed to achieve full extension.[38] Excessive graft tension leads to an overconstrained knee with less anteroposterior translation, internal-external rotation and varus-valgus movement compared with the uninjured knee, resulting clinically in a significant decrease in knee motion.[39] Exceedingly high initial tension may also induce histologic graft changes leading to wear-related graft failure.[39-42]

Behavior of the ACL Reconstructed Knee is Graft Type and Fixation Device-specific

Initial tension applied to a graft during an ACL reconstruction appears to be tissue specific. Stiffness and elasticity vary among graft tissues. The material (stiffness) and geometrical (size and length) properties of the graft influence the amount of tension that needs to be applied.[31] Initial stiffness decreases significantly leading to significant increase in anterior laxity after cyclic loading depending on the stiffness of graft-fixation construct combination.[33] Multiple outcome studies have indicated that hamstring autografts are associated with higher postoperative laxity than bone-tendon-bone (BTB) grafts.[31,43,44] Considering the properties of hamstring grafts (longer tendons, no bone-bone healing), most surgeons reconstruct using higher tensions compared to BTB grafts.[31,45] BTB graft with interference screws has higher stiffness and ultimate failure load than doubled flexor tendon graft fixed with interference screws which in turn has higher stiffness compared to doubled flexor tendon graft fixed with sutures.[35] In case of allografts, there is a substantial decrease in strength during initial phases of healing due to inflammatory response and revascularization. Hence, it seems prudent to fix allografts at a higher initial tension.[46,47]

How much Initial Tension is Sufficient?

Although high initial graft tension can better replicate normal knee kinematics at time-zero, these effects diminish during the early graft healing process. There is no need to over-constrain the knee by using higher initial tension. For example, it has been proved that there is no advantage of overcorrecting AP laxity by 2 mm vis-à-vis restoring it compared to the opposite knee in terms of clinical, functional, patient-reported, and osteoarthritis (OA) imaging outcomes even 84 months after surgery.[48]

For hamstring grafts, though subjective clinical results do not differ, postoperative laxity can be better mitigated, if higher initial tension of 80 N is used compared to 20 N.[49-51] Hamstring grafts fixed with suture-post technique lose around 50% of their initial tension after 1,000 cycles of cyclic loading. To restore anterior translation to within 3 mm of the native ACL condition after cyclic loading, approximately 68 N of initial tension is required using this fixation technique.[36] Considering the tension of the native ACL (16 to 87 N), for a hamstring graft fixed with interference screws, an increase in initial tension above 80 N has no biomechanical advantages.[34]

As the BTB autograft is approximately twice as stiff as the hamstring autograft, less force would be required to restore stability and biomechanics when compared to hamstring autograft.[52,53] When the graft is fixed in extension, higher initial tension of 90 N may better restore anterior laxity than 45 N, though it has no effects on the clinical outcomes.[54] In fact, high initial tension applied to a BTB graft at 30 degrees of flexion can lead to loss of extension postsurgery.

Surveys have revealed that the actual amount of manual tension applied by orthopedic surgeons during ACL reconstruction (ACLR) using a STG graft is 65.8 ± 32 N.[55]

What are the Surgical Steps Vital to Ideal ACL Tensioning and Conditioning?

To minimize graft stretching after reconstruction, pretensioning, conditioning and tensioning of ACL grafts are recommended. To review, "pretensioning" refers to loading of ACL graft that is performed before the graft is pulled into the knee. "Conditioning" refers to cyclic loading of ACL graft that is performed once the graft is fixed at one end (within one bone tunnel) and immediately before final graft fixation at the other bone tunnel. "Tensioning" refers to isometric loading of ACL graft that is performed during final fixation.

Pretensioning

It is reasonable to assume that pretensioning removes some graft creep. Though the amount of tension and technique for pretensioning remains debatable, there are a few things that need to be pointed out. First, the initial tension given (manually or by a tensioning device) will gradually decrease over time as the graft is stretched. Hence, it should not be assumed that a given tension setting on device stretches the graft constantly with a fixed force for the period of pretensioning. Second, pretensioning eliminates creep especially at the suture-graft interface. Hence, it is advantageous to pretension the graft with sutures taken at both ends rather than the graft alone. Approximately 2 mm of graft elongation can occur, particularly in the stitched portion, after pretensioning. Hence, it is important to focus on careful removal of slack from each stitch during suturing.[56] Third, stiffness of the BTB graft is high enough that there may be no obvious utility in pretensioning BTB grafts. That said, viscoelastic creep has been proven in BTB grafts using both an in-vivo and an in-vitro model; 20 lbs (89 N) of pretension leads to around 10% of length change in BTB graft.[57] In the absence of pretensioning, significant postimplantation graft creep will occur. Lastly, in spite of pretensioning there are no studies to disprove recoil of the graft after pretensioning when it is taken off the preparation table to the knee before final fixation. Graft preparation boards with calibrated tension meters are available, but it must be noted that pretensioning reversibly elongates collagen fibers in the graft. These fibers will recoil once the graft is taken in hand for final fixation. Pretensioning to an exact measurement may not be of value at this stage, and is best reserved for final tensioning at the time of graft fixation (Figs. 21.3A and B).

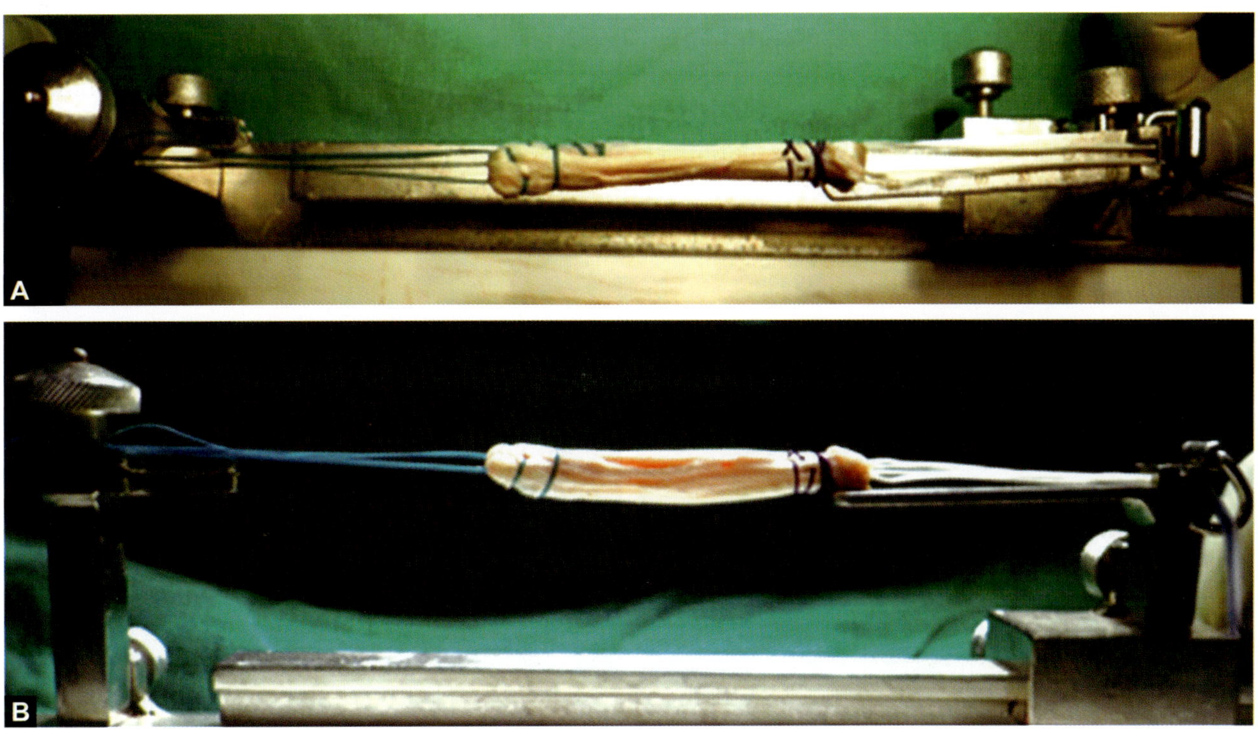

Figs. 21.3A and B: Pretensioning of six-strand hamstring graft (UHMWPE whip-stitches on one end and adjustable cortical loop at the other end) on a graft preparation board.

Conditioning

Conditioning involves taking the knee through a range of motion with constant tension on one end of the graft after it has been fixed at the other end. At the time of operation, "cycling" the knee with the graft tensed will "precondition" the graft, to ensure less graft relaxation after it has been re-tensed and finally fixed.[45] An added advantage of conditioning is that it allows the surgeon to identify force-flexion curve (behavior) of the graft before final fixation. This can enable the surgeon to decide the fixation angle (Fig. 21.4A). Current biomechanical literature demonstrates the potential clinically beneficial effects of pretensioning and conditioning, including reduced graft elongation and greater preservation of graft tension and stiffness following fixation.[58]

Tensioning

Tensioning involves isometric loading of the ACL graft after it has been fixed at one end before final fixation. Surgeons' surveys have revealed that a majority use manual tensioning rather than tensioning device. Factors that affect tensioning protocols include graft type and size, patient age and anthropometry, contralateral knee stability and individual surgeon training and experience.[59,60] Applying the appropriate tension to the final graft reconstruction has traditionally been performed by the surgeon and is based on the surgeon's experience and perception of applied tension. There are inherent problems with manual application of tension to the ACL reconstruction. These include under- or overtightening the reconstruction, inconsistent tension application among subjects, and variable load application among the strands. Commercially available ACL tensioning devices can be applied to the tibial end of the graft. These provide theoretical benefits of applying a stable, known tension force to the graft.[61] This may ensure consistent and higher amount of initial tension compared to a single-handed manual maximum pull used conventionally. Measured tensioning of graft up to 80–90 N (9 kg/20 lbs) may or may not improve side-to-side difference in laxity and it does not improve clinical outcome postoperatively when compared with conventional tensioning maneuvers.[62,63]

Pretensioning (89 N/20 lbs for 20 mins) or preconditioning (cycling 20 times), after 30 minutes, leaves a graft with higher residual tension. Both have an additive effect and result in significantly greater retained

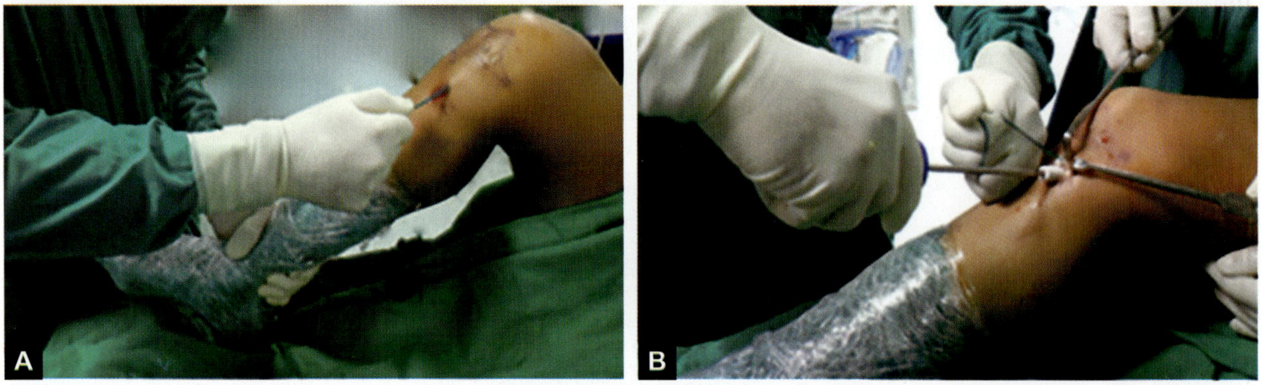

Figs. 21.4A and B: (A) Cyclic conditioning is carried out by the surgeon, maintaining sustained tension on the graft; (B) Fixation of hamstring graft at 30 degrees of flexion with posterior drawer force and single handed manual maximum pull on the graft.

tension than either method performed individually. A simple pull up to 80 N before fixation does not impart sufficient tension to a graft to prevent it from failing. Clinicians must pretension and condition soft tissue grafts before final tensioning and tibial fixation.[3]

Fixation Angle

Fixation angle of ACL has been suggested to influence the performance of an ACL-reconstructed knee.[45] Tunnel placement affects postoperative joint laxity more than initial graft tension, which in-turn is more important than graft fixation angle for graft-tunnel biomechanics.[64] We know from kinematic studies that the forces generated in the graft as well as the native ACL are greatest at full extension and minimal between 30 degrees and 60 degrees of flexion.[16] If a surgeon applies a certain initial tension at around 30 degrees of flexion, graft tension values obtained at more extension and more flexion positions will be greater than the initial tension value. Conversely, if a surgeon applies a certain initial tension at full extension, graft tension values at all flexion positions will be lower than the initial tension value. Increase in graft tension and decrease in anterior laxity can be better produced by changing the fixation angle from 0 degrees to 30 degrees, rather than doubling initial tension from 20 N to 40 N.[30,65]

Fixation at angles greater than 30 degrees of flexion imparts higher initial tension (stability) but can create difficulty in regaining full extension postoperatively. Fixation at complete extension ensures range of motion but can jeopardize stability in flexion.[66] This may be important in patients with preoperative knee hyperextension, and it seems imperative to fix grafts in such patients at 0 degrees rather than at 30 degrees. Fixing the graft in hyperextension is detrimental. Forces generated in the native ACL reach a maximum in hyperextension.[19] Any graft fixed in hyperextension will lose tension as the knee bends and hence the minimum required initial tension may not be achieved.

As mentioned earlier, during cyclic loading, one can check the behavior of the ACL graft. Every graft produces its own individual force-flexion curve based on the position of femoral and tibial tunnels. Once the graft is fixed at one end, exit through the other bone tunnel can be monitored to gauge the graft-motion in tunnel with varying degrees of knee flexion. If the reconstructed tunnels are positioned anatomically, whilst conditioning, the ACL graft will shorten in the tibial tunnel with extension and will marginally move outward in the tibial tunnel with increasing knee flexion. An ACL graft that is isometric will show no significant motion and can be tensioned at any point in the flexion arc. This relationship may change depending on the location of the tibial and femoral tunnels. As long as the pattern of graft-motion in tibial tunnel is similar to the force-flexion curve of the native ACL (less than 2–3 mm of motion), tunnel position can be considered acceptable. Ideally, fixation should be at the knee flexion angle where graft has lengthened compared to the tibial tunnel, as it will then ensure incremental initial tension at other degrees of range of motion. But as we have mentioned earlier, any graft fixed at an angle of more than 30 degrees risks curtailing knee extension postoperatively.

In summary, fixation between 10 degrees and 30 degrees will impart significant initial tension to the ACL graft. Fixation at any flexion angle more than 30 degrees may create difficulty in regaining complete extension after surgery. Fixation in complete extension or hyperextension carries the risk of suboptimal initial tension especially at flexion angles. Clinically, it would seem prudent to fix a hamstring tendon graft at 30 degrees of knee flexion to avoid insufficient tension after surgery. Conversely, a BTB graft can be fixed at full extension to avoid postoperative flexion contracture of the knee due to overtensioning.

Fixation angle must be decided on a case-by-case basis by the surgeon depending on the behavior of the graft during conditioning. With well-placed tunnels, the inflexion point of the ACL graft should be near full extension (10–30 degrees). At this angle, the desired initial tension can be given and the graft fixed (*see* Fig. 21.4B).

Note on Graft Tension for Double-bundle ACL Reconstruction

The ACL does not function as a simple tube of fibers with a constant tension, but rather consists of fiber groups that are subjected to episodes of lengthening and slackening throughout the range of motion.[67] This phenomenon has prompted the functional subdivision of the ACL into an AM and a PL bundle.[68,69] The lengths of the two bundles change with varying degrees of knee flexion, implying that they are not isometric. There is no consensus on the exact pattern of force distribution in the ACL bundles at various knee flexion angles. Most authors agree that the PL bundle shows highest tension at full extension. However, the tension-flexion curve of the AM bundle and what portion of the overall ACL tension it represents remains unclcar.

Bundle-tensioning protocol is a variable that has a significant effect on the bundle-loading patterns in double-bundle ACL reconstruction.[70] Too much tension of the PL bundle has been raised as a potential problem causing extension deficit or decrease of the PL bundle function.[71,72] Tensioning both AM and PL bundles together at 15–20 degrees of flexion best matches the intact knee rotations and anteroposterior laxity throughout the range of motion.[70,73] Protocols that involve fixing both bundles at 30 degrees, either bundle first or AM bundle at 60 degrees over-constrain the knee.[74-76]

Lower graft tensions are required to match intact knee laxity in double-bundle ACL reconstruction. It is recommended that a moderate tensioning force be applied to the PL bundle and a minimal tensioning force to the AM bundle to obtain better knee kinematics.[77] Good clinical outcome has been reported at 2 years postoperatively with 20 N of initial tension.[78] Initial tension less than 20 N is not recommended because it might result in residual pivot shift in some cases.[79] Conversely, 40 N tension applied to each graft at 30° of knee flexion leads to loss of knee extension in comparison to 30 N tension applied to each graft at 10°.[80] The minimum required tension in both bundles to effect rotational stability (to negate a pivot-shift phenomenon) is an average of 24 N (total AM + PL) and it is much lesser than the minimum required tension in case of a single bundle ACLR.[81]

THE IDEAL TENSIONING AND CONDITIONING PROTOCOL (THE WAY WE DO IT)

- Once the graft is harvested, in case of a hamstring tendon after cleaning off muscle fibers, it is mounted on the graft board and stretched between two posts. This imparts some tension, elongating crimped fibers, whilst whip-stitches are taken at the ends. In case of a BTB or quadriceps tendon graft, once harvested, preparation is done without any pretensioning.
- After whip-stitching ends, if suspensory fixation is planned on the femoral side, adjustable or fixed loop device of choice is taken on the prep table. Depending on the hamstring graft configuration (three, four, five or six strand), the tendons are looped/tied around the device. Multiple tendon grafts may be homogenized using sutures. BTB and quadriceps tendon grafts are generally fixed with interference

fixation at both ends and rarely with suspensory fixation at the femoral end. Hence, BTB grafts most commonly have high molecular weight polyethylene sutures running through pin-sized tunnels in the bone blocks at both ends. Quadriceps tendon grafts have bone tunnel-sutures at one end and whip-stitches at the other (that may be tied to a cortical-loop device).

- The next step, after sizing the graft, is pretensioning. In case of a hamstring graft, whilst the cortical loop is attached to a special post on the graft preparation board, the other end with sutures is fixed to another post. In case of a BTB or quadriceps tendon, graft the two suture ends are tied around two posts. These two posts are then distracted manually to hold the harvested ligament taut. Graft preparation boards with a calibrated tension meter are available, but we do not use these routinely. At this juncture, the graft is covered with a vancomycin soaked gauze till the bone tunnels are drilled and the knee is ready for graft fixation.
- Once the graft is fixed at the femoral end, the knee is taken through a complete range of motion at least ten times. During this step, two things are done additionally. First, isometric tension is maintained at the tibial end of the graft throughout the cyclic loading process. Second, the tibial tunnel exit is palpated to check, if the graft excursion is less than 2–3 mm and follows the anatomic tension-flexion curve. This step, called conditioning, is always carried out irrespective of graft type.
- The last and most important step is tensioning at a particular fixation angle. All grafts are fixed with a manual maximum pull instead of a tensioning device. A posterior drawer force is applied on the proximal tibia at the same time. Hamstring grafts are fixed at 30 degrees of flexion, BTB and quadriceps tendon grafts are fixed at 0–10 degrees with metal or biointerference screws. In patients older than 50 years, the graft is fixed at full extension, irrespective of graft type. In younger patients, an adjustable cortical loop device is used at the femoral end preferably because it allows further tensioning of the graft after tibial fixation. The goal in these cases is to match the anterior laxity of the contralateral knee.

SUMMARY

Initial tension affects the biology of the graft and is a time-dependent interplay of biomechanical forces and host incorporation. A number of factors affect graft tension including initial tension (pretensioning, conditioning and tensioning), tunnel placement, graft type, size and fixation type. Historically, much debate has existed in literature regarding these issues. The authors seek to lend clarity to this confusing topic and have defined their ideal evidence-based tensioning and conditioning protocol.

PEARLS AND PITFALLS

- Pretensioning stretches the suture-tendon interface more than the tendon itself. Whip-stitches must be checked carefully before the graft is taken off the table. Sometimes, if the graft has been prepared inappropriately, the sutures may cut through and come off on isometric tensioning.
- Pretensioning may reduce the graft diameter by half a size and unless checked, this may lead to larger bone tunnels than needed, hindering secure graft fixation.
- If there is excessive graft excursion during cyclic conditioning, it may hint improper bone tunnel placement.
- Sometimes the initial tension in the ACL graft may be inadequate even after well-fixed final tibial fixation. In such cases, an adjustable cortical-loop device on the femur can help increase the initial tension. We have occasionally used an additional interference screw on the intra-articular side of the femoral tunnel. This may help to increase tension in the graft.

REFERENCES

1. Sherman SL, Chalmers PN, Yanke AB, et al. Graft tensioning during knee ligament reconstruction: principles and practice. J Am Acad Orthop Surg. 2012;20(10):633-45.
2. Jones KG. Reconstruction of the anterior cruciate ligament. J Bone Joint Surg Am. 1963;45(5):925-32.
3. Pilia M, Murray M, Guda T, et al. Pretensioning of Soft Tissue Grafts in Anterior Cruciate Ligament Reconstruction. Orthopedics. 2015;38(7):e582-7.
4. Brand J, Weiler A, Caborn DNM, et al. Graft fixation in cruciate ligament reconstruction. Am J Sports Med. 2000;28(5):761-74.
5. Frisén M, Mägi M, Sonnerup L, et al. Rheological analysis of soft collagenous tissue. Part II: experimental evaluations and verifications. J Biomech. 1969;2(1):21-8.
6. Noyes FR, Delucas JL, Torvik PJ. Biomechanics of anterior cruciate ligament failure. J Bone Joint Surg Am. 1974;56(2):236-53.
7. Dargel J, Gotter M, Mader K, et al. Biomechanics of the anterior cruciate ligament and implications for surgical reconstruction. Strategies Trauma Limb Reconstr. 2007;2(1):1-12.
8. Frank C, McDonald D, Bray D, et al. Collagen fibril diameters in the healing adult rabbit medial collateral ligament. Connect Tissue Res. 1992;27(4):251-63.
9. Harrington IJ. A bioengineering analysis of force actions at the knee in normal and pathological gait. Biomed Eng. 1976;11(5):167-72.
10. Morrison J. Function of the knee joint in various activities. Biomed Eng. 1976;4(12):573-80.
11. Woo SLY, Hollis JM, Adams DJ, et al. Tensile properties of the human femur-anterior cruciate ligament-tibia complex. Am J Sports Med. 1991;19(3):217-25.
12. Noyes FR, Grood ES. The strength of the anterior cruciate ligament in humans and Rhesus monkeys. J Bone Joint Surg Am. 1976;58(8):1074-82.
13. Woo S, Wu C, Dede O, et al. Biomechanics and anterior cruciate ligament reconstruction. J Orthop Surg Res. 2006;1:2.
14. Petersen W, Zantop T. Anatomy of the anterior cruciate ligament with regard to its two bundles. Clin Orthop Relat Res. 2007;454:35-47.
15. Takeda Y, Xerogeanes JW, Livesay GA, et al. Biomechanical function of the human anterior cruciate ligament. Arthroscopy. 1994;10(2):140-7.
16. Fleming B, Beynnon BD, Johnson RJ, et al. Isometric versus tension measurements. Am J Sports Med. 1993;21(1):82-8.
17. Beynnon B, Howe JG, Pope MH, et al. The measurement of anterior cruciate ligament strain in vivo. Int Orthop. 1992;16(1):1-12.
18. Wascher DC, Markolf KL, Shapiro MS, et al. Direct in vitro measurement of forces in the cruciate ligaments. Part I. J Bone Joint Surg Am. 1993;75(3):377-86.
19. Markolf KL, Gorek JF, Kabo JM, et al. Direct measurement of resultant forces in the anterior cruciate ligament. An in vitro study performed with a new experimental technique. J Bone Joint Surg Am. 1990;72(4):557-67.
20. Paulos L, Noyes FR, Grood E, et al. Knee rehabilitation after anterior cruciate ligament reconstruction and repair. Am J Sports Med. 1981;9(3):140-9.
21. Cooper DE, Deng XH, Burstein AL, et al. The strength of the central third patellar tendon graft: A biomechanical study. Am J Sports Med. 1993;21(6):818-24.
22. Hamner DL, Brown CH, Steiner ME, et al. Hamstring tendon grafts for reconstruction of the anterior cruciate ligament. J Bone Joint Surg Am. 1999;81(4):549-57.
23. Staubli HU, Schatzmann L, Brunner P, et al. Quadriceps tendon and patellar ligament: Cryosectional anatomy and structural properties in young adults. Knee Surg Sports Traumatol Arthrosc. 1996;4(2):100-10.
24. Schmitt-Sody M, Kirchhoff C, Luciani E, et al. Dynamic in vitro analysis of tractile forces of the anterior cruciate ligament (ACL) transplant using patellar and semitendinosus muscle tendon: a cadaver study. Arch Orthop Trauma Surg. 2014;135(1):29-39.
25. Hefzy MS, Grood ES, Noyes FR. Factors affecting the region of most isometric femoral attachments. Am J Sports Med. 1989;17(2):208-16.

26. Musahl V, Plakseychuk A, VanScyoc A, et al. Varying femoral tunnels between the anatomical footprint and isometric positions: effect on kinematics of the anterior cruciate ligament-reconstructed knee. Am J Sports Med. 2005;33(5):712-8.
27. Arnold MP, Verdonschot N, van Kampen A. The normal anterior cruciate ligament as a model for tensioning strategies in anterior cruciate ligament grafts. Am J Sports Med. 2005;33(2):277-83.
28. Arnold MP, Verdonschot N, van Kampen A. ACL graft can replicate the normal ligament's tension curve. Knee Surg Sports Traumatol Arthrosc. 2005;13(8):625-31.
29. Lubowitz JH. Anatomic ACL reconstruction produces greater graft length change during knee range-of-motion than transtibial technique. Knee Surg Sports Traumatol Arthrosc. 2013;22(5):1190-5.
30. Bylski-Austrow DI, Grood ES, Hefzy MS, et al. Anterior cruciate ligament replacements: A mechanical study of femoral attachment location, flexion angle at tensioning, and initial tension. J Orthop Res. 1990;8(4):522-31.
31. Burks RT, Leland R. Determination of graft tension before fixation in anterior cruciate ligament reconstruction. Arthroscopy. 1988;4(4):260-6.
32. Fleming B, Beynnon B, Howe J, et al. Effect of tension and placement of a prosthetic anterior cruciate ligament on the anteroposterior laxity of the knee. J Orthop Res. 1992;10(2):177-86.
33. Yamanaka M, Yasuda K, Tohyama H, et al. The effect of cyclic displacement on the biomechanical characteristics of anterior cruciate ligament reconstructions. Am J Sports Med. 1999;27(6):772-7.
34. Numazaki H, Tohyama H, Nakano H, et al. The effect of initial graft tension in anterior cruciate ligament reconstruction on the mechanical behaviors of the femur-graft-tibia complex during cyclic loading. Am J Sports Med. 2002;30(6):800-5.
35. Nakano H, Yasuda K, Tohyama H, et al. Interference screw fixation of doubled flexor tendon graft in anterior cruciate ligament reconstruction—biomechanical evaluation with cyclic elongation. Clin Biomech. 2000;15(3):188-95.
36. Boylan D, Greis PE, West JR, et al. Effects of initial graft tension on knee stability after anterior cruciate ligament reconstruction using hamstring tendons: a cadaver study. Arthroscopy. 2003;19(7):700-5.
37. Arnold MP, Lie DT, Verdonschot N, et al. The remains of anterior cruciate ligament graft tension after cyclic knee motion. Am J Sports Med. 2005;33(4):536-42.
38. Melby A, Noble JS, Askew MJ, et al. The effects of graft tensioning on the laxity and kinematics of the anterior cruciate ligament reconstructed knee. Arthroscopy. 1991;7(3):257-66.
39. Andersen HN, Jørgensen U. The immediate postoperative kinematic state after anterior cruciate ligament reconstruction with increasing peroperative tension. Knee Surg Sports Traumatol Arthrosc. 1998;6(1):S62-9.
40. Katsuragi R, Yasuda K, Tsujino J, et al. The effect of nonphysiologically high initial tension on the mechanical properties of in situ frozen anterior cruciate ligament in a canine model. Am J Sports Med. 2000;28(1):47-56.
41. Graf BK, Henry J, Rothenberg M, et al. Anterior cruciate ligament reconstruction with patellar tendon. Am J Sports Med. 1994;22(1):131-5.
42. Yoshiya S, Andrish JT, Manley MT, et al. Graft tension in anterior cruciate ligament reconstruction: An in vivo study in dogs. Am J Sports Med. 1987;15(5):464-70.
43. Feller JA, Webster KE. A randomized comparison of patellar tendon and hamstring tendon anterior cruciate ligament reconstruction. Am J Sports Med. 2003;31(4):564-73.
44. Freedman K, D'Amato M, Nedeff D, et al. Arthroscopic anterior cruciate ligament reconstruction: a meta-analysis comparing patellar tendon and hamstring tendon autografts. Am J Sports Med. 2003;31(1):2-11.
45. Amis AA, Jakob RP. Anterior cruciate ligament graft positioning, tensioning and twisting. Knee Surg Sports Traumatol Arthrosc. 1998;6(1):S2-12.
46. Jackson DW, Grood ES, Wilcox P, et al. The effects of processing techniques on the mechanical properties of bone-anterior cruciate ligament-bone allografts. Am J Sports Med. 1988;16(2):101-5.
47. Jackson DW, Grood ES, Cohn BT, et al. The effects of in situ freezing on the anterior cruciate ligament. An experimental study in goats. J Bone Joint Surg Am. 1991;73(2):201-13.
48. Akelman MR, Fadale PD, Hulstyn MJ, et al. Effect of matching or overconstraining knee laxity during anterior cruciate ligament reconstruction on knee osteoarthritis and clinical outcomes. Am J Sports Med. 2016;44(7):1660-70.

49. Yasuda K, Tsujino J, Tanabe Y, et al. Effects of initial graft tension on clinical outcome after anterior cruciate ligament reconstruction. Am J Sports Med. 1997;25(1):99-106.
50. Kim SG, Kurosawa H, Sakuraba K, et al. The effect of initial graft tension on postoperative clinical outcome in anterior cruciate ligament reconstruction with semitendinosus tendon. Arch Orthop Trauma Surg. 2005;126(4):260-4.
51. Arneja S, McConkey MO, Mulpuri K, et al. Graft tensioning in anterior cruciate ligament reconstruction: a systematic review of randomized controlled trials. Arthroscopy. 2009;25(2):200-7.
52. Peña E, Martínez MA, Calvo B, et al. A finite element simulation of the effect of graft stiffness and graft tensioning in ACL reconstruction. Clin Biomech. 2005;20(6):636-44.
53. Suggs J, Wang C, Li G. The effect of graft stiffness on knee joint biomechanics after ACL reconstruction—a 3D computational simulation. Clin Biomech. 2003;18(1):35-43.
54. Nicholas SJ, D'Amato MJ, Mullaney MJ, et al. A prospectively randomized double-blind study on the effect of initial graft tension on knee stability after anterior cruciate ligament reconstruction. Am J Sports Med. 2004;32(8):1-6.
55. Cunningham R, West JR, Greis PE, et al. A survey of the tension applied to a doubled hamstring tendon graft for reconstruction of the anterior cruciate ligament. Arthroscopy. 2002;18(9):983-8.
56. Fujii M, Furumatsu T, Miyazawa S, et al. Features of human autologous hamstring graft elongation after pre-tensioning in anterior cruciate ligament reconstruction. Int Orthop. 2016;40(12):2553-8.
57. Howard ME, Cawley PW, Losse GM, et al. Bone—patellar tendon—bone grafts for anterior cruciate ligament reconstruction: The effects of graft pretensioning. Arthroscopy. 1996;12(3):287-92.
58. Jisa KA, Williams BT, Jaglowski JR, et al. Lack of consensus regarding pretensioning and preconditioning protocols for soft tissue graft reconstruction of the anterior cruciate ligament. Knee Surg Sports Traumatol Arthrosc. 2015;24(9):2884-91.
59. McRae SM, Chahal J, Leiter JR, et al. Survey study of members of the Canadian Orthopaedic Association on the natural history and treatment of anterior cruciate ligament injury. Clin J Sport Med. 2011;21(3):249-58.
60. Kirwan GW, Bourke MG, Chipchase L, et al. Graft tensioning practices in anterior cruciate ligament reconstruction amongst orthopaedic surgeons in Australia: a national survey. Arch Orthop Trauma Surg. 2015;135(12):1733-41.
61. O'Neill BJ, Byrne FJ, Hirpara KM, et al. Anterior cruciate ligament graft tensioning. is the maximal sustained one-handed pull technique reproducible? BMC Res Notes. 2011;4(1):244.
62. Grunau PD, Arneja S, Leith JM. A randomized clinical trial to assess the clinical effectiveness of a measured objective tensioning device in hamstring anterior cruciate ligament reconstruction. Am J Sports Med. 2016;44(6):1482-6.
63. Kirwan GW, Bourke MG, Chipchase L, et al. Initial graft tension and the effect on postoperative patient functional outcomes in anterior cruciate ligament reconstruction. Arthroscopy. 2013;29(5):934-41.
64. Dhaher YY, Salehghaffari S, Adouni M. Anterior laxity, graft-tunnel interaction and surgical design variations during anterior cruciate ligament reconstruction: A probabilistic simulation of the surgery. J Biomech. 2016;49(13):3009-16.
65. Gertel TH, Lew WD, Lewis JL, et al. Effect of anterior cruciate ligament graft tensioning direction, magnitude, and flexion angle on knee biomechanics. Am J Sports Med. 1993;21(4):572-81.
66. Asahina S, Muneta T, Ishibashi T, et al. Effects of knee flexion angle at graft fixation on the outcome of anterior cruciate ligament reconstruction. Arthroscopy. 1996;12(1):70-5.
67. Amis AA. The functions of the fibre bundles of the anterior cruciate ligament in anterior drawer, rotational laxity and the pivot shift. Knee Surg Sports Traumatol Arthrosc. 2012;20(4):613-20.
68. Christel PS, Akgun U, Yasar T, et al. The contribution of each anterior cruciate ligament bundle to the Lachman test: a cadaver investigation. J Bone Joint Surg Br. 2012;94-B(1):68-74.
69. Fleming BC, Beynnon BD, Nichols CE, et al. An in vivo comparison of anterior tibial translation and strain in the anteromedial band of the anterior cruciate ligament. J Biomech. 1993;26(1):51-8.
70. Muneta T, Koga H, Ju YJ, et al. Effects of different initial bundle tensioning strategies on the outcome of double-bundle ACL reconstruction: a cohort study. Sports Med Arthrosc Rehabil Ther Technol. 2011;3(1):15.

71. Asagumo H, Kimura M, Kobayashi Y, et al. Anatomic reconstruction of the anterior cruciate ligament using double-bundle hamstring tendons: surgical techniques, clinical outcomes, and complications. Arthroscopy. 2007;23(6): 602-9.
72. Otsubo H, Shino K, Nakamura N, et al. Arthroscopic evaluation of ACL grafts reconstructed with the anatomical two-bundle technique using hamstring tendon autograft. Knee Surg Sports Traumatol Arthrosc. 2007;15(6): 720-8.
73. Vercillo F, Woo SLY, Noorani SY, et al. Determination of a safe range of knee flexion angles for fixation of the grafts in double-bundle anterior cruciate ligament reconstruction: a human cadaveric study. Am J Sports Med. 2007;35(9):1513-20.
74. Cuomo P, Rama KR, Bull AM, et al. The effects of different tensioning strategies on knee laxity and graft tension after double-bundle anterior cruciate ligament reconstruction. Am J Sports Med. 2007;35(12):2083-90.
75. Murray PJ, Alexander JW, Gold JE, et al. Anatomic double-bundle anterior cruciate ligament reconstruction: kinematics and knee flexion angle–graft tension relation. Arthroscopy. 2010; 26(2):202-13.
76. Miura K. Effects of Knee Flexion Angles for Graft Fixation on Force Distribution in Double-Bundle Anterior Cruciate Ligament Grafts. Am J Sport Med. 2006;34(4):577-85.
77. Hoshino Y, Kuroda R, Nagamune K, et al. The effect of graft tensioning in anatomic 2-bundle ACL reconstruction on knee joint kinematics. Knee Surg Sport Traumatol Arthrosc. 2006;15(5):508-14.
78. Mae T, Shino K, Matsumoto N, et al. Anatomic double-bundle anterior cruciate ligament reconstruction using hamstring tendons with minimally required initial tension. Arthroscopy. 2010;26(10):1289-95.
79. Koga H, Muneta T, Yagishita K, et al. Effect of initial graft tension on knee stability and graft tension pattern in double-bundle anterior cruciate ligament reconstruction. Arthroscopy. 2015;31(9):1756-63.
80. Kondo E, Yasuda K, Kitamura N, et al. Effects of initial graft tension on clinical outcome after anatomic double-bundle anterior cruciate ligament reconstruction: comparison of two graft tension protocols. BMC Musculoskelet Disord. 2016;17(1):65.
81. Nakamura K, Koga H, Sekiya I, et al. Dynamic evaluation of pivot-shift phenomenon in double-bundle anterior cruciate ligament reconstruction using triaxial accelerometer. Arthroscopy. 2016;32(12):2532-8.

CHAPTER

22

All-inside ACL Reconstruction

SR Sundararajan, Amit Kumar Jha, Balaji Sambandam, S Rajasekaran

INTRODUCTION

Anterior cruciate ligament (ACL) reconstruction techniques have evolved over the years due to a better understanding of ACL anatomy of the femoral and tibial insertions of its two bundles. In the past decade, primary focus has been on anatomical ACL reconstruction with femoral tunnel placement at the native footprint to restore normal kinematics and function of the knee. The femoral tunnel traditionally has been created by a transtibial technique. Recently, with increase in anatomic ACL reconstruction, several authors have advocated independent femoral tunnel drilling using the anteromedial (AM) portal technique.[1-3] This technique, however, is associated with several potential pitfalls like socket blowout or difficulty in visualizing the position of the guide wire when the knee is brought to the hyperflexion position.[4] Hence, in order to avoid these pitfalls, the creation of the ACL femoral tunnel using an outside-in technique has been recommended by some authors.[5,6] The traditional outside-in technique for creating the ACL femoral socket has fallen out of favor since it involves lateral-distal femoral muscle splitting and being a more invasive technique.[7,8] However, with advances in instrumentation, minimally invasive procedure for ACL reconstruction has been developed called the all-inside technique. In this technique, specifically designed narrow-diameter guide pins that may be transformed into retrograde drills are used,[6,9] allowing "no-incision" outside-in technique for creating the ACL femoral socket. A tibial socket is made instead of tibial tunnel and graft is fixed with adjustable loop cortical button on both femoral and tibial sides. Hence, complications related to tibial tunnel and graft fixation with interference screw are also avoided.

ADVANTAGES OF THE ALL-INSIDE ACL RECONSTRUCTION TECHNIQUE

- ACL femoral socket is created in the comfortable position of 90 degrees knee flexion and allows for independent anatomic femoral tunnel placement.
- Longer socket compared with the AM portal technique can be made by adjusting outside in jig[10] as this technique allows measurement of the femoral intraosseous distance before socket creation, by using standard outside-in femoral guide and guide pin sleeves.
- Premeasurement is a safety feature of the outside-in technique because a short distance may allow less graft tissue be contained within the femoral socket.[11]
- All-epiphyseal pediatric ACL reconstruction without damaging physis can be performed with this technique.

- Lower Visual Analog Scale (VAS) pain score compared to AM portal technique as there is no breach in outer tibial cortex.[12]
- Improved cosmesis and no graft-related morbidity when allograft used.
- Proper visualization of femoral footprint as AM portal acts as viewing portal and jig is passed through AL portal.

In addition, technical developments, which simplify all-inside ACL reconstruction, are:

- Retrograde drilling
- Second generation buttons have graft loops that are adjustable in length, such that after the button flips and becomes fixed on the cortex, the graft loop can be tightened, pulling the graft into the socket in a manner that completely fills the socket with graft tissue. Second-generation adjustable graft loop buttons are unique in the sense that further tightening increases the graft tension thereby allowing us to tension the graft even after fixation in the socket.
- Use of cannulas for maintaining portals and preventing soft tissue from becoming intertwined in sutures while passing graft through AM portal.

SPECIAL EQUIPMENT

- Graft-preparation station and high-strength suture; e.g. No. 2 FiberWire® (Arthrex, Naples, FL) (Fig. 22.1)

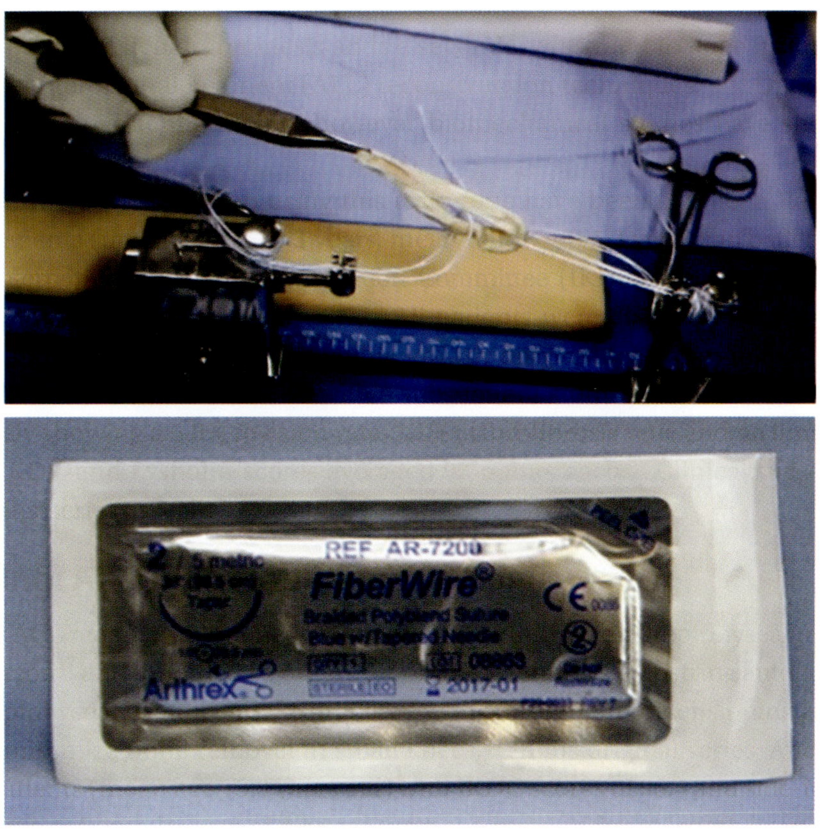

Fig. 22.1: Graft-preparation station and high-strength suture [e.g. No. 2 FiberWire® (Arthrex)].

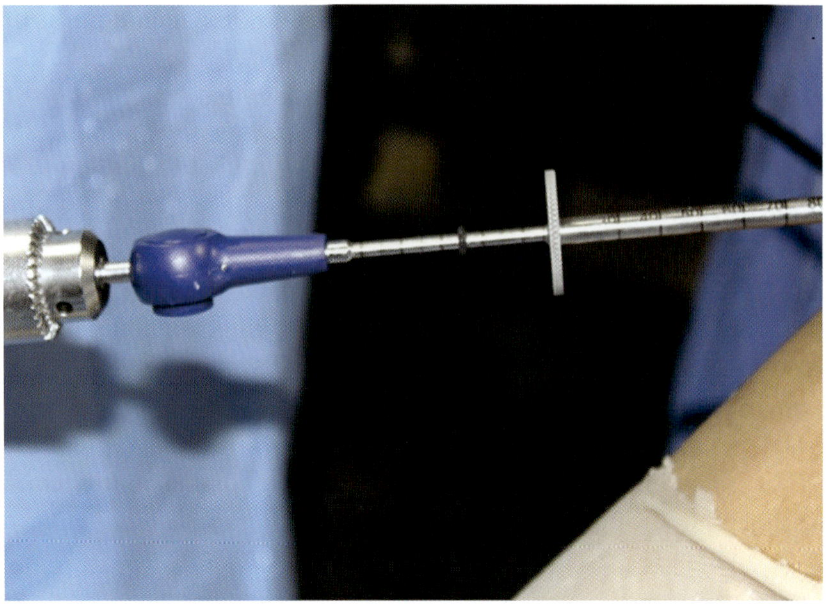

Fig. 22.2: FlipCutter® and FlipCutter® guide pin sleeve.

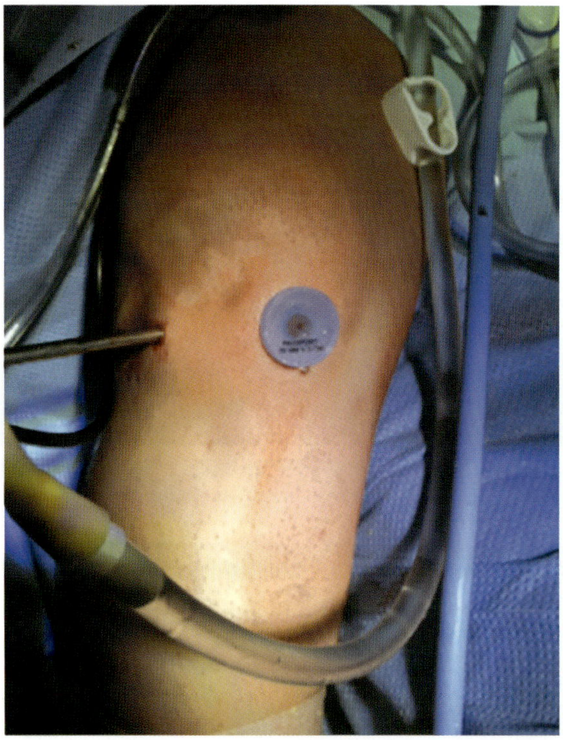

Fig. 22.3: PassPort® Cannula (Arthrex).

- FlipCutter® and FlipCutter® guide pin sleeve (Arthrex, Naples, FL) (Fig. 22.2)
- PassPort® Cannula (Arthrex, Naples, FL) (Fig. 22.3)

ALL-INSIDE ACL RECONSTRUCTION WITH GRAFTLINK® TECHNIQUE STEP-BY-STEP

Graft Selection

Autograft

Most often semitendinosus graft alone is sufficient as a quadrupled graft of minimum 65–70 mm length is required. In cases where the semitendinosus is short or of inadequate diameter, gracilis can be secondarily harvested.

Allograft

"No-incision" graft choice with no graft harvest-site morbidity. Usually tibialis posterior and peroneus longus tendons are used. However, allograft has its own merits and demerits.

Graft Length

It is very important to understand before preparing the graft in all-inside technique that sockets are created and not full bone tunnel. Therefore, to tension the graft, it must not bottom out in the sockets. So, the total graft length must be less than the sum of femoral socket length plus intra-articular graft distance plus tibial socket length. This prevents bottoming out of the graft in the sockets and graft loosening. A graft length of not more than 75 mm, after tensioning, is a general guideline, and this distance is adjusted according to patient size.

Graft Preparation

- Placing two TightRope® RT (Arthrex, Naples, FL) over the posts of an ACL graft preparation stand so that the loops face each other.
- Passing the graft through loop so that it forms quadrupled strand.
- Both free ends of graft stitched to each other with No. 0 FiberWire, so that the graft forms a closed loop with TightRope® RT on both sides (Fig. 22.4).

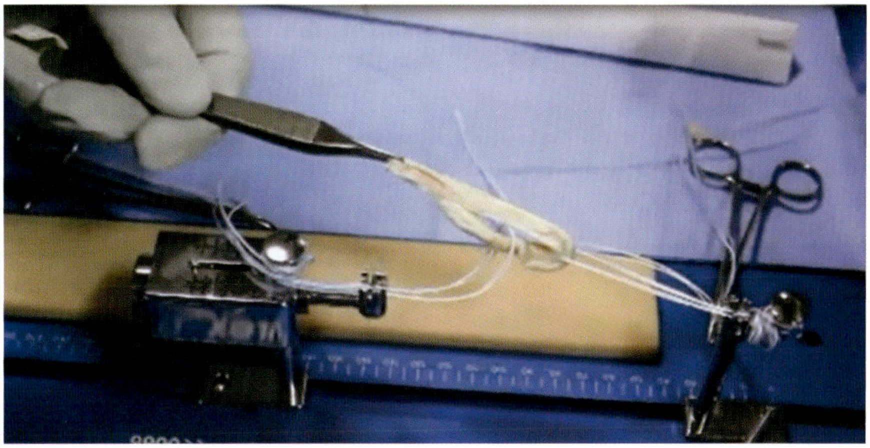

Fig. 22.4: Free ends of the graft being stitched with No. 0 FiberWire®.

- Both femoral and tibial ends of graft stitched approximately 1.5 cm from ends in the following manner:
    - First bite taken into two of the four strands from center to outer strands (3-4) as shown in Figure 22.5A.
    - Then in reverse way bite taken through all strands (4-3-2-1) and again through all strands (1-2-3-4) as shown in Figures 22.5B and C.

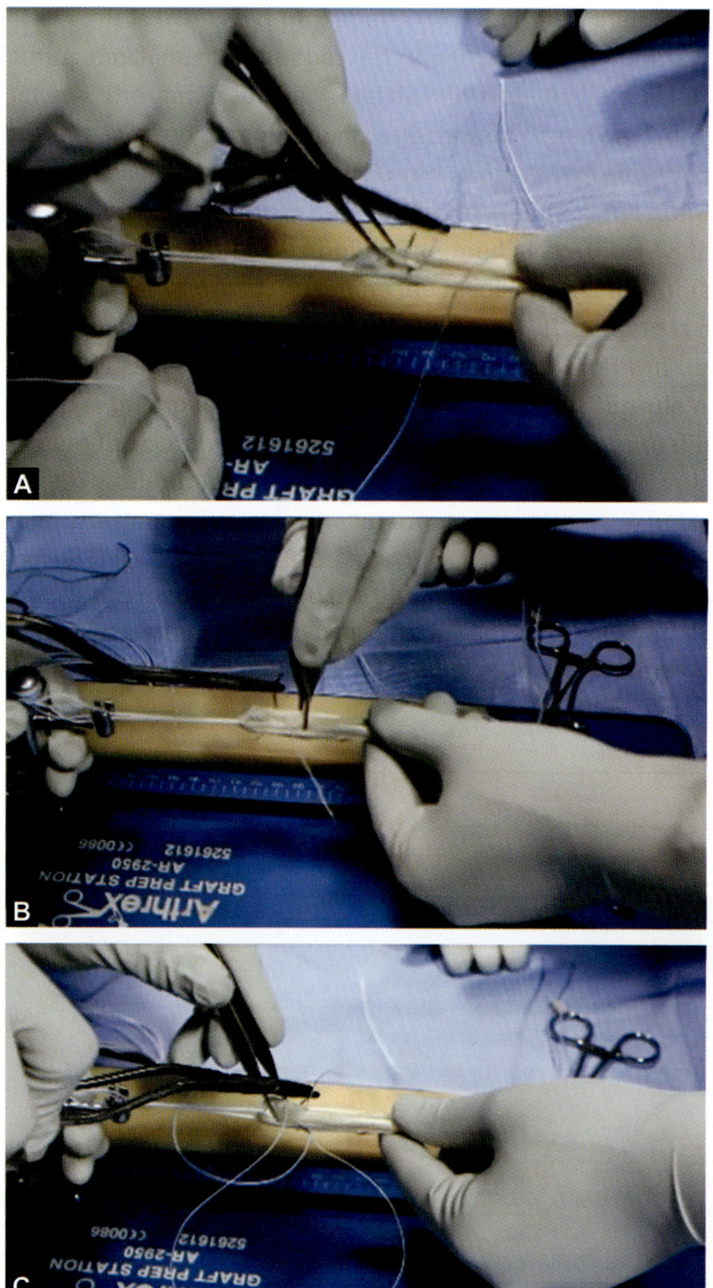

Figs. 22.5A to C: (A) First bite taken into two of the four strands from center to outer strands; (B) The needle is then reversed to take a bite through all four strands; (C) The needle is reversed again and a bite is taken through all four strands.

- FiberWire® wrapped three turns around all four strands and bite taken through two strands (4–3) in such a way that needle end of FiberWire® comes to the center and knotting done and smaller end of suture is cut (Figs. 22.6A and B).
- The knot is buried by taking bite in two strands into out (2–1) and FiberWire® cut flush with the graft (Fig. 22.7).

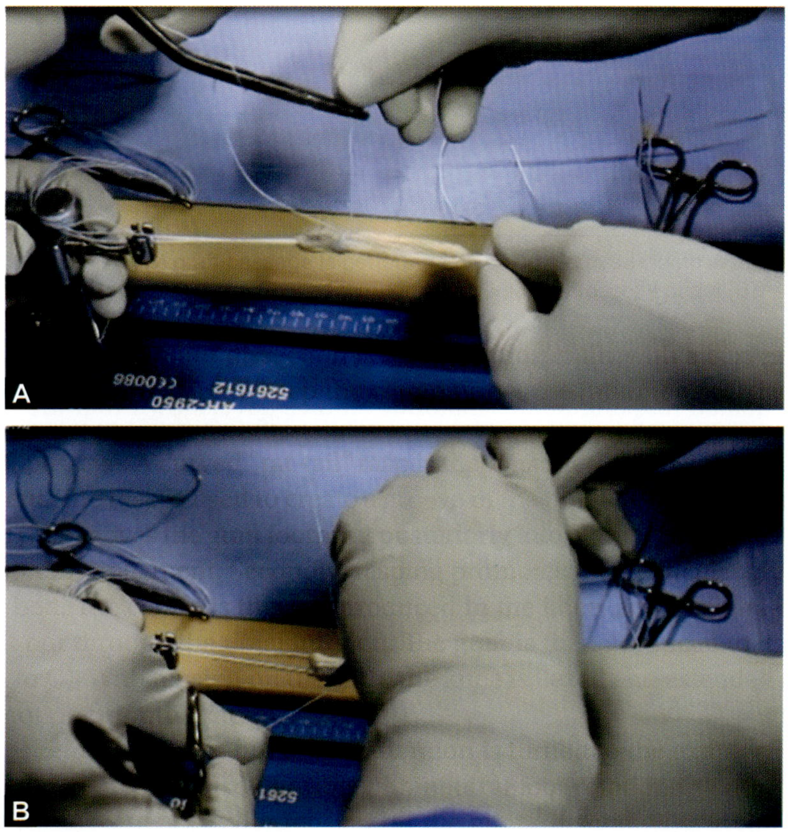

Figs. 22.6A and B: The FiberWire® ends are knotted after taking three turns around the graft; (B) Cutting of shorter end of FiberWire® after knotting.

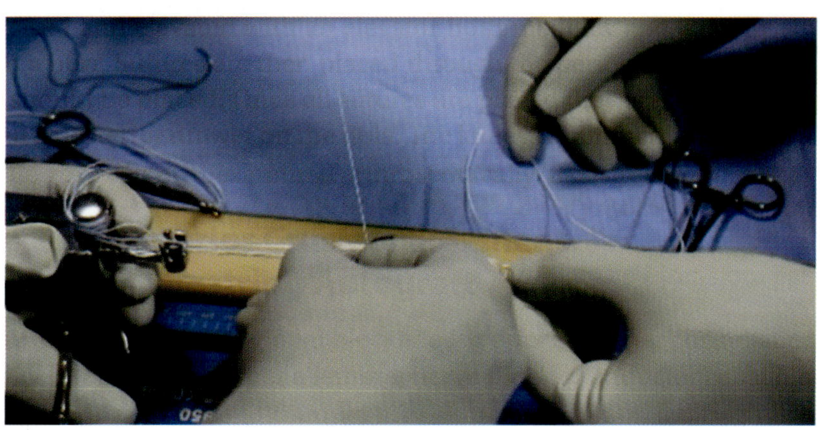

Fig. 22.7: Cutting the FiberWire® after burying the knot by passing the needle through two strands from center to outside.

Femoral Socket Creation

It is essential to precisely identify the anatomic ACL footprint center on both the femoral and tibial sides.[13-16] Soft-tissue notchplasty is performed and some patients may need bony notchplasty when there is a small notch orifice. Ideal is to mark the footprint anatomy with radiofrequency for proper placement of the jig. AM portal viewing provides an improved perspective for analyzing the ACL femoral footprint anatomy and to adjust the mark to ensure precise identification of center of the footprint.

Positioning the Femoral Jig

Surgeons have their choice of point-to-point marking hooks (Fig. 22.8A), or "footprint" marking hooks (Fig. 22.8B) which allow visualization of the round socket before drilling.

In cases where the *native ACL stump is visible*, the footprint guides facilitate recreating native femoral positioning by replicating tunnel shape and size before drilling. The low profile tip of the guide is placed through the lateral portal for best possiblc visualization of the socket edges in relation to the cartilage border and posterior wall as shown in Figures 22.9A to C.

In cases where the *ACL stump is not visible*, the direct measurement technique may be used with the assistance of the graduated marking hook. Anatomic studies have shown that the average center of the ACL footprint, or the bifurcate ridge, is located approximately half (43%) of the distance from the proximal cartilage border to the distal cartilage border[17] as shown in Figure 22.10.

With the knee flexed to 90°, the notch can be measured using the graduated FlipCutter® marking hook. The guide should be placed through the lateral portal and held parallel to the long axis of the femur.

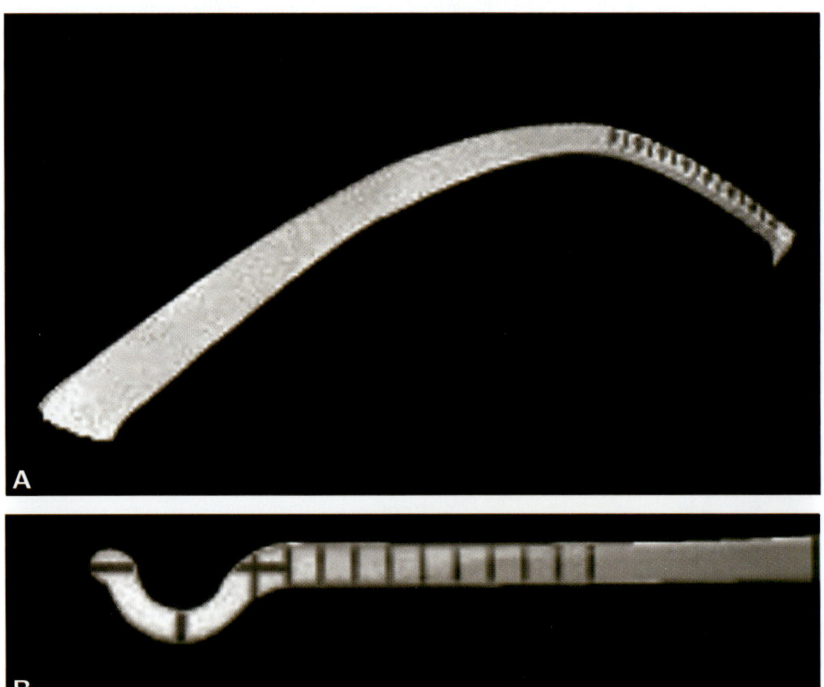

Figs. 22.8A and B: (A) Point-to-point marking hook; (B) "Footprint" marking hook.

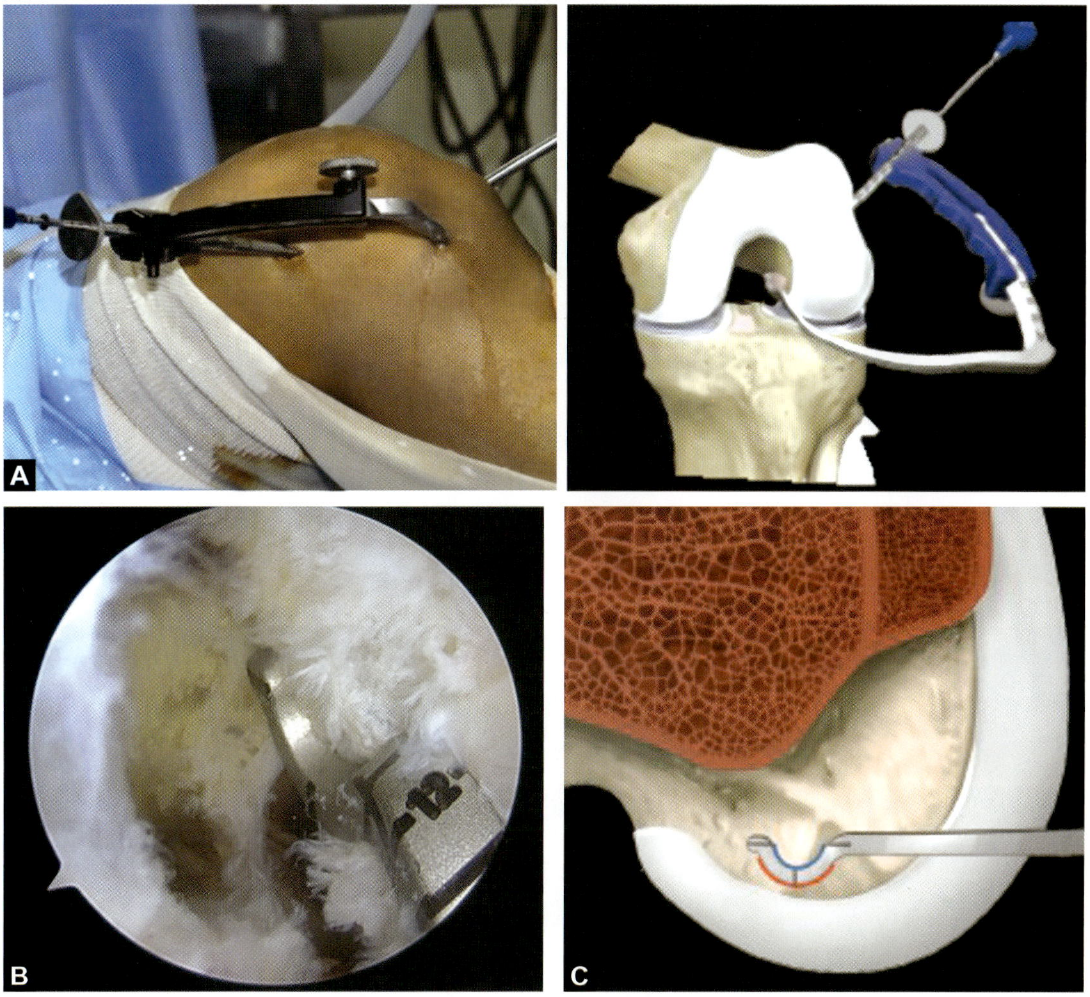

Figs. 22.9A to C: (A) Positioning of jig through anterolateral portal (external view); (B and C) Arthroscopic view of jig placement at femoral footprint.

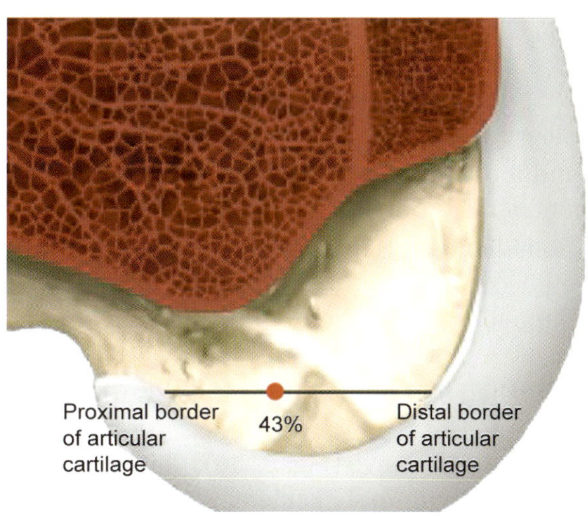

Fig. 22.10: ACL femoral footprint center.

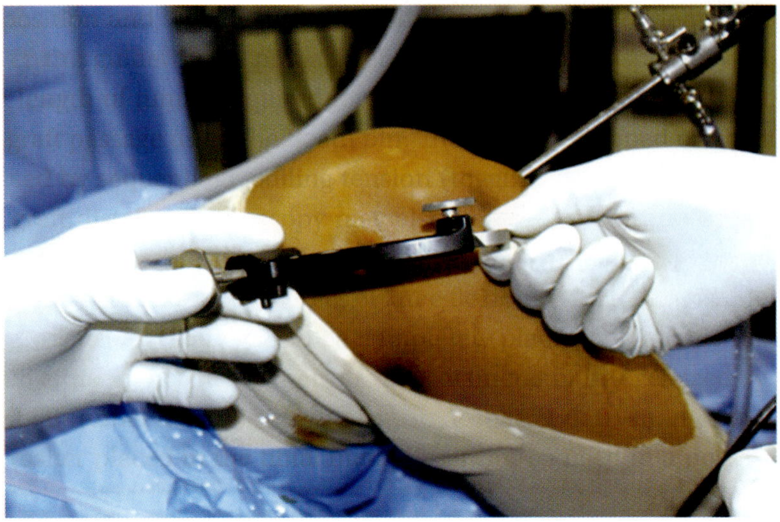

Fig. 22.11: Cannulated guide pin sleeve of FlipCutter® is pushed hard onto the lateral femoral cortex.

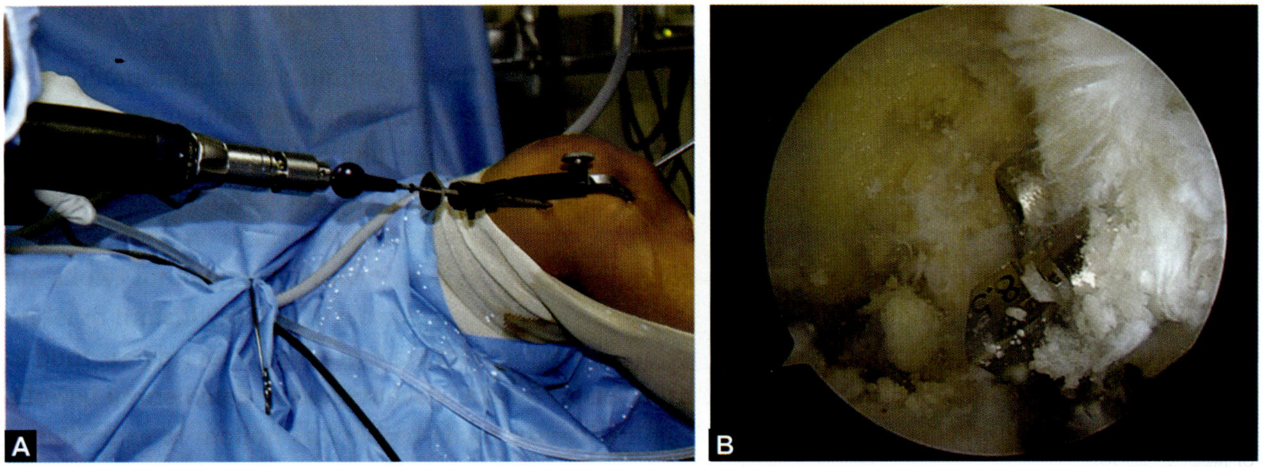

Figs. 22.12A and B: (A) Drilling FlipCutter® into joint (external view); (B) Arthroscopic view showing FlipCutter® entering through femoral footprint.

- The FlipCutter® guide pin sleeve is advanced to the level of the skin and at that point a stab incision is made through the skin and iliotibial band. The cannulated guide pin sleeve for the FlipCutter® is pushed hard on to bone over lateral femur as shown in Figure 22.11.
- FlipCutter® of same size as graft diameter is drilled into joint and the jig is removed as shown in Figures 22.12A and B.
- The 7 mm drill sleeve tip is tapped into bone lightly with a mallet (Fig. 22.13) to prevent cortical blow-out while retrograde drilling.
- Button on the FlipCutter® is pushed and blue hub is slid forward to flip blade into cutting position as in Figures 22.14A and B.
- Depth marker is set to base of the drill sleeve (Fig. 22.15). Before this, it must be confirmed that blade of drill is in touch with bone to get accurate socket length. In case where we preserve stump, that extra length of stump size must to be drilled, otherwise the socket length will be smaller than desired.

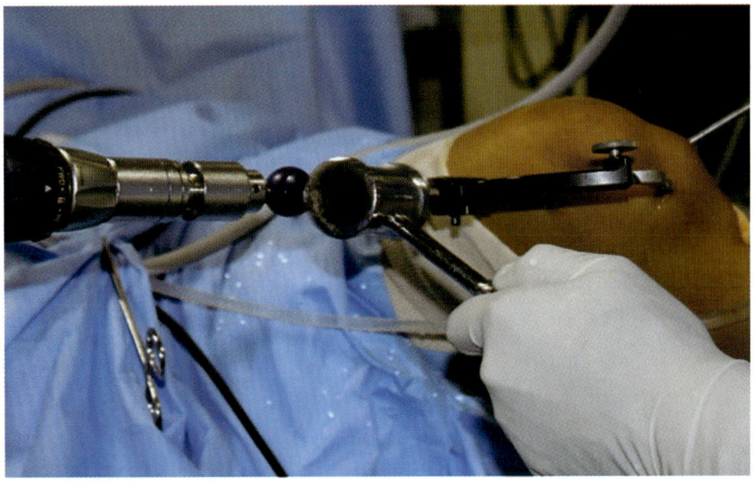

Fig. 22.13: Tapping the 7 mm drill sleeve tip into bone lightly with a mallet.

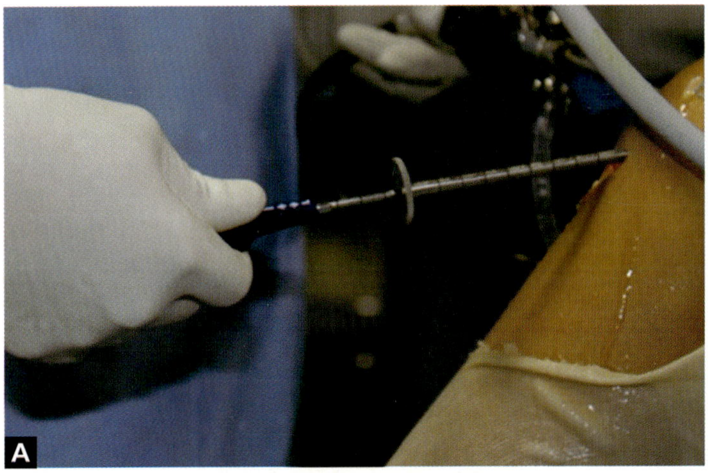

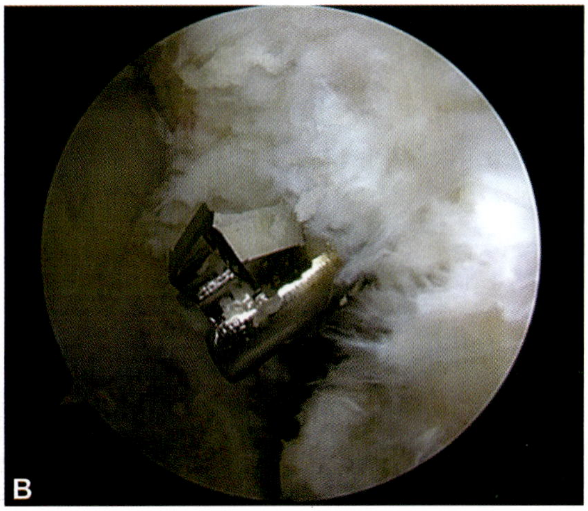

Figs. 22.14A and B: (A) Button is pushed and blue hub is slid forward to flip blade into cutting position; (B) Arthroscopic view of flipped blade.

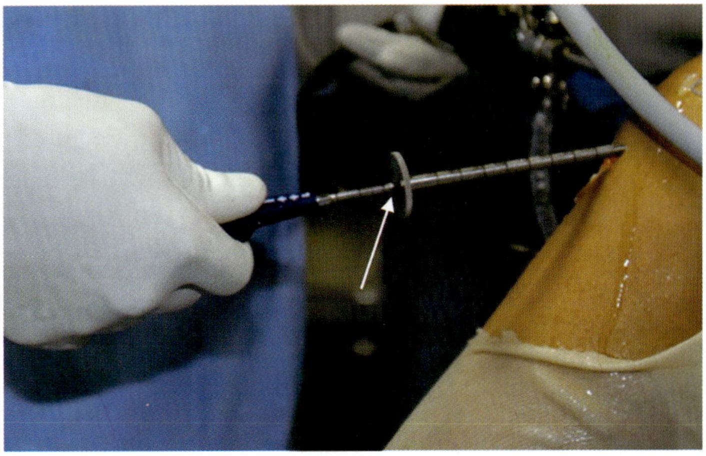

Fig. 22.15: Depth marker (shown with white arrow) is set to base of the drill sleeve.

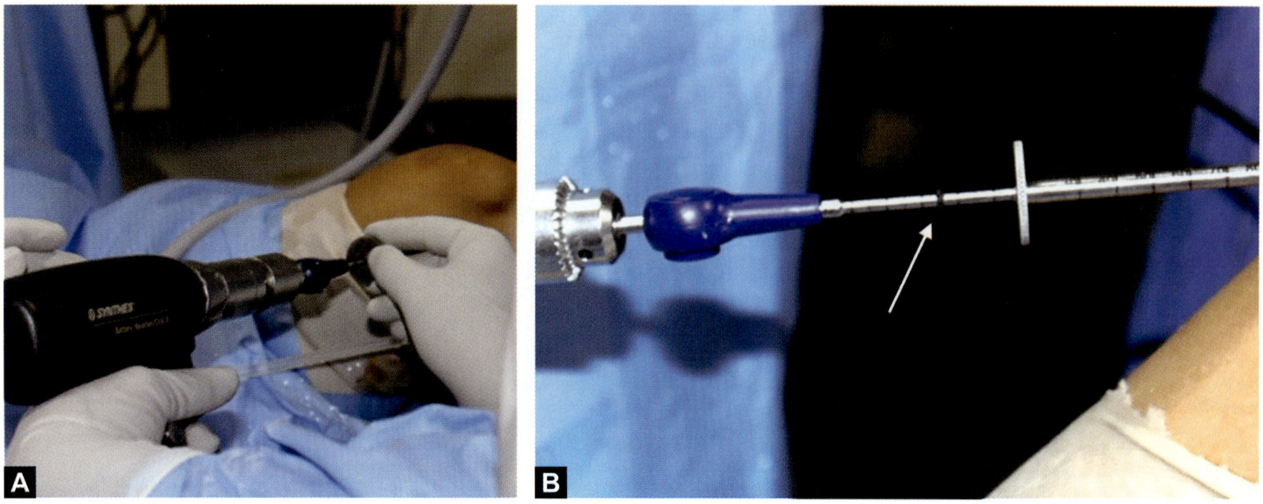

Figs. 22.16A and B: (A) Forward pressure is applied to hold the sleeve while drilling; (B) Socket length may be read off on the pin by seeing position of black rubber marker (white arrow).

- Drilling is done until FlipCutter® "bottoms out" on the drill sleeve, while applying forward pressure to hold onto sleeve (Fig. 22.16A). This ensures creation of a socket, preventing a lateral cortex blow-out. Socket length may be read off on the pin (Fig. 22.16B).
- Forward drilling then performed to visualize the flipped blade in the joint. The blade is straightened by pushing the button and sliding blue hub back. The FlipCutter® is removed and the sleeve held in place.
- A loop of FiberWire® (Arthrex) is advanced through the cannulated guide pin sleeve with help of open eyelet guide pin (Figs. 22.17A and B). The arthroscope is shifted to the anterolateral portal and the loop is retrieved through the AM portal. This femoral graft passing FiberWire® loop is docked with a small clamp during tibial surgery.

Tibial Socket Creation

With the arthroscope in the anterolateral portal, the FlipCutter® ACL tibial marking hook is locked on the FlipCutter® guide ring at an angle of approximately 55–60° and placed at tibial foot print (Fig. 22.18). Guide position and angle are optimized to maximize tibial intraosseous distance so that the graft does not bottom out during tensioning. Distance may be read on the FlipCutter® guide pin sleeve before drilling. As a preventative measure, if the distance is short, the guide should be readjusted before drilling. Tibial socket creation is completed with the FlipCutter® following the same steps as described in the "Femoral Socket Creation" section.

Marking the Graft

The first distance that should be measured and marked (Fig. 22.19) on the GraftLink® construct is the femoral aperture-cortex distance. This distance should be marked on the adjustable graft loop, measuring from the tip of the cortical suspensory button, while the surgeon holds the button in a "pre-flipped" position. During graft

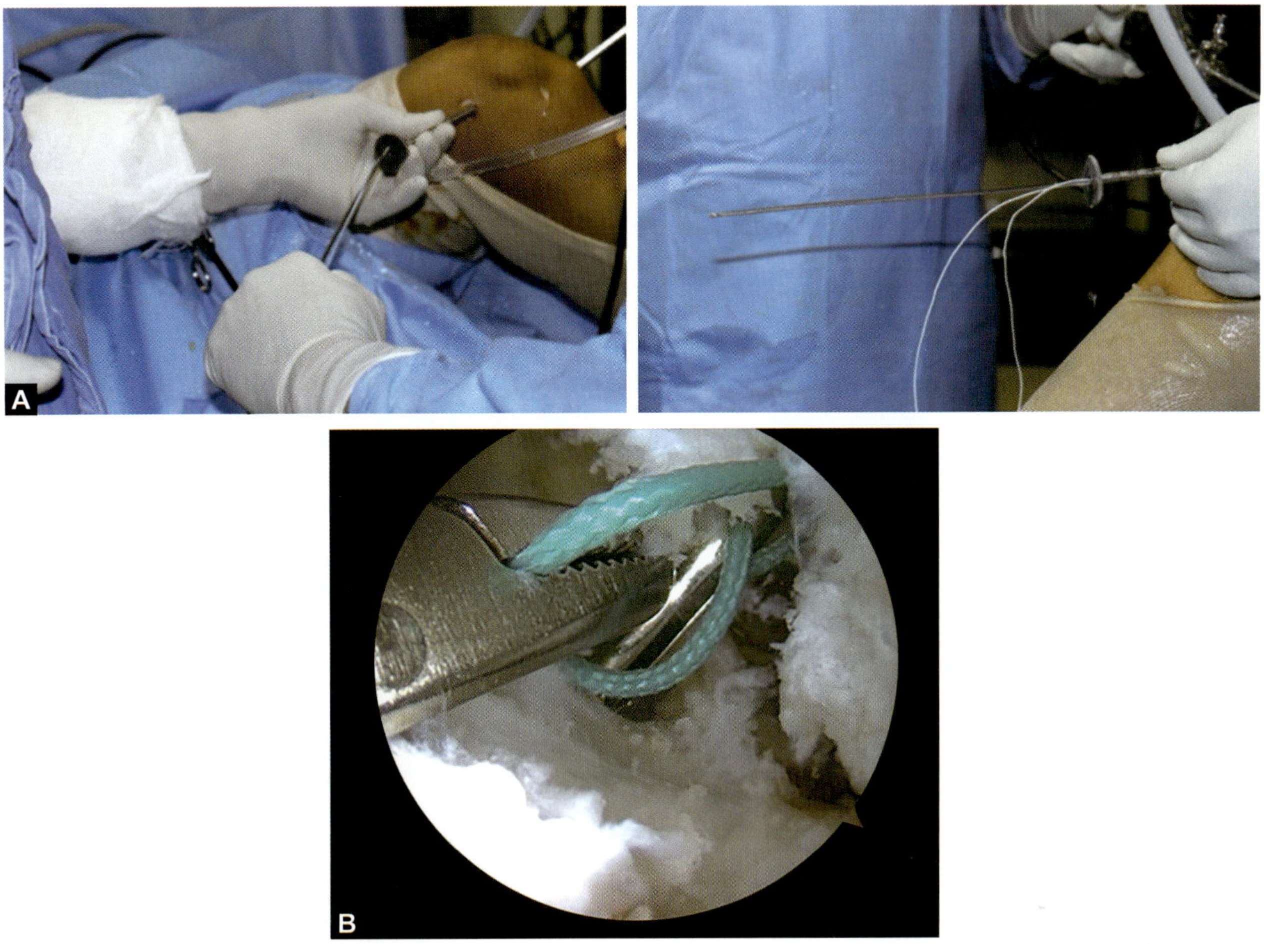

Figs. 22.17A and B: (A) A FiberWire® loop is advanced through the cannulated guide pin sleeve with help of open eyelet guide pin; (B) Arthroscopic view showing femoral graft—passing FiberWire® loop retrieval.

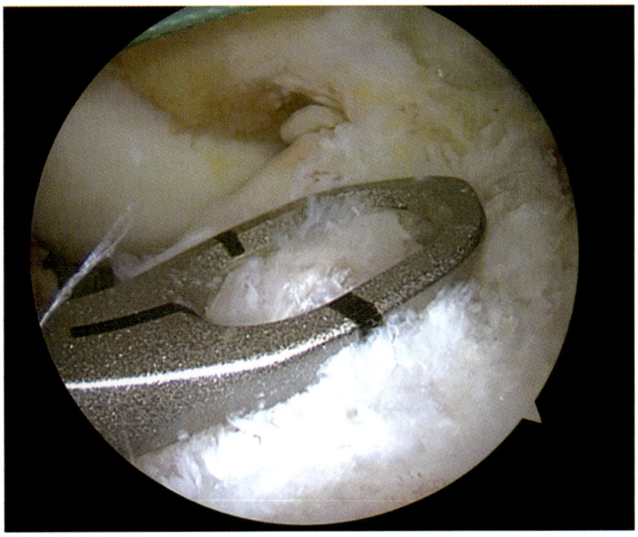

Fig. 22.18: Arthroscopic view showing the jig at tibial footprint center.

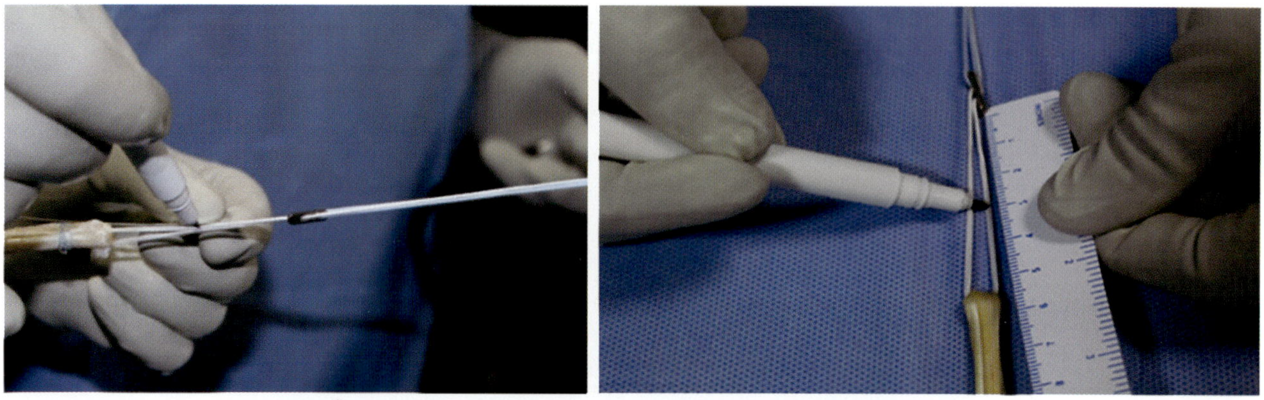

Fig. 22.19: Marking on GraftLink® corresponding to the femoral aperture-cortex distance.

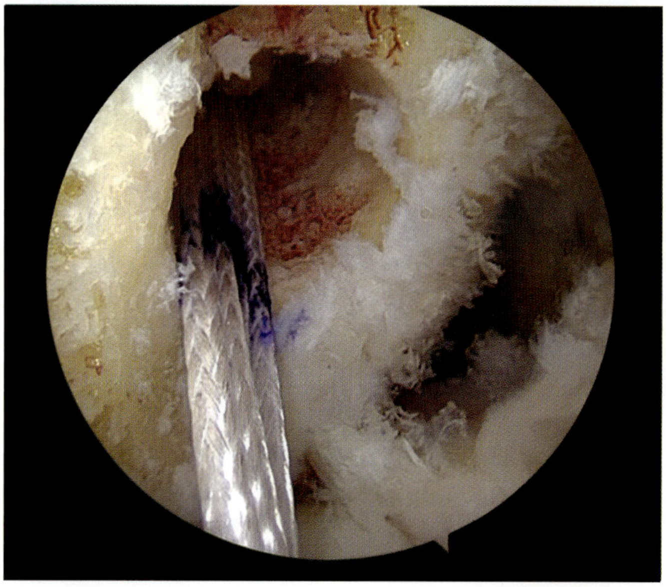

Fig. 22.20: Point when the mark on the loop reaches the entry of the socket, the button flips over the outer cortex.

passage, when the mark on the adjustable graft loop reaches the femoral socket orifice, this indicates that the button is in position to flip (Fig. 22.20).

The second distance that should be measured and marked on the GraftLink® construct is the length of graft within the femoral socket. The goal is to maximize collagen in the socket but ensure that the graft is not bottoming out during tensioning. A typical amount of graft in the femoral socket is 25 mm. This distance is marked on the graft itself, measuring from the femoral end. During graft passage, when the mark on the graft reaches the femoral socket orifice, this indicates that femoral graft tensioning is complete.

This is repeated for the tibial side of the graft.

Graft Passage

A cannula (PassPort®, Arthrex) prevents soft tissue interposition and is essential because the graft is passed through the AM arthroscopic portal. If a cannula is not used then both femoral and tibial

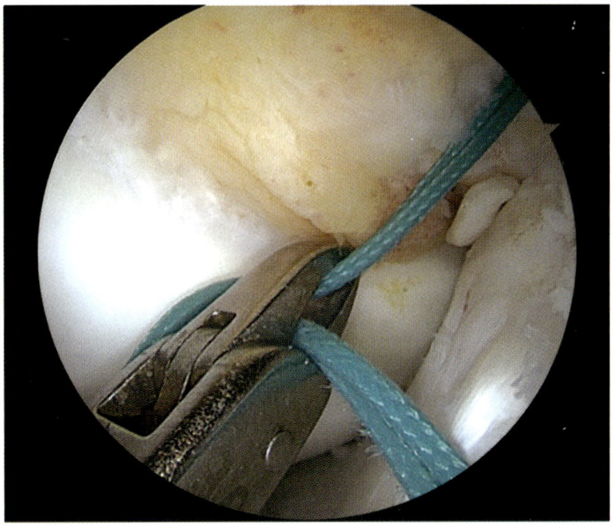

Fig. 22.21: Graft passing suture loops of femur and tibia are retrieved simultaneously through anteromedial (AM) portal to prevent soft tissue entanglement while passing graft.

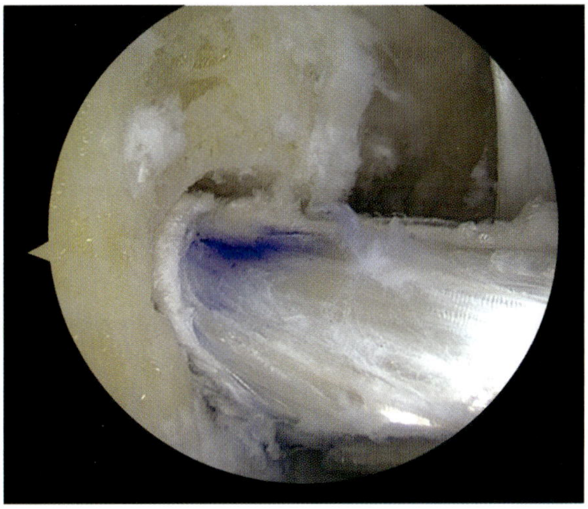

Fig. 22.22: Marking on the graft has reached the entry of femoral socket indicating that the graft has filled the socket completely.

graft passing FibreWire® loops are retrieved simultaneously through AM portal to prevent soft tissue entanglement (Fig. 22.21).

Graft Fixation

The femoral graft-passing suture loop is pulled through the distal-lateral femoral stab incision until the mark on the graft loop reaches the socket orifice under direct arthroscopic visualization, indicating that the button has flipped over the femoral cortex proximally. Once the button flips, we pull the white sutures on the TightRope® RT until the mark on the graft reaches the socket orifice which suggests that graft had filled the femoral socket (Fig. 22.22).

The *flip-then-fill technique* is repeated on the tibial side.

Graft Tensioning

The knee is moved through its range of motion, and additional tension may be applied by pulling the femoral or tibial pull sutures by hand. Knots may be tied to at both ends to increase the tension.

Rehabilitation

Rehabilitation is the same as standard ACL rehabilitation with any other technique.

PEARLS

- The total graft length must be less than the sum of femoral socket length plus intra-articular graft distance plus tibial socket length. Therefore, length of the graft should be measured after tensioning and accordingly sockets must be prepared. Otherwise, there will be a mismatch between total graft length and socket length and bottoming out. To prevent bottoming out of graft in socket and loosening, it is safer to create an extra 5 mm socket length on femoral side and final tightening of graft from femoral side done only after fixing the graft on the tibial side.
- Socket diameter should be a snug fit to ensure biological graft incorporation. If the graft is too large, it could get stuck at the socket orifices after the button is flipped, and this represents an intraoperative problem.
  Bailout solutions include:
  - If the adjustable loop is visible, cutting the loop arthroscopically allows the button to be pulled out of the thigh with passing sutures;
  - The other option is open button removal by extending the distal-lateral femoral stab incision.

  After removal of button, the graft can be retrieved and trimmed or the socket can be redrilled to a larger size. Therefore, "one should never undersize the socket diameter."
- After drilling the socket till passage of suture loop, the drill sleeve must be held in place. Otherwise, it becomes difficult to locate the tunnel on the lateral femoral or medial tibial cortex.

REFERENCES

1. Kim HS, Seon JK, Jo AR. Current trends in anterior cruciate ligament reconstruction. Knee Surg Relat Res. 2013;25: 165-73.
2. Mulcahey MK, David TS, Epstein DM, et al. Transtibial versus anteromedial portal anterior cruciate ligament reconstruction using soft-tissue graft and expandable fixation. Arthroscopy. 2014;30:1461-7.
3. Harner CD, Honkamp NJ, Ranawat AS. Anteromedial portal technique for creating the anterior cruciate ligament femoral tunnel. Arthroscopy. 2008;24:113-5.
4. Lubowitz JH. Anteromedial portal technique for the anterior cruciate ligament femoral socket: Pitfalls and solutions. Arthroscopy. 2009;25:95-101.
5. Lubowitz JH, Ahmad CS, Anderson K. All-inside anterior cruciate ligament graft-link technique: Second generation, no-incision anterior cruciate ligament reconstruction. Arthroscopy. 2011;27: 717-27.
6. Kim SG, Kurosawa H, Sakuraba K, et al. Development and application of an inside-to-out drill bit for anterior cruciate ligament reconstruction. Arthroscopy. 2005;21:1012.
7. Harner C, Marks P, Fu F, et al. Anterior cruciate ligament reconstruction: Endoscopic versus two-incision technique. Arthroscopy.1994;10:502-12.
8. Yu J, Garrett W. Femoral tunnel placement in anterior cruciate ligament reconstruction. Oper Tech Sports Med. 2006;14:45-9.
9. Lubowitz JH, Konicek J. Anterior cruciate ligament femoral tunnel length: Cadaveric analysis comparing anteromedial portal versus outside-in technique. Arthroscopy. 2010;26:1357-62.
10. Basdekis G, Abisafi C, Christel P. Influence of knee flexion angle on femoral tunnel characteristics when drilled through the anteromedial portal during anterior cruciate ligament reconstruction. Arthroscopy. 2008;24: 459-64.

11. Zantop T, Ferretti M, Bell K, et al. Effect of tunnel-graft length on the biomechanics of anterior cruciate ligament-reconstructed knees intra-articular study in a goat model. Am J Sports Med. 2008;36:2158-66.
12. Lubotiz JH, Schwartzberg R, Smith P, et al. Randomized controlled trial comparing all-inside anterior cruciate ligament reconstruction technique with anterior cruciate ligament reconstruction with a full tibial tunnel. Arthroscopy. 2013;29(7):1195-200.
13. Colombet P, Robinson J, Christel P, et al. Morphology of anterior cruciate ligament attachments for anatomic reconstruction: A cadaveric dissection and radiographic study. Arthroscopy. 2006;22: 984-92.
14. Ho J, Gardiner A, Shah V, et al. Equal kinematics between central anatomic single-bundle and double-bundle anterior cruciate ligament reconstructions. Arthroscopy. 2009;25:464-72.
15. Kaz R, Starman JS, Fu FH. Anatomic double-bundle anterior cruciate ligament reconstruction revision surgery. Arthroscopy. 2007;23:1250.e1-e3.
16. Lubowitz J, Poehling G. Watch your footprint: Anatomic ACL reconstruction. Arthroscopy. 2009;25:1059-60.
17. Piefer JW, Pflugner TR, Hwang MD, et al. Anterior cruciate ligament femoral footprint anatomy: systematic review of the 21st century literature. Arthroscopy. 2012;28(6):872-81.

CHAPTER 23

Anterior Cruciate Ligament Reconstruction in Skeletally Immature Patients

Michael P McClincy, Mininder S Kocher

INTRODUCTION AND EPIDEMIOLOGY

Anterior cruciate ligament (ACL) tears were once considered rare in skeletally immature athletes, however due to the dramatic rise in youth athletic participation, early sports specialization, and year-round training schedules they are now increasingly recognized in younger athletic populations. A recent epidemiological study documented a threefold increase in the rate of ACL reconstruction in patients under the age of 20 years over a two-decade timespan between 1990 and 2009. This same population currently represents the largest per capita demographic of ACL reconstructions.[1] Other studies have documented similar results, demonstrating a 900% increase in ambulatory ACL procedures in adolescent patients from 1994 to 2006.[2,3]

Historically, pediatric ACL ruptures underwent nonoperative management until skeletal maturity, followed by traditional ACL reconstruction to avoid interference with normal skeletal growth. However, more recent literature has highlighted the perils of nonoperative or delayed surgical treatment on the pediatric or adolescent knee. Vavken and Murray reviewed 47 studies focusing on the operative and nonoperative management outcomes of ACL injuries in pediatric patients and showed operative reconstruction to have superior outcomes with regard to patient outcomes, future instability, and development of secondary injuries.[4] Studies have showed a time sensitive effect on delayed ACL reconstruction in pediatric patients in the development of secondary injuries.[5,6] Lawrence et al. showed delaying reconstruction more than 12 weeks was associated with a fourfold increase in medial meniscal tears, a 5.6-fold increase in medial compartment chondral injury, and an 11.5-fold increase in lateral compartment chondral injury. They also noted a continuous time-dependent relationship between surgical delay and development of medial meniscal or lateral/patellofemoral chondral injuries, with a recent series noting a 6% increased risk of meniscal tear per month of ACL reconstruction delay.[5,7] In light of these findings, surgical techniques and instrumentation have evolved, in order to accommodate the unique anatomy of skeletally immature patients.

MANAGEMENT OF PEDIATRIC ANTERIOR CRUCIATE LIGAMENT INJURIES: REVIEW OF LITERATURE

In caring for pediatric and adolescent athletes, ACL reconstruction strategies must respect growing physes. Minimal growth (<1 cm per limb segment) remains around the knee after the age of 12–13 years in girls (i.e. 1 year after menarche) and the age of 14 years in boys.[8] The true prevalence of growth disturbance following a standard ACL reconstruction in skeletally-immature athletes is likely misrepresented in the literature, as only small case series have reported on growth disturbance after ACL reconstruction.[9-15] A survey collected from members of the Herodicus Society and ACL Study Group identified 15 cases of postoperative deformity due to physeal injury, included genu valgum (femoral), tibial recurvatum and leg length discrepancy.[16] This survey, which tracked the outcomes of highly experienced surgeons, noted complications across a number of reconstruction techniques. More recent case reports and imaging studies demonstrate the potential for variably amounts of growth disturbance after a variety of reconstruction techniques, some of which include pediatric-specific modifications.[17-26] These growth disturbances resulted in limb length discrepancy and/or angular deformity due to physeal arrest, retardation, tethering, or overgrowth. Below, the commonly used techniques for pediatric ACL reconstruction are highlighted with a review of their literature regarding pertinent outcomes and complications.

Physeal-Sparing: Iliotibial Band Combined Extra- and Intra-articular Reconstruction

In prepubescent children (Tanner stage 1–2; skeletal age ≤11 years in females, ≤12 years in males), a modified MacIntosh combined intra-articular and extra-articular iliotibial band (ITB) reconstruction described by Micheli[27] and further characterized by Kocher[28] may be performed. This technique has many advantages in that it obviates the need for bone tunnels and their associated risk of physeal injury, it simplifies revision reconstructions in that it avoids the commonly used autograft tissue and preserves native bone stock, and the extra-articular tenodesis adds a secondary restraint to knee instability similar to the currently described anterolateral ligament (ALL) reconstruction techniques.[29-31] Opponents of this technique cite its nonanatomic configuration, however biomechanical studies have shown restoration of kinematic constraint.[32]

Outcomes after ACL reconstruction using this technique have been excellent. Re-tear rate was 4.5% in a cohort of 44 patients (mean age of 10.3 years, mean follow-up 5.3 years); in patients with intact grafts at follow-up, the International Knee Documentation Committee (IKDC) subjective knee score was 96.7 ±6.0 and the Lysholm knee score was 95.7±6.7.[28] All patients were able to return to their preoperative sporting activities, and no clinical or radiographic growth disturbances were noted. These results have been maintained in the longer-term as well with a subsequent study of 237 patients at an average of 6.2 years postoperatively showing a 5.8% revision rate, 2.1% arthrofibrosis rate, and no limb length or angular deformities. Pedi-IKDC and Lysholm scores averaged 93 points each.[33] Clinical success has been replicated in other smaller series as well.[34,35]

Physeal-Sparing: All-Epiphyseal

Another option for ACL reconstruction in prepubescent children is an all-epiphyseal technique originally described by Anderson[17] and modified by others[19,36,37] which employs hamstring autograft and all-epiphyseal sockets with epiphyseal fixation. Grafts prepared with subsequent pretensioning and circumferential compression may minimize bone removal in small knees.[38] In his original series, Anderson reported on 12 prepubescent patients (mean age 13.3 years old) with IKDC scores of 96.5 and side-to-side KT-1000 difference of 1.5 mm at a mean follow-up of 4.1 years without any significant length or angular limb deformity.[17] Cassard et al. noted 100% return to activities in a series of 28 subjects at 2.8 years, however this outcome was not reported in other studies.[39] Complications have been reported in the orthopedic literature which consists mostly of small and short-term series. Graft rupture rates varying from 4% to 17% have been reported.[17,19,20,39,40] A magnetic resonance imaging (MRI) study noted physeal compromise in 10/15 tibiae (67%) and 1/23 femora (4%) due to epiphyseal drilling, without clinical growth disturbances at 1 year.[41] There have, however, been reports of limb length and angular deformity after epiphyseal-only tunnel drilling, with few cases requiring surgical correction.[13,17,19,20]

Physeal Respecting: Partial Transphyseal Reconstruction

In borderline pubescent children who are nearing skeletal maturity but have limited remaining growth (e.g. Tanner stage 3), a partial-transphyseal reconstruction has been described.[24,42] In this technique, a physeal-avoiding over-the-top position or all-epiphyseal femoral tunnel is used in conjunction with a transphyseal, vertical, centrally-located tibial tunnel. This technique aims to avoid injury to the lateral distal femoral physis and resultant angular deformity while minimizing changes to the tibial tunnel preparation. Few small series have demonstrated clinical outcomes using this technique, with no significant length or angular deformity but graft rupture and subsequent cartilage/meniscal injury rates of 20–25%.[24,42]

Physeal Respecting: Transphyseal Reconstruction

In older children and adolescents with some growth remaining (Tanner stage ≥3; skeletal age ≥12 years in females, ≥13 years in males), "physeal-respecting" transphyseal reconstruction may be performed by removing an acceptable amount of physeal tissue and utilizing soft-tissue grafts with metaphyseal fixation[43-45] (Fig. 23.1). In this technique, both the tibial and femoral tunnels are created in the standard, transphyseal fashion with care to violate as little physeal tissue as possible to avoid growth disturbance. Recent clinical data suggests that transtibial ACL tunnel drilling techniques may remove less physeal tissue than independent drilling, however an independent tunnel may be created with a more vertical trajectory to accomplish the same goal.[46] Animal studies indicate that removal of less than 7% of the area of the physeal plate is not associated with an increased risk of growth disturbance; however, the applicability of this data to humans remains uncertain.[47-49]

Kocher reported the use of transphyseal ACL reconstruction in 61 knees in skeletally immature pubescent adolescents (Tanner stage 3), evaluated at a mean of 3.6 years postoperatively. This technique had a 3% revision rate; in the remaining patients the IKDC subjective knee score was 90 and the Lysholm knee score was 91. No limb length or angular deformities arose.[45] This is in line with other reports of transphyseal ACL reconstructions.[14,18,22,23,50-54] Leg length discrepancy has been reported in up to 30% of patients, however it rarely exceeds 1 cm in size.[14,18,21-23,54,55] At a mean follow-up of 2–4 years, IKDC and Lysholm scores in the 90s have been reported,[18,21-23,45,50,54] with durable results as long as 6–10 years postoperatively.[22,51] There is typically a low rate of revision surgery (0–14%) which is often due to reinjury after return to full sports participation.[51,55,56]

AUTHOR'S PREFERRED SURGICAL TECHNIQUES

Anterior cruciate ligament reconstruction techniques are chosen based on a multitude of considerations for each individual patient, including age (both chronologic and skeletal), gender, and anticipated growth

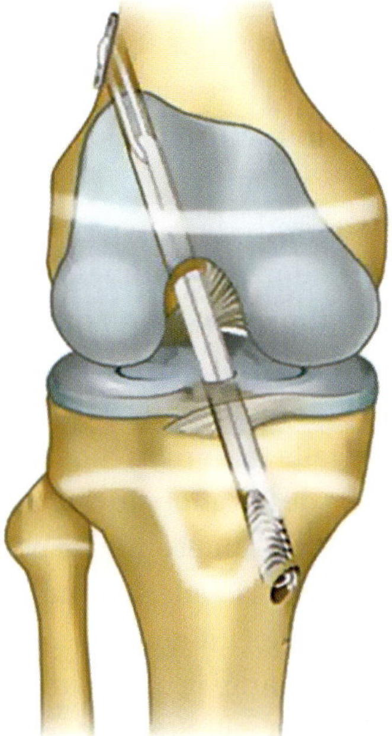

Fig. 23.1: The transphyseal anterior cruciate ligament (ACL) reconstruction with Hamstring autograft and metaphyseal fixation (physeal respecting).

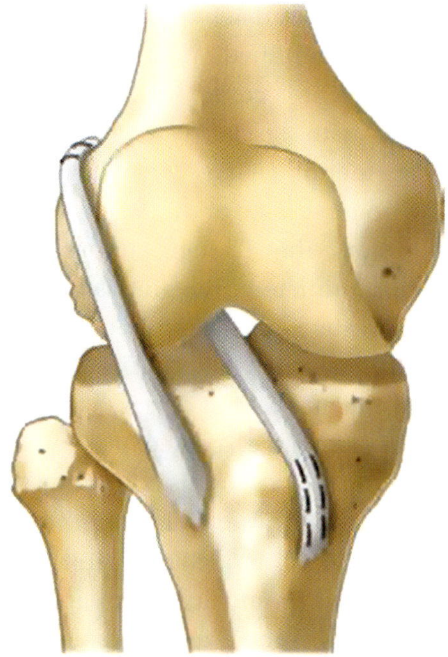

Fig. 23.2: The modified Macintosh iliotibial band (ITB) anterior cruciate ligament (ACL) reconstruction.

remaining. Generally, in prepubescent patients with significant growth remaining (Tanner stage 1–2; skeletal age ≤11 years in girls or ≤12 years in boys), we perform a physeal-sparing ACL reconstruction with ITB autograft (Fig. 23.2).[27,28] In pubescent patients with growth remaining (Tanner stage ≥3; skeletal age ≥12 years in girls or ≥13 years in boys), we perform a transphyseal ACL reconstruction with hamstring autograft and metaphyseal fixation (Fig. 23.1).[45] Descriptions for both of these techniques are detailed in the following sections.

Anterior Cruciate Ligament Reconstruction without Bone Tunnels

A combined general anesthetic with regional blockade is performed after consultation with the anesthesiologist, which consists of either a fascia iliaca block or a combination of femoral and lateral femoral cutaneous nerve block, both of which provided added anesthesia to the distal lateral thigh. Depending on surgeon, anesthesiologist, and family preference, an indwelling catheter may be left in place overnight to provide sustained analgesia.

After an examination under anesthesia, a nonsterile tourniquet may be placed high on the thigh. To ensure adequate access to the upper thigh during ITB graft harvest, the tourniquet should not be inflated until the graft is successfully harvested. Surgery begins with ITB harvest through a longitudinal-oblique incision which starts at the lateral joint line (a point midway between Gerdy's tubercle and the lateral epicondyle) and extends to the anterior border of the ITB, which is commonly palpable with the knee in 90° of flexion. A long, broad Cobb elevator is used to elevate the subcutaneous tissue off the superficial surface of the ITB a minimum of 15 cm up the thigh.

Distally, at a point about 1–2 cm proximal to the lateral epicondyle, the anterior and posterior borders of the ITB are identified. Anteriorly, the ITB is confluent with the fascia of the vastus lateralis; however, a transition point is commonly identified where the dense and opaque ITB tissue transitions to a more transparent vastus fascia. Posteriorly, the ITB blends into the posterior intermuscular septum. Once these borders are identified, the ITB is incised near either border leaving a few millimeters of intact ITB on either side. The undersurface of the ITB is then freed from underlying tissue with the use of wood-handled or Cobb elevators. The ITB incisions are continued proximally with curved meniscotomes for a distance of at least 15 centimeters. The graft is truncated proximally with a curved meniscotome or an open-ended tendon harvester with cutting mechanism. After harvest, the free end is tubularized with a nonabsorbable suture in a whip-stitch pattern. The graft is further freed distally from the lateral joint capsule to the level of the lateral epicondyle, but care is taken to maintain its attachment distally to Gerdy's tubercle (Figs. 23.3A and B). The graft is then placed back into the harvest wound to prevent desiccation during arthroscopy.

Diagnostic arthroscopy is performed through standard anterolateral and anteromedial portals and any meniscal or chondral work is performed at this point. The medial portal is widened and a large curved clamp is introduced through the medial portal. Widening the medial portal facilitates easier clamp spreading and prevents traumatic and irregular enlargement of the portal. The clamp is placed through the soft-tissue remnants at the proximal aspect of the over-the-top position which will function as a graft "sling" after passage, and the clamp is then pushed through the posterolateral capsule of the knee and into the ITB defect on the lateral knee. The clamp is opened and closed several times to dilate the passageway and allow for easy graft passage. The suture attached to the free end of the graft is placed in the clamps and brought back into the knee. The graft is typically drawn into the over-the-top position and the sutures are brought out the medial portal (Figs. 23.4A and B).

Next, a longitudinal incision is made medial to the tibial tubercle and distal to the tibial epiphysis near the superior border of the pes anserinus tendon insertion. Practically speaking, this incision typically lies directly distal to the anteromedial arthroscopy portal. Dissection is carried down to, but not through, the

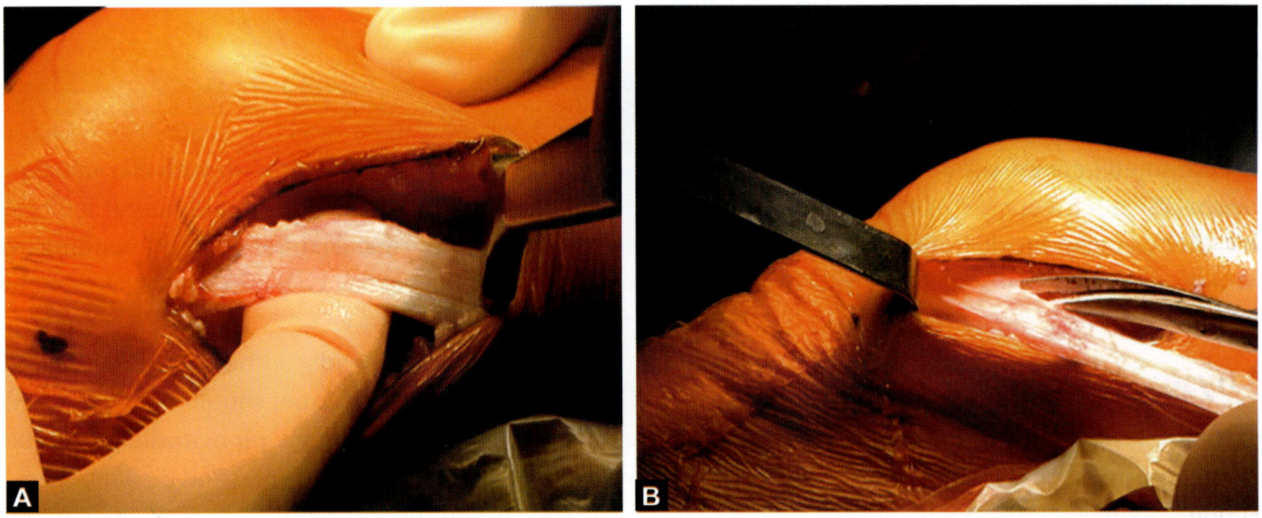

Figs. 23.3A and B: Iliotibial band (ITB) graft harvest. Isolation of the midportion of the ITB (A) is followed by proximal detachment and dissection distally to the Gerdy tubercle (B). The graft is then tubularized proximally with sutures that are used to pass the graft.[28]

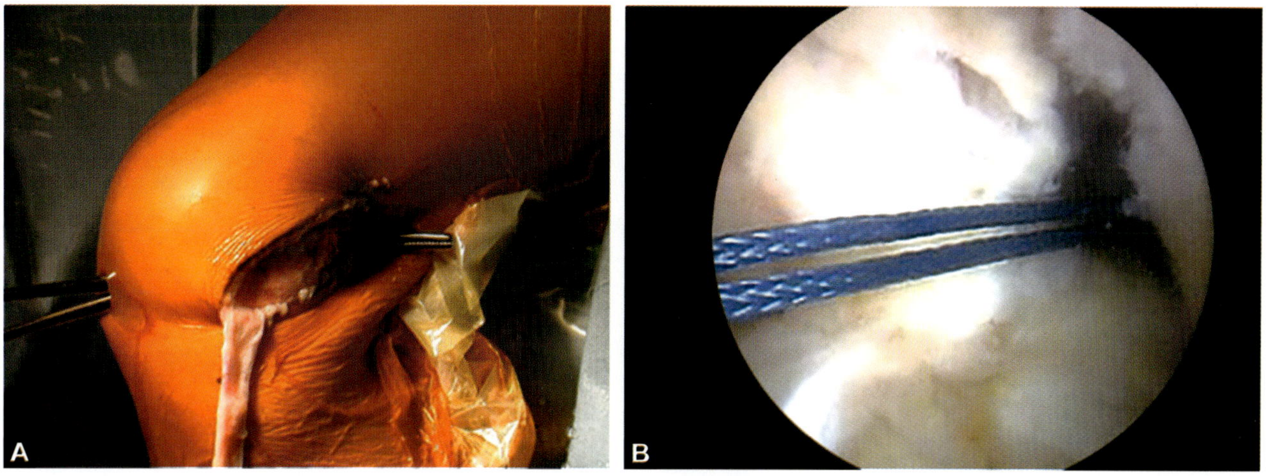

Figs. 23.4A and B: Iliotibial band (ITB) graft passage is performed by using a curved clamp in the over-the-top position (A). The sutures are then passed intra-articularly and pulled through the medial arthroscopy portal (B).[28]

tibial periosteum. At this point, blunt dissection is directed proximally with a curved clamp (i.e. Schnidt tonsil forcep) into the knee, with care to keep the clamp under the intermeniscal ligament. The clamp is serially opened and closed in this position to dilate the pathway, which facilitates both tibial preparation and subsequent graft passage. A curved "rat-tail" rasp is then inserted, following the same path under the intermeniscal ligament. The rasp is used to create a groove in the tibial ACL footprint with two goals. First, rasping the proximal tibia moves the graft footprint posteriorly into a more anatomically appropriate position to avoid extension impingement. Secondly, rasping promotes intra-articular graft healing by exposing a bleeding bony bed. The clamp is then reintroduced in the knee, and the intra-articular sutures are grasped and brought out through the tibial incision. The graft is then advanced to its final intra-articular position (Figs. 23.5A to C). With tension on the graft, the knee is flexed and extended to confirm impingement-free range of motion prior to fixation.

The arthroscope is removed at this point, and attention is turned to the extra-articular tenodesis. The knee is allowed to hang in 90° of relaxed flexion with neutral foot rotation in order to prevent overconstraint of the lateral compartment.[32] With tension on the graft, the graft is sewn into the periosteum of the lateral femoral condyle and the intermuscular septum (Fig. 23.6) with a heavy nonabsorbable suture, using at least two or three figure-of-eight stitches to complete the extra-articular tenodesis.

After completion of the tenodesis, the leg is placed into extension (Fig. 23.7). The periosteum in the tibial incision is incised and elevated with an elevator both medially and laterally. The underlying bone is decorticated with a burr. Sutures are then placed through the periosteal flaps and graft but not tied. At least three sutures should be placed. Once all sutures are placed they are tied sequentially with firm tension on the graft and a posterior drawer on the tibia. The knee is examined to confirm a negative Lachman examination, and the graft can be reexamined arthroscopically, if desired.

Physeal Respecting Anterior Cruciate Ligament Reconstruction with Hamstring Autograft

A combined general anesthetic with regional blockade is performed after consultation with the anesthesiologist, which typically consists of either a femoral nerve block or adductor canal block. After an examination under anesthesia, a nonsterile tourniquet may be placed high on the thigh and is inflated prior to initial incision.

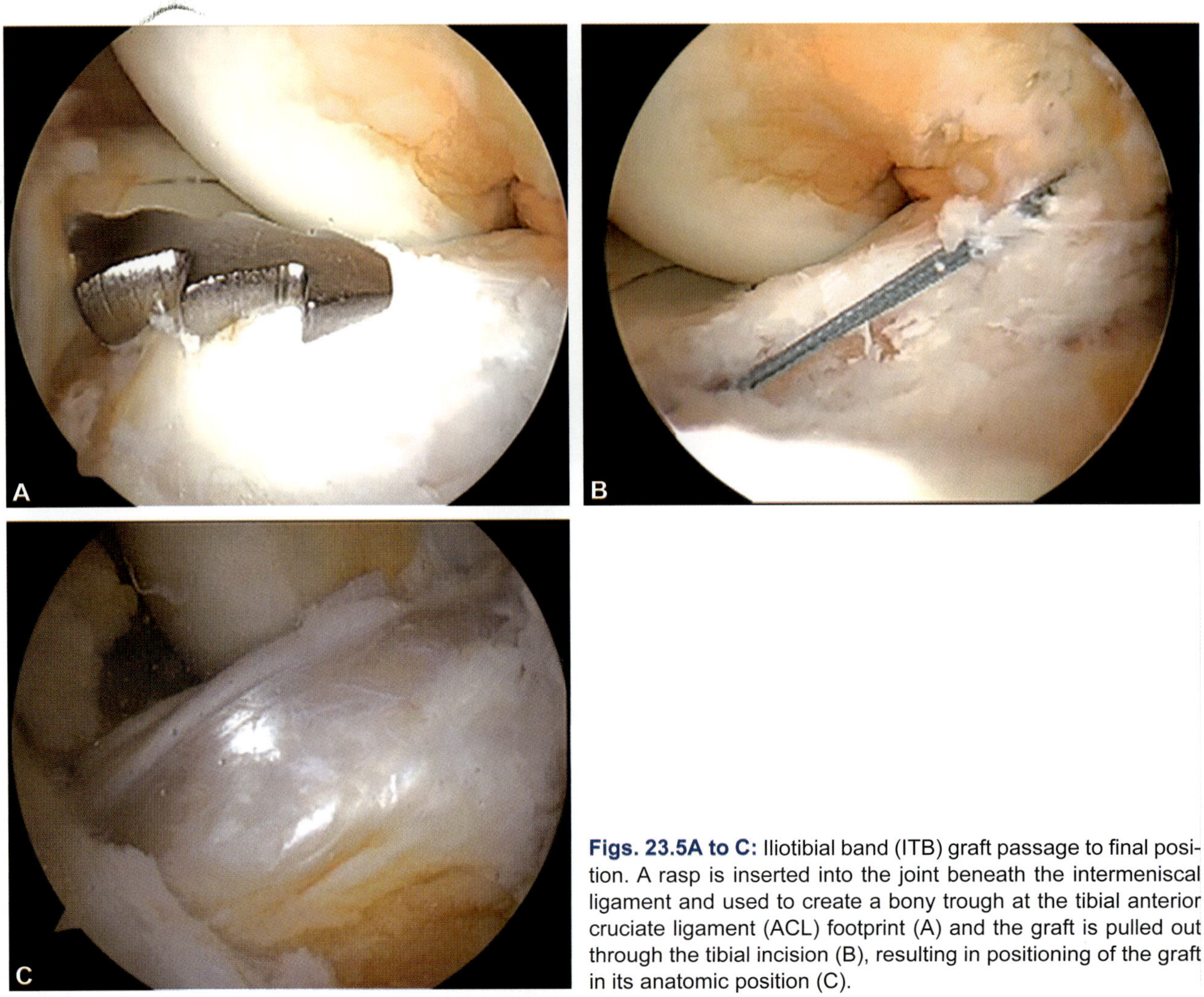

Figs. 23.5A to C: Iliotibial band (ITB) graft passage to final position. A rasp is inserted into the joint beneath the intermeniscal ligament and used to create a bony trough at the tibial anterior cruciate ligament (ACL) footprint (A) and the graft is pulled out through the tibial incision (B), resulting in positioning of the graft in its anatomic position (C).

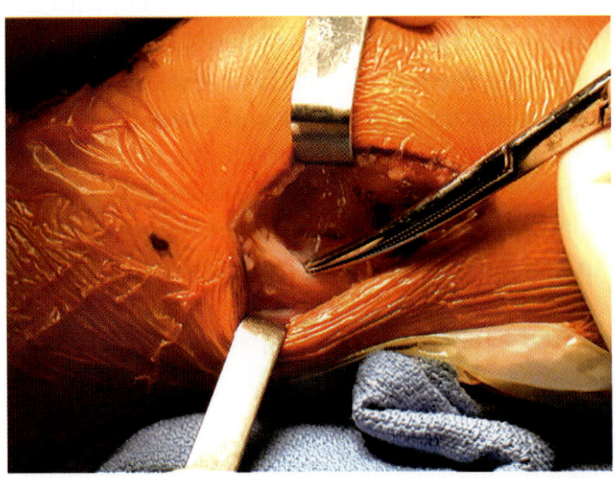

Fig. 23.6: With tension on the graft, the graft is sewn into the periosteum of the lateral femoral condyle and the intermuscular septum (identified with clamp) with a heavy nonabsorbable suture using at least two figure-of-eight stitches to achieve an extra-articular tenodesis.[28]

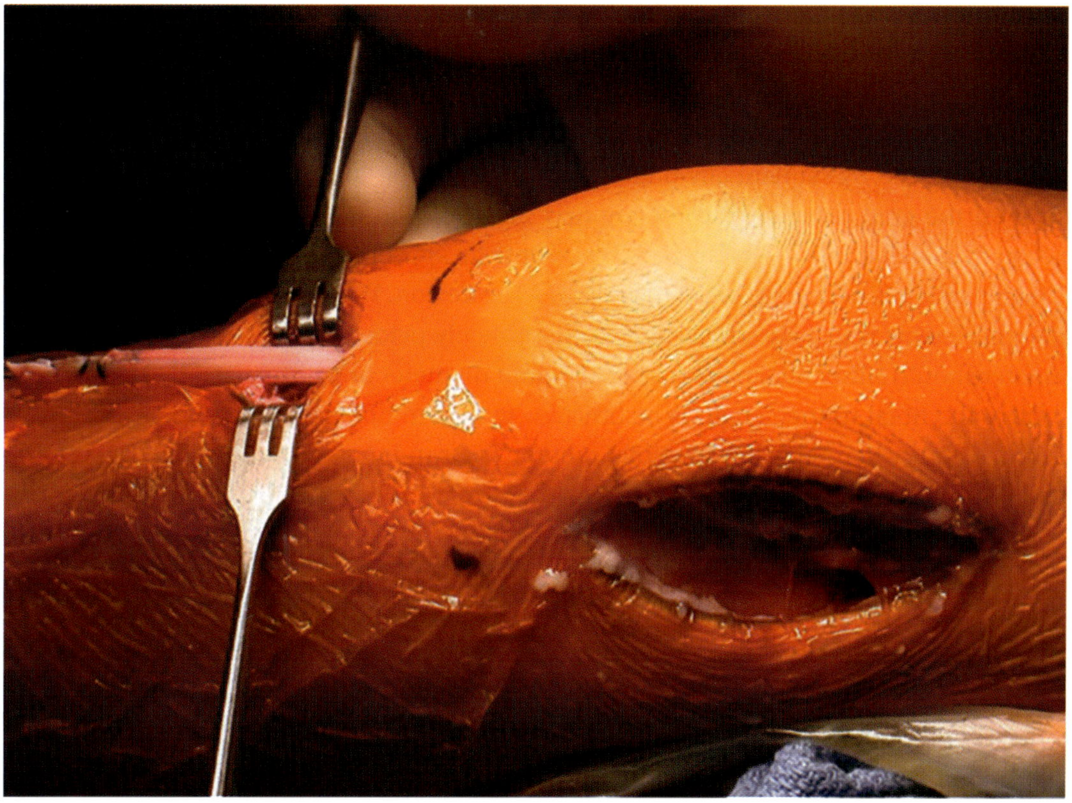

Fig. 23.7: After extra-articular tenodesis, the iliotibial band (ITB) autograft is tensioned through the medial tibial incision with the leg held in extension, and the graft is sutured to the tibial metaphyseal periosteum to complete the intra-articular graft fixation.

The semitendinosus and gracilis tendons are harvested through a longitudinal incision centered on the pes anserinus. They are each doubled to produce a quadrupled graft and sized using standard instruments. The quadrupled graft is then placed on a 15-mm fixed-loop suspensory cortical fixation device and pretensioned on a graft preparation board.

Diagnostic arthroscopy and any meniscal or chondral work is performed through standard anterolateral and anteromedial portals. A gentle notchplasty can be performed in cases with concern for notch stenosis; however, it is essential to avoid vigorous resection deep in the notch given the proximity of the distal femoral growth plate to the over-the-top position.

Bone tunnel drilling is typically done using a transtibial technique in order to obtain a central tunnel across the physis. The tibial guide is set to 55° to ensure a long metaphyseal tunnel distal to the physis. To ensure that the tibial tunnel does not violate the tibial tubercle apophysis, the guide pin is inserted just anterior to the medial collateral ligament fibers at the tibial cortex. This location is typically 1 cm anterior to the posteromedial border of the tibia. The guide pin is placed in the posterior-central portion of the tibial ACL footprint to allow easy access to the over-the-top position. The tibial tunnel is reamed over the guide pin with the appropriate-sized rigid reamer to match the size of the hamstring graft.

An over-the-top femoral guide is selected next. The guide size is determined by the width of the prepared ACL graft based on the formula [0.5 × graft diameter (in mm) + 1] to allow a 1.0–1.5-mm back wall. The appropriate femoral guide is inserted through the tibial tunnel and positioned with its aiming arm in the over-the-top position and a guide pin is drilled through the lateral femoral condyle. The femoral tunnel is reamed over the guidewire in preparation to support the suspensory fixation construct, taking into account the length of tunnel required for flipping the cortical button on its fixed loop. Passing sutures are used for graft passage using the Beath pin. The button is flipped on the lateral femoral cortex and security is assessed by sequentially pulling tension (toggling) the passing sutures as well as pulling firm tension on the graft distally. Fluoroscopy may also be used to confirm appropriate button placement. The graft is visualized arthroscopically to confirm appropriate position and impingement-free motion. Tibial fixation is performed at 20 degrees of knee flexion. With the transtibial technique, a 20–25-mm interference screw is usually sufficient to be completely placed and still be distal to the physis. The screw diameter should either match the tunnel and graft diameter or be oversized by 1 mm in softer bone. In cases where the tibial tunnel length is insufficient to accommodate an interference screw, a 4.5 mm cortical screw with washer placed in the tibial metaphysis can be used in a postfixation method for the ACL graft.

POSTOPERATIVE MANAGEMENT

Rehabilitation is largely similar for both ITB ACL reconstructions and for transphyseal hamstring autograft reconstructions. The main difference between the two techniques following surgery is the management of weight bearing and range of motion activities in the first 6 weeks postoperatively. Patients who undergo ITB ACL reconstruction maintain touchdown weight bearing (20% of body weight) for 6 weeks with range of motion limited to 0–30° for 2 weeks followed by 0–90° through week 6. This schedule allows for adequate protection of implant-free periosteal fixation of the ITB autograft. Patients who undergo transphyseal ACL reconstruction with hamstring autograft remain partial weight bearing (50% of body weight) for 2 weeks and are then progressed to weight bearing as tolerated, with 0–90° of motion allowed immediately postoperatively. After 6 weeks, both rehabilitation protocols consist of progression to full range of motion and closed-chain strengthening, with straight-line jogging initiated at 10 weeks postoperatively.

Running and agility training are started at 12 weeks and progressed toward sport-specific training and jump-landing. Patients are evaluated with an ACL return-to-play (RTP) assessment at 6 months, including range of motion, strength, thigh girth, balance, and functional testing. Any identified deficits are targeted. RTP is gradual and initiated at 6–9 months depending on RTP assessment. Patients wear a functional ACL brace for use during exercise and sports out to 2 years postoperatively. Two years after surgery, bracing becomes optional but is encouraged for younger, prepubescent patients and those who compete in high-risk sports. Patients are typically followed with annual clinical examinations until skeletal maturity to ensure lower extremity growth is progressing in a normal fashion. Alignment radiographs are not routinely obtained but are used in cases where growth disturbances are suspected.

CONCLUSION

Anterior cruciate ligament tears are increasingly recognized in skeletally immature athletes. Nonoperative management until skeletal maturity through activity restriction is unrealistic and generally cautioned due to the link between delayed ACL reconstruction and the development of secondary injuries in this cohort.[5-7] In light of these considerations, surgical techniques and instrumentation have evolved in order to accommodate the unique anatomy of skeletally immature patients. In caring for pediatric athletes with ACL injuries, a multitude of considerations must be made for each individual patient, including age (both chronologic and skeletal), gender, and anticipated growth remaining, to ensure a successful ACL reconstruction and maintenance of growth potential.

PEARLS AND PITFALLS

During the ITB ACL reconstruction procedure, three steps are the most critical and require the greatest technical consideration.

1. During graft harvest, it is essential to obtain as lengthy an ITB graft as possible. The meniscotomes to create the anterior and posterior borders should typically be buried in the lateral wound as they are passed proximally to ensure adequate length. In the event that the graft is difficult to detach from the proximal remnant of the ITB, a proximal counterincision may be made to connect the anterior and posterior meniscotome cuts and free the graft. Again, ensuring adequate access to this location is important during extremity draping. In the event that the ITB autograft is of insufficient size, the autograft may be tubularized over a 7 mm allograft hamstring tendon to add further length or girth, if desired.[34]
2. During femoral graft passage, the posterolateral capsule is on occasion difficult to penetrate with the blunt large curved clamp. In these instances, a more pointed instrument (i.e. Schnidt tonsil clamp) can be used to penetrate the capsule, after which the large curved clamp can be reinserted and passed into the ITB defect on the lateral thigh.
3. During tibial graft passage, clamp insertion under the intermeniscal ligament can be tedious. Typically, the clamp should be directed directly proximal along the medial tibial incision into the knee to replicate the ACLs native trajectory from the lateral femoral condyle to its interspinous insertion.

During the transphyseal hamstring autograft ACL reconstruction, many of the expected intraoperative issues will mirror that of a standard hamstring autograft ACL reconstruction. One technical consideration that must be stressed is the means of fixation on both the tibial and femoral sides. As mentioned above, the femur is typically fixated with a cortical button on a fixed loop to provide graft suspension within the tunnel. In cases where the femoral cortex is violated during tunnel preparation, an extended cortical button construct should also be available in all of these cases, as interference screws will almost uniformly cross the physis if used. On the tibial side, a short interference screw is often an acceptable means of fixation, but in cases of an unexpectedly short tunnel, a 4.5 mm cortical screw with washer placed in the metaphysis is the recommended form of fixation.

REFERENCES

1. Dodwell ER, Lamont LE, Green DW, et al. 20 years of pediatric anterior cruciate ligament reconstruction in New York State. Am J Sports Med. 2014;42(3):675-80.

2. Buller LT, Best MJ, Baraga MG, et al. Trends in anterior cruciate ligament reconstruction in the United States. Orthop J Sports Med. 2015;3(1):2325967114563664.
3. Werner BC, Yang S, Looney AM, et al. Trends in Pediatric and Adolescent Anterior Cruciate Ligament Injury and Reconstruction. J Pediatr Orthop. 2016;36(5):447-52.
4. Vavken P, Murray MM. Treating anterior cruciate ligament tears in skeletally immature patients. Arthroscopy. 2011;27(5):704-16.
5. Lawrence JT, Argawal N, Ganley TJ. Degeneration of the knee joint in skeletally immature patients with a diagnosis of an anterior cruciate ligament tear: is there harm in delay of treatment? Am J Sports Med. 2011;39(12):2582-7.
6. Magnussen RA, Pedroza AD, Donaldson CT, et al. Time from ACL injury to reconstruction and the prevalence of additional intra-articular pathology: is patient age an important factor? Knee Surg Sports Traumatol Arthrosc. 2013;21(9):2029-34.
7. Vavken P, Tepolt FA, Kocher MS. Concurrent meniscal and chondral injuries in pediatric and adolescent patients undergoing ACL reconstruction. J Pediatr Orthop. 2016.
8. Kelly PM, Dimeglio A. Lower-limb growth: how predictable are predictions? J Child Orthop. 2008;2(6):407-15.
9. Chotel F, Henry J, Seil R, et al. Growth disturbances without growth arrest after ACL reconstruction in children. Knee Surg Sports Traumatol Arthrosc. 2010;18(11):1496-500.
10. Chotel F, Seil R. Growth disturbances after transphyseal ACL reconstruction in skeletally immature patients: who is more at risk? Young child or adolescent? J Pediatr Orthop. 2013;33(5):585-6.
11. Higuchi T, Hara K, Tsuji Y, et al. Transepiphyseal reconstruction of the anterior cruciate ligament in skeletally immature athletes: an MRI evaluation for epiphyseal narrowing. J Pediatr Orthop Part B. 2009;18(6):330-4.
12. Koman JD, Sanders JO. Valgus deformity after reconstruction of the anterior cruciate ligament in a skeletally immature patient. A case report. J Bone Joint Surg Am. 1999;81(5):711-5.
13. Lawrence JT, West RL, Garrett WE. Growth disturbance following ACL reconstruction with use of an epiphyseal femoral tunnel: a case report. J Bone Joint Surg Am. 2011;93(8):e39.
14. Lipscomb AB, Anderson AF. Tears of the anterior cruciate ligament in adolescents. J Bone Joint Surg Am. 1986;68(1): 19-28.
15. Robert HE, Casin C. Valgus and flexion deformity after reconstruction of the anterior cruciate ligament in a skeletally immature patient. Knee Surg Sports Traumatol Arthrosc. 2010;18(10):1369-73.
16. Kocher MS, Saxon HS, Hovis WD, et al. Management and complications of anterior cruciate ligament injuries in skeletally immature patients: survey of the Herodicus Society and the ACL Study Group. J Pediatr Orthop. 2002;22(4): 452-7.
17. Anderson AF. Transepiphyseal replacement of the anterior cruciate ligament in skeletally immature patients. A preliminary report. J Bone Joint Surg Am. 2003;85-A(7):1255-63.
18. Cohen M, Ferretti M, Quarteiro M, et al. Transphyseal anterior cruciate ligament reconstruction in patients with open physes. Arthroscopy. 2009;25(8):831-8.
19. Cruz AI Jr, Fabricant PD, McGraw M, et al. All-Epiphyseal ACL Reconstruction in children: Review of safety and early complications. J Pediatr Orthop. 2017;37(3):204-9.
20. Koch PP, Fucentese SF, Blatter SC. Complications after epiphyseal reconstruction of the anterior cruciate ligament in prepubescent children. Knee Surg Sports Traumatol Arthrosc. 2016;24(9):2736-40.
21. Kohl S, Stutz C, Decker S, et al. Mid-term results of transphyseal anterior cruciate ligament reconstruction in children and adolescents. Knee. 2014;21(1):80-5.
22. Kumar S, Ahearne D, Hunt DM. Transphyseal anterior cruciate ligament reconstruction in the skeletally immature: follow-up to a minimum of sixteen years of age. J Bone Joint Surg Am. 2013;95(1):e1.
23. Liddle AD, Imbuldeniya AM, Hunt DM. Transphyseal reconstruction of the anterior cruciate ligament in prepubescent children. J Bone Joint Surg Br. 2008;90(10):1317-22.
24. Lo IK, Kirkley A, Fowler PJ, et al. The outcome of operatively treated anterior cruciate ligament disruptions in the skeletally immature child. Arthroscopy. 1997;13(5):627-34.

25. Shifflett GD, Green DW, Widmann RF, et al. Growth arrest following ACL reconstruction with hamstring autograft in skeletally immature patients: A review of 4 cases. J Pediatr Orthop. 2016;36(4):355-61.
26. Yoo WJ, Kocher MS, Micheli LJ. Growth plate disturbance after transphyseal reconstruction of the anterior cruciate ligament in skeletally immature adolescent patients: an MR imaging study. J Pediatr Orthop. 2011;31(6):691-6.
27. Micheli LJ, Rask B, Gerberg L. Anterior cruciate ligament reconstruction in patients who are prepubescent. Clin Orthop Relat Res. 1999(364):40-7.
28. Kocher MS, Garg S, Micheli LJ. Physeal sparing reconstruction of the anterior cruciate ligament in skeletally immature prepubescent children and adolescents. J Bone Joint Surg Am. 2005;87(11): 2371-9.
29. Claes S, Vereecke E, Maes M, et al. Anatomy of the anterolateral ligament of the knee. J Anat. 2013;223(4):321-8.
30. Parsons EM, Gee AO, Spiekerman C, et al. The biomechanical function of the anterolateral ligament of the knee. Am J Sports Med. 2015;43(3):669-74.
31. Vincent JP, Magnussen RA, Gezmez F, et al. The anterolateral ligament of the human knee: an anatomic and histologic study. Knee Surg Sports Traumatol Arthrosc. 2012;20(1):147-52.
32. Kennedy A, Coughlin DG, Metzger MF, et al. Biomechanical evaluation of pediatric anterior cruciate ligament reconstruction techniques. Am J Sports Med. 2011;39(5):964-71.
33. Kocher MS, Heyworth BE, Tepolt F, et al. Outcomes of physeal sparing ACL reconstruction with IT band in skeletally immature children. [Submitted for publication].
34. Faneli D, Henrikus W. Pediatric ACL reconstruction with iliotibial band autograft. Presented at the 3rd Annual Meeting of the Pediatric Research in Sports Medicine Society. San Diego, CA; January 28-30, 2016.
35. Willimon SC, Jones CR, Herzog MM, et al. Micheli anterior cruciate ligament reconstruction in skeletally immature youths: A retrospective case series with a mean 3-year follow-up. Am J Sports Med. 2015;43(12):2974-81.
36. Lawrence JT, Bowers AL, Belding J, et al. All-epiphyseal anterior cruciate ligament reconstruction in skeletally immature patients. Clin Orthop Relat Res. 2010;468(7):1971-77.
37. McCarthy MM, Graziano J, Green DW, et al. All-epiphyseal, all-inside anterior cruciate ligament reconstruction technique for skeletally immature patients. Arthrosc Tech. 2012;1(2):e231-9.
38. Cruz AI Jr, Fabricant PD, Seeley MA, et al. Change in size of hamstring grafts during preparation for ACL reconstruction: Effect of tension and circumferential compression on graft diameter. J Bone Joint Surg Am. 2016;98(6):484-9.
39. Cassard X, Cavaignac E, Maubisson L, et al. Anterior cruciate ligament reconstruction in children with a quadrupled semitendinosus graft: preliminary results with minimum 2 years of follow-up. J Pediatr Orthop. 2014;34(1):70-7.
40. Cordasco FA, Mayer SW, Green DW. All-inside, all-epiphyseal anterior cruciate ligament reconstruction in skeletally immature athletes. Am J Sports Med. 2016:363546516677723.
41. Nawabi DH, Jones KJ, Lurie B, et al. All-inside, physeal-sparing anterior cruciate ligament reconstruction does not significantly compromise the physis in skeletally immature athletes: a postoperative physeal magnetic resonance imaging analysis. Am J Sports Med. 2014;42(12):2933-40.
42. Demange MK, Camanho GL. Nonanatomic anterior cruciate ligament reconstruction with double-stranded semitendinosus grafts in children with open physes: minimum 15-year follow-up. Am J Sports Med. 2014;42(12):2926-32.
43. Fabricant PD, Jones KJ, Delos D, et al. Reconstruction of the anterior cruciate ligament in the skeletally immature athlete: a review of current concepts: AAOS exhibit selection. J Bone Joint Surg Am. 2013;95(5):e28.
44. Gausden EB, Calcei JG, Fabricant PD, et al. Surgical options for anterior cruciate ligament reconstruction in the young child. Curr Opin Pediatr. 2015;27(1):82-91.
45. Kocher MS, Smith JT, Zoric BJ, et al. Transphyseal anterior cruciate ligament reconstruction in skeletally immature pubescent adolescents. J Bone Joint Surg Am. 2007;89(12):2632-9.
46. Cruz AI Jr, Lakomkin N, Fabricant PD, et al. Transphyseal ACL reconstruction in skeletally immature patients: Does independent femoral tunnel drilling place the physis at greater risk compared with transtibial drilling? Orthop J Sports Med. 2016;4(6):2325967116650432.
47. Janarv PM, Wikstrom B, Hirsch G. The influence of transphyseal drilling and tendon grafting on bone growth: an experimental study in the rabbit. J Pediatr Orthop. 1998;18(2):149-54.

48. Makela EA, Vainionpaa S, Vihtonen K, et al. The effect of trauma to the lower femoral epiphyseal plate. An experimental study in rabbits. J Bone Joint Surg Br. 1988;70(2):187-91.
49. Stadelmaier DM, Arnoczky SP, Dodds J, et al. The effect of drilling and soft tissue grafting across open growth plates. A histologic study. Am J Sports Med. 1995;23(4):431-5.
50. Aronowitz ER, Ganley TJ, Goode JR, et al. Anterior cruciate ligament reconstruction in adolescents with open physes. Am J Sports Med. 2000;28(2):168-75.
51. Calvo R, Figueroa D, Gili F, et al. Transphyseal anterior cruciate ligament reconstruction in patients with open physes: 10-year follow-up study. Am J Sports Med. 2015;43(2):289-94.
52. Courvoisier A, Grimaldi M, Plaweski S. Good surgical outcome of transphyseal ACL reconstruction in skeletally immature patients using four-strand hamstring graft. Knee Surg Sports Traumatol Arthrosc. 2011;19(4):588-91.
53. Hui C, Roe J, Ferguson D, et al. Outcome of anatomic transphyseal anterior cruciate ligament reconstruction in Tanner stage 1 and 2 patients with open physes. Am J Sports Med. 2012;40(5): 1093-8.
54. McIntosh AL, Dahm DL, Stuart MJ. Anterior cruciate ligament reconstruction in the skeletally immature patient. Arthroscopy. 2006;22(12):1325-30.
55. Seon JK, Song EK, Yoon TR, et al. Transphyseal reconstruction of the anterior cruciate ligament using hamstring autograft in skeletally immature adolescents. J Korean Med Sci. 2005;20(6):1034-8.
56. Lemaitre G, Salle de Chou E, Pineau V, et al. ACL reconstruction in children: a transphyseal technique. Orthop Traumatol Surg Res. 2014;100(4 Suppl):S261-5.

CHAPTER

24

Remnant Preservation Techniques in Anterior Cruciate Ligament Reconstruction

Sanesh Vijay Tuteja, Bertrand Sonnery-Cottet

INTRODUCTION

Although a successful result following an anterior cruciate ligament reconstruction (ACLR) depends on multiple factors, graft incorporation in the form of revascularization and ligamentization is proposed to be an important factor for restoration of graft strength.[1-8]

The mechanism of graft failure in an ACLR can be grossly divided into those related to the surgical technique, due to failure of graft incorporation, and those following trauma.[9] In spite of constant improvements in the surgical techniques, graft rupture rates continue to be reported between 3% and 10%.[10-13] There is therefore a lot of emphasis on optimizing the graft integration and preservation of local biology.

Crain et al.[14] in 2005 identified four patterns of ACL remnant morphology on arthroscopic exploration. Although the remnant maintains a physical bridge between the tibia and the femur, it contributes little to maintaining the anterolateral rotational stability of the knee joint, as the femoral attachment of such a stump is almost always abnormally positioned. These therefore are akin to a complete ACL tear.

Preserving the ACL remnant may offer multiple advantages (Table 24.1) ranging from mechanical, improving postoperative proprioception,[15] or biological by enhancing the healing potential, owing to an intact vascular support by the synovial sheath.[16-18]

Table 24.1: Advantages and disadvantages of remnant preservation.

	Advantages[1-8]	*Disadvantages*[19]
1.	Accelerated revascularization and ligamentization	Incorrect tibial tunnel placement
2.	Preservation of the proprioceptive nerve fibers	Cyclops formation
3.	Enhanced biological environment for healing	Technically demanding
4.	Maintenance of the anchor point at the native tibial attachment	
5.	Lower incidence of tibial bone tunnel enlargement	

RATIONALE

Histological examination of human ACL remnants demonstrates an intrinsic healing potential,[20] by retaining the vascularity that is provided by the synovial layer and fibroblasts that have the ability to synthesize collagen.[21]

Graft revascularization and synovialization are known to be crucial for both consolidation of the tendon graft and for restoration of graft strength.[22,23] The initial strength and fixation of the graft could be responsible for early failure but does not explain late graft ruptures.[24] Therefore, the lack of biological integration of the graft could be responsible for this kind of failure.

Murray and Spector[25] demonstrated that cells in the human ACL retain their ability to migrate into an adjacent scaffold in vitro, which begins 4 weeks after a complete rupture. ACL remnants may accelerate the cellular proliferation and revascularization of the grafted tendon.[26] In a canine model study, Matsumoto et al.[27] noted that the remnant ACL tissue when sutured to the tibial side of the graft contributed to early tendon-bone healing in ACL reconstruction. The authors further concluded that the ruptured ACL tissue had a therapeutic potential in promoting an appropriate environment for tendon-to-bone healing in bone tunnels of ACL reconstruction.

The outcomes of studies investigating ACL augmentation in patients with preserved remnants have been encouraging. Nevertheless, there are few studies comparing this technique to a standard ACL reconstruction.[1,28-31]

Preservation of the ACL remnant may in addition contribute to anterior knee stability[32] and improvement in the biomechanical strength of the construct in the immediate postoperative period.[33,34] Biomechanical testing has shown that failure to load was significantly higher in the augmentation group compared with the conventional reconstruction group.[35] The presence of proprioceptive neuroreceptors in the ACL remnant and their possible reinnervation of ACL grafts have been published by many authors.[3,36,37] Mechanoreceptors in the native ACL bundles are proposed to play a role in preserving and restoring joint stability. Therefore, it may be expected that the more the tibial remnant is kept intact, the better is the preservation of proprioceptive function.[5,38]

REVIEW OF SOME COMMONLY PERFORMED ACL AUGMENTATION PROCEDURES[39-41]

It may sometimes become difficult to ascertain if the remaining bundle represents a partial or complete tear of the ACL. The decision depends on a thorough consideration of physical examination, magnetic resonance imaging (MRI), and arthroscopic findings.[35] An examination under general anesthesia is advisable for all patients (Lachman's and Pivot-shift test).

Quantitative evaluation of anteroposterior knee laxity can be an indicator for this decision. A partial rupture of the ACL may be suspected when the side-to-side difference in the anterior displacement of the tibia is less than about 5 mm and a delayed, but firm end point is noted.[39] MRI also provides valuable information, especially about the femoral attachment of ACL.

An ACL augmentation procedure may be performed on patients having a remnant ACL tissue that is of either types 1, 2, or 3 as classified by Crain et al.[14] Patients with no identifiable remnant ACL tissue may be managed alternatively with a standard ACL reconstruction (type 4: resorption). Having said that, the final decision can be made after an arthroscopic examination of the injured knee and confirmation of the status of the injured ACL.

A standard anterolateral (AL) visualization portal and an anteromedial (AM) instrumentation portal may be used. Additionally, an accessory AM portal located approximately 2.5–3 cm medial to the medial border of the patellar tendon may be used.[41] This far AM (FAM) portal can be used for instrumentation, allowing the standard AM portal to be used to visualize the lateral wall of the intercondylar notch.[39]

As with any ACL reconstruction, a routine diagnostic round must be performed with a 30°, 4 mm arthroscope. Careful probing may be needed to assess the ACL remnant pattern; more so on the femoral side as most ACL tears occur in the proximal half, close to the femoral attachment. Partial rupture of the ACL may be suspected when continuity of a part of the ligament is observed between the anatomic footprint of the ACL on the lateral femoral condyle and the tibia. Furthermore, some authors have suggested that an arthroscopic examination at various knee-flexion angles must be performed to consider the different tension patterns of the two bundles.[42-45] Any additional meniscal or osteochondral pathologies identified during the arthroscopic must be managed accordingly.

The semitendinosus tendon may be harvested through a longitudinal skin incision and a tendon stripper. A rough estimate to identify the location of the pes anserinus is four finger-breadths below the medial joint line and one finger-breath medial to the crest of the tibia. The muscle tissue of the harvested tendon is removed and tripled or quadrupled to obtain a graft diameter of 8–11 mm. An appropriate size of a suspensory fixation device is connected to the graft on the femoral side and an interference screw or staple may be used on the tibial side. Kazusa et al.[39] suggested the use of a polyester tape with interference screw system for fixation of the graft on the tibia. Alternatively, the use of artificial ligaments like LARS or Telos has been suggested by Ahn et al.[41] In cases of double-bundle augmentation, the semitendinosus tendon could be divided in half. Each tendon is then doubled, and grafts are prepared accordingly.[39]

The ACL remnant is often scarred to the posterolateral (PL) corner of the tibial footprint. If so, the frayed soft tissue is elevated with a curette and debrided. A suture hook with a no. 0 polydioxanone synthetic (PDS) suture may be inserted into the AM portal and passed through the remnant ACL tissue. Two to three such stitches on the remnant ACL tissue is recommended.[41] The remnant stump is retracted medially for better visualization, through the accessory AM portal. This ensures an anatomic placement of the tibial tunnel and pullout repair to be performed easily by lengthening of the remnant tissue.[41] Clearance of the lateral wall of the intercondylar notch with a small bone curette and rasps was recommended by Takazawa et al.[40] with the aim of preserving as much of the remnant as possible.

The femoral tunnels can be created using either the transtibial or the transportal technique and utilizing the FAM portal. The transportal technique is preferred by many authors[39,40] as this technique allows more maneuverability for accurate anatomic positioning of the femoral tunnel during drilling as compared to the transtibial technique. Kazusa et al.[39] recommended that excision of the femoral stump using a motorized shaver system must be kept to a minimum. In addition, a notchplasty must be avoided to retain as much of the remnant as possible. The targeted point for the femoral tunnel can be marked with a microfracture awl with the knee in 90° of flexion followed by inserting a 2.4-mm guidewire from the FAM portal into the femoral footprint through the previously marked point. A guide pin is then inserted from the FAM portal to create a femoral tunnel with 110° to 120° of knee flexion. A 4.5-mm cannulated drill is used to drill a through and through tunnel. A femoral socket is drilled to a depth of 10–20 mm, with a diameter equal to that of the graft. It must be ensured that the tunnel is positioned behind the ridge, while the remnant is retracted away. Intraoperative radiographs may be used to confirm the location of the guidewire tip.[40,46]

While performing a single-bundle augmentation for PL bundle ruptures, the position of the central portion of the femoral tunnel must be placed between 2 o'clock and 2:30 o'clock (left knee) or between 9:30

o'clock and 10 o'clock (right knee).[47] The marked position must be such that approximately one-quarter of the femoral tunnel opening should include the femoral attachment of the AM bundle. In cases of AM bundle ruptures, the aim is to position the center of the femoral tunnel between 1:30 o'clock and 2 o'clock (left knee) or between 10 o'clock and 10:30 o'clock (right knee).[47] The marked position in this case must be such that approximately one-quarter of the femoral tunnel opening should include the femoral attachment of the PL bundle. Whereas, for a double-bundle reconstruction, the centers of the femoral tunnel openings should be placed posterior to resident's ridge.[48]

To establish a femoral tunnel using the transtibial technique, the marked point must be near the 10-o'clock position for a right knee or 2 o'clock for a left knee. The entry point is then made at the more medial side of the tibia. When the optimal position is achieved, the guide pin is overdrilled with an appropriately sized cannulated drill. The accessory AM portal in this technique can be used for traction on the sutured remnant tissue to avoid injury during tunnel formation and provide a better visual field. A poor visual field and damage to the remnant tissue would be inevitable if the femoral tunnel is made through the accessory AM portal. However, some authors[39] have suggested that the FAM portal technique is as effective as the transtibial technique and results in good restoration of joint stability and knee scores, despite a shorter femoral tunnel length and an inferoposterior position of the suspensory fixation device.[49]

The tibial attachment of the ACL remnant is a useful landmark for orientation because the tibial insertion of the ACL is normal in most of the cases. For preparing the tibial tunnel, the tip of the tibial guide system is inserted through the AM portal and put through the central portion of the remnant tissue. The tip of the tibial guide is positioned toward the central portion of the remnant tissue through the elevated posterolateral corner.[6]

Alternatively, the ACL remnant may be longitudinally slit and the tip is placed in the center of the slit. The guide is set to an angle of 40° to 45° in the sagittal plane. A 2.4-mm guide pin is inserted through the guide. A tibial bone tunnel is made using a cannulated reamer of the same diameter as that of the distal portion of the graft. The reamer is advanced carefully to minimize damage to the remnant. After removing the bony debris in both tunnels, a loop of suture is passed from the tibial tunnel, PL to the remnant, to the femur side, and the graft railroaded over it.

Kazusa el al.[39] made a longitudinal slit in the center of the ACL remnant through the AM portal. This, the authors believed, enhanced the visualization of the tip of the guidewire. In addition, while using the transtibial technique, it is difficult to find the tip of the guidewire for the PL bundle in the slit, because this technique requires the wire to be inserted at a shallower angle to the tibial plateau. As a result, the wire for the PL bundle will be parallel to the preserved ACL remnant. The use of an image intensifier is required for intraoperative localization of the wire when using the transtibial technique. However, it has several risks including radiation exposure, extended time of surgery, increased infection rates, and lower accuracy of measuring the distance between the wires than arthroscopy. The FAM portal technique does not impose any restrictions on the angle of the tibial tunnel. Increasing the inclination of the tibial tunnels to 65°, therefore allows better visualization of the tips of the guidewires.

In single-bundle reconstructions, the tip of the drill guide is positioned in the center of the tibial insertion of the whole ACL for PL bundle reconstructions. Whereas, in cases of AM bundle reconstructions, the tibial tunnel opening should be positioned as anterior as possible within the tibial footprint of the ACL.[47]

The position of the guidewire in this case is checked with the knee extended to see if the guidewire impinges on the roof of the intercondylar notch. The tunnels are then prepared with a 2.0-mm Kirschner wire inserted using the drill guide.

For double-bundle reconstructions, the guidewire for the AM bundle should be inserted first to facilitate the tibial tunnel opening of the AM bundle to be positioned as anterior as possible within the tibial footprint of the ACL.[48] The guidewire for the PL bundle must then be positioned 8 mm posterior to the first wire to keep 2–3 mm thick of bony wall between the tibial bone tunnels.

During graft passage, the remnant tissue is retracted to the medial side by use of a probe to allow entry of the graft into the femoral tunnel. The graft may be fixed with any of the available fixation devices. After fixation any additional sutures on the remnant can be taken using an absorbable PDS suture.

Although the postoperative rehabilitation protocols differ with the type of surgery and fixation, there is broad consensus that all patients must begin active range-of-motion, isometric muscle strengthening, and closed kinetic chain exercises from the first postoperative day.

Postoperative knee bracing was not prescribed by Takazawa et al.,[40] and they allowed all the patients to bear full weight immediately. In contrast, Ahn et al.,[41] advocated the use of crutches and partial weight bearing from 3 days to 6 weeks after surgery. They additionally used an ACL limited-motion brace, and joint motion exercise was carried out at 15° increments per week. At 4 weeks and 6 weeks after surgery, 90° and 135° of motion, respectively, were allowed.

In addition, patients have to be educated on performing proprioceptive balancing exercise at 3 months after surgery. Jogging is encouraged after 2 months, and open kinetic chain exercises are allowed after 3 months. Jump landing, twisting, and cutting exercises should be allowed at 4 months, and straight-line sprinting and other competitive exercises may be allowed at 6 months. At 9 months after surgery, changing the direction while running (cutting) is permissible. Subsequently, return to full sports activities are permitted in a stepwise manner.

SINGLE ANTEROMEDIAL BUNDLE BIOLOGICAL AUGMENTATION (SAMBBA) TECHNIQUE[50]

Surgical Setup

The patient is placed in the supine position, with a lateral post just proximal to the knee, at the level of the padded tourniquet, and a foot roll positioned with the knee at 90° of flexion. This allows the knee to be moved freely through its range of movement while preventing the hip from externally rotating.

Graft Harvesting

Our chosen graft for the ACL reconstruction is the semitendinosus (ST) tendon. The goal is to obtain a graft that is of 8–10 mm in diameter and 12-cm in length, measuring from its tibial insertion on the pes anserinus [usually a tripled ST graft]. The graft is harvested with an open-ended tendon stripper, which allows the tibial insertion to be preserved, thereby improving fixation and vascularity of the graft.[51] Once harvested, the graft is evaluated to determine whether an 8–10 mm graft diameter with a 12 cm length can be obtained. Tripling or quadrupling the graft over two suture loops to perform this evaluation helps us determine the required diameter of the bony tunnel.

Femoral Guide Placement

The arthroscope is placed in the lateral gutter, and the best entry point for the femoral tunnel is determined with a standard needle. A small stab incision in then made at this chosen site. A 4-mm shaver is introduced through the stab incision in the lateral gutter, and the synovial tissue situated between the lateral cortex and the fascia lata is debrided for better visualization of the button-flipping process over the lateral femoral cortex. The femoral tunnel is prepared with an outside-in femoral guide (Arthrex). A minimal notch debridement is performed (Fig. 24.1A). The femoral guide system is introduced through the AM portal and the tip is placed at the femoral footprint of the ACL. The sleeve of the guide is then pushed through the stab incision at the chosen entrance point in the lateral gutter. A 20 mm femoral socket is created with a FlipCutter II device (Arthrex) with the size determined by the previously estimated diameter of the graft (Fig. 24.1B).

Tibial Tunnel Placement and Drilling

With the knee in 30° of flexion, the tibial ACL remnant is inspected. If fixed to the posterior cruciate ligament or a nonanatomic site on the femoral condyle; it is carefully mobilized, preserving its entire synovial cover and tibial attachment. The tibial guide is introduced through the AM portal and positioned so that the guidewire either splits or stays within the center of the ACL tibial stump (Fig. 24.1C). When the location of the guidewire is satisfactory, the tunnel is drilled with increasing drill-bit diameters, stopping as soon as the bone of the tibial plateau is breached. It must be ensured that the drill remains strictly within the ACL remnant to conserve residual tissue. A shaver is passed through the tibial tunnel and into the remnant to emerge at its upper end so that the remnant is hollowed out for passage of the graft. The interior of the synovial sleeve is debrided to avoid overpacking of the intercondylar notch, which may cause anterior impingement and an extension deficit.

Graft Length Measurement and Graft Preparation

Accurate graft length measurement is required to be able to tension the graft from its tibial insertion to the bottom of the femoral socket; the prepared graft should be slightly shorter than this distance. A FiberStick (Arthrex) is passed through the femoral and tibial sockets to measure this distance. The proximal tip of the FiberStick is blocked at the proximal margin of the femoral socket, and a forceps is clamped onto the FiberStick at the level of the graft's tibial insertion (Fig. 24.2).

The length between the forceps and the proximal margin of the FiberStick is equal to the distance between the graft's tibial insertion and the proximal end of the femoral socket (Fig. 24.1D). The graft is prepared with a length 5 mm shorter than the aforementioned distance to obtain adequate graft tensioning (Fig. 24.3). A marking pen is used (Fig. 24.3A) to mark the previously measured graft length minus 0.5 cm. For example, if the graft length is 12.5 cm, a pen mark is placed 12 cm from the ST tibial insertion. A second pen mark is placed 4 cm from the tibial insertion to obtain a minimum length of 8 cm for the tripled or quadrupled graft portion. The graft is then doubled (Fig. 24.3B), tripled (Fig. 24.3C), and possibly quadrupled (Fig. 24.3D) over a TightRope RT suspensory fixation device (Arthrex) between these two pen marks, and the looped graft is sutured to itself (Figs. 24.1E and 24.3E).

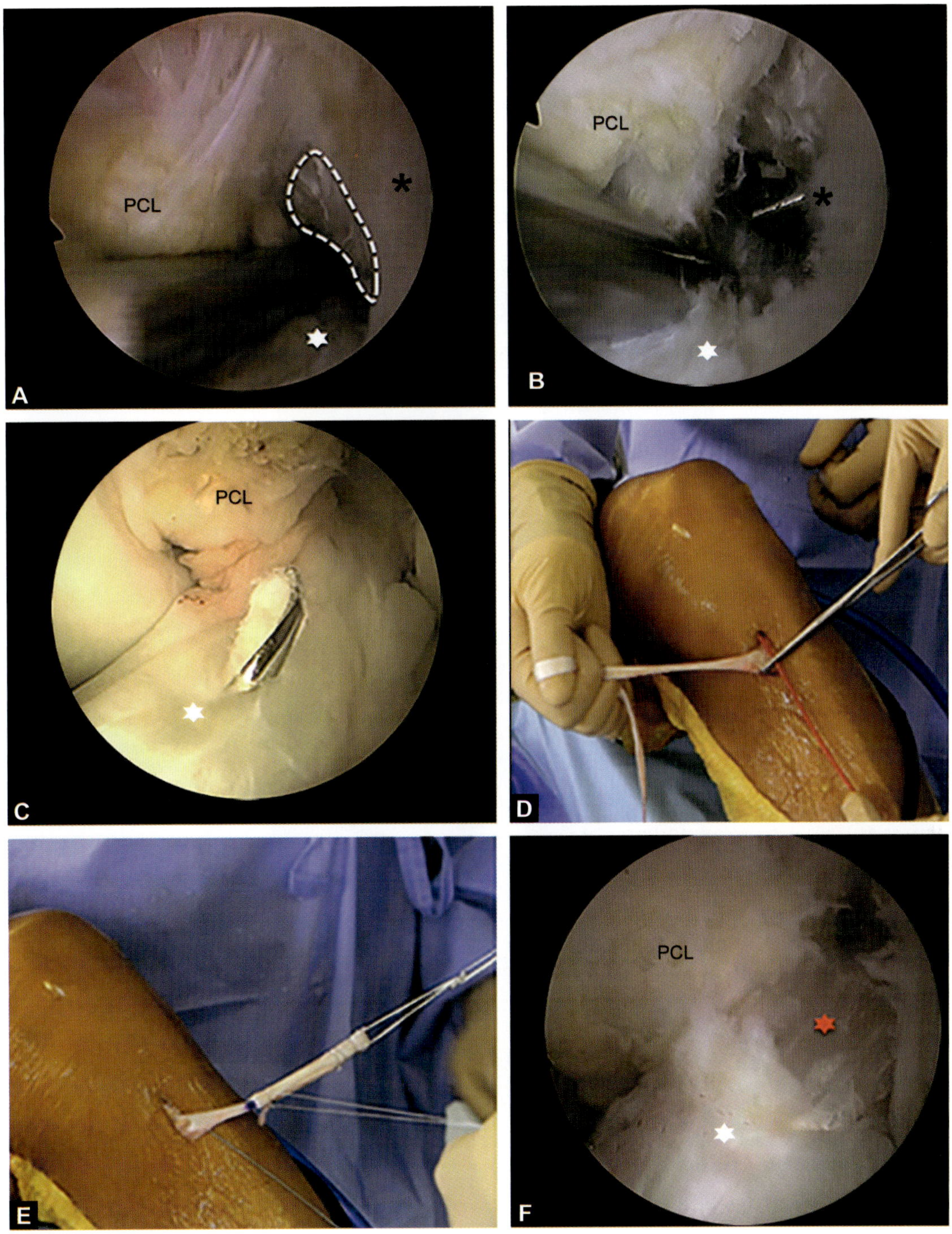

Figs. 24.1A to F: Intraoperative images showing steps during single anteromedial bundle biological augmentation technique in a left knee undergoing ACL reconstruction. (A) Arthroscopic view showing area for minimal notch debridement in anteromedial ACL bundle. (B) Arthroscopic view showing FlipCutter emerging in area of anteromedial bundle. (C) Arthroscopic view showing tibial pin positioned in center of remnant ACL stump. (D) Intraoperative photograph showing use of FiberStick to measure graft length. (E) Intraoperative photograph showing quadrupled ST graft, loaded with TightRope RT, ready for passage into prepared graft tunnel. (F) Arthroscopic view showing final image of ST graft emerging from within ACL remnant toward its femoral socket. The black asterisks indicate the lateral femoral condyle; white asterisks, ACL remnant; white dotted line, area for minimal debridement of anteromedial bundle; and red asterisk, ST graft.
(PCL: Posterior cruciate ligament; ACL: Anterior cruciate ligament; ST graft: Split-thickness graft).

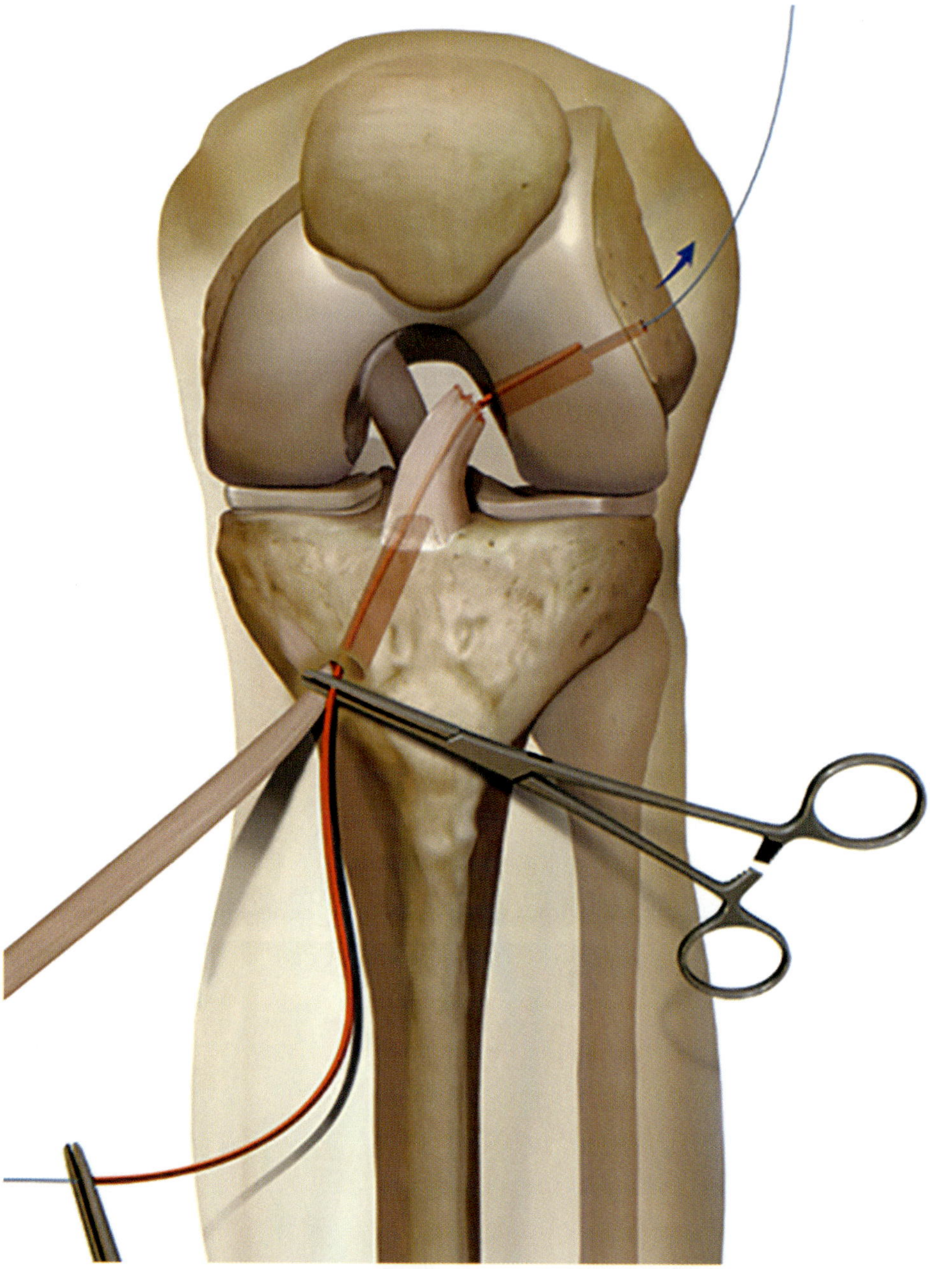

Fig. 24.2: Measurement of graft length. A FiberStick is passed through the path of the graft to measure the distance between the graft's tibial insertion and the proximal margin of the femoral socket.

Graft Passage

Leaving the knee at 90° of flexion, the graft is routed from the tibia to the femur (Fig. 24.1F). Introducing the arthroscope into the lateral gutter of the knee joint allows visualization of the exit point of the button on the lateral cortex of the femur and control of the passage of the TightRope button through the pinhole. The graft is secured on the femoral side with the TightRope tensioning mechanism. The graft is secured on the tibial side with a screw fixation in the standard fashion.

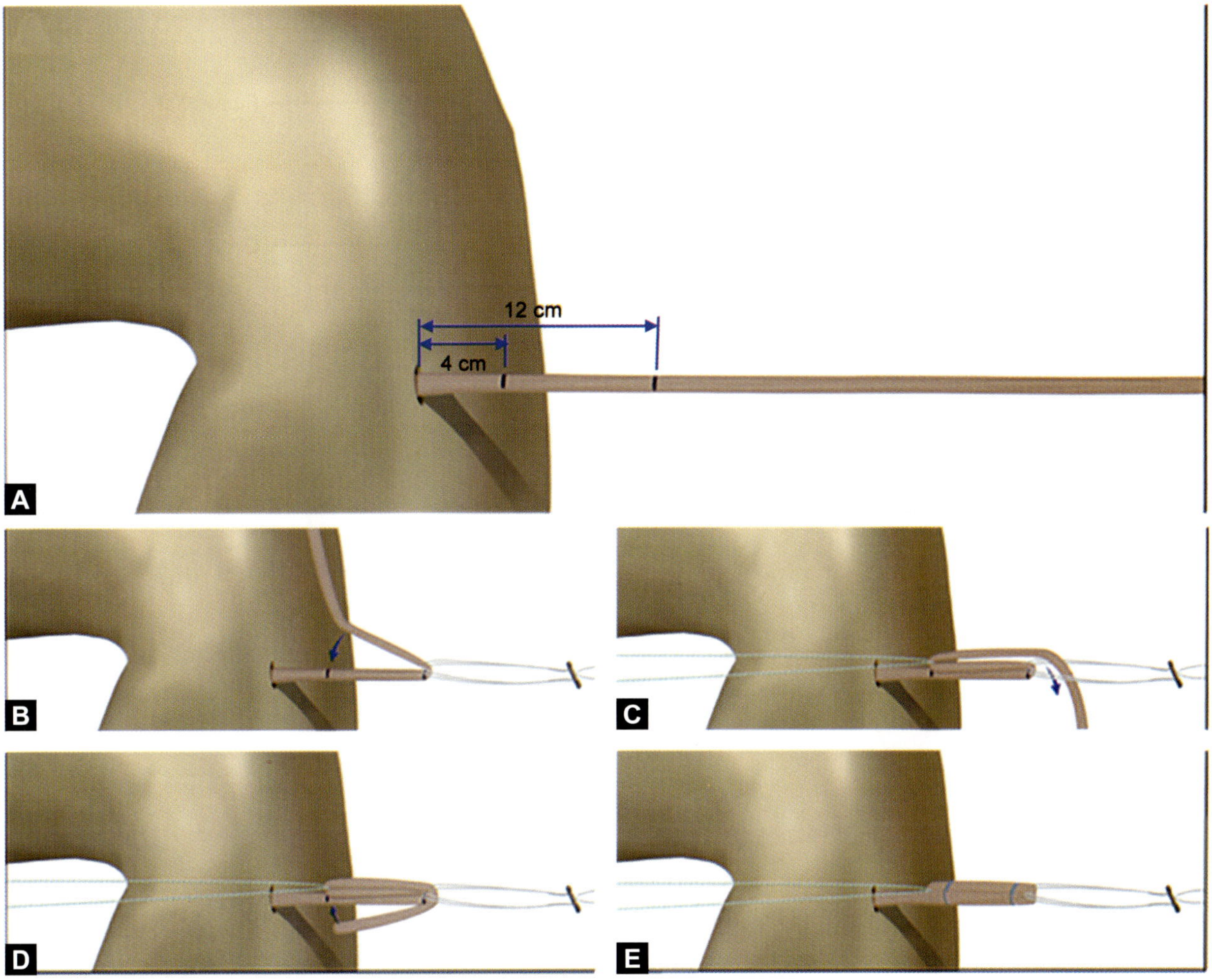

Figs. 24.3A to E: Steps in preparation of ST (split-thickness) graft: (A) Pen marks are placed at the previously measured graft length, minus 0.5 cm, and at a point closer to the tibial insertion of the semitendinosus tendon to obtain a minimum graft length of 8 cm for the tripled or quadrupled graft portion. The graft is (B) doubled, (C) then tripled, and (D) finally (if required), quadrupled over a TightRope RT between these two pen marks. (E) The looped graft is sutured to itself.

Remnant Fixation

We have noted that in acute ACL tears, the tibial remnant can be very soft and can slip down to the tibial insertion of the graft, causing soft-tissue impingement with the intercondylar notch. In these cases, the synovial sheath is secured to the proximal part of the graft by using a single polydioxanone no. 1 suture. Once the graft is secured, it lies within the intact ACL stump with a good synovial coverage all around the graft.

Advantages of Single Anteromedial Bundle Biological Augmentation

We believe that this technique of remnant preserving ACL reconstruction is both reliable and tissue conserving. It additionally uses the native graft vascularity to enhance the healing process. The ST graft

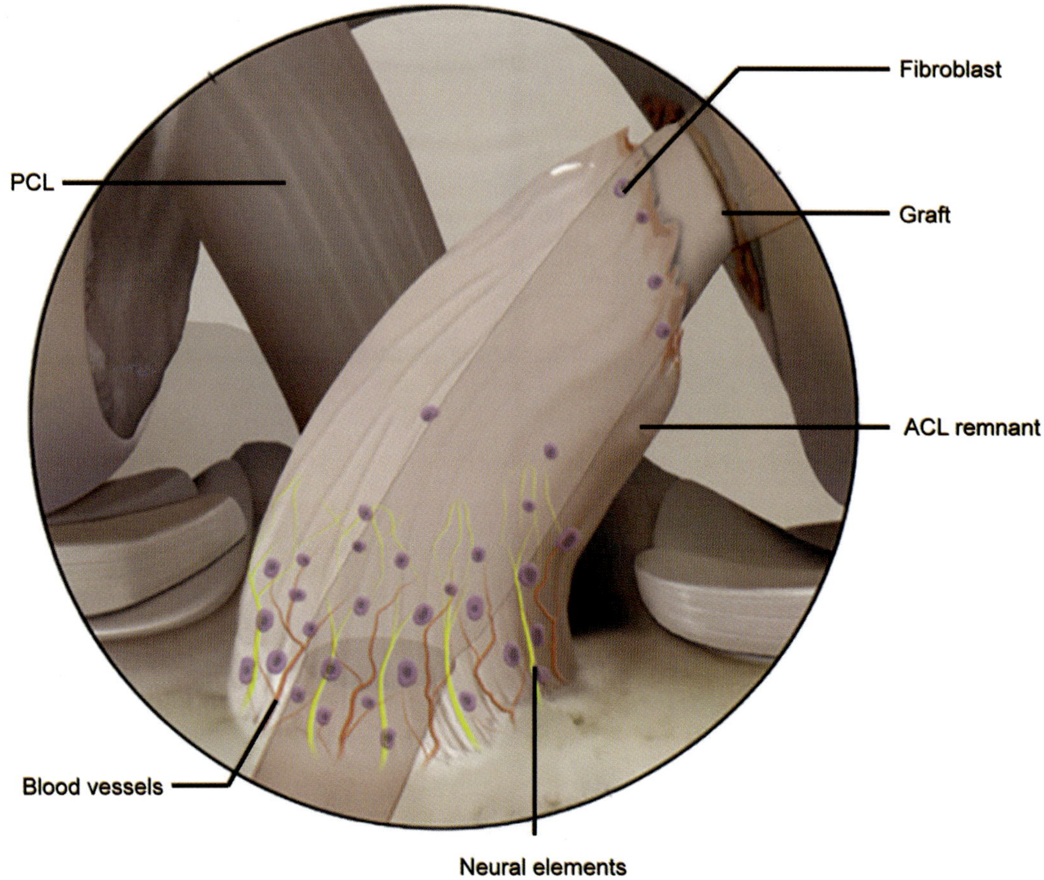

Fig. 24.4: ST graft within ACL remnant, which includes blood vessels, neural elements, and competent fibroblasts. (PCL: Posterior cruciate ligament; ACL: Anterior cruciate ligament; ST graft: Split-thickness graft).

is placed within the ACL remnant rich in blood vessels, neural elements, and competent fibroblasts (Fig. 24.4). Retaining the tibial attachment of the ST graft, we believe bypasses the stages of avascular necrosis and revascularization that occur with the use of a free tendon autograft.

The use of an outside-in technique for the femoral socket allows femoral tunnel placement with only minimal notch debridement. This retrograde drilling process enables the creation of a femoral socket rather than a transcondylar femoral tunnel. Not only does this preserves bone stock, but also permits the retention of the remnant with minimal notch debridement. In comparison, the inside-out technique requires some major debridement to visualize the femoral insertion of the ACL and risks damage to the notch and the articular cartilage during reaming. Moreover, the transportal technique using the accessory AM portal requires hyperflexion of the knee which can sometimes result in a poor visual field, and attempts at remnant preservation in hyperflexion of the knee can make the surgery technically challenging.

Additionally, drilling the tibial tunnel with increasing diameters of the drill-bits along with the use of a 4-mm shaver passed into the ACL remnant facilitates preservation of residual ACL tissue.

Table 24.2: Complications: prevention and course corrections.[50]

S. no.	*Surgical step*	*Pitfalls*	*Pearls*	*Bail outs*
1.	Tendon graft harvesting	▪ Premature amputation of the tendon	When harvesting the semitendinosus tendon to preserve the tibial insertion, use a right-angled clamp to retract the tendon and cut the two expansions before using the stripper.	▪ Instead of using only the semitendinosus, the gracilis tendon is harvested in addition and is used to prepare the graft
		▪ Avulsion of the tibial insertion		▪ Fix the avulsed tendon to the bone under the pes anserinus with two SwiveLock (4.75 mm) (Arthrex) anchors
2.	Notch debridement	Aggressive notchplasty leads to damage to remnant	Use a small shaver (4 mm in diameter) for cautious debridement. Only debride the proximal notch just enough to visualize the femoral insertion of the ACL	Nothing much can be done once the remnant is damaged. Hence emphasis must be placed on minimal debridement in the intercondylar notch
3.	Tibial tunnel placement	Errors in placement of the guide pin through the stump of the remnant	Use a guide with a ring-shaped target for better visualization of the guide pin inside the ACL stump	The key point is to drill the tibial tunnel in incremental diameter reamers (initially 6 mm followed by 8 mm, then 9 mm, and so on)
		Unsatisfactory position of the tibial guide pin	When drilling the tibial tunnel, first reposition the guide pin manually through the tunnel and then push it through the entire length of the ACL remnant before enlarging the tunnel by increasing the drill-bit diameter in 1-mm increments	
4.	Creating a hollow stump	Avulsion or damage to the remnant ACL stump	When drilling to enlarge the tibial tunnel, ensure that the entire tip of the drill has passed through the intraarticular cortex. Using low speed (revolutions per minute), the ACL remnant should move rhythmically as the drill gently turns inside it.	Nothing much can be done once the remnant is damaged. Hence, emphasis must be placed on gently carrying out low speed drilling.
5.	Suspensory fixation device (TightRope RT) deployment	Soft tissue interposition between the button and lateral femoral cortex	Deploy the femoral button under direct vision by placing the arthroscope in the lateral gutter	Reposition of the button and arthroscopic confirmation of correct placement
6.	Graft placement	Overstuffing of the notch resulting in anterior impingement	Using a graft of 8–10 mm diameter. Minimal notch debridement	An additional notchplasty and arthroscopic assessment of the knee in full extension

(ACL: Anterior cruciate ligament).

Conflict of interest and source of funding

BSC is a paid consultant, receives research support, and has made presentations for Arthrex.

REFERENCES

1. Adachi N, Ochi M, Uchio Y, et al. Anterior cruciate ligament augmentation under arthroscopy. A minimum 2-year follow-up in 40 patients. Arch Orthop Trauma Surg. 2000;120:128-33.
2. Gohil S, Annear PO, Breidahl W. Anterior cruciate ligament reconstruction using autologous double hamstrings: a comparison of standard versus minimal debridement techniques using MRI to assess revascularisation. A randomised prospective study with a one-year follow-up. J Bone Joint Surg Br. 2007;89:1165-71.
3. Junkin DM Jr, Johnson DL. ACL tibial remnant, to save or not? Orthopedics. 2008;31:154-9.
4. Kim SJ, Jo SB, Kim TW, et al. A modified arthroscopic anterior cruciate ligament double-bundle reconstruction technique with autogenous quadriceps tendon graft: remnant-preserving technique. Arch Orthop Trauma Surg. 2009;129:403-7.
5. Lee BI, Kwon SW, Kim JB, et al. Comparison of clinical results according to amount of preserved remnant in arthroscopic anterior cruciate ligament reconstruction using quadrupled hamstring graft. Arthroscopy. 2008;24:560-8.
6. Ahn JH, Lee YS, Ha HC. Anterior cruciate ligament reconstruction with preservation of remnant bundle using hamstring autograft: technical note. Arch Orthop Trauma Surg. 2009;129:1011-5.
7. Garrett WE Jr, Swiontkowski MF, Weinstein JN, et al. American Board of Orthopaedic Surgery Practice of the Orthopaedic Surgeon: Part-II, certification examination case mix. J Bone Joint Surg Am. 2006;88:660-7.
8. Kocher MS, Steadman JR, Briggs K, et al. Determinants of patient satisfaction with outcome after anterior cruciate ligament reconstruction. J Bone Joint Surg Am. 2002;84:1560-72.
9. Johnson DL, Coen MJ. Revision ACL surgery. Etiology, indications, techniques, and results. Am J Knee Surg. 1995;8: 155-67.
10. Fu FH, Shen W, Starman JS, et al. Primary anatomic double-bundle anterior cruciate ligament reconstruction: a preliminary 2-year prospective study. Am J Sports Med. 2008;36:1263-74.
11. Salmon L, Russell V, Musgrove T, et al. Incidence and risk factors for graft rupture and contralateral rupture after anterior cruciate ligament reconstruction. Arthroscopy. 2005;21:948-57.
12. Wright RW, Dunn WR, Amendola A, et al. Risk of tearing the intact anterior cruciate ligament in the contralateral knee and rupturing the anterior cruciate ligament graft during the first 2 years after anterior cruciate ligament reconstruction: a prospective MOON cohort study. Am J Sports Med. 2007;35:1131-34.
13. Shelbourne KD, Gray T, Haro M. Incidence of subsequent injury to either knee within 5 years after anterior cruciate ligament reconstruction with patellar tendon autograft. Am J Sports Med. 2009;37:246-51.
14. Crain EH, Fithian DC, Paxton EW, et al. Variation in anterior cruciate ligament scar pattern: does the scar pattern affect anterior laxity in anterior cruciate ligament-deficient knees? Arthroscopy. 2005;21:19-24.
15. Ochi M, Iwasa J, Uchio Y, et al. The regeneration of sensory neurones in the reconstruction of the anterior cruciate ligament. J Bone Joint Surg Br. 1999;81(5):902-6.
16. Arnoczky SP, Tarvin GB, Marshall JL. Anterior cruciate ligament replacement using patellar tendon. An evaluation of graft revascularization in the dog. J Bone Joint Surg Am. 1982;64:217-24.
17. Murray MM, Martin SD, Martin TL, et al. Histological changes in the human anterior cruciate ligament after rupture. J Bone Joint Surg Am. 2000;82:1387-97.
18. Howell SM, Knox KE, Farley TE, et al. Revascularization of a human anterior cruciate ligament graft during the first 2 years of implantation. Am J Sports Med. 1995;23(1):42-9.
19. Jackson DW, Schaefer RK. Cyclops syndrome: loss of extension following intra-articular anterior cruciate ligament reconstruction. Arthroscopy. 1990;6:171-8.
20. Haus BM, Mastrangelo AN, Murray MM. Effect of anterior cruciate healing on the uninjured ligament insertion site. J Orthop Res. 2012;30:86-94.
21. Vavken P, Murray MM. The potential for primary repair of the ACL. Sports Med Arthrosc. 2011;19:44-9.
22. Weiler A, Peters G, Mäurer J, et al. Biomechanical properties and vascularity of an anterior cruciate ligament graft can be predicted by contrast-enhanced magnetic resonance imaging: a 2-year study in sheep. Am J Sports Med. 2001;29(6):751-61.

23. Zaffagnini S, De Pasquale V, Marchesini Reggiani L, et al. Neoligamentization process of BTPB used for ACL graft: histological evaluation from 6 months to 10 years. Knee. 2007;14(2):87-93.
24. Papageorgiou CD, Ma CB, Abramowitch SD, et al. A multidisciplinary study of the healing of an intraarticular anterior cruciate ligament graft in a goat model. Am J Sports Med. 2001;29(5):620-6.
25. Murray MM, Spector M. The migration of cells from the ruptured human anterior cruciate ligament into collagen-glycosaminoglycan regeneration templates in vitro. Biomaterials. 2001;22:2393-402.
26. Ohsawa T, Kimura M, Kobayashi Y, et al. Arthroscopic evaluation of preserved ligament remnant after selective anteromedial or posterolateral bundle anterior cruciate ligament reconstruction. Arthroscopy. 2012;28:807-17.
27. Matsumoto T, Kubo S, Sasaki K, et al. Acceleration of tendon-bone healing of anterior cruciate ligament graft using autologous ruptured tissue. Am J Sports Med. 2012;40:1296-302.
28. Pujol N, Colombet P, Potel JF, et al. Anterior cruciate ligament reconstruction in partial tear: selective anteromedial bundle reconstruction conserving the posterolateral remnant versus single-bundle anatomic ACL reconstruction: preliminary 1-year results of a prospective randomized study. Orthop Traumatol Surg Res. 2012;98:S171-7.
29. Papalia R, Franceschi F, Zampogna B, et al. Surgical management of partial tears of the anterior cruciate ligament. Knee Surg Sports Traumatol Arthrosc. 2014;22(1):154-65.
30. Hu J, Qu J, Xu D, et al. Clinical outcomes of remnant preserving augmentation in anterior cruciate ligament reconstruction: a systematic review. Knee Surg Sports Traumatol Arthrosc. 2014;22(9):1976-85.
31. Demirag B, Ermutlu C, Aydemir F, et al. A comparison of clinical outcome of augmentation and standard reconstruction techniques for partial anterior cruciate ligament tears. Eklem Hastalik Cerrahisi. 2012;23:140-4.
32. Maestro A, uárez-Suárez MA, Rodríguez-López L, et al. Stability evaluation after isolated reconstruction of anteromedial or posterolateral bundle in symptomatic partial tears of anterior cruciate ligament. Eur J Orthop Surg Traumatol. 2013;23:471-80.
33. Ochi M, Iwasa J, Uchio Y, et al. Induction of somatosensory evoked potentials by mechanical stimulation in reconstructed anterior cruciate ligaments. J Bone Joint Surg Br. 2002; 84:761-6.
34. Nakamae A, Ochi M, Deie M, et al. Biomechanical function of anterior cruciate ligament remnants: how long do they contribute to knee stability after injury in patients with complete tears? Arthroscopy. 2010;26:1577-85.
35. Mifune Y, Ota S, Takayama K, et al. Therapeutic advantage in selective ligament augmentation for partial tears of the anterior cruciate ligament: results in an animal model. Am J Sports Med. 2013;41:365-73.
36. Johansson H, Sjolander P, Sojka P. Receptors in the knee joint ligaments and their role in the biomechanics of the joint. Crit Rev Biomed Eng. 1991;18:341-68.
37. Lee BI, Min KD, Choi HS, et al. Immunohistochemical study of mechanoreceptors in the tibial remnant of the ruptured anterior cruciate ligament in human knees. Knee Surg Sports Traumatol Arthrosc. 2009;17:1095-101.
38. Chouteau J, Testa R, Viste A, et al. Knee rotational laxity and proprioceptive function 2 years after partial ACL reconstruction. Knee Surg Sports Traumatol Arthrosc. 2012;20:762-6.
39. Kazusa H, Nakamae A, Ochi M. Augmentation technique for anterior cruciate ligament injury. Clin Sports Med. 2013;32(1):127-40.
40. Takazawa Y, Ikeda H, Kawasaki T, et al. ACL reconstruction preserving the ACL remnant achieves good clinical outcomes and can reduce subsequent graft rupture. Orthop J Sports Med. 2013;1(4):2325967113505076.
41. Ahn JH, Wang JH, Lee YS, et al. Anterior cruciate ligament reconstruction using remnant preservation and a femoral tensioning technique: clinical and magnetic resonance imaging results. Arthroscopy. 2011;27:1079-89.
42. Siebold R, Fu FH. Assessment and augmentation of symptomatic anteromedial or posterolateral bundle tears of the anterior cruciate ligament. Arthroscopy. 2008;24:1289-98.
43. Petersen W, Zantop T. Partial rupture of the anterior cruciate ligament. Arthroscopy. 2006;22:1143-5.
44. Sonnery-Cottet B, Chambat P. Arthroscopic identification of the anterior cruciate ligament posterolateral bundle: the figure-of-four position. Arthroscopy. 2007;23:1128.e1-3.
45. Sonnery-Cottet B, Barth J, Graveleau N, et al. Arthroscopic identification of isolated tear of the posterolateral bundle of the anterior cruciate ligament. Arthroscopy. 2009;25:728-32.
46. Howell SM, Hull ML. Checkpoints for judging tunnel and anterior cruciate ligament graft placement. J Knee Surg. 2009;22(02):161-70.
47. Nakamae A, Deie M, Adachi N, et al. Augmentation procedure for partial rupture of the anterior cruciate ligament. Tech Knee Surg. 2010;9:194-200.

48. Ochi M, Abouheif MM, Kongcharoensombat W, et al. Double bundle arthroscopic anterior cruciate ligament reconstruction with remnant preserving technique using a hamstring autograft. Sports Med Arthrosc Rehabil Ther Technol. 2011;3:30.
49. Nakamae A, Ochi M, Adachi N, et al. Clinical comparisons between the transtibial technique and the far anteromedial portal technique for posterolateral femoral tunnel drilling in anatomic double bundle anterior cruciate ligament reconstruction. Arthroscopy. 2012;28:658-66.
50. Sonnery-Cottet B, Freychet B, Murphy CG, et al. Anterior cruciate ligament reconstruction and preservation: the single-anteromedial bundle biological augmentation (SAMBBA) technique. Arthrosc Tech. 2014;3(6):e689-93.
51. Papachristou G, Nikolaou V, Efstathopoulos N, et al. ACL reconstruction with semitendinosus tendon autograft without detachment of its tibial insertion: a histologic study in a rabbit model. Knee Surg Sports Traumatol Arthrosc. 2007;15:1175-80.

CHAPTER

25

Anterior Cruciate Ligament Augmentation

Humza Shaikh, Marcio Albers, Weimin Zhu, Freddie H Fu

INTRODUCTION

The anterior cruciate ligament reconstruction (ACLR) is amongst the most common procedures in orthopedics, with nearly 130,000 ACL reconstructions (ACLR) performed annually in the United States.[1] Isolated ACL injuries can be either complete or partial, with partial tears occurring 10–35% of the time.[2,3] Of these, typically only 5–10% of single bundle tears become symptomatic.[4,5] Though studies report that 38–50% of partial lesions evolve into complete tears, treatment of partial ACL tears, in particular using the ACL augmentation technique, is controversial and this injury continues to pose a dilemma for orthopedic surgeons.[6,7]

DIAGNOSIS OF PARTIAL ANTERIOR CRUCIATE LIGAMENT TEARS

From a clinical perspective, no consensus definition regarding partial tears has been reached. Descriptions of partial tears vary from intrasubstance hemorrhage, to total rupture of the anteromedial (AM) or posterolateral (PL) bundle.[5,8,9] Others define ACL tears according to the percentage of torn fibers. Arbitrarily, 25%–75% of torn fibers have been considered partial tears, while others have defined high-grade versus low-grade ACL tears according to a 50% cutoff.[6,10-14] Direct identification of the torn ACL bundle can further aid in classification of these injuries, with diagnosis by physical examination, magnetic resonance imaging (MRI), and arthroscopy.

Nonetheless, partial tears of the ACL should be defined by the functional stability and degree of laxity as measured by specific clinical tests, rather than asymptomatic findings on MRI or arthroscopy.[15]

Physical Examination

Partial ACL tears are diagnosed by comparison to the contralateral, uninjured knee, most consistently with an asymmetric Lachman test, a low-grade KT-1,000 arthrometer measurement (≤3 mm difference), and a negative or only slightly positive (0 or 1+) pivot-shift under anesthesia.[4,16-18] Studies have also suggested that, regardless of grade, any asymmetric positive pivot shift is consistent with functional instability and should be treated as a complete ACL tear.[18,19]

Despite the sensitivity of these examinations, other studies have found that single bundle tears cannot be reliable detected on physical examination. Cadaveric studies have shown that abnormal knee laxity is only appreciable after significant ACL injury.[15] One such study found that physical examination could only identify partial ACL tears when more than 75% of the ligament had failed, in particular, complete PL bundle plus half AM bundle rupture.[15] This suggests that 50% of the ACL is enough to maintain normal findings on physical examination.[15] Another cadaveric study found it impossible to detect differences between an AM bundle partial tear and an intact ACL using clinical examination and KT-1000 arthrometery.[20] Thus, it may be difficult to distinguish a partial tear of the ACL from an intact ACL based on physical examination alone.[15,20,21] Regardless, an asymmetric Lachman test or KT-1000 arthrometry is indicative of an ACL injury that requires further evaluation.

Magnetic Resonance Imaging Evaluation

MRI is helpful in differentiating between complete and partial ACL tears. However, given the low sensitivity and specificity for diagnosing single bundle tears, MRI findings cannot be solely used to make a final diagnosis.[14,22,23] MRI findings indicative of partial tears include the presence of high signal intensity within the ligament, without disruption of its continuity and orientation[24,25] (Figs. 25.1A and B). Primary signs (those involving the ACL itself) and secondary signs (associated abnormalities) are used to determine the extent of injury. Primary signs include: mass effect, loss of ligament continuity, increased MRI signal intensity within the ligament, and abnormal ligament contour. Secondary signs include osteochondral defects, posterior cruciate ligament (PCL) buckling, anterior

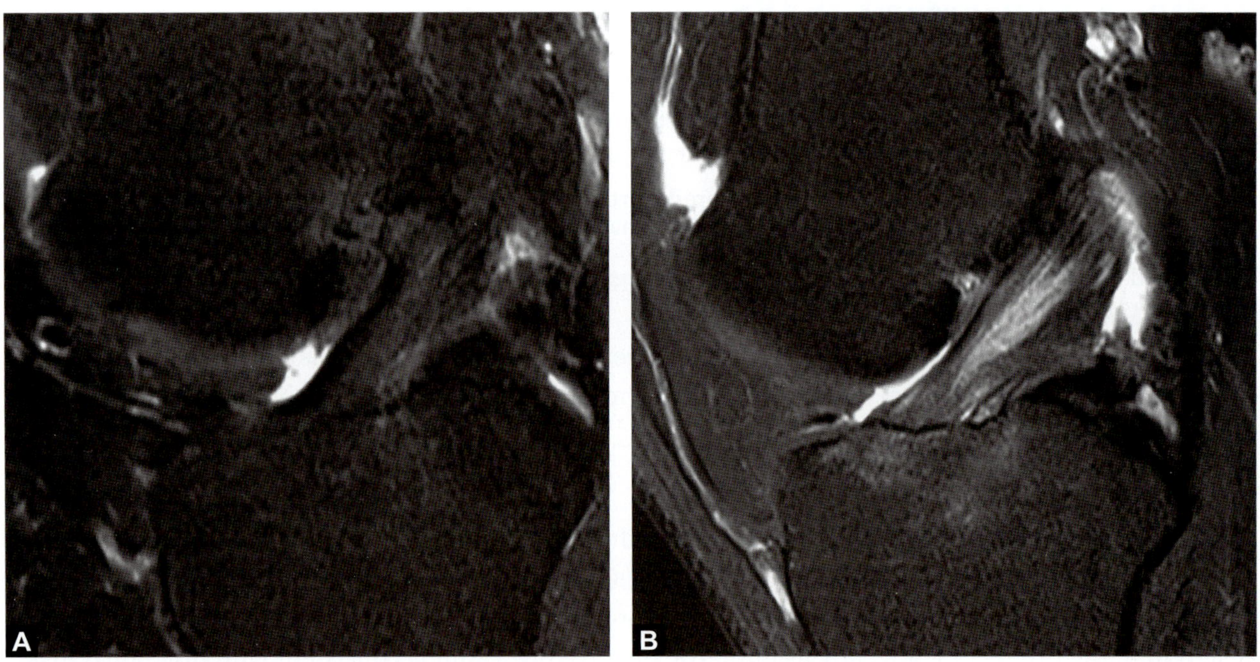

Figs. 25.1A and B: Sagittal T2 fat saturated MRI shows (A) a posterolateral (PL) bundle hemorrhage with conservation of the anteromedial (AM) bundle and (B) an isolated AM tear.

tibial translation, and a deep lateral femoral notch.[25] These primary signs are seen in 33–43% of patients with a partial ACL rupture.[6] Unfortunately, secondary signs do little to improve the detection of partial tears.[22] MRI has been found to have a 55% sensitivity and a 75% specificity for the diagnosis of partial tears of the ACL when the diagnosis is based on one or more of the following criteria: abnormal intrasubstance signal intensity with intact fibers, bowing or undulation of intact fibers, no visualization on the T1-weighted image with intact fibers seen on inverse-recovery or T2-weighted pulse sequences, and the absence of secondary signs.[23]

Given the oblique course of the ACL, additional parasagittal and paracoronal planes have been examined to improve ACL visualization.[24] However, these additional oblique views are of marginal value for improving MRIs diagnostic accuracy in single bundle ACL tears.[14,24,26] As such, MRI can only be used to supplement other clinical findings when diagnosing partial tears of the ACL.

Arthroscopic Evaluation

Since diagnosis of partial ACL tears by office examination is unreliable, definitive diagnosis typically relies on arthroscopy.[6,9,20,27-31] Intraoperative testing of the ACL to assess for relies on arthroscopic visualization of the ACL during anterior tibial translation and internal/external rotation of the leg to assess for laxity and ligamentous damage. However, accurate grading of ACL injuries is difficult for several reasons. For instance, healthy appearing ACL tissue may mask significant injury. The ligament may appear intact despite experiencing plastic deformation, being lax and structurally nonfunctional. Partial injury without synovial sheath injury may give the ligament the appearance of minimal injury. Finally, a completely torn ACL may adhere to the intercondylar notch or PCL by scar tissue, giving a normal appearance to the damaged ligament.[32]

Thus, while arthroscopy best assesses an injured ACL, like the other modalities it should also not be the lone diagnostic tool. The ultimate purpose of arthroscopy is to confirm ACL pathology after a complete clinical evaluation and examination under anesthesia.

TREATMENT OF PARTIAL ANTERIOR CRUCIATE LIGAMENT TEARS

Individualized, Anatomic Anterior Cruciate Ligament Reconstruction

The concept of individualized, anatomic ACLR relies on four principles. The first principle is to restore the two functional bundles of the ACL. The second principle is that tunnels placed within the native ACL footprint should restore the ACL insertion sites on the tibia and femur. The third principle is that each bundle should adhere to the correct tensioning pattern. The fourth and final principle is individualized surgery for each patient considering his specific anatomy and needs.[33] This concept applies to single-bundle, double-bundle ACLR, ACL revision surgery, and ACL augmentation.

Anterior Cruciate Ligament Augmentation Surgery

Treatment should be individualized to the patient's activity level. Those with a low-demand lifestyle (low risk) usually have minimal symptoms, a negative pivot-shift test, and can be effectively managed nonoperatively. Those with a high-demand lifestyle (high risk) are more likely to have symptomatic instability, a positive pivot-shift test, and require operative treatment. Treatment of partial ACL ruptures must be customized to the unique clinical presentation, physical activity requirements, and associated injuries.

Studies have shown that anywhere from 12–86% of partial tears progress to complete tears.[6] These patients can present with worsening knee laxity, a positive pivot shift test in 25% of cases, and a higher rate of meniscal and cartilage lesions.[6,11,21,34,35] As compared to complete ACL ruptures, patients with partial tears experience a significantly longer delay between injury and surgery, exacerbating these complications.[36,37] In order to diminish these complications, the clinical course of partial ACL tears supports ACL augmentation surgery.

Guidelines for Selecting Treatment

The first step in the operative management of partial ACL tears is examination under anesthesia for the confirmation of diagnosis. Pivot shift test sensitivity can improve from 24% to 92% under these conditions, making it the most important diagnostic tool for the evaluation of functional status and the rotational stability of residual ACL fibers.[14,16,17]

Our experience has been that a negative pivot shift test during the office clinical examination in the setting of history and imaging indicative of a partial ACL injury may warrant an examination under anesthesia. If the pivot shift test remains negative during examination under anesthesia but the surgeon maintains a high level of suspicion, he may proceed with diagnostic arthroscopy to rule out intraarticular pathology possibly confounding pivot shift test results. This includes displaced ACL tissue, displaced menisci, or osteochondral fragments. Once these injuries are addressed and if the ACL appears healthy on direct visualization, the pivot shift test can be repeated. If all confounding injuries have been ruled out and the pivot shift test remains negative, further management should be nonoperative. However, if repeat pivot shift test is positive, then the patient is a candidate for ACL augmentation surgery.

Remnant Preservation

Anterior cruciate ligament remnant preservation confers a number of advantages over standard reconstruction surgery. Studies suggest improved biomechanical, vascular, and proprioceptive outcomes, with maintenance of a landmark for graft tunnel positioning.[38-42]

Anterior cruciate ligament remnants have been variably described. Most commonly, scar tissue attaches the ACL proximally to the PCL.[43] Occasionally, the remnant remains adhered to the femur, attached to a different femoral attachment site than the native ACL. This remnant may maintain some of the native ACLs biomechanical restraint against AP laxity, potentially decreasing anterior translation.[44,45] This added biomechanical strength in the immediate postoperative period may help protect the graft.

Additionally, remnant preservation may confer a healing advantage by providing vascular support for the new graft. Blood supply is of critical importance in preventing native ACL insufficiency, and its preservation supports the healing process of the graft.[46,47]

Preservation of the ACL remnant may also help maintain proprioceptive innervation of the ACL. Somatosensory evoked potentials have been described in approximately 50% of ACL remnants, and Golgi tendon organ-like mechanoreceptors have been described in the synovial membrane.[48-52] These mechanoreceptors are linked to the ACLs proprioceptive function; their preservation may improve joint position sense, allowing improved postoperative rehabilitation and a safer return to sports.[38,39]

ANTERIOR CRUCIATE LIGAMENT AUGMENTATION SURGICAL TECHNIQUE

Anterior cruciate ligament augmentation is now considered the standard surgical treatment for unstable partial tears of the ACL. This procedure is performed by selectively reconstructing the AM or PL bundle while preserving the intact remnant.

The ACL augmentation surgical technique follows the individualized, anatomic ACLR concept. Graft choice, rehabilitation protocol, and return to sports timing are all tailored to the specific injury pattern. Individual arthroscopic analysis determines notch cleaning, tunnel positioning, drill guide use, and graft size.

The patient is placed supine on the operating table, the injured knee is stabilized in a leg holder with a nonsterile tourniquet around the upper thigh, allowing range of motion (ROM) from 0° to 120°.[4,53] A three-portal technique is recommended, with a high anterolateral portal, central portal, and accessory medial portal. This approach improves visualization of all knee structures, allowing precise placement of the femoral and tibial tunnels.

After debridement of Hoffa's fat pad with an arthroscopic shaver, a global evaluation is performed to assess cartilage and meniscus health. ACL remnant analysis is then performed with careful evaluation of the native tibial and femoral footprints. Examination of the ruptured bundle is important and care must be taken to debride scar tissue attachments with a nonmotorized instrument. The integrity of the intact fibers is then tested using a probe, with an anterior drawer test performed by the first assistant with accompanying direct visualization of the ACL. The diagnosis of a partial tear is confirmed by arthroscopic visualization and probing, correlating the findings with the clinical examination under anesthesia (Figs. 25.2A and B).

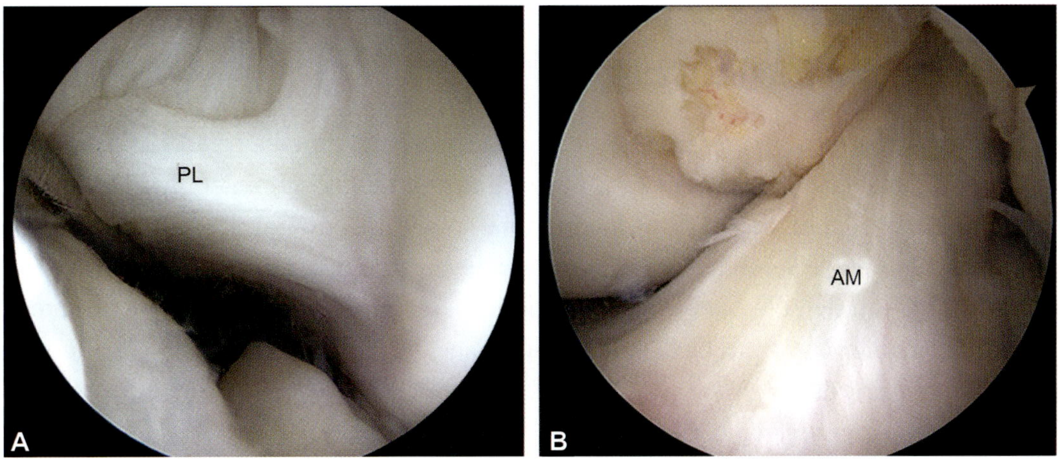

Figs. 25.2A and B: Scope views showing (A) posterolateral (PL) bundle insufficiency during probing; (B) intact anteromedial (AM) bundle.

The AM bundle is probed through the anterolateral portal, with the knee at 60° to 90° flexion and neutral rotation. In some cases, it is difficult to distinguish between PCL adherence and an intact native AM bundle. Given the low position of the PL bundle insertion on the lateral femoral condyle, direct observation is better through the central or accessory medial portal.[4] Ideally, the PL bundle is examined with the knee at 80° flexion, in varus and with external rotation of the hip (figure-of-four position).[53] The knee is then moved through its complete ROM, examining tension on each bundle.

The vascularity of the remnant should also be noted as this helps determine the biological environment of the future graft and gives clues about graft healing potential.[39]

Graft Selection

Graft selection should be individualized to the patient's activity level and based on the surgeon's experience.[37] Most surgeons prefer hamstring tendon (doubled semitendinosus) for ACL augmentation.[5,53-58] Graft selection in an augmentation case is influenced by the difficulty associated with graft passage in the joint. The space left in the notch by the intact bundle means a 7–8 mm graft is typically ideal.[53,57]

Anteromedial Bundle Reconstruction

Anteromedial bundle reconstruction begins with careful debridement of the ACL, avoiding damage to the intact PL bundle. The tibial drill guide is set to 55° and the tunnel's distal entrance should be marked 1.5 cm medial to the anterior tibial tuberosity.[4] With the knee maximally flexed and using the tibial remnant as a landmark, a K-wire is inserted 4–5 mm lateral to the medial tibial spine and 4–5 mm posterior to the anterior rim of the ACL stump. To prevent impingement with the intercondylar notch, the anterior femoral fibers of the remnant should serve as the anterior border. The knee can be brought to full extension with the K-wire in the joint to test for impingement. The femoral AM tunnel is then drilled through the accessory medial portal with a headed reamer. Final drill progression must be done by hand, at low speed, to prevent damage to the bundle remnant. The drill can also be inserted using a cannula to avoid PL fiber damage. Finally, the graft is passed through the tunnels (Fig. 25.3A).

Posterolateral Bundle Reconstruction

During PL bundle reconstruction, the tibial tunnel is positioned more medially, 3.5 cm medial to the tibial tuberosity with the tibial drill guide set to 45°.[4] Intraarticular guide position should correspond with the posterior tibial remnant, 5 mm medial to the lateral tibial spine. The femoral side is then marked based on the ACL remnant, on average 5 mm posterior to the shallow articular cartilage of the lateral femoral condyle.[4] Drilling is done through the accessory medial portal, just above the anterior horn of the medial meniscus. Using a headed reamer, care must be taken not to damage the medial condyle. An outside-in technique can be used to prevent any damage of the AM bundle. Anatomic placement of the PL bundle graft helps the AM bundle regain its native tension (Fig. 25.3B).

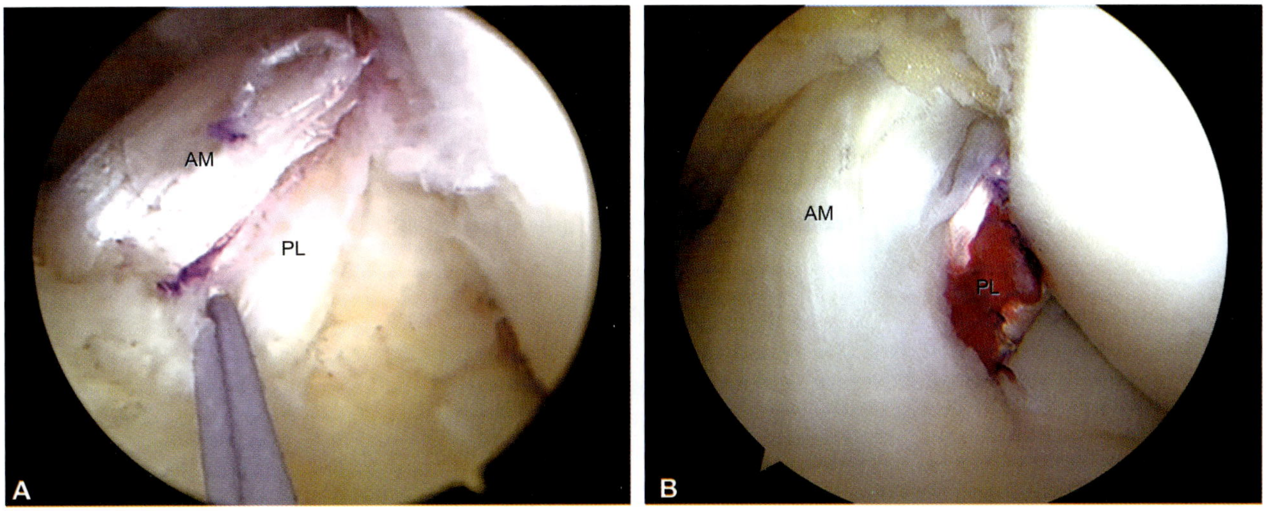

Figs. 25.3A and B: Scope view from the anterolateral portal which (A) shows the posterolateral (PL) graft in place with intact anteromedial (AM) bundle tightened and (B) shows AM graft in place, while PL bundle is conserved.

Graft Fixation

For the inside-out technique, the femoral side is commonly fixed with a suspensory device while the tibial side is fixed with a biologically inert screw.[4,55,59] For the outside-in technique, inert screws are used in both tunnels.[60] Fixation is done after preconditioning and cycling—the PL bundle is fixed at 0° while the AM bundle is fixed at 45°, replicating the native ACL biomechanical properties.[4,61-63] Once the graft is fixed, the knee is ranged through its full arc, ensuring the graft does not impinge on the intercondylar notch roof, the PCL, and the lateral edge of the medial condyle. When placed anatomically, augmentation surgery reconstructs an ACL that resembles and mimics the native ACL.

REHABILITATION

Rehabilitation following ACL augmentation surgery follows the same principles that guide traditional ACLR rehabilitation.

Immediately postoperation, the knee is immobilized in a brace. Patients are discharged the same day with adequate pain medication and an icing device.

During the 1st week(s), focus should be placed on reducing pain and swelling, restoring full ROM, and regaining quadriceps muscle strength. The day after surgery, patients begin to perform ankle pumps, straight leg raises, quadriceps sets, gastrocnemius stretches, and heel slides. At the end of the 1st week, continuous passive motion is initiated with progression to full extension.

Depending on the progress made, crutches and brace are typically weaned after 6 weeks. Once quadriceps muscle strength returns, straight line walking can be initiated at 6 weeks, with progression to jogging in a straight line and stationary biking at 3 months. Pivoting and cutting exercises are not initiated until at least 6 months, and return to sport is generally no sooner than 9 months postoperatively.

Patient progression through the rehabilitation phases is dependent on the patient's readiness as determined through periodic evaluation by the physical therapist and the surgeon. Clinical findings and rehabilitation tests should be monitored in this process. Periodic evaluation by MRI to assess graft healing can also be instituted, particularly if the patient desires an earlier return to sports.[64]

CONCLUSION

Though the frequency of the partial tears ranges from 10% to 35%, the incidence of symptomatic anteromedial (AM) or posterolateral (PL) bundle tears is between 5% and 10%. The diagnosis of symptomatic AM or PL bundle tear relies on a combination of the patient's history, clinical examination, MRI, and arthroscopic evaluation. To guide successful treatment, partial tears should be evaluated on the basis of functional symptoms, not solely on structural deficiencies. Examination under anesthesia is indicated for this purpose, with the pivot shift test remaining the most important for evaluation of ACL function. The final operative treatment decision must be taken after thorough arthroscopic testing, in which each bundle is evaluated independently.

Based on the individualized, anatomic ACLR concept, the ACL augmentation technique reconstructs the injured bundle while sparing the intact fibers. Several factors may support preserving the intact ACL remnant instead of debriding it. These include better orientation of the graft, mechanical stability, vascularization, proprioceptive innervation, faster remodeling of the ACL graft, and ultimately, a faster and safer rehabilitation for the patient.

REFERENCES

1. Mall NA, Chalmers PN, Moric M, et al. Incidence and trends of anterior cruciate ligament reconstruction in the United States. Am J Sports Med. 2014;42(10):2363-70.
2. Noyes FR, Bassett RW, Grood ES, et al. Arthroscopy in acute traumatic hemarthrosis of the knee. Incidence of anterior cruciate tears and other injuries. J Bone Joint Surg Am. 1980;62(5):687-95, 757.
3. Liljedahl SO, Lindvall N, Wetterfors J. Early diagnosis and treatment of acute ruptures of the anterior cruciate ligament; a clinical and arthrographic study of forty-eight cases. J Bone Joint Surg Am. 1965;47(8):1503-13.
4. Siebold R, Fu FH. Assessment and augmentation of symptomatic anteromedial or posterolateral bundle tears of the anterior cruciate ligament. Arthroscopy. 2008;24(11):1289-98.
5. Ochi M, Adachi N, Deie M, et al. Anterior cruciate ligament augmentation procedure with a 1-incision technique: anteromedial bundle or posterolateral bundle reconstruction. Arthroscopy. 2006;22(4):463, e461-5.
6. Noyes FR, Mooar LA, Moorman CT, 3rd, et al. Partial tears of the anterior cruciate ligament. Progression to complete ligament deficiency. J Bone Joint Surg Br. 1989;71(5):825-33.
7. Fruensgaard S, Johannsen HV. Incomplete ruptures of the anterior cruciate ligament. J Bone Joint Surg Br. 1989;71(3):526-30.
8. Odensten M, Lysholm J, Gillquist J. The course of partial anterior cruciate ligament ruptures. Am J Sports Med. 1985;13(3):183-6.
9. Farquharson-Roberts MA, Osborne AH. Partial rupture of the anterior cruciate ligament of the knee. J Bone Joint Surg Br. 1983;65(1):32-4.
10. Messner K, Maletius W. Eighteen- to twenty-five-year follow-up after acute partial anterior cruciate ligament rupture. Am J Sports Med. 1999;27(4):455-9.
11. Lehnert M, Eisenschenk A, Zellner A. Results of conservative treatment of partial tears of the anterior cruciate ligament. Int Orthop. 1993;17(4):219-23.

12. Kocher MS, Micheli LJ, Zurakowski D, et al. Partial tears of the anterior cruciate ligament in children and adolescents. Am J Sports Med. 2002;30(5):697-703.
13. Lamar DS, Bartolozzi AR, Freedman KB, et al. Thermal modification of partial tears of the anterior cruciate ligament. Arthroscopy. 2005;21(7):809-14.
14. Hong SH, Choi JY, Lee GK, et al. Grading of anterior cruciate ligament injury. Diagnostic efficacy of oblique coronal magnetic resonance imaging of the knee. J Comput Assist Tomogr. 2003;27(5):814-9.
15. Hole RL, Lintner DM, Kamaric E, et al. Increased tibial translation after partial sectioning of the anterior cruciate ligament. The posterolateral bundle. Am J Sports Med. 1996;24(4):556-60.
16. Lubowitz JH, Bernardini BJ, Reid JB, 3rd. Current concepts review: comprehensive physical examination for instability of the knee. Am J Sports Med. 2008;36(3):577-94.
17. Bach BR, Jr., Warren RF, Wickiewicz TL. The pivot shift phenomenon: results and description of a modified clinical test for anterior cruciate ligament insufficiency. Am J Sports Med. 1988;16(6):571-6.
18. Bach BR, Jr., Warren RF, Flynn WM, et al. Arthrometric evaluation of knees that have a torn anterior cruciate ligament. J Bone Joint Surg Am. 1990;72(9):1299-306.
19. DeFranco MJ, Bach BR, Jr. A comprehensive review of partial anterior cruciate ligament tears. J Bone Joint Surg Am. 2009;91(1):198-208.
20. Lintner DM, Kamaric E, Moseley JB, et al. Partial tears of the anterior cruciate ligament. Are they clinically detectable? Am J Sports Med. 1995;23(1):111-8.
21. Fritschy D, Panoussopoulos A, Wallensten R, et al. Can we predict the outcome of a partial rupture of the anterior cruciate ligament? A prospective study of 43 cases. Knee Surg Sports Traumatol Arthrosc. 1997;5(1):2-5.
22. Yao L, Gentili A, Petrus L, et al. Partial ACL rupture: an MR diagnosis? Skeletal Radiol. 1995;24(4):247-51.
23. Umans H, Wimpfheimer O, Haramati N, et al. Diagnosis of partial tears of the anterior cruciate ligament of the knee: value of MR imaging. AJR Am J Roentgenol. 1995;165(4):893-7.
24. Duc SR, Zanetti M, Kramer J, et al. Magnetic resonance imaging of anterior cruciate ligament tears: evaluation of standard orthogonal and tailored paracoronal images. Acta Radiol. 2005;46(7):729-33.
25. Walker CW, Moore TE. Imaging of skeletal and soft tissue injuries in and around the knee. Radiol Clin North Am. 1997;35(3):631-53.
26. Staeubli HU, Adam O, Becker W, et al. Anterior cruciate ligament and intercondylar notch in the coronal oblique plane: anatomy complemented by magnetic resonance imaging in cruciate ligament-intact knees. Arthroscopy. 1999;15(4):349-59.
27. O'Connor RL. Arthroscopy in the diagnosis and treatment of acute ligament injuries of the knee. J Bone Joint Surg Am. 1974;56(2):333-7.
28. Noyes FR, Barber-Westin SD. Arthroscopic repair of meniscal tears extending into the avascular zone in patients younger than twenty years of age. Am J Sports Med. 2002;30(4):589-600.
29. McDaniel WJ. Isolated partial tear of the anterior cruciate ligament. Clin Orthop Relat Res. 1976(115):209-12.
30. DeHaven KE. Diagnosis of acute knee injuries with hemarthrosis. Am J Sports Med. 1980;8(1):9-14.
31. Finsterbush A, Frankl U, Mann G. Fat pad adhesion to partially torn anterior cruciate ligament: a cause of knee locking. Am J Sports Med. 1989;17(1):92-5.
32. Bach BR, Jr., Warren RF. "Empty wall" and "vertical strut" signs of ACL insufficiency. Arthroscopy. 1989;5(2):137-40.
33. Shen W, Forsythe B, Ingham SM, et al. Application of the anatomic double-bundle reconstruction concept to revision and augmentation anterior cruciate ligament surgeries. J Bone Joint Surg Am. 2008;90(Suppl 4):20-34.
34. Pujol N, Colombet P, Cucurulo T, et al. Natural history of partial anterior cruciate ligament tears: a systematic literature review. Orthop Traumatol Surg Res. 2012;98(8 Suppl):S160-4.
35. Buckley SL, Barrack RL, Alexander AH. The natural history of conservatively treated partial anterior cruciate ligament tears. Am J Sports Med. 1989;17(2):221-5.
36. Panisset JC, Duraffour H, Vasconcelos W, et al. Clinical, radiological and arthroscopic analysis of the ACL tear. A prospective study of 418 cases. Rev Chir Orthop Reparatrice Appar Mot. 2008;94(8 Suppl):362-8.

37. Dejour D, Potel JF, Gaudot F, et al. The ACL tear from the pre-operative analysis to a 2-year follow-up, influence of the graft choice on the subjective and objective evaluation. Rev Chir Orthop Reparatrice Appar Mot. 2008;94(8 Suppl):356-61.
38. Adachi N, Ochi M, Uchio Y, et al. Mechanoreceptors in the anterior cruciate ligament contribute to the joint position sense. Acta Orthop Scand. 2002;73(3):330-4.
39. Georgoulis AD, Pappa L, Moebius U, et al. The presence of proprioceptive mechanoreceptors in the remnants of the ruptured ACL as a possible source of re-innervation of the ACL autograft. Knee Surg Sports Traumatol Arthrosc. 2001;9(6):364-8.
40. Ochi M, Iwasa J, Uchio Y, et al. Induction of somatosensory evoked potentials by mechanical stimulation in reconstructed anterior cruciate ligaments. J Bone Joint Surg Br. 2002;84(5):761-6.
41. Ochi M, Iwasa J, Uchio Y, et al. The regeneration of sensory neurones in the reconstruction of the anterior cruciate ligament. J Bone Joint Surg Br. 1999;81(5):902-6.
42. Dejour D, Ntagiopoulos PG, Saggin PR, et al. The diagnostic value of clinical tests, magnetic resonance imaging, and instrumented laxity in the differentiation of complete versus partial anterior cruciate ligament tears. Arthroscopy. 2013;29(3):491-9.
43. Crain EH, Fithian DC, Paxton EW, et al. Variation in anterior cruciate ligament scar pattern: does the scar pattern affect anterior laxity in anterior cruciate ligament-deficient knees? Arthroscopy. 2005;21(1):19-24.
44. Liu W, Maitland ME, Bell GD. A modeling study of partial ACL injury: simulated KT-2000 arthrometer tests. J Biomech Eng. 2002;124(3):294-301.
45. Colombet P, Dejour D, Panisset JC, et al. Current concept of partial anterior cruciate ligament ruptures. Orthop Traumatol Surg Res. 2010;96(8 Suppl):S109-18.
46. Dodds JA, Arnoczky SP. Anatomy of the anterior cruciate ligament: a blueprint for repair and reconstruction. Arthroscopy. 1994;10(2):132-9.
47. Bray RC, Leonard CA, Salo PT. Vascular physiology and long-term healing of partial ligament tears. J Orthop Res. 2002;20(5):984-9.
48. Schutte MJ, Dabezies EJ, Zimny ML, et al. Neural anatomy of the human anterior cruciate ligament. J Bone Joint Surg Am. 1987;69(2):243-7.
49. Boisgard S, Levai JP, Geiger B, et al. Study of the variations in length of the anterior cruciate ligament during flexion of the knee: use of a 3D model reconstructed from MRI sections. Surg Radiol Anat. 1999;21(5):313-7.
50. Barrack RL, Buckley SL, Bruckner JD, et al. Partial versus complete acute anterior cruciate ligament tears. The results of nonoperative treatment. J Bone Joint Surg Br. 1990;72(4):622-4.
51. Denti M, Monteleone M, Berardi A, et al. Anterior cruciate ligament mechanoreceptors. Histologic studies on lesions and reconstruction. Clin Orthop Relat Res. 1994(308):29-32.
52. Schultz RA, Miller DC, Kerr CS, et al. Mechanoreceptors in human cruciate ligaments. A histological study. J Bone Joint Surg Am. 1984;66(7):1072-6.
53. Sonnery-Cottet B, Barth J, Graveleau N, et al. Arthroscopic identification of isolated tear of the posterolateral bundle of the anterior cruciate ligament. Arthroscopy. 2009;25(7):728-32.
54. Armour T, Forwell L, Litchfield R, et al. Isokinetic evaluation of internal/external tibial rotation strength after the use of hamstring tendons for anterior cruciate ligament reconstruction. Am J Sports Med. 2004;32(7):1639-43.
55. Adachi N, Ochi M, Uchio Y, et al. Anterior cruciate ligament augmentation under arthroscopy. A minimum 2-year follow-up in 40 patients. Arch Orthop Trauma Surg. 2000;120(3-4):128-33.
56. Veselko M, Rotter A, Tonin M. Cyclops syndrome occurring after partial rupture of the anterior cruciate ligament not treated by surgical reconstruction. Arthroscopy. 2000;16(3):328-31.
57. Buda R, Di Caprio F, Giuriati L, et al. Partial ACL tears augmented with distally inserted hamstring tendons and over-the-top fixation: an MRI evaluation. Knee. 2008;15(2):111-6.
58. Buda R, Ferruzzi A, Vannini F, et al. Augmentation technique with semitendinosus and gracilis tendons in chronic partial lesions of the ACL: clinical and arthrometric analysis. Knee Surg Sports Traumatol Arthrosc. 2006;14(11):1101-7.

59. Ochi M, Adachi N, Uchio Y, et al. A minimum 2-year follow-up after selective anteromedial or posterolateral bundle anterior cruciate ligament reconstruction. Arthroscopy. 2009;25(2):117-22.
60. Sonnery-Cottet B, Lavoie F, Ogassawara R, et al. Selective anteromedial bundle reconstruction in partial ACL tears: a series of 36 patients with mean 24 months follow-up. Knee Surg Sports Traumatol Arthrosc. 2010;18(1):47-51.
61. Nicholas SJ, D'Amato MJ, Mullaney MJ, et al. A prospectively randomized double-blind study on the effect of initial graft tension on knee stability after anterior cruciate ligament reconstruction. Am J Sports Med. 2004;32(8):1881-6.
62. Austin JC, Phornphutkul C, Wojtys EM. Loss of knee extension after anterior cruciate ligament reconstruction: effects of knee position and graft tensioning. J Bone Joint Surg Am. 2007;89(7):1565-74.
63. van Kampen A, Wymenga AB, van der Heide HJ, et al. The effect of different graft tensioning in anterior cruciate ligament reconstruction: a prospective randomized study. Arthroscopy. 1998;14(8):845-50.
64. Miyawaki M, Hensler D, Illingworth KD, et al. Signal intensity on magnetic resonance imaging after allograft double-bundle anterior cruciate ligament reconstruction. Knee Surg Sports Traumatol Arthrosc. 2014;22(5):1002-8.

CHAPTER

26

Primary ACL Repair

Sachin Tapasvi, Anshu Shekhar, Prashanth Gorur

INTRODUCTION

The treatment of anterior cruciate ligament (ACL) injuries has evolved from conservative management to ACL repairs and extra-articular procedures in 1970s to open intra-articular reconstructions with various grafts in 1980s to the current "gold standard" of anatomic and individualized arthroscopic reconstruction.[1] The aim of the treatment, however, continues to be the same, i.e. to provide a stable joint allowing the patient to return to his preinjury level of activity, improve knee-related quality of life and avoid late sequelae of an ACL deficient knee. Although ACL reconstruction gives predictable and good results with objective and subjective scores, it seldom "feels" normal and had a host of problems like donor site morbidity, failure of graft, mismatch between footprint and graft diameter, lack of proprioception.[2–4]

Advantages of a primary acute arthroscopic ACL repair are theoretically:[5,6]

- Less invasive
- Avoids graft donor site morbidity
- Retains native ACL anatomy, collagen orientation and bundles especially at the footprint
- Possibly retains proprioceptive functions which protects the knee from secondary changes
- Preserves the complex biomechanical properties of the ligament allowing faster recovery
- Physeal sparing option in pediatric patients.

REVIEW OF THE EVOLUTION OF ANTERIOR CRUCIATE LIGAMENT REPAIR

The first repair of the ACL in the English literature is attributed to AW Mayo Robson in 1895. In his report, he described the care of a miner who underwent suture repair of both the ACL and posterior cruciate ligament 3 years after his original injury. The case report stated that 6 years later, the patient was able to walk without a limp, described his knee as "perfectly strong" and he had not missed a day of work due to his knee injury, certainly an outcome of "good patient satisfaction".[7] In 1938, Palmer described the failure of spontaneous healing of a complete ACL tear and subsequent importance of repair. He advocated that early repair was critical to healing and used a repair technique using silk sutures and drawing them through a femoral tunnel.[8] Following on Palmer's work, O'Donoghue reported his technique of ACL repair in the 1950s. His technique consisted of a suture weave through the tibial stump, which then again had the ends passed through a tunnel in the femur and tied. O'Donoghue immobilized his patients for 4 weeks in 30° of flexion.[9] Both Palmer and O'Donoghue stressed the importance of early repair of the ACL.

In the 1970s, John Feagin continued the clinical studies of primary repair of the ACL. During his 4-year-tour at Keller Army Hospital at West Point, he became team physician for the Army football and basketball teams and noted that the natural history of an untreated ACL tear was not usually conducive to continuation of the active lifestyle of a cadet or officer. He began operating on acute ACL tears and repairing them. Feagin noted that these acute tears were often Z-shaped, with the posterolateral (PL) bundle proximally torn and the anteromedial (AM) bundle often torn more distally. Along with Walter Curl, Feagin reported on their experience with primary suture repair for ACL injuries in West Point cadets. Feagin advocated use of a Dexon suture woven through the tibial stump and passed up through bone tunnels in the femur. He immobilized his patients for 6 weeks after surgery in 30° of flexion. The 5-year follow-up results had 71% of patients with pain, 66% with swelling, 71% with stiffness and 94% with knee instability.[10] John Marshall reported a suture repair technique using multiple loop-varying depth sutures in both the femoral and tibial cruciate stump, using polyester sutures and individually tensioning each suture. Marshall's studies appeared more promising, with a 2.5-year follow-up study where no patients with repair had giving way symptoms or needed subsequent meniscal surgery (even though 93% of them were active in sports).[11]

After these initial reports of suture repair, two randomized clinical trials were reported in the 1980s. In 1985, Odensten et al. published the first prospective, randomized trial of suture repair versus nonoperative therapy for ACL injuries. At 18 months from surgery, the authors reported no significant difference between operated and nonoperated knees in terms of overall outcome scores; however, 95% patients in the repaired group had a stable knee at follow-up (with a negative pivot shift or Slocum's test), while only 11% in the nonoperated group had a stable knee. In addition, the patients who did not have a repair needed meniscal surgery twice as often as patients undergoing suture repair in the first 18 months after injury.[12] The other study by Sandberg et al. reported results similar to those of Odensten, but they concluded that there was no functional difference between nonoperative and repair groups. This, in spite of their objective data showing decrease in instability and need for meniscal surgery later.[13] Thus, while both of these studies concluded that functional performance was comparable between the two groups; other important characteristics (stable knee, preservation of the menisci) appeared to be better in the group undergoing primary repair.

Although the results of the first primary open ACL suture repair techniques were initially promising, inconsistent long-term results with high re-rupture rates of as high as 24–36% and the inconsistent improvements in anteroposterior laxity led to the abandonment of these techniques.[14-16] However, with improved understanding of the biology, biomechanics and injury patterns of the ACL, there has been a paradigm shift in the concept of performing an ACL repair. The most remarkable of these is perhaps selecting the ideal patient with a tear pattern most amenable to repair. Sherman et al. classified ACL tears into four types. Type 1 in their classification was "an avulsion of the entire ligament off the femoral insertion, without a major bone fragment, leaving no remnant of proximal tissue"[17] (*for details refer to Chapter 9*). In their cohort, better objective outcomes were seen with this group. Zantop et al. described that approximately 12% of ACL tears are proximal avulsions with an intact stump.[18] Steadman et al.

suggested that proximal lesions have a higher healing potential than mid-substance ruptures of the ACL.[19] Nguyen et al. investigated the intrinsic healing response of the ACL using standard histology and immunostaining of α-smooth muscle actin and collagen type 3. They concluded that the histologic features of the proximal third of the ACL and the medial collateral ligament were similar and a similar healing response can be expected.[20]

Current literature advocates careful selection of patients for arthroscopic ACL repair. This includes patients with femoral-sided avulsion injuries guided by preoperative imaging and excellent tissue quality on arthroscopic examination. DiFelice et al. suggested that advances in imaging, surgical techniques, and hardware may allow us to select a specific patient cohort who will benefit from repair. In his small case series of 11 patients with proximal avulsion tears, the ACL was reattached to bone using 4.75 mm BioComposite SwiveLock® suture anchors (Arthrex, Naples, FL). At mean follow-up of 41 months, the mean International Knee Documentation Committee (IKDC) score was 86, the mean Lysholm score was 93 and the mean Cincinnati score was 91. These results are certainly encouraging.[6] Weninger et al. described a double-bundle repair of proximal ACL tears using 2.9 mm PushLock® (Arthrex, Naples, FL) suture anchors.[21] Achtnich et al. compared clinical and radiologic results of primary ACL suture anchor repair and microfracturing with anatomic ACL single-bundle reconstruction in patients with acute proximal ACL avulsion tears. They found no significant differences in knee stability between the groups on clinical examination, Lachman and pivot-shift tests, or KT-1000 side-to-side measurements. They reported no failures in the primary ACL reconstruction group whereas three patients in the ACL refixation group showed recurrent instability and were considered failures (15%) but this was not statistically significant. They concluded that proximal refixation of the ACL using 2.9 mm PushLock® (Arthrex) suture anchors and microfracturing restores knee stability and results in comparable functional outcomes to a control group treated with single-bundle ACL reconstruction.[16] McKay et al. reported the results of ACL repair with internal brace ligament augmentation (IBLA) in 68 patients. There were four reinterventions including one for re-rupture, and one each for surgery for arthrofibrosis, meniscal tear and chondral pathology. Arthroscopy in these three patients revealed a healed ACL. They concluded that early functional outcome and failure data that demonstrates the technique of ACL repair with IBLA is comparable with early results from ACL reconstruction, with the greatest improvements seen in return to sporting activity.[22] Thus, combined with direct suture repair of proximal ACL tears, microfracture improves the biological healing response by recruitment of marrow elements at the repair site, and augmentation with high strength suture tape provides mechanical protection to the repair in the initial healing phase. Both these interventions could help improve the success of this procedure.

INDICATIONS*

- Acute femoral avulsion type ACL injury (Type I Sherman)
- Subsynovial ACL tear or stretch injury
- Partial ACL tear (isolated AM/PL bundle injury)
- Pediatric patients.

* The quality of tissue must be excellent with no fraying of the stump end.

CONTRAINDICATIONS

- Chronic tear with stump resorption
- Mid-substance tears
- Poor tissue quality.

SURGICAL TECHNIQUE

General Preparation

Patient is placed in supine position. A high thigh tourniquet is applied with side support and table flat. Examination under anesthesia is performed to confirm the laxity and quantify the same. MRI imaging is carefully studied to detect a proximal avulsion (Figs. 26.1A to C). All patients planned for a repair must be counseled about this procedure, and also an informed consent is obtained to proceed to a standard anatomic reconstruction, if the tear is deemed unsuitable for repair. After preparation, tourniquet is inflated and a high anterolateral (AL) portal and standard AM portals are created. A diagnostic round in performed to confirm the diagnosis of ACL tear and other associated pathologies. Careful probing of the stump is carried out to confirm a femoral sided avulsion and quality of the tissue (Fig. 26.2). Presence of the synovial sheath over the ACL indicates a low velocity trauma. At this point, a central portal (CP) through the medial third of patella tendon is created, which allows excellent visualization of the femoral insertion site (FIS) (Fig. 26.3).[23] Decision to perform a primary repair is taken, if the tissue quality is deemed excellent.

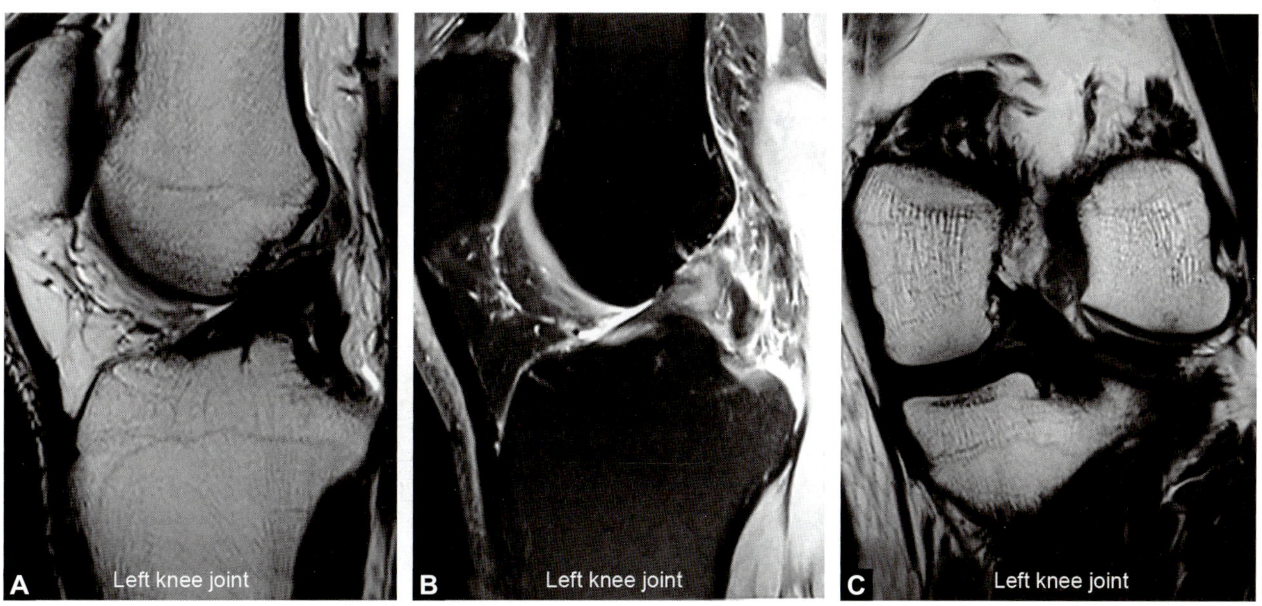

Figs. 26.1A to C: (A) T2 sagittal; (B) Proton-density fat saturated sagittal; (C) Proton-density coronal magnetic resonance images of left knee showing proximal avulsion of the anterior cruciate ligament with minimal marrow edema.

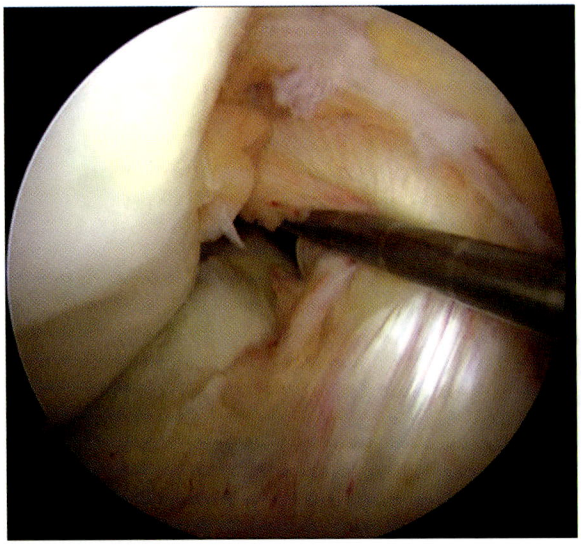

Fig. 26.2: The anterior cruciate ligament being probed to confirm the presence and characterize the site of the tear, viewing from the anterolateral portal.

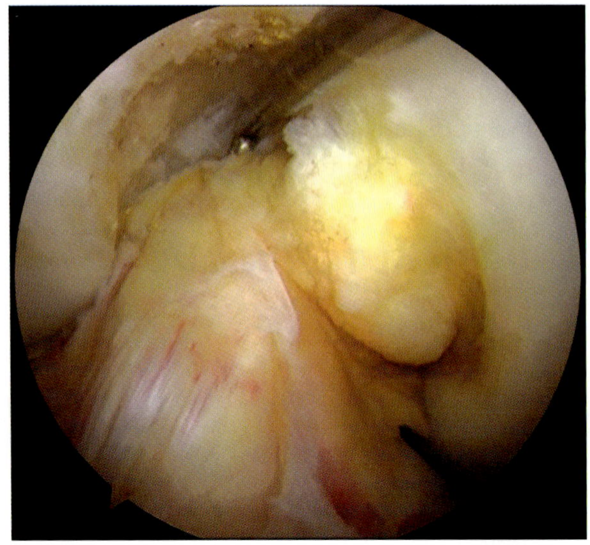

Fig. 26.3: Viewing from the central portal greatly improves the visualization of the femoral insertion site. Note the probe at the femoral end of anterior cruciate ligament showing a complete avulsion.

Preparing the Notch and Anterior Cruciate Ligament Stump

1. A bony notchplasty is not routinely done unless the notch is deemed too narrow, especially in female patients. Soft tissue around the FIS is cleared using a shaver.
2. Three to four holes are created around the FIS with a microfracture awl to potentiate healing of the ACL stump (Fig. 26.4).

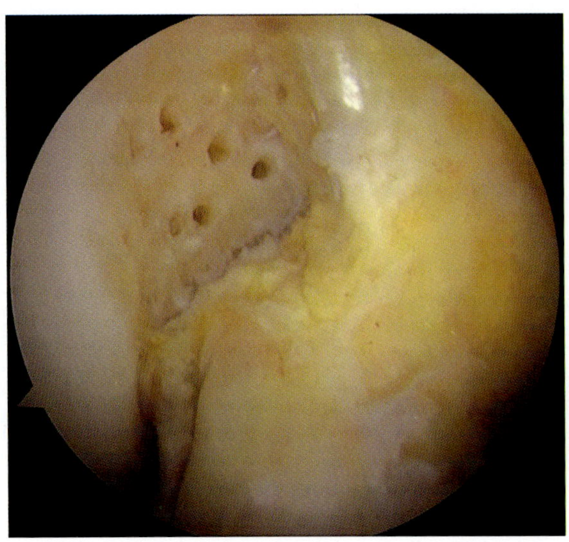

Fig. 26.4: Microfractures near the anterior cruciate ligament femoral footprint, viewed from the central portal. This procedure enhances healing response by recruitment of marrow elements.

3. The ACL stump is sutured with No. 2 FiberWire® (Arthrex, Naples, FL) using a Labral Scorpion™ loaded with SureFire® Scorpion™ needle (Arthrex, Naples, FL) suture passer instrument through the AM portal. This instrument allows grasping the tissue, suture passage and retrieval in a single step, thus minimizing tissue trauma. Suturing is begun distally and advanced proximally taking cruciate stitches so that two to three passes are taken through the ACL with each limb of the suture, to hold the tissue firmly (Figs. 26.5A and B). Utmost care is taken to avoid taking a bite though a previously passed stitch and thus lacerating the suture in the process.
4. The two ends of the suture are then retrieved through the AM portal.

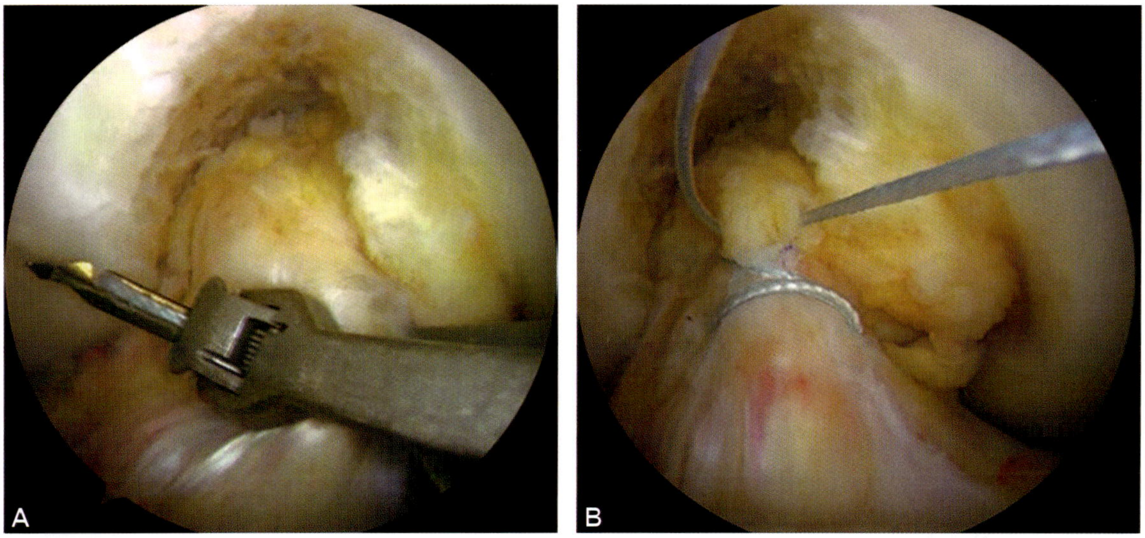

Figs. 26.5A and B: (A) Suturing of the anterior cruciate ligament is begun distally with a Labral Scorpion™ (Arthrex) self-retrieving suture passer loaded with No. 2 FiberWire®; (B) The suturing is progressed proximally using cruciate stitches.

Insertion of the Stump at the Femoral Insertion Site and Augmentation

1. The FIS is identified accurately by viewing from the CP. A pilot hole is created at the anatomic mid-bundle position using an awl for the SwiveLock® anchor introduced from an accessory low medial portal to obtain a straight trajectory (Fig. 26.6).
2. The two ends of FiberWire® along with a FiberTape® (Arthrex, Naples, FL) are loaded into the eyelet of a 4.75 mm PEEK SwiveLock® SP self-punching anchor (Arthrex, Naples, FL). This additional augmentation with the FiberTape® is like an InternalBrace™ and protects the repair till healing has occurred, by providing initial stability.
3. The driver is introduced through the accessory medial portal and inserted into the pilot hole by tapping till the anchor tip is seen, while ensuring that there is no slack in any suture by pulling them individually.
4. The anchor is inserted by turning the handle in a clockwise manner while viewing from the CP and knee in 90° flexion and application of posterior drawer force to keep the ACL in tension (Figs. 26.7A and B).

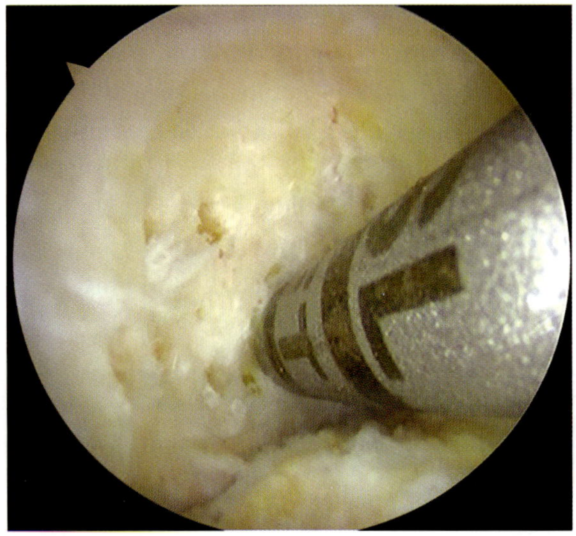

Fig. 26.6: Entry hole for 4.75 mm SwiveLock® suture anchor being created at the center of the femoral footprint using an awl.

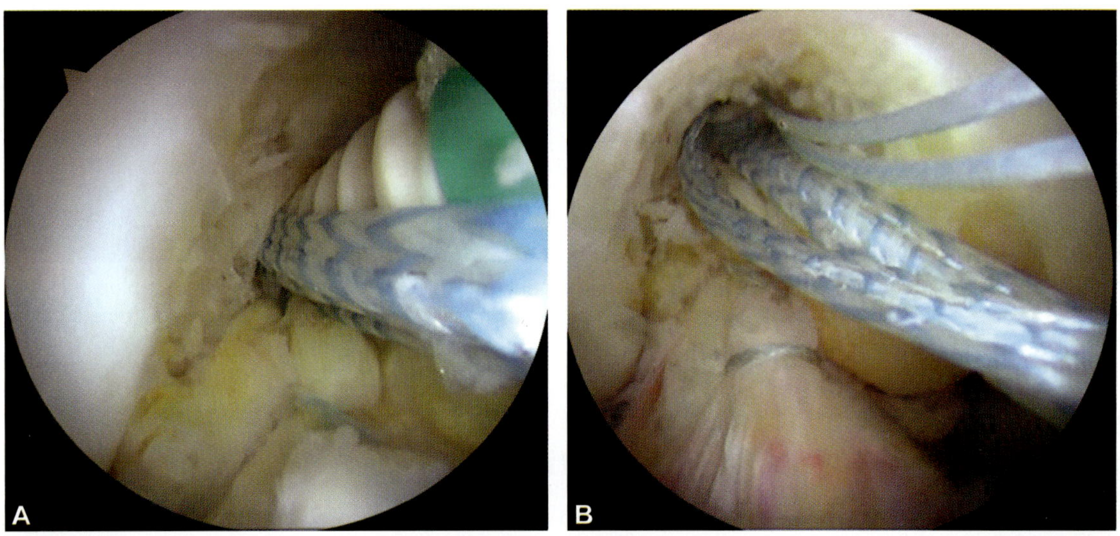

Figs. 26.7A and B: (A) SwiveLock® anchor loaded with No. 2 FiberWire® and a FiberTape® being inserted into the center of femoral footprint; (B) The anterior cruciate ligament is anchored at its femoral attachment site.

5. The driver is removed after the anchor is fully inserted and the tip retention suture is removed. The ends of FiberWire® are cut flush using an open-ended suture cutter.
6. Firm fixation of the stump is confirmed by probing.
7. The arthroscope is then shifted to the AL portal and ACL tibial insertion visualized. A pilot hole is created at the center of the tibial footprint using the AWL for SwiveLock®.
8. The two ends of the FiberTape® are then loaded onto another 4.75 mm PEEK SwiveLock® SP self-punching anchor. This is then inserted into the tibial socket in a similar manner (Fig. 26.8).
9. The knee is extended to confirm that there is no impingement. A final probing is done to confirm the strength and tension of the entire construct (Figs. 26.9A and B).

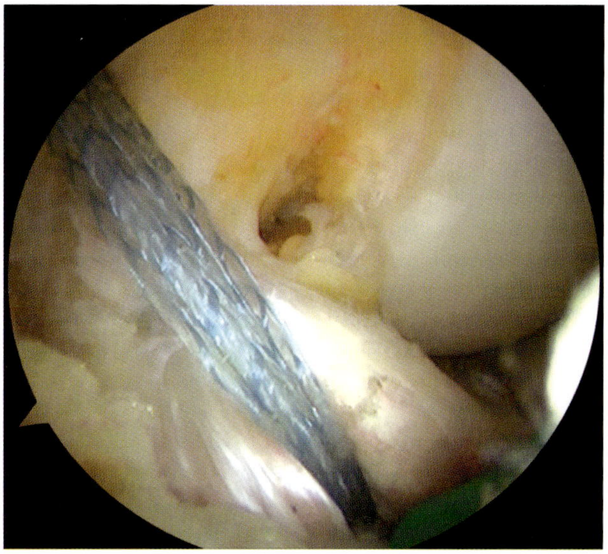

Fig. 26.8: Another 4.75 mm SwiveLock® anchor loaded with the FiberTape® being inserted at the tibial attachment of the anterior cruciate ligament while viewing from the anterolateral portal.

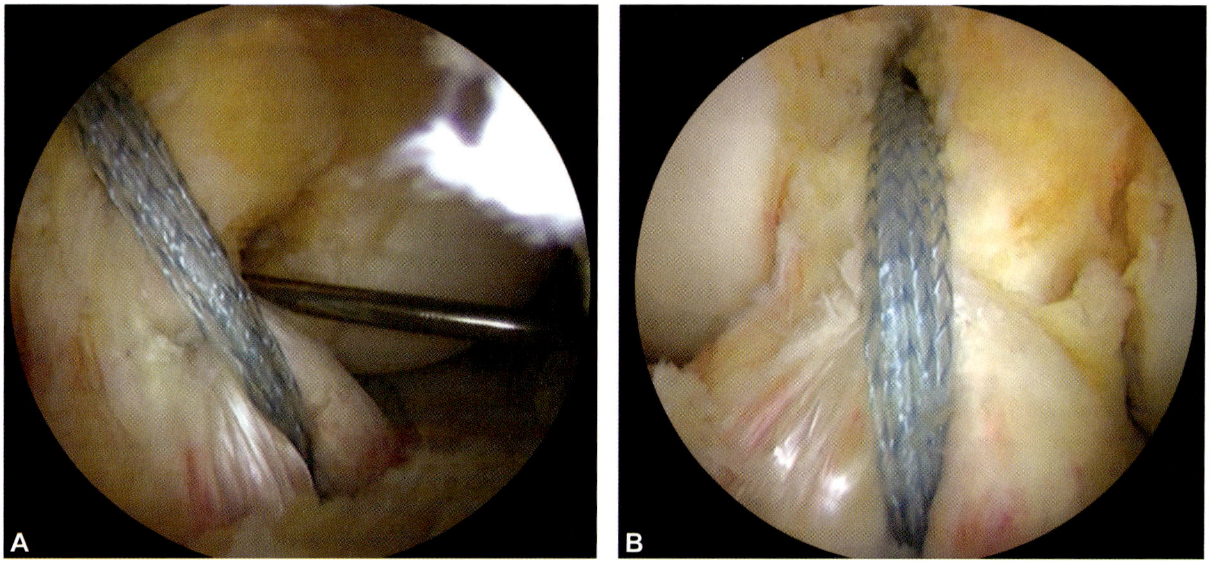

Figs. 26.9A and B: (A) Probing of the repair construct while viewing from the anterolateral portal to confirm adequate tension; (B) Note the anterior cruciate ligament attached at the femoral footprint along with the FiberTape® augmentation from femur to tibia, viewed from anteromedial portal.

REHABILITATION

A knee brace locked in extension is applied for 4 weeks. Weight bearing as tolerated is allowed immediately. Isometric exercises are begun along with early gentle range of motion. Cryotherapy is given for 3 weeks to control edema and pain. A hinge knee brace without lock is allowed after 4 weeks and strengthening, stability training and proprioception exercises are begun. Sports specific training is started after 6 months and return to sports is allowed after 9 months.

PEARLS AND PITFALLS

- Careful assessment of the ACL for suitability for repair determines outcome. Proximal avulsions with excellent tissue quality only are suitable for repair. In case of doubt, perform a standard anatomic ACL reconstruction with remnant preservation.
- A CP greatly improves visualization of the FIS of ACL.
- Only high strength suture material must be used, preferably with a self-retrieving suture passing instrument.
- A low accessory medial portal provides a straight trajectory for insertion of the suture anchor.
- Creation of a pilot hole allows easy insertion of the anchor and prevents dislodgement of the tip in hard bone.
- Augmentation with high strength suture tape provides initial stability, protects the repair and allows early range of motion.

REFERENCES

1. Irarrázaval S, Kurosaka M, Cohen M, et al. Anterior cruciate ligament reconstruction. J ISAKOS. 2016;1(1):38-52.
2. Co FH, Skinner HB, Cannon WD. Effect of reconstruction of the anterior cruciate ligament on proprioception of the knee and the heel strike transient. J Orthop Res. 1993;11(5):696-704.
3. Fridén T, Roberts D, Ageberg E, et al. Review of knee proprioception and the relation to extremity function after an anterior cruciate ligament rupture. J Orthop Sports Phys Ther. 2001;31(10):567-76.
4. Valeriani M, Restuccia D, Lazzaro V, et al. Clinical and neurophysiological abnormalities before and after reconstruction of the anterior cruciate ligament of the knee. Acta Neurol Scand. 1999;99(5):303-7.
5. Proffen BL, Sieker JT, Murray MM. Bio-enhanced repair of the anterior cruciate ligament. Arthroscopy. 2015; 31(5):990-7.
6. DiFelice GS, Villegas C, Taylor S. Anterior cruciate ligament preservation: early results of a novel arthroscopic technique for suture anchor primary anterior cruciate ligament repair. Arthroscopy. 2015;31(11):2162-71.
7. Robson AW. VI. Ruptured Crucial Ligaments and their Repair by Operation. Ann Surg. 1903;37(5):716-8.
8. Palmer I. On the injuries to the ligaments of the knee joint. Clin Orthop Relat Res. 1983;172:5-10.
9. O'Donoghue DH. Surgical treatment of fresh injuries to the major ligaments of the knee. J Bone Joint Surg Am. 1950;32(4):721-38.
10. Feagin JA, Curl WW. Isolated tear of the anterior cruciate ligament: 5-year follow-up study. Am J Sports Med. 1976;4(3):95-100.
11. Marshall JL, Warren RF, Wickiewicz TL. Primary surgical treatment of anterior cruciate ligament lesions. Am J Sports Med. 1982;10(2):103-7.
12. Odensten M, Hamberg PER, Nordin M, et al. Surgical or conservative treatment of the acutely torn anterior cruciate ligament. Clin Orthop Relat Res. 1985;(198):87-93.
13. Sandberg R, Balkfors B, Nilsson B, et al. Operative versus non-operative treatment of recent injuries to the ligaments of the knee. A prospective randomized study. J Bone Joint Surg Am. 1987;69(8):1120-6.
14. Jorjani J, Altmann D, Auen R, et al. Mittel- bis langfristige Ergebnisse nach vorderer Kreuzbandruptur und Versorgung in Healing-Response-Technik. Z Orthop Unfall. 2013;151(06):570-9.
15. Kubik-Huch R, Pfirrmann C, Grehn H, et al. Proximal anterior cruciate ligament tears: the healing response technique versus conservative treatment. J Knee Surg. 2012;26(04):263-72.
16. Achtnich A, Herbst E, Forkel P, et al. Acute Proximal anterior cruciate ligament tears: outcomes after arthroscopic suture anchor repair versus anatomic single-bundle reconstruction. Arthroscopy. 2016;32(12):2562-9.
17. Sherman MF, Lieber L, Bonamo JR, et al. The long-term follow up of primary anterior cruciate ligament repair: Defining a rationale for augmentation. Am J Sports Med. 1991;19(3):243-55.
18. Zantop T, Brucker PU, Vidal A, et al. Intra-articular rupture pattern of the ACL. Clin Orthop Relat Res. 2007;454:48-53.
19. Steadman JR, Cameron-Donaldson ML, Briggs KK, et al. A minimally invasive technique ("healing response") to treat proximal ACL injuries in skeletally immature athletes. J Knee Surg. 2006;19(1):8-13.

20. Nguyen DT, Ramwadhdoebe TH, van der Hart CP, et al. Intrinsic healing response of the human anterior cruciate ligament: an histological study of reattached ACL remnants. J Orthop Res. 2013;32(2):296-301.
21. Weninger P, Wepner F, Kissler F, et al. Anatomic double-bundle reinsertion after acute proximal anterior cruciate ligament injury using knotless pushlock anchors. Arthrosc Tech. 2015;4(1):e1-6.
22. MacKay G, Anthony IC, Jenkins PJ, et al. Anterior cruciate ligament repair revisited. Preliminary results of primary repair with internal brace ligament augmentation: a case series. Orthop Muscul Syst. 2015;04(02):188.
23. Araujo PH, van Eck CF, Macalena JA, et al. Advances in the three-portal technique for anatomical single- or double-bundle ACL reconstruction. Knee Surg Sports Traumatol Arthrosc. 2011;19(8):1239-42.

CHAPTER

27

Fixation of ACL Avulsion with Screws

Abhay Narvekar

INTRODUCTION

Fractures of the intercondylar eminence of the tibia were first described by Poncet in 1875 (Burstein, Viola and Fulkerson 1988)[1] and have been considered to be the childhood equivalent of anterior cruciate ligament (ACL) ruptures in adults. It was only in 1959 that Meyers and McKeever described the surgical management of type 2 injuries of tibial spine.[2] This injury is well documented in children and adults. It usually occurs in individuals between the ages of 8 years and 14 years.[3] In children, the most common cause is sports injury whereas in adults, it is because of road traffic accidents.[4,5] In older patients, tibial eminence fractures are often combined with lesions of the menisci, capsule, or collateral ligaments.[6]

MECHANISM OF INJURY

- It commonly occurs as a result of deceleration, internal rotation, and excessive hyperextension, or deceleration, valgus and internal rotation.[7,8]
- In children, it is either due to a direct blow on the lowermost part of the femur or forceful hyperextension with rotation.[9-11]
- It is more common in children because of weakness of incompletely ossified tibial eminence in comparison to strong and elastic ACL.[6]

APPLIED ANATOMY

The tibial eminence is anatomically divided into four distinct regions by the medial and lateral intercondylar spines and anterior and posterior recesses.[12,13] It serves as the insertion point for the anterior and posterior cruciate ligaments and the menisci.[14,15] The ACL inserts on the tibial eminence at the anterior intercondylar area in the recess anterior to the medial tibial spine. Hence, tibial spine avulsion is a misnomer as the avulsion is in the recess and not on any spine. The intermeniscal ligament traverses between the medial and lateral menisci anterior to the tibial eminence where it is vulnerable to entrapment within these fractures, thereby blocking reduction.[16-18]

CLASSIFICATION

Meyers' and McKeever's Classification (1959);[2] Modified by Zaricznyj in 1977[7] (Fig. 27.1)

- *Type I* fractures are non-displaced or associated with minimal displacement of the anterior margin
- *Type II* fractures have superior displacement of their anterior aspect with an intact posterior hinge, resembling a bird's beak
- *Type III* fractures are completely displaced. They have been subclassified:[19]
  - *Type IIIA* involves the ACL insertion only.
  - *Type IIIB* includes the entire intercondylar eminence.
- *Type IV*: Comminuted avulsion (Zaricznyj).[7]

EVALUATION

Patients present with a painful swollen knee and complain of difficulties in bearing weight.[20] Lachman's and other tests for ACL insufficiency are positive. A complete neurologic and vascular examination must be performed.[21]

IMAGING

Radiographs

Standard anteroposterior (AP), lateral and notch view is helpful for diagnosis (Figs. 27.2A and B). In skeletally immature patients, size of the fragment is larger than what it appears on the radiograph because of the cartilaginous portion.

CT Scan

It helps to delineate fracture anatomy and degree of comminution.[22]

MRI Scan

It helps in diagnosing associated injuries like meniscus, cartilage and other ligamentous injury.[11,23,24]

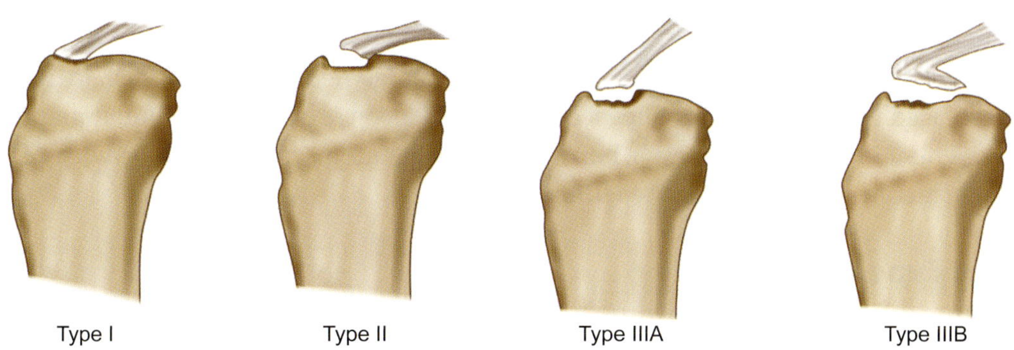

Fig. 27.1: Classification of anterior cruciate ligament avulsions.

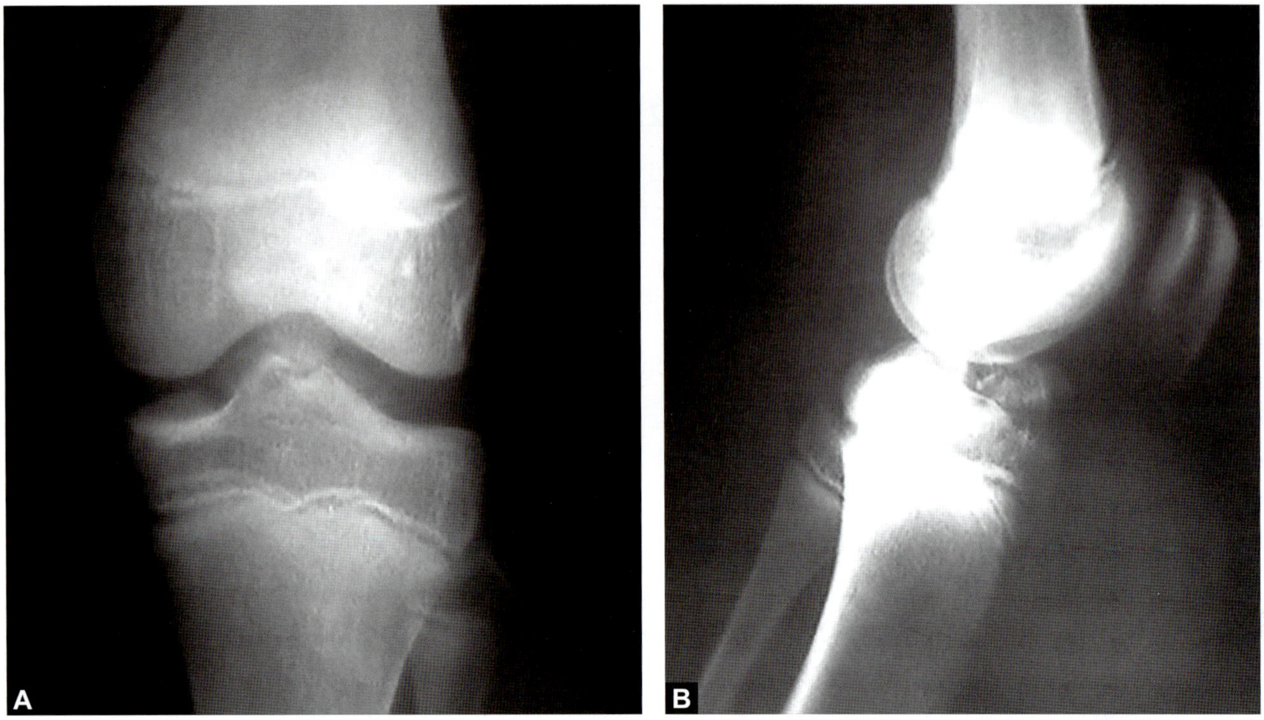

Figs. 27.2A and B: Plain radiographs showing anterior cruciate ligament avulsion in anteroposterior and lateral views.

TREATMENT

Type I

If the hemarthrosis is tense, then aspiration followed by immobilization in a long straight knee brace for 4 weeks is advised. Static quadriceps, straight leg raises and non-weight bearing ambulation are encouraged in the brace. Repeat radiograph is taken every 2 weeks to assess the fracture position and aggressive physiotherapy started after 6 weeks.[22,25]

Type II

If reduction is achieved in extension then it is treated as type I. If reduction is not achieved, then arthroscopic reduction and internal fixation (ARIF) is the best treatment.

Arthroscopic reduction of tibial eminence fractures has gained popularity due to its successful outcomes, decreased invasiveness, and improved recovery time. It is common to find entrapment of the anterior intermeniscal ligament,[26] anterior horn of the medial meniscus or anterior horn of the lateral meniscus in the fracture site preventing the reduction.

Type III and Type IV

Treatment of displaced tibial spine avulsion fractures has evolved over a period of time from conservative management to open reduction and internal fixation to ARIF.[25]

Many different types of fixation methods have been described including screw, suture, anchor, and suture-button fixation. The two most popular techniques employed are suture and screw fixation.

There are only few comparative studies in literature to recommend which is the best technique of fixation for these fractures. Seon and Park did a clinical comparative study of screw and suture fiction of tibial spine avulsion fractures and concluded that there is no significant clinical difference in terms of clinical outcome and stability.[27,28] Bong and coworkers in their biomechanical comparative study of screw versus FiberWire® (Arthrex, Naples, FL) fixation concluded that FiberWire® fixation was significantly stronger than cannulated screw fixation.[29,30] Biomechanical comparison of four different methods of fixation was done by Mahar and colleagues on immature bovine knees.[31] They concluded that two single-armed No. 2 Ethibond sutures, three bioabsorbable nails, a single resorbable screw, or a single metal screw do not have any significant mechanical advantage over the other. Tsukada and coworkers did a biomechanical comparative study of antegrade screw fixation, retrograde screw fixation, and pull-out suture fixation.[32] They compared the initial fixation strength in response to a cyclic tensile load and found that antegrade screw is most effective in providing initial fixation strength.

SURGICAL TECHNIQUE

Arthroscopic Reduction and Antegrade Cancellous Screw Fixation: The Way I Do It

1. Patient is supine.
2. The leg is in the leg holder. The foot end of the table is dropped so that the knee can be flexed to more than 100°.
3. A diagnostic arthroscopy is done using standard anteromedial and anterolateral portals.
4. The hemarthrosis is drained. Associated meniscal and cartilage lesions are addressed.
5. The fracture surfaces are freshened using a motorized shaver. The inter meniscus ligament is identified. Very often it is in between the fracture surfaces and needs to be delivered out before the fracture fragments can be reduced.
6. The type of fracture, whether comminuted or single fragment, is identified. One needs to probe the fragment to identify any additional fragments within the attached ACL fibers.
7. The fragment size should be around 10 mm to accommodate a 4.0 mm cannulated cancellous screw without fracturing it.
8. Identify the anterior extent of the avulsed fragment. If the anterior extent of the fragment is too posterior, i.e. close to the intercondylar notch, it would not be suitable for screw fixation as the screw head would impinge on the notch and precipitate a resultant flexion deformity.
9. The avulsed fragment is reduced. Reduction is achieved in extension. The reduction is maintained by drilling a "K" wire transpatellar tendon, just distal to the lower pole of the patella. This wire is fairly tangential to the fracture. It should be introduced into the distal tibia only a small distance as the popliteal structures are directly posterior.
10. Once the fracture is held temporarily with this wire, the knee can be flexed without loss of reduction (Fig. 27.3).
11. With a 16-gauge Venflon™ needle as a guide, a midpatellar medial portal is created such that there is adequate clearance from the curve of the femoral condyle.

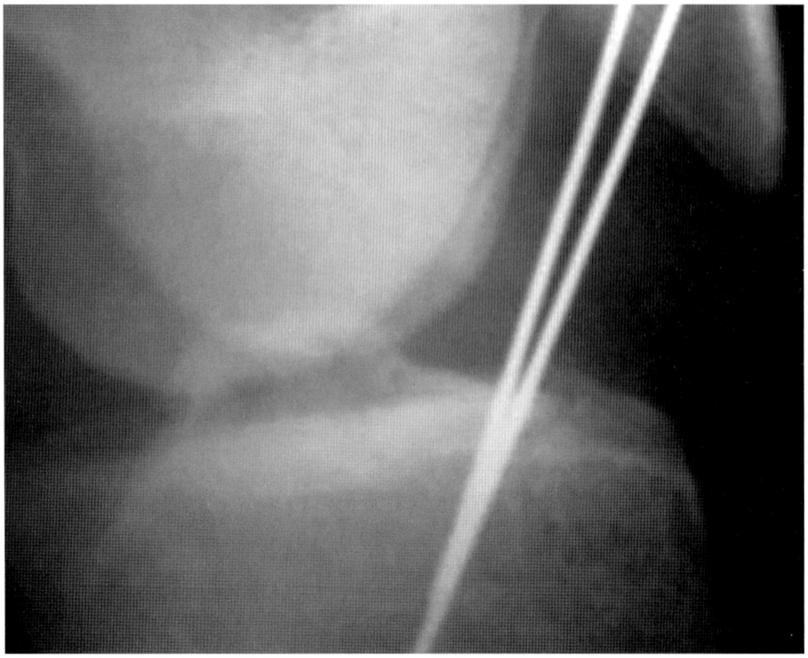

Fig. 27.3: Trial reduction with K wires and confirming reduction.

12. The wire of the cannulated screw is then introduced from a new superomedial portal. If the epiphysis is closed, then one needs to be more perpendicular to the tibial plateau and the wire is drilled facing the foot end of the patient. If the epiphysis is open, the wire needs to be more tangential. To avoid the epiphyseal plate, one can drill facing the head end of the patient.
13. Anatomically, the anterior horn of the lateral meniscus is continuous with the anterior fibers of the ACL. The fragment invariably hinges on this soft tissue. Hence, once the medial side of the fragment is fixed, the construct becomes stable. Lateral fixation may not be required.
14. In case the fragment is large enough to accommodate two screws, the medial screw is followed by the lateral screw.
15. The screw is introduced as close to the center as possible and as anterior as possible so that the head of the screw does not impinge on the notch roof. A notchplasty would then be necessary. It should be done as a last resort.
16. The fragment is then drilled with a cannulated drill bit followed by the tap and then the screw.
17. The screw need not purchase the posterior tibial cortex as per the principle of the "tent peg". Also the dead man's angle, as described by Stephen Burkhart,[33] requires the screw to be inserted at a 45° or less angle to the ACL so as to increase its pullout strength (Figs. 27.4A and B).
18. The head of the screw acts as a washer. Hence, unless there is some comminution, a washer is never used.
19. The knee is brought through a full range of motion to assess the impingement, if any, tension of the ACL, and the stability of the fracture (Fig. 27.5).
20. In comminuted fractures, the main fragment containing major portion of the ACL is fixed with a screw. Other smaller fragments very often fall in place. A hybrid repair with pullout stitch using one or two No. 2 FibreWire® (Arthrex, Naples, FL) through the tibial end of the substance of the ACL can be added to the screw fixation.

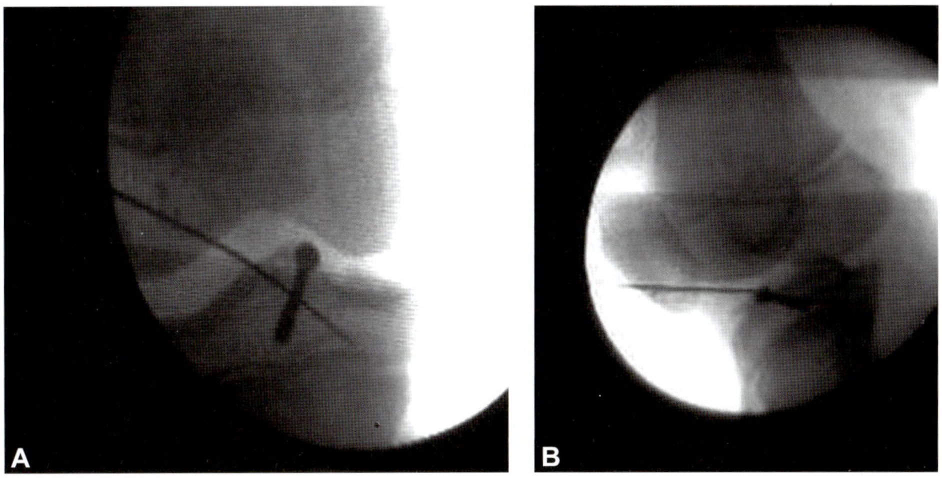

Figs. 27.4A and B: Intraoperative fluoroscopic images of fixation in a patient with open physis, avoiding the physeal plate.

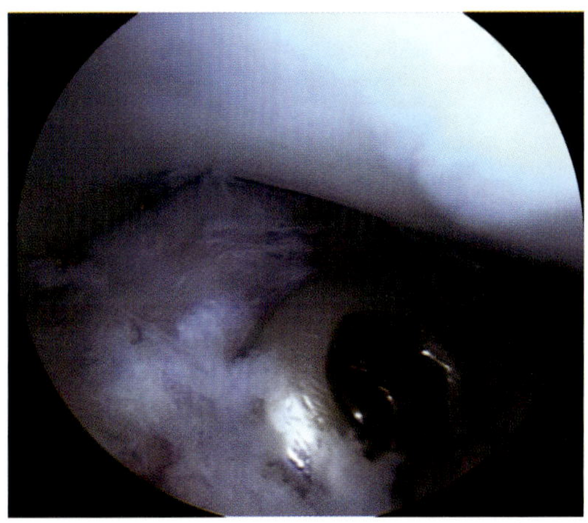

Fig. 27.5: Arthroscopy image of a central and anterior screw not impinging the femoral condyle.

POSTOPERATIVE REGIME

- Patient is kept in a long straight knee brace. Static knee exercises and ankle pumps are started immediate postoperatively.
- Straight leg raises in brace, non-weight bearing ambulation on crutches is started from the following day.
- Depending on the fixation, gentle knee movements are started by 2 weeks and closed kinetic chain flexion at 3 weeks.
- Bedside bending is started at 4–5 weeks and active extension at 6 weeks.
- Patient is non-weight bearing for 6 weeks. Once there is full active extension, partial weight bearing and progressively full weight bearing is permitted.
- Patient uses the straight knee brace in between exercise sessions so as to avoid fixed flexion deformity and is encouraged to use it at night too.
- Hinged knee brace is used after 4–6 weeks.
- Progressive strengthening program, proprioception and perturbations are started at 6 weeks.

- Walking in water and other aquatic exercises are started at 6 weeks.
- Running and agility activities are started after 4 months. Sports participation is started around 6 months when other criteria for sports participation are fulfilled.

PITFALLS

- Placement of the screw should be such that whereas it has good purchase on the fragment, it should not impinge on the femoral condyle or notch. Hence, after introducing the K wire of the screw, a careful trial extension of the knee helps to get this information. In case of impingement, a different site can then be chosen.
- If there is comminution, either on probing or while drilling, a different method of fixation should be used.
- In children, the wire or screw should not penetrate the epiphyseal plate; hence it has to be drilled at a more acute angle to the ACL, yet should not be too tangential to the fragment. Intraoperative fluoroscopy is vital for this (Figs. 27.6A and B).
- The wire for the screw from the superomedial portal should have the desired angle and should be adequately distanced from the cartilage of the condyle so the screw head does not scuff it (Figs. 27.7A and B).
- Patient is advised to get the screw removed after 4–5 months. Removal should be earlier if the epiphyseal plate is inadvertently violated.

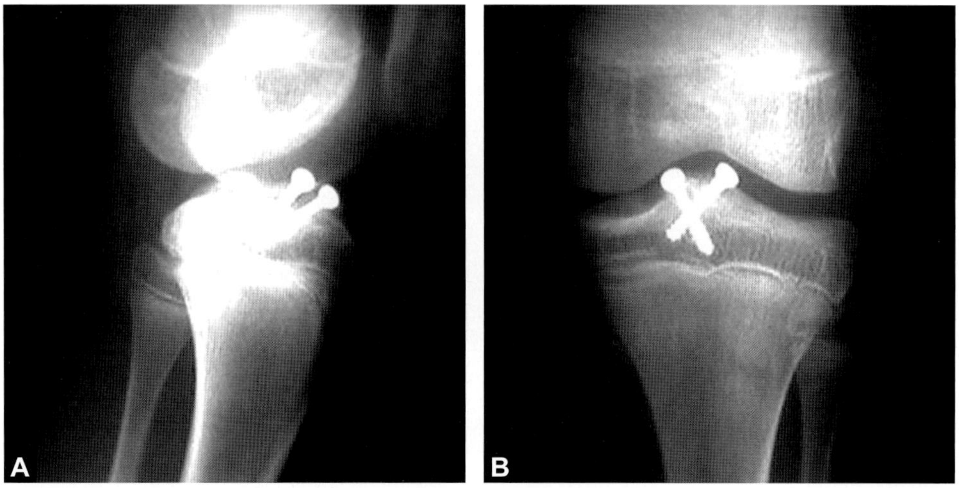

Figs. 27.6A and B: Lateral and anteroposterior radiographs of the fixation in a pediatric patient with open physis, not crossing the epiphyseal plate.

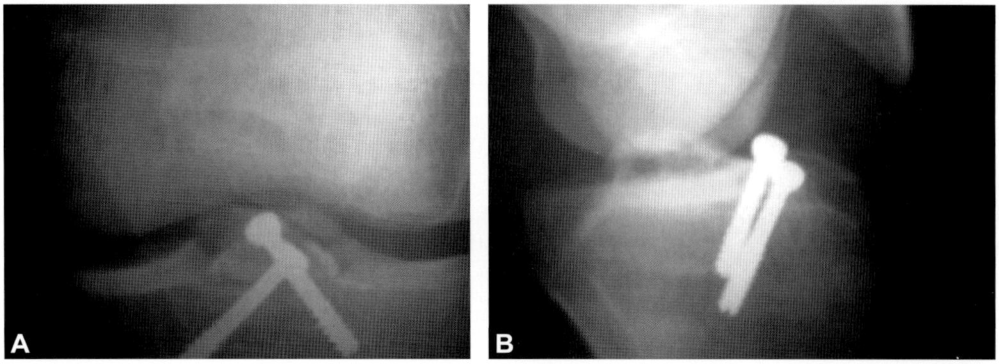

Figs. 27.7A and B: Anteroposterior and lateral radiographs of screw fixation of a comminuted fracture wherein the major fragments are fixed. Note that the screws are more vertical as the epiphyseal plate is fused.

Table 27.1: Summary of advantages, disadvantages and considerations to take into account for repair of tibial eminence fractures.

	Advantages	*Disadvantages*	*Considerations*
Suture fixation	▪ Allows for fixation of fractures with small fragments of bone. ▪ Can be used for all fracture patterns ▪ Does not rely on bone fragment for fixation	▪ Permanent suture might cause tethering of growth physis ▪ Prominent suture might need second surgery for removal ▪ Involves second incision over bone cortex of tibia to the sutures.	▪ Suture through ACL substance or bony fracture has unclear long term affects ▪ Absorbable suture vs permanent suture has risks and benefits to both
Screw fixation	▪ Provides direct compressive fixation across fracture ▪ Avoids placing suture through ACL	▪ Fractures fragment may be too small to accommodate screw ▪ Second surgery might be needed for removal of hardware ▪ Growth disturbance due to damaged growth physis if screw is too long	▪ Cannulated vs non-cannulated screw ▪ One screw vs two screw fixation (one screw is more acceptable in more recent literature)

(ACL: Anterior cruciate ligament).

CONCLUSION

Anterior tibial spine avulsion fractures are common in children. They are easily managed with arthroscopic fixation with cannulated cancellous 4.0 mm screws that can be used without violating the epiphyseal plate, yet give adequate stability. They, however, are better removed 6 months later. Fixation with a screw is a simple, quick and reliable method of treating selected tibial eminence fractures (Table 27.1).[34] Comminuted fractures need to be treated with some sort of pullout stitches or with use of anchors.

REFERENCES

1. Poncet A. Arrachement de l'epine du tibia a l'insertion du ligament croise antérieur. Bull Mem Soc Chir Paris. 1875;1:883-4.
2. Meyers MH, McKeever FM. Fracture of the intercondylar eminence of the tibia. J Bone Jt Surg. 1959;41(2):209-22.
3. Grönkvist H, Hirsch G, Johansson L. Fracture of the anterior tibial spine in children. J Pediatr Orthop. 1984;4:465-8.
4. Wiley JJ, Baxter MP. Tibial spine fractures in children. Clin Orthop Rel Res. 1990;255:54-60.
5. Anderson CN, Anderson AF. Tibial eminence fracture. Clin Sports Med. 2011;30(4):727-42.
6. Luhmann S. Acute traumatic knee effusions in children and adolescents. J Pediatr Orthop 2003;23:199-202.
7. Zaricznyj B. Avulsion fracture of the tibial eminence treated by open reduction and pinning. J Bone Joint Surg Am. 1997;59:1111-4.
8. Roth PB. Fracture of the spine of the tibia. J Bone Joint Surg Am. 1928;10(3):509-18.
9. Casalonga A, Bourelle S, Chalencon F, et al. Tibial intercondylar eminence fractures in children: the long-term perspective. Orthop Traumatol Surg Res. 2010;96:525-30.
10. Kocher M, Micheli LJ, Gerbino P, et al. Tibial eminence fractures in children: prevalence of meniscal entrapment. Am J Sports Med. 2003;31(3):404-7.
11. Wilfinger C, Castellani C, Raith J, et al. Nonoperative treatment of tibial spine fractures in children-38 patients with a minimum follow-up of 1 year. J Orthop Trauma. 2009;23(7):519-24.
12. Agur A, Lee M. Grant's Atlas of Anatomy, 9th Edition. Baltimore: Williams and Wilkins; 1991.
13. Clemente C. Anatomy: A Regional Atlas of the Human Body, 4th Edition. Baltimore: Williams and Wilkins; 1997. pp. 387-8.
14. Girgis F. The cruciate ligaments of the knee joint. anatomical, functional and experimental analysis. Clin Orthop Relat Res. 1975;(106):216-31.

15. Petersen W. Anatomy of the anterior cruciate ligament with regard to its two bundles. Clin Orthop Relat Res. 2007;454:35-47.
16. Harner C. Quantitative analysis of human cruciate ligament insertions. Arthroscopy. 1999;15(7):741-9.
17. Messner K. The menisci of the knee joint. Anatomical and functional characteristics, and a rationale for clinical treatment. J Anat. 1998;193(Pt 2):161-78.
18. Accousti WK, Willis RB. Tibial eminence fractures. Orthop Clin North Am. 2003;34:365-75.
19. Mclennan JG. Lessons learned after second-look arthroscopy in type III fractures of the tibial spine. J Pediatr Orthop. 1995;15(1):59-62.
20. Perugia D, Basiglini L, Vadalà A, et al. Clinical and radiological results of arthroscopically treated tibial spine fractures in childhood. Int Orthop. 2009;33(1):243-8.
21. Wiss DA, Watson JT. Fractures of the tibial plateau. In: Rockwood CA, Green DP, Bucholz RW, Heckman JD (Eds). Rockwood and Green's Fractures in Adults. Philadelphia: Lippincott-Raven; 1996. pp. 1920-53.
22. Griffith J, Antonio GE, Tong CW, et al. Cruciate ligament avulsion fractures. Arthroscopy. 2004;20(8):803-12.
23. Toye L, Cummings P, Armendariz G. Adult tibial intercondylar eminence fracture: evaluation with MR imaging. Skeletal Radiol. 2002;31(1):46-8.
24. Prince J, Laor T, Bean J. MRI of anterior cruciate ligament injuries and associated findings in the pediatric knee: changes with skeletal maturation. AJR Am J Roentgenol. 2005;185(3):756-62.
25. Fyfe IS, Jackson JP. Tibial intercondylar fractures in children: a review of the classification and the treatement of malunion. Injury. 1981;13:165-9.
26. Senekovic V, Veselko M. Anterograde arthroscopic fixation of avulsion fractures of the tibial eminence with a cannulated screw: five-year results. Arthroscopy. 2003;19(1):54-61.
27. Anderson AF, Anderson CN. Anterior cruciate ligament injuries with bony avulsion. In: Lieberman JR, Berry DJ, Azar FM (Eds). AAOS Advanced Reconstruction: Knee. Rosemont: American Academy of Orthopaedic Surgeons; 2011. pp. 603-12.
28. Seon J, Park SJ, Lee KB, et al. A clinical comparison of screw and suture fixation of anterior cruciate ligament tibial avulsion fractures. Am J Sports Med. 2009;37(12):2334-9.
29. Eggers A, Becker C, Weimann A, et al. Biomechanical evaluation of different fixation methods for tibial eminence fractures. Am J Sports Med. 2007;35(3):404-10.
30. Bong M, Romero A, Kubiak E, et al. Suture versus screw fixation of displaced tibial eminence fractures: a biomechanical comparison. Arthroscopy. 2005;21(10):1172-6.
31. Mahar A, Duncan D, Oka R, et al. Biomechanical comparison of four different fixation techniques for pediatric tibial eminence avulsion fractures. J Pediatr Orthop. 2008;28(2):159-62.
32. Tsukada H, Ishibashi Y, Tsuda E, et al. A biomechanical comparison of repair techniques for anterior cruciate ligament tibial avulsion fracture under cyclic loading. Arthroscopy. 2005;21(10):1197-201.
33. Burkhart SS. The dead man theory of suture anchors: observations along a south texas fence line. Arthroscopy. 1995;11(1):119-23.
34. Anciano Granadillo V. Comparison of two fixation methods in treating displaced pediatric tibial eminence fractures at Boston Children's Hospital. Doctoral dissertation. Harvard Medical School; 2015.

CHAPTER

28

Fixation of ACL Avulsion Using a Suture-bridge Technique

Roshan Wade, Chaitanya Waghchoure

INTRODUCTION

Poncet first described anterior cruciate ligament (ACL) avulsion fracture, also called as tibial eminence fracture or tibial spine fracture, in 1875.[1] It is bony avulsion of ACL from its tibial insertion on the intercondylar eminence. ACL avulsion is an uncommon injury seen more often in children (8–14 years old) and young population compared to adults; accounting for less than 5% of ACL injuries in adults.[2,3] The mechanism of injury is similar to that of ACL injuries and can occur in contact sports, skiing, accidents, and falls.[4,5] Sudden deceleration and hyperextension of the knee with a rotational force or valgus lead to transverse shear forces at the tibial spine causing ACL avulsion fractures[4,6,7] (Fig. 28.1). Associated injuries to menisci, collateral ligaments or cartilage are not uncommon, more so in adults.[3,4,8,9]

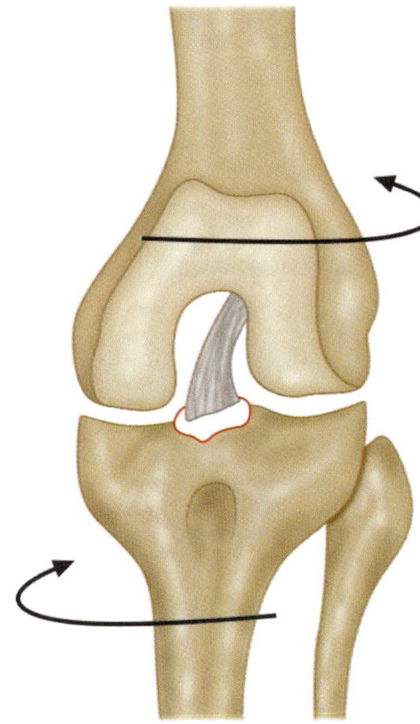

Fig. 28.1: Mechanism of injury.

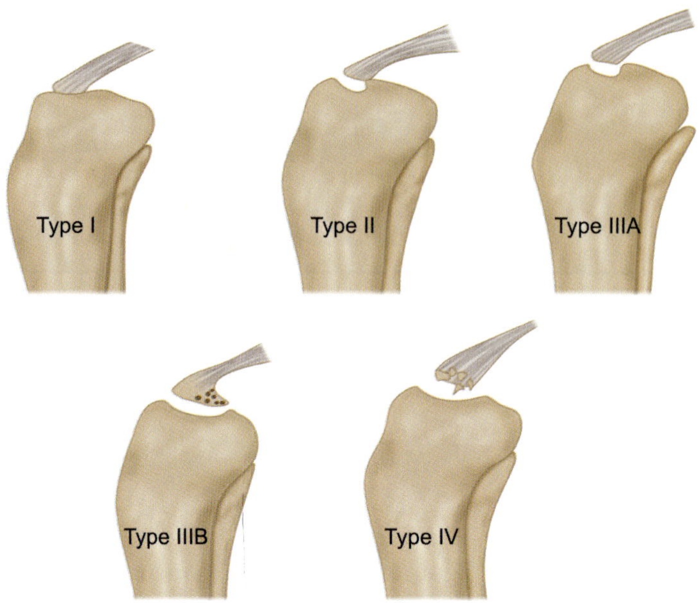

Fig. 28.2: Classification of anterior cruciate ligament avulsion.

CLASSIFICATION

Myeres and McKeever classified these fractures in 1959 into three types[10,11] (Fig. 28.2). *Type I* fractures represent undisplaced or minimally displaced avulsion fracture of the eminence. *Type II* is partially displaced fracture where the anterior third to half of the avulsed bone is elevated with an intact posterior hinge. This produces a "bird-beak" appearance on lateral radiograph. In *Type IIIA*, there is a complete displacement of the fragment, elevating it both anteriorly and posteriorly. *Type IIIB* has upward rotation of the displaced fragment. Zaricznyj updated the classification by adding *Type IV*, which is a displaced comminuted fracture.[12]

IMAGING

Standard radiographs of knee, anteroposterior and lateral views are used (Fig. 28.3). Particularly for assessing the degree of displacement of the fragment, a true lateral view is very helpful. Computed tomography (CT) scan delineates the fracture personality, especially the comminution and displacement of fragments. Magnetic resonance imaging (MRI) provides additional information on associated injuries to menisci, cartilage, and ligaments.

TREATMENT

Type I fractures can be managed conservatively with immobilization.[11] Displaced ACL avulsion fractures lead to instability and sometimes, anterior impingement. Degenerative changes in ACL have been shown during the chronic course of such fractures because of laxity or decreased tension in the ligament.[13] The rates of nonunion and arthrofibrosis are also higher with the conservatively managed displaced fractures.[14]

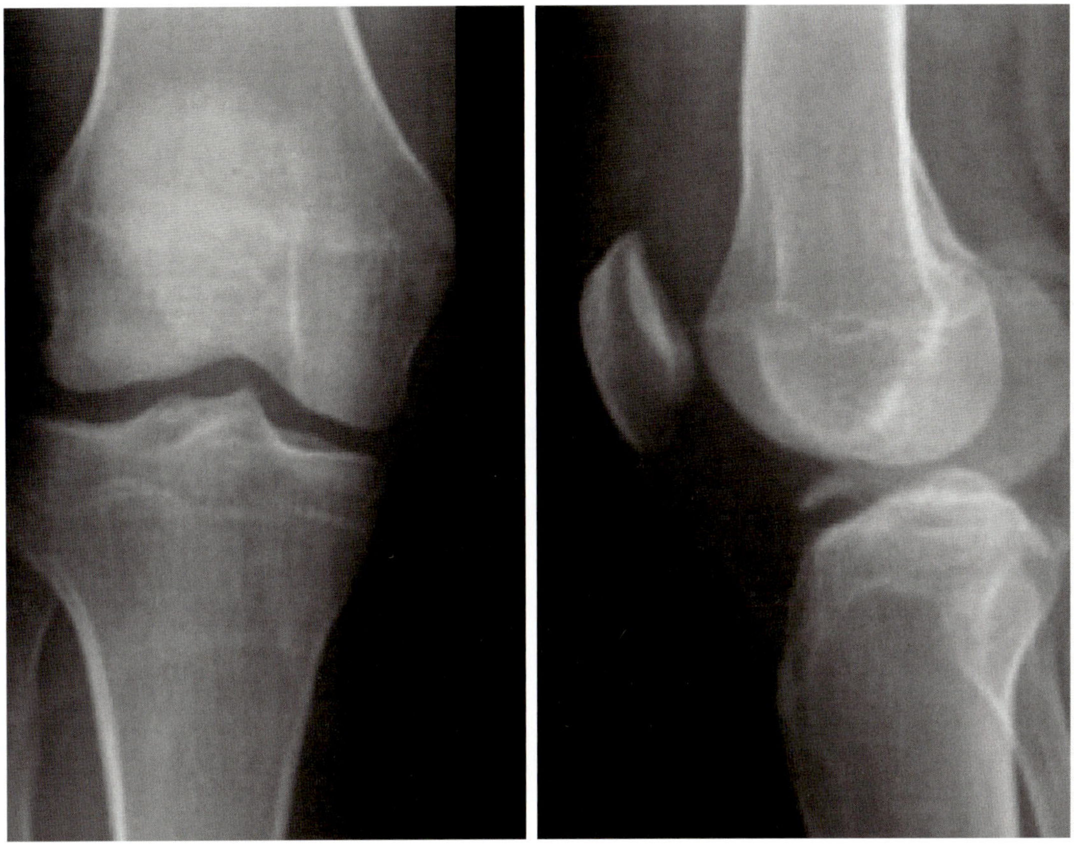

Fig. 28.3: Plain radiograph to diagnose the fracture and displacement.

Thus, anatomic arthroscopic reduction and internal fixation (ARIF) at the earliest has become a gold standard for displaced ACL avulsion fractures (*Types II, III,* and *IV*) to effectively restore normal knee biomechanics.[3,14] Various methods have been described using wires, screws, staples, button, anchors, and sutures for fixing these fractures.

The suture-bridge technique has become a preferred technique amidst the available options due to its operative simplicity and advantages. Firstly, it needs no second surgery for prominent hardware removal. Secondly, by passing intraligamentous sutures in ACL instead of avulsed bone, an even reduction can be achieved. Also, multiple sutures in different configurations can be used to gain a secure fixation of comminuted fracture or small fragment, thus avoiding the potential risk of fracture fragmentation seen with screw fixation.

Surgical Techniques for Suture-bridge Fixation

Depending on the number of tunnels, mainly two types of suture techniques can be followed: two-tunnel technique and four-tunnel technique. Various suture configurations are possible using these techniques. Broadly, they can be classified as "transligamentous configuration" and "lasso-loop configuration". In two-tunnel technique, a transligamentous transverse bridge or a lasso-loop suture configuration can be used, while in four-tunnel technique, a transligamentous transverse bridge or a transligamentous crisscross suture configuration can be applied (Figs. 28.4A to D).

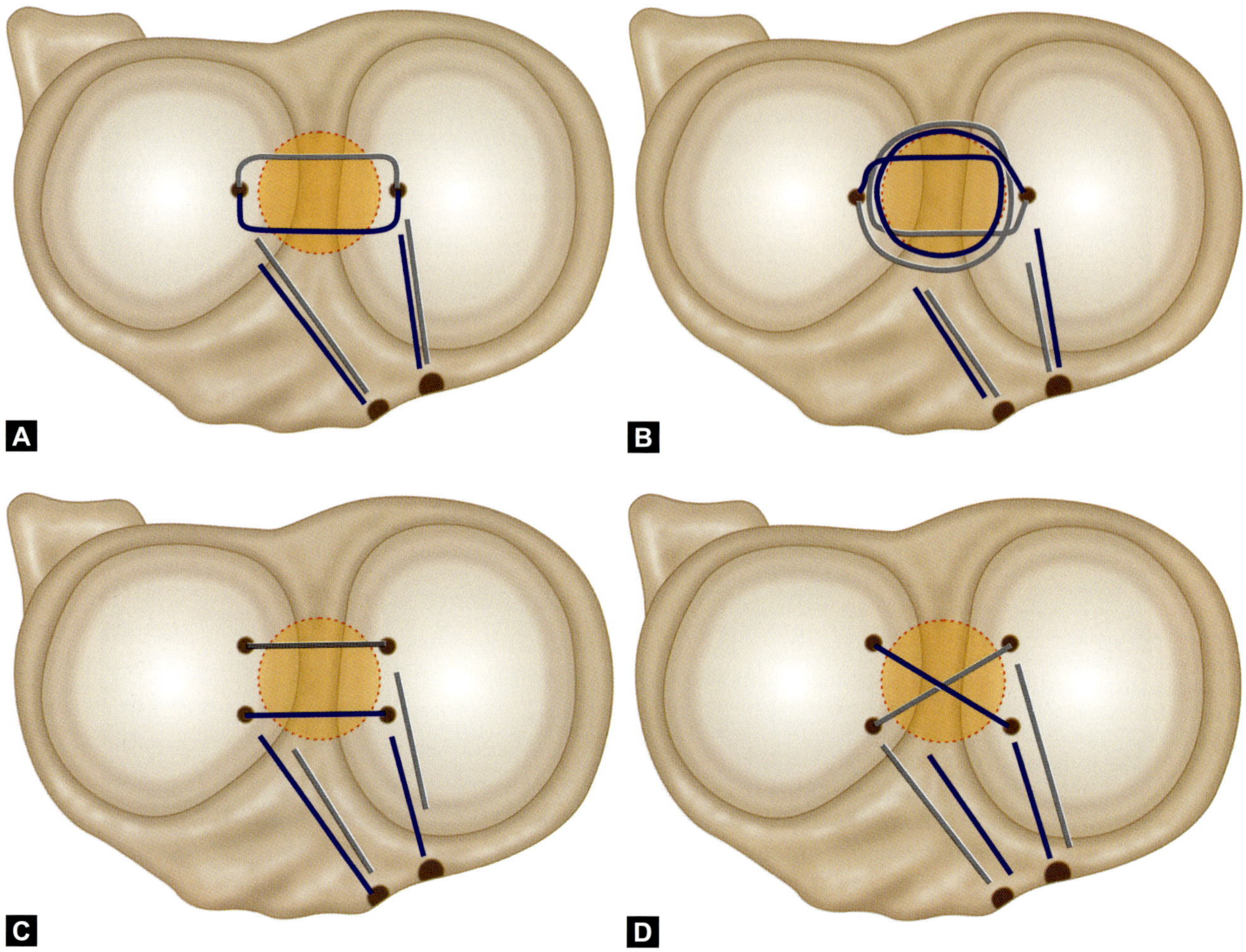

Figs. 28.4A to D: (A) Transverse two-tunnel; (B) lasso-loop two-tunnel; (C) transverse four-tunnel, and (D) crisscross four-tunnel axial schematic configurations.

Two-tunnel Technique

In this technique, the main principle is to pass sutures through the anterior and posterior part of the ACL substance and pull them through the two tunnels made on either side of the fracture crater, which is then fixed over the anteromedial (AM) cortex of proximal tibia. This provides indirect concentric reduction of bony fragment. As two nonabsorbable synthetic sutures are passed through the osteoligamentous junction, it provides maximum cut-through resistance.

The patient is positioned supine on the operating table and a standard leg holder and a thigh tourniquet is applied. Three anterior knee portals are used: anterolateral (AL), anteromedial, and superomedial. Diagnostic arthroscopy is performed to evaluate the knee joint and hematoma is evacuated. Associated injuries to menisci, other ligaments, cartilage or fracture extension into the condyles is to be identified and addressed. The first step in achieving good reduction is to debride the crater of tibial spine and the undersurface of fracture fragment with oscillating shaver. Frequently, the intermeniscal ligament tends to interpose between the fracture fragment and the crater. This needs to be retracted using a probe through AM portal to achieve the anatomical reduction of the fracture. Cutting of this ligament should be avoided as it provides stability to the anterior horns of both menisci. A 1.2-mm K-wire is then passed through the superomedial portal into the anterior central portion of the fragment to maintain the reduction provisionally.

A 2-cm vertical incision is made over the AM surface of the tibia just below the level of tibial tuberosity. Two 2.2-mm drill pins are placed 1–2 mm outside the medial and lateral margins of the fracture crater using a tip aiming ACL tibial drill guide (ACUFEX Director, Smith & Nephew, Andover, MA) through the AM portal (Fig. 28.5). A 6-mm cannula is then placed in the AM portal for effective suture management. At first, a No. 1 polydioxanone suture (PDS) (Ethicon) is passed through the AM portal into the posterior fibers of the ACL close to the osteoligamentous junction with the help of a 90° ACCU-PASS® (Smith & Nephew, Andover, MA) or a 90° SPECTRUM® suture passer (Conmed Linvatec) (Fig. 28.6A). Both the ends of the suture are then retrieved into the cannula placed in AM portal. This PDS suture is used to shuttle a No. 2 ULTRABRAID® (Smith & Nephew, Andover, MA) through the posterior fibers of ACL (Fig. 28.6B). Alternatively, No. 2 FiberWire® or FiberTape® (Arthrex, Naples, FL) can be used. Similar steps are followed for passing a second PDS suture and then another different colored nonabsorbable suture is shuttled through the anterior fibers of ACL. This creates transverse suture-bridge going across the anterior and posterior fibers of ACL from medial to lateral side (*see* Fig. 28.4A). Once the sutures are shuttled, a 4-mm cannulated drill is then used to create the tunnels over the guide pins on either side of the crater for pull-through sutures. Care needs to be taken to maintain a minimum of 10-mm bony bridge between the two tunnels on the metaphyseal cortex. These 4-mm tunnels allow easy passage of suture retrieval devices like simple suture retriever or suture hook (Conmed Linvatec). Medial ends of both the nonabsorbable sutures are pulled out through the medial tunnel, whereas the lateral ends of the sutures are retrieved through the lateral tunnel using the suture retrieval device (Fig. 28.7).

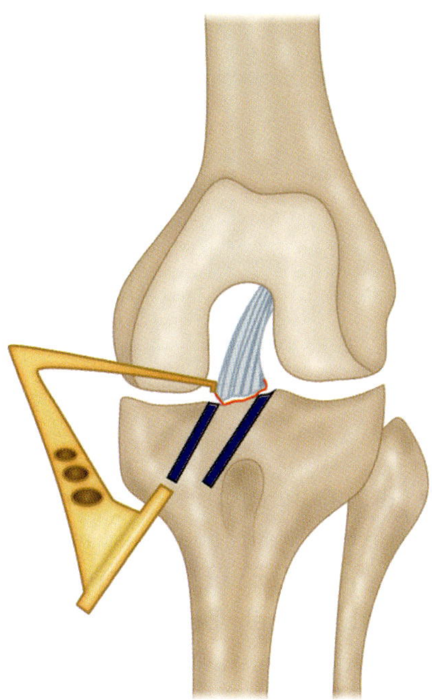

Fig. 28.5: Using an anterior cruciate ligament aimer guide to place accurate tunnels for suture passage.

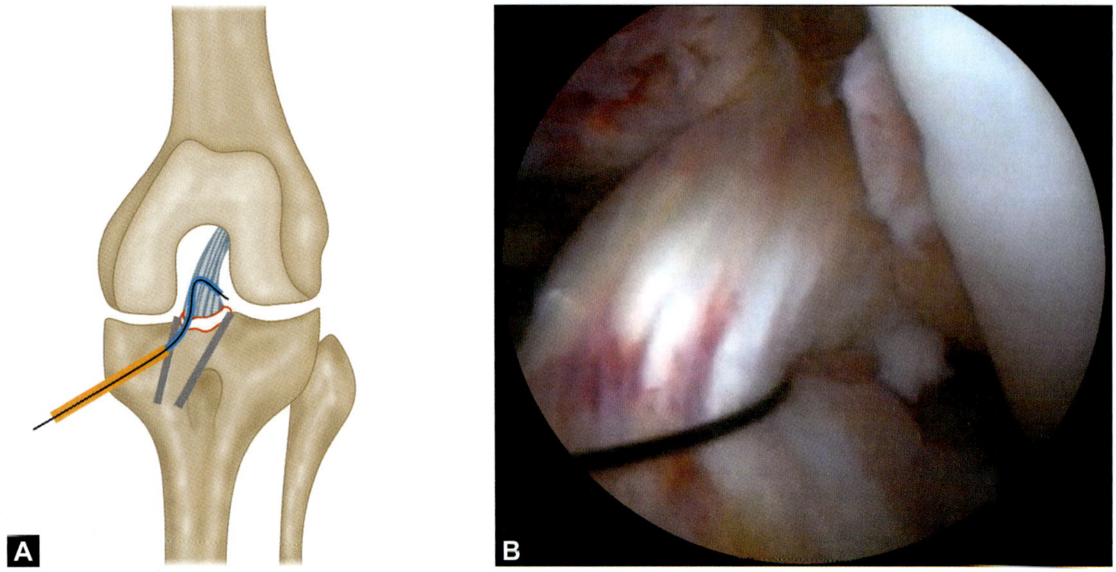

Figs. 28.6A and B: (A) Schematic representation and (B) arthroscopic view of suture shuttling.

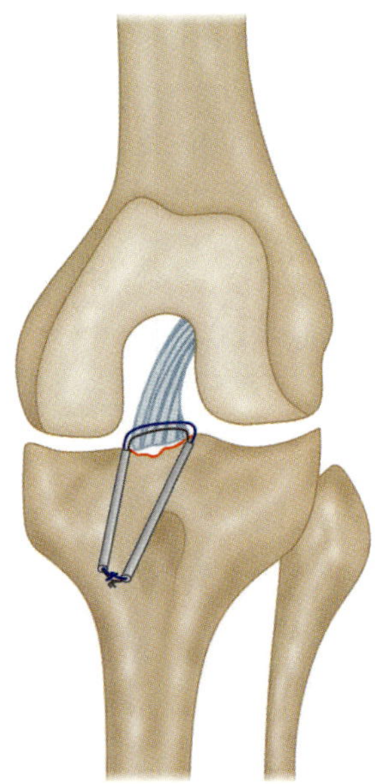

Fig. 28.7: Transverse two-tunnel technique coronal schematic configuration.

In lasso-loop configuration, one end of the suture is passing through the anterior fibers is retrieved through the ipsilateral tunnel, while the other end is looped around the ACL stump and then retrieved through the contralateral tunnel. Similarly, suture passed through posterior fibers is looped around the ACL and then pulled through contralateral tunnel, thus creating a lasso (*see* Fig. 28.4B). After confirming the concentric anatomical reduction of the fracture and tension to the ACL, retrieved sutures are tied with each other over the AM tibial cortex (Fig. 28.8). Additionally, an image intensifier or radiograph can be used to check the adequacy of reduction (Fig. 28.9).

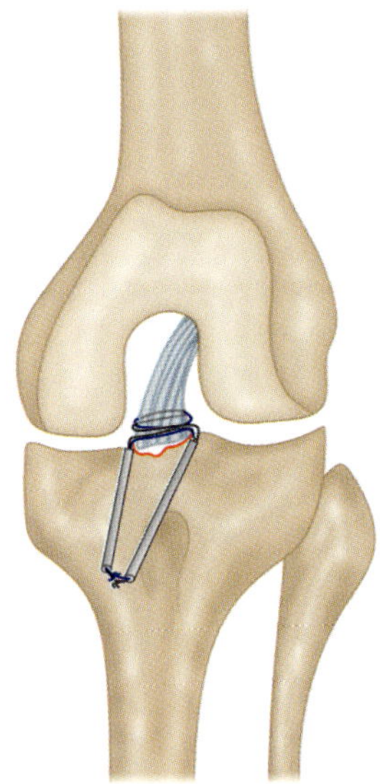

Fig. 28.8: Lasso-loop two-tunnel technique coronal schematic configuration.

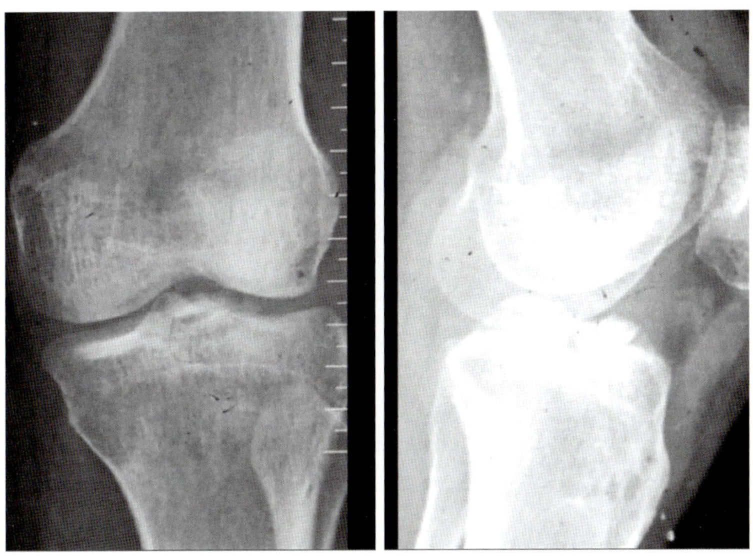

Fig. 28.9: Postoperative radiographs showing good reduction.

Four-tunnel Technique

This technique has been well described by Boutsiadis et al.[15] and has an added advantage of four-point stabilization to secure small fragments or slightly comminuted fragments in multiple planes. Four tunnels are placed anteromedially, anterolaterally, posteromedially, and posterolaterally around the tibial crater. Two posterior tunnels are made using ACL tibial guide set at 55°, while the anterior two tunnels are placed at 45° to avoid coalescence between the anterior and posterior tunnels (Fig. 28.10). Again, a bony bridge of 10 mm has to be maintained between the four tunnels over the tibial cortex. In this technique, sutures can

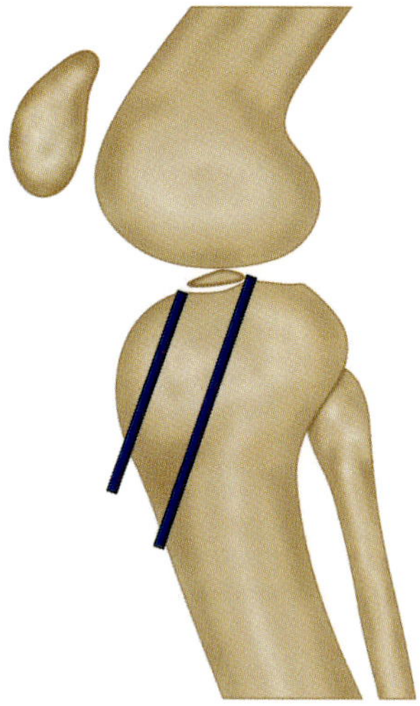

Fig. 28.10: Four-tunnel technique saggital schematic representation.

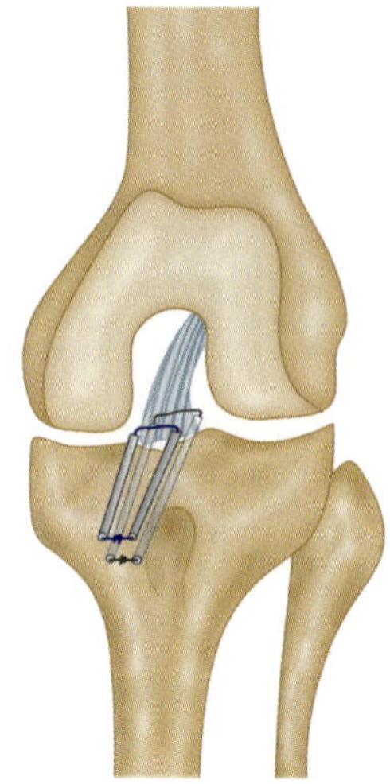

Fig. 28.11: Tranverse four-tunnel technique coronal schematic configuration.

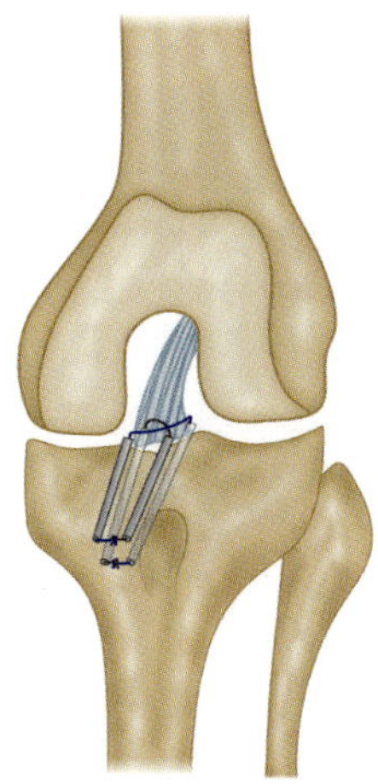

Fig. 28.12: Crisscross four-tunnel technique coronal schematic configuration.

either be shuttled through the ACL in anterior and posterior fibers to form transverse bridge configuration (Figs. 28.4C and 28.11), or can be placed diagonally across the four tunnels in a crisscross manner (Figs. 28.4D and 28.12). These various permutations and combinations using multiple sutures increase the contact forces across the entire fracture area allowing good bone-to-bone healing.

REHABILITATION PROTOCOL

The protocol for these fractures is almost similar to that of ACL reconstruction. A hinged knee brace locked at 0° flexion is used for the first 4 weeks while allowing isometric strengthening exercises, straight-leg raises, and passive or active-assisted range of motion (ROM) from 0° to 60° flexion in prone position. Weight bearing is allowed as per the pain tolerance in the first few days gradually extending to full weight bearing using brace in extension. At 4 weeks, brace can be removed and ROM is increased from 0° to 120°

till the end of 8 weeks. Closed-chain quadriceps exercises are also incorporated. Treadmill running can be started at 8 weeks with further strengthening exercises. After 12 weeks, agility training and sports specific training can be started provided the muscle strength regained is 85% of normal knee. Complete recovery is expected within 6 months.

COMPLICATIONS

Blowout of the anterior tibial cortex or coalescence of the cortical holes can occur, if the tunnels are not spaced out adequately. This complication can be addressed by using a suture disk or ENDOBUTTON® (Smith & Nephew, Andover, MA) over the tibial cortex to secure the sutures.

Asymptomatic residual laxity can be seen in both operative and nonoperative treatments, and can be attributed to the ligament elongation at the time of injury.[16,17]

Stiffness is one of the most common issues, which can be seen in case of prolonged immobilization.[17,18] This can be easily avoided by rigid fixation of the fracture and aggressive rehabilitation.

Nonunion with laxity can occur due to interposition of the intermeniscal ligament or inadequate debridement of the fragment or fracture crater.[16,18,19] Nonunions can be treated with debridement of fibrous tissue and ARIF.[20,21]

Malunion of fractures can occur due to incomplete reduction or malreduction of fracture leading to anterior impingement and thus, loss of extension. However, in case of significant loss of knee extension, it is advisable to recreate the fracture and refix it.[21] Sometimes, femoral notchplasty can be added.

PEARLS AND PITFALLS

- Surgical simplicity and variability makes suture-bridge a preferred technique for treating displaced ACL avulsion fractures. Also, it is devoid of complications seen with screw fixation, including fragment fractures and need for prominent hardware removal.
- The associated injuries need to be identified and addressed before fixing the ACL avulsion fracture.
- The suture-bridge technique can be used to fix *Types II* and *III* as well as *Type IV* ACL avulsion fractures securely.
- Various suture configurations, passing separately through the AM and AL bundle of ACL, help in indirect concentric reduction of the avulsed fragment or fragments and therefore allowing anatomic repair.
- To facilitate the accurate reduction of fracture, retraction of the interposed anterior intermeniscal ligament is a crucial step.
- Use of different colored sutures allows better suture management.
- Spacing out of the tunnels over the cortex of the tibia is essential to avoid the complication of blowout of cortex.
- Stiffness of knee is not uncommon, and can be prevented with aggressive rehabilitation protocol.

REFERENCES

1. Poncet A. Arrachement de l'epine du tibia a l'insertion du ligament croise anterieur. Bull Mem Soc Chir Paris. 1875;1:883-4.
2. Garcia A, Neer CS. Isolated fractures of the intercondylar eminence of the tibia. Am J Surg. 1958;95(4):593-8.
3. Kendall NS, Hsu SY, Chan KM. Fracture of the tibial spine in adults and children. J Bone Joint Surg Br. 1992;74(6):848-52.
4. Lubowitz JH, Grauer JD. Arthroscopic treatment of anterior cruciate ligament avulsion. Clin Orthop Relat Res. 1993;294:242-6.
5. Grönkvist H, Hirsch G, Johansson L. Fracture of the anterior tibial spine in children. J Pediatr Orthop. 1984;4(4):465-8.
6. Accousti WK, Willis RB. Tibial eminence fractures. Orthop Clin North Am. 2003;34(3):365-75.
7. Ahmad CS, Stein BE, Jeshuran W, et al. Anterior cruciate ligament function after tibial eminence fracture in skeletally mature patients. Am J Sports Med. 2001;29(3):339-45.
8. McLennan JG. Lessons learned after second-look arthroscopy in type III fractures of the tibial spine. J Pediatr Orthop. 1995;15(1):59-62.

9. Monto RR, Cameron-Donaldson ML, Close MA, et al. Magnetic resonance imaging in the evaluation of tibial eminence fractures in adults. J Knee Surg. 2006;19(3):187-90.
10. Meyers MH, McKeever FM. Fracture of the intercondylar eminence of the tibia. J Bone Joint Surg Am. 1959;41-A(2): 209-22.
11. Meyers MH, McKeever FM. Fracture of the intercondylar eminence of the tibia. J Bone Joint Surg Am. 1970;52(8): 1677-84.
12. Zaricznyj B. Avulsion fracture of the tibial eminence. J Bone Joint Surg Am. 1977;59(8):1111-4.
13. Horibe S, Shi K, Mitsuoka T, et al. Nonunited avulsion fractures of the intercondylar eminence of the tibia. Arthroscopy. 2000;16(7):757-62.
14. Gans I, Baldwin KD, Ganley TJ. Treatment and management outcomes of tibial eminence fractures in pediatric patients. Am J Sports Med. 2014;42(7):1743-50.
15. Boutsiadis A, Karataglis D, Agathangelidis F, et al. Arthroscopic 4-point suture fixation of anterior cruciate ligament tibial avulsion fractures. Arthrosc Tech. 2014;3(6):e683-7.
16. Hunter RE, Willis JA. Arthroscopic fixation of avulsion fractures of the tibial eminence: technique and outcome. Arthroscopy. 2004;20(2):113-21.
17. Baxter MP, Wiley JJ. Fractures of the tibial spine in children. An evaluation of knee stability. J Bone Joint Surg Br. 1988;70(2):228-30.
18. Perugia D, Basiglini L, Vadalà A, et al. Clinical and radiological results of arthroscopically treated tibial spine fractures in childhood. Int Orthop. 2009;33(1):243-8.
19. Kocher MS, Foreman ES, Micheli LJ. Laxity and functional outcome after arthroscopic reduction and internal fixation of displaced tibial spine fractures in children. Arthroscopy. 2003;19(10):1085-90.
20. Zhao J, Huangfu X. Arthroscopic treatment of nonunited anterior cruciate ligament tibial avulsion fracture with figure-of-8 suture fixation technique. Arthroscopy. 2007;23(4):405-10.
21. Panni AS, Milano G, Tartarone M, et al. Arthroscopic treatment of malunited and nonunited avulsion fractures of the anterior tibial spine. Arthroscopy. 1998;14(3):233-40.

CHAPTER

29 Lateral Extra-articular Tenodesis

Pederzini LA, Cheli AF, Serafini F, Nicoletta F

INTRODUCTION AND BACKGROUND

The concept of anterolateral and rotatory instability of the knee following anterior cruciate ligament (ACL) injuries is old and so is the use of a lateral extra-articular tenodesis (LET) to address it. Several LET techniques were described in the past by pioneering surgeons and were used in isolation even before the advent of intra-articular ACL reconstructions techniques. LET techniques were disregarded by most surgeons after the advent of arthroscopic ACL surgery, when the intra-articular reconstruction took center role, and it was believed that the extra-articular component was unnecessary.[1] Although controversies still exist regarding anterolateral capsular and ligamentous structures of the knee, a better understanding of its anatomy and function has recently renewed the popularity of this topic in literature.

Isolated LET are nowadays unanimously considered obsolete, but many surgeons are currently combining a lateral tenodesis with traditional ACL reconstruction in selected cases, in an attempt to better control the residual rotatory instability sometimes observed after ACL reconstructions and to reduce its failure rate.

Literature has suggested a 19% incidence of pivot shifts grade II/III after ACL reconstruction with either hamstring (HS) (single and double bundles) or patellar tendon graft and a reinjury rate of greater than 20% in the age group younger than 20 years.[2,3] Furthermore, residual rotational instability after ACL reconstruction is thought to be a cause of recurrent injuries.[4] Despite the evolving ACL surgery, and the significant improvement in the last decades, with a substantial shift from non-anatomic to anatomic reconstructions, the problem has probably still to be completely solved. Hence, the hypothesis that rotational stability may not be completely restored by use of standard intra-articular reconstruction alone.

Nowadays, the so-called anterolateral ligament (ALL) of the knee has aroused a lot of talk in orthopedics. In a recent editorial [*Knee Surg Sports Traumatol Arthrosc (2016)*], Fu and colleagues stated the following:

"While performing anatomic dissections on 24 different animal species, we have consistently found a double lateral collateral ligament (LCL) in three types of primates; however, an anterolateral ligament (ALL) was never seen in any of the examined species. This suggests a negative selection against this feature in our own evolution. We have also dissected several fetuses aged 18–22 weeks, and again no distinguishable anterolateral ligament was identified within the capsule."

These lines perfectly sum up the incessantly growing interest these days in the orthopedic literature, regarding the anatomy of the anterolateral structures of the knee and their possible contribution to knee rotatory stability.

HISTORICAL ASPECTS

In 1879, the French surgeon Paul Segond described *a pearly, resistant, fibrous band* inserting on the anterolateral aspect of the proximal tibia. A connection of this structure to the avulsion fracture of the anterolateral proximal tibial plateau was called Segond's fracture.[5,6] The anatomy of the anterolateral portion of the knee has experienced a long history of anatomic descriptions and studies and it has been referred to with different names until a recently renewed interest in it (*see* later). In 2007 Vieira et al. first coined the term ALL.[7] Since then the highly speculated and variable structure at the anterolateral aspect of the knee has been largely known as the ALL, with its popularity crossing the borders of the medical world. After being apparently forgotten for 20 years (from 1987 to 2007) this anatomical structure is now being reconsidered for its important role: it seems to act as a limiter of tibial internal rotation (IR) (Table 29.1).

In 1920 Hey Groves described the so called "jerk" as a movement of the tibia over the femur observed in the ACL deficient knees. In 1972, the term "pivot shift" was used for the first time to describe a test to manually reproduce and observe the "jerk" phenomenon during physical examination.[8,9]

It is still highly disputed, if and to what extent the ALL takes part in the development of what is called the pivot shift. To the actual knowledge it seems like the ALL supports the anterolateral capsule of the knee and can thus be compared to the glenohumeral ligaments of the shoulder.

ANTEROLATERAL ANATOMY OF THE KNEE

Although the effects of an LET on knee stability have been largely known since many years, the real anatomy and biomechanics of the anterolateral structures of the knee have remained largely unknown until recently. Renewed interest on the lateral structures of the knee, as supposed to be able to participate in controlling rotatory stability of the knee, has pushed anatomical studies further. A systematic review claims the presence of the ALL in 96% of all investigated knees. On the other hand, unilateral appearance of the ligament between right and left sides has also been noted. This could relate to possible limb dominance.[18] Lutz et al. claimed the ALL as part of the "triangular capsular ligament complex" formed together with the lateral collateral ligament (LCL).[19] Claes et al. identified a strong connection between the ALL and the periphery of the middle third of the lateral meniscal body, and suggested to divide the ALL into a meniscofemoral and a meniscotibial band.[17]

Helito et al. noticed a bifurcation after approximately half of the course of the ALL, splitting it into two parts and creating a more proximal insertion to the anterior horn of the lateral meniscus (thus, it is possible to hypothesize that the ALL may participate in the genesis of lateral meniscus tears, especially peripheral

Table 29.1: Summary of the history of anatomical description of the anterolateral structure of the knee, differently named during years by several authors. .

Author	*Description*
Segond[6] 1879	Pearly, resistant, fibrous band
Last[10] 1948	Short lateral ligament
Hughston[11] 1976 Laprade et al., Sanchez et al.	Mid-third lateral capsular ligament
Johnson[12] 1979 Dietz et al.	Lateral capsular ligament complex
Fulkerson and Gossling[13] 1980 Goldman et al.	Anterior slip of the LCL
Terry et al.[14] 1986	Capsulo-osseous layer of the ITT/some sort of anterolateral ligament
Irvine et al.[15] 1987 Campos et al.	Anterior oblique band
Vieira et al.[7] 2007	ALL as part of the ITT
Vincent et al.[16] 2012	ALL as a capsular structure/thickening
Claes et al.[17] 2013	ALL as an extra-capsular distinctive structure

(LCL: Lateral collateral ligament; ITT: Iliotibial tract; ALL: Anterolateral ligament).

rim detachment tears) and a more distal insertion on the proximal tibia.[20] The femoral attachment has been described between the LCL and the popliteus tendon (PT), being closer to the LCL. The tibial attachment has been described halfway between the fibular head (FH) and the Gerdy's tubercle (GT), being a little closer to the FH[20-22] (Figs. 29.1A and B).

Histological appearance of anterolateral capsule of the knee is that of a collagenous organized structure with a collagen fibers pattern apparently organized in different bundles. A large amount of peripheral nerves and mechanoreceptors suggested a potential proprioceptive role of this area.[21,23] Anterolateral capsule of the knee histology was compared with that of the LCL. The LCL showed a clear linear alignment of collagen fibers, while the anterolateral capsule showed some alignment but not pronounced enough to constitute a true ligament.[24] According to several authors the ALL can be seen on magnetic resonance imaging (MRI). The meniscal portion is the easiest to identify (94.8%). A 3.0 T study with 0.4 mm slice thickness and fat suppression images is recommended.[23-26] Ultrasonographic and arthroscopic visualization of the ALL have also been reported.[27,28]

BIOMECHANICS AND FUNCTION OF ANTEROLATERAL STRUCTURES OF THE KNEE

Studies have shown that the posterolateral (PL) bundle of the ACL contributes little to the rotational stability of the knee and even some double-bundled reconstructions do not restore normal knee kinematics under simulated pivot shift; this function might be performed by knee peripheral structures.[17,29,30]

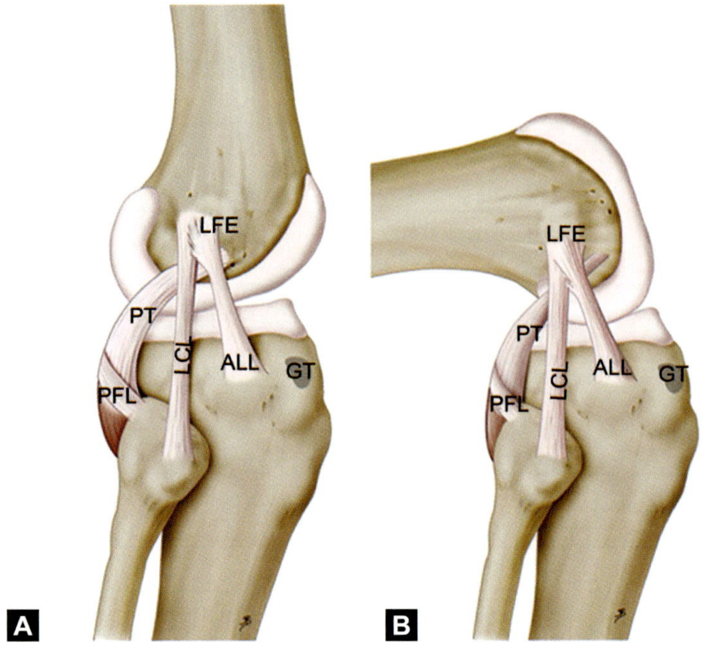

Figs. 29.1A and B: Schematic anatomy of the anterolateral ligament.[17]
(LFE: Lateral femoral epicondyle. PT: Popliteus tendon. LCL: Lateral collateral ligament. PFL: Popliteofibular ligament. ALL: Anterolateral ligament. GT: Gerdy's tubercle).

Interestingly, while some isolated ACL injuries can result in a pivot shift, others do not. Furthermore an isolated injury to the lateral structures can also produce the pivot shift without a torn ACL.[31-34] This may explain why sometimes pivot shift remains positive after ACL reconstruction.

As recent anatomical studies have defined a possible new ligamentous structure with its own function (the ALL), biomechanical studies have followed.

Anterolateral ligament has been described to show a behavior close to isometricity between 0° and 60° of flexion; then the ligament slackens when the knee is flexed further to 90°; it is lengthened and tightened with tibial IR. An increased tightening of the ALL in IR has been noted to correspond with an increased slackening of the ACL.[35-37]

According to an in vitro study, isolated ACL resection could only produce a pivot shift no higher than grade I, whereas the additional ALL resection resulted in a high-grade (grade II or III) pivot shift.[29] Particularly, cutting the PL bundle did not increase anterior translation and rotation of the knee. Cutting the ALL showed increased anterior translation at 60° and IR at 30°, 45°, and 60°. The authors concluded that cutting the ALL increased tibial rotation and could be related to the pivot-shift phenomenon.

Current consensus among experts is that the anterolateral structures of the knee or ALL mainly function as additional rotational stabilizers of the knee.

COMMON SURGICAL TECHNIQUES FOR LATERAL EXTRA-ARTICULAR TENODESIS

Lateral extra-articular tenodesis is thought to be analogous to the recently developed ALL reconstruction, in terms of controlling anterolateral rotational instability; however, the two differ anatomically. Many LET

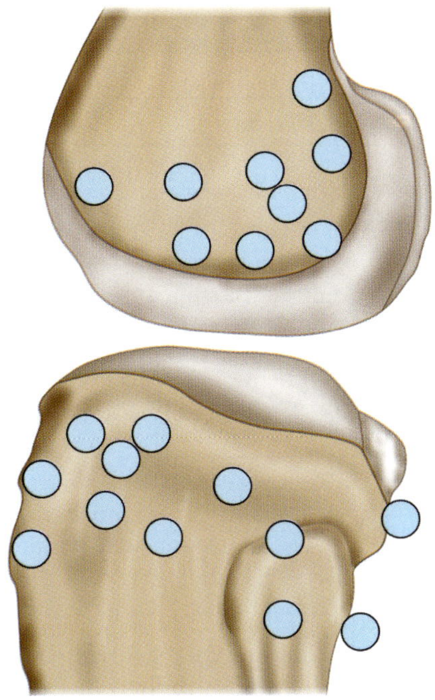

Fig. 29.2: Different proximal and distal insertion points for different lateral extra-articular tenodesis procedures described in literature.

techniques incorporate a proximal fixation point close to the femoral epicondyle and are fixed distally at or around the GT, often running deep to the LCL.[1]

Most of the techniques traditionally described for LET use different grafts that are placed in a variety of anatomic locations (Fig. 29.2), they are not anatomic and should not be considered as anatomic ALL reconstructions. Recently, after detailed anatomical and biomechanical studies, surgeons are attracted by the seductive idea of performing a real anatomic reconstruction rather than a functional tenodesis or augmentation only.

Since the first description of an extra-articular procedure by Lemaire in 1967,[38] a lot of different techniques and modifications of the original technique have emerged (Table 29.2 and Fig. 29.3). Common aim of all procedures is to achieve a better control of tibial IR, than with ACL reconstruction alone.

Other techniques have also been proposed and described in literature.[39-41]

LITERATURE EVIDENCE

Combined procedures (ACL reconstruction + LET/ALL reconstruction) are becoming more popular today, after more detailed anatomical studies on the anterolateral structures of the knee, but still few studies with direct comparison between ACL reconstruction alone and combined augmentation and between different LET techniques have been conducted.

Biomechanical Comparative Studies

In 2007, Monaco et al. compared lateral tenodesis plus single bundle ACL reconstruction (Group A) with anatomic double bundle ACL reconstruction (Group B); a significant reduction in IR of the tibia was found

Table 29.2: Brief history of techniques for anterolateral extra-articular stabilization of the knee (LET).[42]

Isolated LET	
Author	*Technique*
Lemaire	ITB is prepared femoral (18 × 1 cm) with preservation of the tibial insertion and then shuttled under the LCL and pulled through a lateral femoral tunnel and again shuttled under the LCL and sutured to the tibial insertion/passed in a tibial tunnel. Fixation at 30° of flexion and neutral rotation.*Modifications*: Neyret et al.; Lazzarone et al.; Wagner and Weiler; Dejour et al. (with free gracilis graft)
Slocum-Larsen	The distal flap of the pes anserinus conjoined tendons (sartorius, gracilis, and semitendinosus) is folded and sutured upwards to the tibial joint line to enhance its effect on tibial internal rotation instead of flexion
MacIntosh I	"Lateral substitution reconstruction"; ITB graft (20 cm × 2 cm) with suture fixation to the proximal tibia, shuttled under the LCL and sutured to the intermuscular septum.*Modifications*: Amirault et al.; Ireland and Trickey; Dandy; Arnold et al.; Christel and Dijan (graft is shorter and not passed under LCL)
Losee	"Sling and reef" procedure: ITB is prepared femoral with preservation of the tibial insertion and then shuttled under the LCL and through the lateral gastrocnemius, then sutured to the LCL and pulled back anterior and sutured to the tibial insertion. *Modifications*: Frank and Jackson
Ellison	"Dynamic distal ITB transfer". Rerouting of the distally prepared ITB (left attached proximally) under the LCL with a reefing of the anterolateral capsule; dynamic LET relying on ITB contraction (tensor fascia lata) and refixation in its old bed.*Modifications*: Reid et al.; Kennedy et al.
Andrews	"Isometric lateral plasty"; ITB is split into two isometric bundles distally (one tight in flexion, the other in extension), sutured up against the distal femur twisted 180° and tied medially creating a "neo" ligament
Patella	"One-loop plasty": ITB graft looped below the capsule through a femoral tunnel and proximally fixed with a staple and distally in a tibial corticocancellous groove
MacIntosh II/III[43]	Similar to MacIntosh I, but the graftis prolonged intra-articularly via the over-the-top position, then through the notch and then through a tibial tunnel In MacIntosh III (Marshall-MacIntosh), the same is achieved in opposite direction by using the central third of the entire extensor mechanism (patellar tendon + quadriceps tendon) as a graft.
Marcacci[44]	The gracilis and semitendinosus tendons are harvested preserving the distal insertion (Figs. 29.5A to F). The graft is then passed through a tibial tunnel and in an over-the-top position on the femoral side using a lateral incision to the distal femur. Proximal fixation at lateral femoral condyle and distal fixation at Gerdy's tubercle are achieved with staples. Extra-articular portion of the graft is passed under ITB.
Claes[17]	Minimally invasive tenodesis with a gracilis graft with anatomical anchor fixation over the lateral femoral epicondyle and the anterolateral proximal tibial plateau

Contd...

Contd...

Author	*Technique*
Helito[45]	Triple semitendinosus and single gracilis graft prepared for combined ACL and ALL reconstruction. The part used to reconstruct the ACL is a quadruple graft, and the remaining part of the gracilis is used to reconstruct the ALL. ALL femoral point is halfway on the Blumensaat line, 3–4 mm below it. Tibial insertion is between the fibular head and Gerdy's tubercle, 5–10 mm below the joint line. Fixation is achieved with two anchors. Tibial fixation is performed with knee between 60° and 90°. According to the size of the graft, it is possible to render the ALL thicker by returning it underneath the iliotibial tract.
Colombet[46]	The graft used is similar to Helito but intra-articular portion is only doubled; the route of the graft is similar to Marcacci, but the graft is passed into a femoral out-in tunnel and then rerouted under ITB and fixed at a tunnel in proximity of Gerdy's tubercle; fixation is achieved with anchors in both tunnels.
Neyret[47-49]	ACL reconstruction is performed routinely with BTB graft; a free gracilis tendon graft is passed in the femoral bone block (prior its passage inside the femoral tunnel); the two free ends of gracilis are used for LET and passed under LCL and then passed into a drill hole at Gerdy's tubercle, coming from lateral to medial and the two limbs are sutured to one another.

(LET: Lateral extra-articular tenodesis; ITB: Iliotibial band; LCL: Lateral collateral ligament; ACL: Anterior cruciate ligament; ALL: Anterolateral ligament; BTB: Bone-tendon-bone).

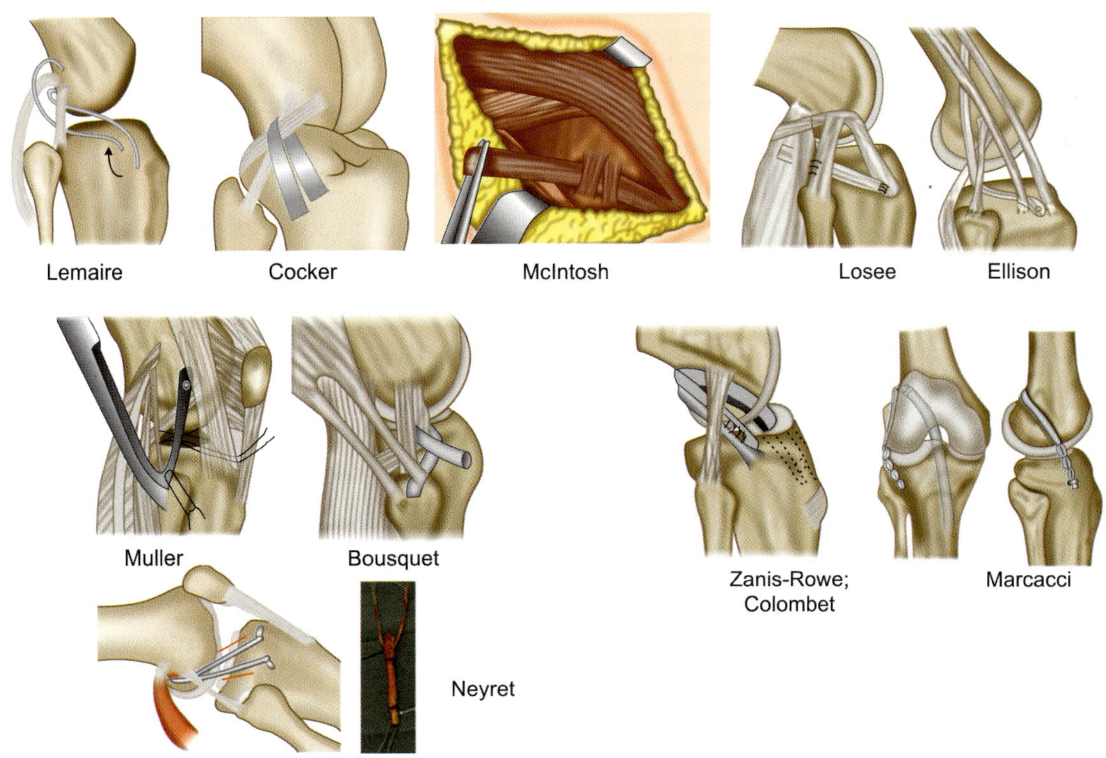

Fig. 29.3: Drawings showing some of the possible techniques for lateral extra-articular tenodesis.

in group A compared with group B. Particularly, comparing the group A after the single bundle reconstruction and the group B after the anteromedial (AM) bundle only fixation, no differences were found in anteroposterior (AP) displacement, IR, and external rotation (ER) of the tibia. Comparing the group A after the addition of the lateral tenodesis and group B after the PL bundle fixation (AM + PL) no differences were found in AP tibial displacement and in ER of tibia. However, a significant reduction in tibial IR was found in group A after the addition of the lateral tenodesis with respect to the group B after the addition of the PL bundle.[50]

In 2012, Zaffagnini et al. assessed in vivo static and dynamic biomechanics of the knee, comparing the Marcacci technique with anatomic double-bundle technique; the lateral augmentation used in Marcacci technique resulted to be able to better control the lateral compartment during drawer test (static). On the other hand, pivot-shift phenomenon was better controlled by anatomic double-bundle reconstruction (dynamic).[51]

In 2014, Monaco et al. evaluated the role of lateral tenodesis on the pivot shift. 20 patients underwent anatomic single-bundle ACL reconstruction with the addition of extra-articular reconstruction. In group A, intra-articular reconstruction was performed first and lateral tenodesis thereafter; in group B, lateral tenodesis was performed first. Extra-articular reconstruction had little effect in reducing anterior tibial translation at 30° of flexion, but it was more effective than intra-articular reconstruction in reducing axial tibial rotation. The authors concluded that anatomic ACL reconstruction and lateral tenodesis were synergic in controlling the pivot-shift phenomenon.[52]

Clinical Comparative Studies

In 2006, Zaffagnini et al. clinically compared the Marcacci technique with the single-bundle patellar tendon (PT) and with the four strand HS techniques at 5 years of follow-up. Stability was significantly better controlled (instrumented Lachman and pivot shift), and subjective scores were significantly higher with PT and Marcacci technique compared to HS technique. Return to sport was faster with Marcacci technique. They concluded that PT and Marcacci techniques can be equivalent options for ACL reconstruction.[53]

In 2009, Marcacci et al. evaluated the outcomes of 54 consecutive high-level athletes operated with their technique at 13-year follow-up. The authors concluded that the technique showed satisfactory results, with maintenance of knee stability at long term. Knee osteoarthritis after the Marcacci technique does not appear to be greater than after conventional ACL reconstruction procedures.[54]

In 2012, Dejour et al. compared three groups of patients treated with double-bundle ACL reconstruction, bone-patellar tendon-bone (BPTB), and bone-patellar tendon-bone in addition with a modified Lemaire's procedures (BPTB + L) at 2 years minimum of follow-up. There was no statistical difference between the groups in terms of pivot shift and subjective/objective International Knee Documentation Committee (IKDC) scores.[55] Improved pivot-shift stability in the combined procedure was expected given the role of extra-articular repair as a secondary restraint to rotational control. The improvement may also be related to the protective effect of the extra-articular procedure during the ligamentization process. The forces may be partially dissipated by the extra-articular procedure thereby preventing some elongation and optimizing the biomechanical environment for ligamentization. As the healing phase process is known to take longer for HS compared to patellar tendon, the addition of an LET to ACL reconstruction with HS may be of greater benefit. Engebretsen et al. showed that the addition of an LET to ACL reconstruction reduced the stress on the ACL graft by 43% in a cadaveric study.[56,57] It may also act as an extra restraint on return to activity in high contact or high level sport.

Review and Meta-analysis

A systematic review conducted by Hewison et al.[1] of different studies dealing with combined extra-articular anterolateral stabilization and intra-articular ACL reconstruction [8 randomized controlled trials (RCTs) and 21 nonrandomized studies] showed that the combination provides a statistically significant better reduction of the pivot-shift phenomenon. The supposed risk of lateral overconstraint and subsequent lateral osteoarthritis was found to be not significant in this review.[58]

Rezende et al.[59] performed a meta-analysis including eight RCTs. They concluded combined intra-articular and extra-articular ACL reconstruction provided marginally improved knee stability and comparable failure rates but no difference in patient reported functional outcomes scores. Complications and adverse events such as knee stiffness may be underreported. Further, they noticed how primary aspects in ACL surgery, such as fixation methods, correct tunnel placement, and postoperative programs, possibly have greater influence in final clinical results and should be addressed before considering the combined procedure. In contrast to other studies, they found no difference between the two groups regarding knee stiffness, development of osteoarthritis, and infection rate. Data suggested that the addition of the extra-articular procedure provided superior stability to ACL procedures with HS grafts. In contrast, ACL procedures with BPTB grafts did not show stability improvement when comparing combined ACL reconstruction with isolated intra-articular reconstruction.

Song et al. conducted a systematic review that included seven studies.[60] Among the five comparative studies, the prevalence of residual pivot shift was significantly lower in patients with LET plus ACL reconstruction than those with isolated ACL reconstruction. However, the distribution of objective IKDC scores and anterior knee stability showed no significant differences between groups at short-term follow-up. They concluded that the combination of LET and intra-articular ACL reconstruction was effective in eliminating the high-grade pivot-shift phenomenon.

OUR EXPERIENCE

In our current practice, possible indications for additional extra-articular anterolateral tenodesis or reconstruction are: rotatory instability in high pivoting sports (soccer, rugby, skiing, etc.); more than 5 mm anterior translation (especially if predominantly lateral) in the Lachman test or anterior drawer test; a high-grade pivot shift; ACL graft failure with rotatory instability.

The senior author routinely decides the eventual planning of an additional LET based on the following summarized criteria:

- Our accepted indications for ACL augmentation with LET/ALL reconstruction:
  - High grade preoperative pivot shift (II or III)
  - Demanding athletes (participating in contact/high pivoting or high level sports), as a backup/protection/load shearing (especially for HS)
  - Chronic ACL insufficiency
  - Hyperlax patients
  - Revision cases (in which no clear reason for failure can be identified)
- How we select a possible candidate for the addition of LET on the basis of preoperative physical examination:
  - Increased tibial internal rotation or predominant lateral compartment translation at drawer test compared to uninjured side
  - Increase in total axial rotation of the healthy knee during the examination along with a decrease in endpoint stiffness at maximum internal rotation (as suggested by computed biomechanical studies conducted by Neyret et al. in 2015).

It should be noted that patients affected by PL corner injury are a contraindication to the addition of any lateral procedure as the PL corner injury has to be addressed separately. Hence, it is mandatory to always rule out a possible posterolateral rotatory instability (PLRI).[61]

In our experience we tried to dissect the anterolateral portion of the knee in several specimens: we were not able to always identify a proper ALL on all knees and sometimes the structure identified was, in our opinion, too thin and too ill defined to represent a true ligament with a proper function (Fig. 29.4). Based on this experience on cadavers and after few not completely satisfying ALL anatomical reconstructions (because of residual flexion deficit), we recently changed our surgical choice to augment intra-articular ACL reconstruc-

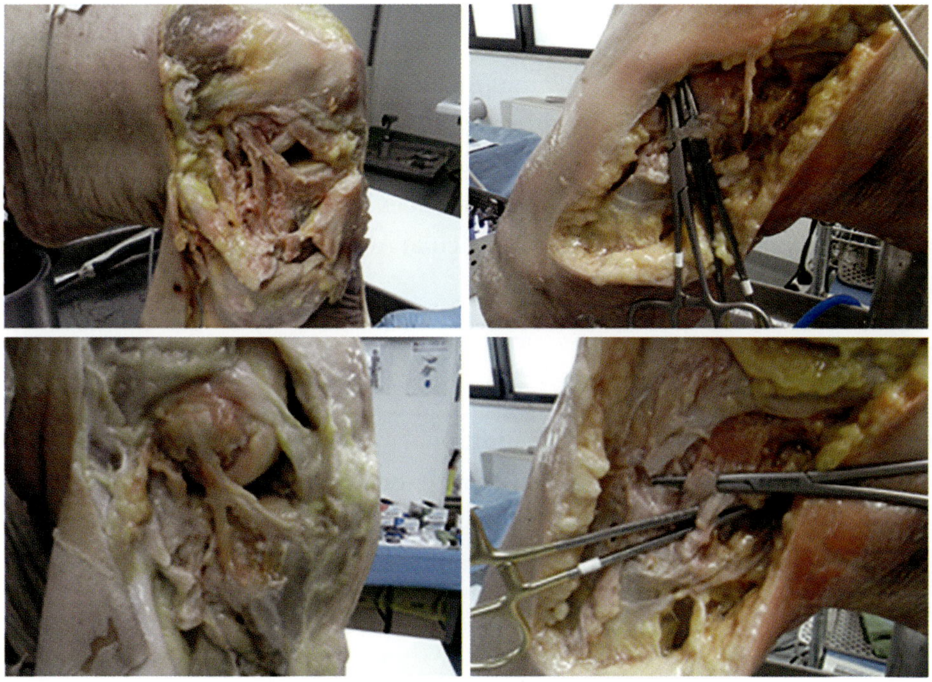

Fig. 29.4: Examples of anatomical specimens dissected attempting the isolation of the anterolateral ligament.

tion when required. We shifted to an LET based on an augmentation with iliotibial band (ITB) as previously described by A. Wiliams (Fortius Clinic, London) during European Society of Sports Traumatology, Knee Surgery and Arthroscopy (ESSKA), Barcelona in 2016 and International Society of Arthroscopy, Knee Surgery and Orthopaedic Sports Medicine (ISAKOS) Congress, Lyon in 2015.

Twenty five patients were operated with this LET procedure + ACL reconstruction with BTB showing a negative pivot shift at an early 18 months follow-up, with no flexion deficit compared to uninjured side (unpublished data).

SURGICAL TECHNIQUE

A 12-cm long and 1-cm wide strip of ITB is harvested, keeping its distal insertion on GT intact. The free end is whip-stitched and the strip is then passed under the LCL and fixed using a double-loaded suture anchor (GII™ QUICK-ANCHOR® Plus—DePuy Mitek; Nickel-Titanium alloy; 8.8 mm × 2.4 mm with ORTHOCORD® partially absorbable suture) at the PL aspect of the lateral femoral condyle, in order to constrain the lateral ITB. The residual portion of the strip is then pulled distally and sutured on itself just distal to the LCL (Figs. 29.5A to K).

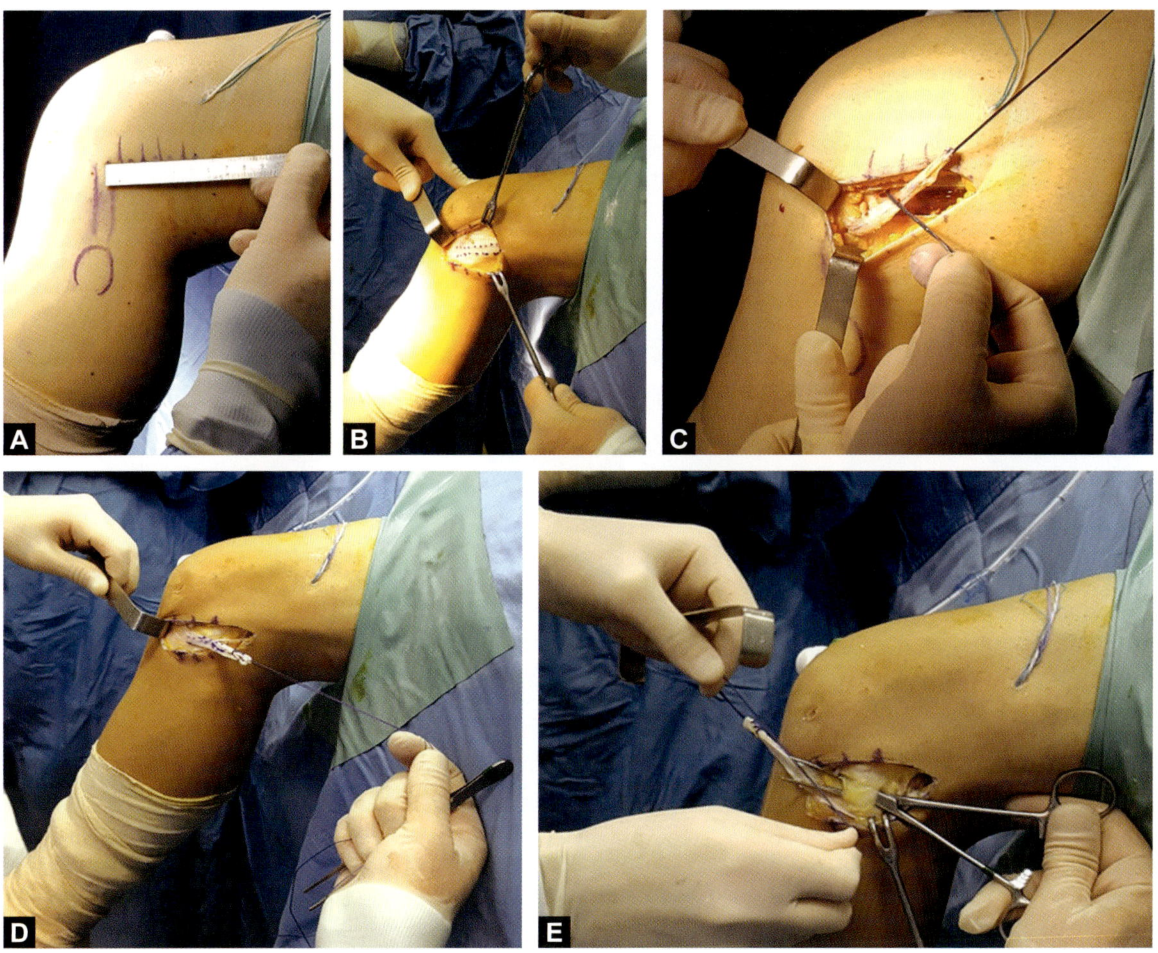

Figs. 29.5A to E

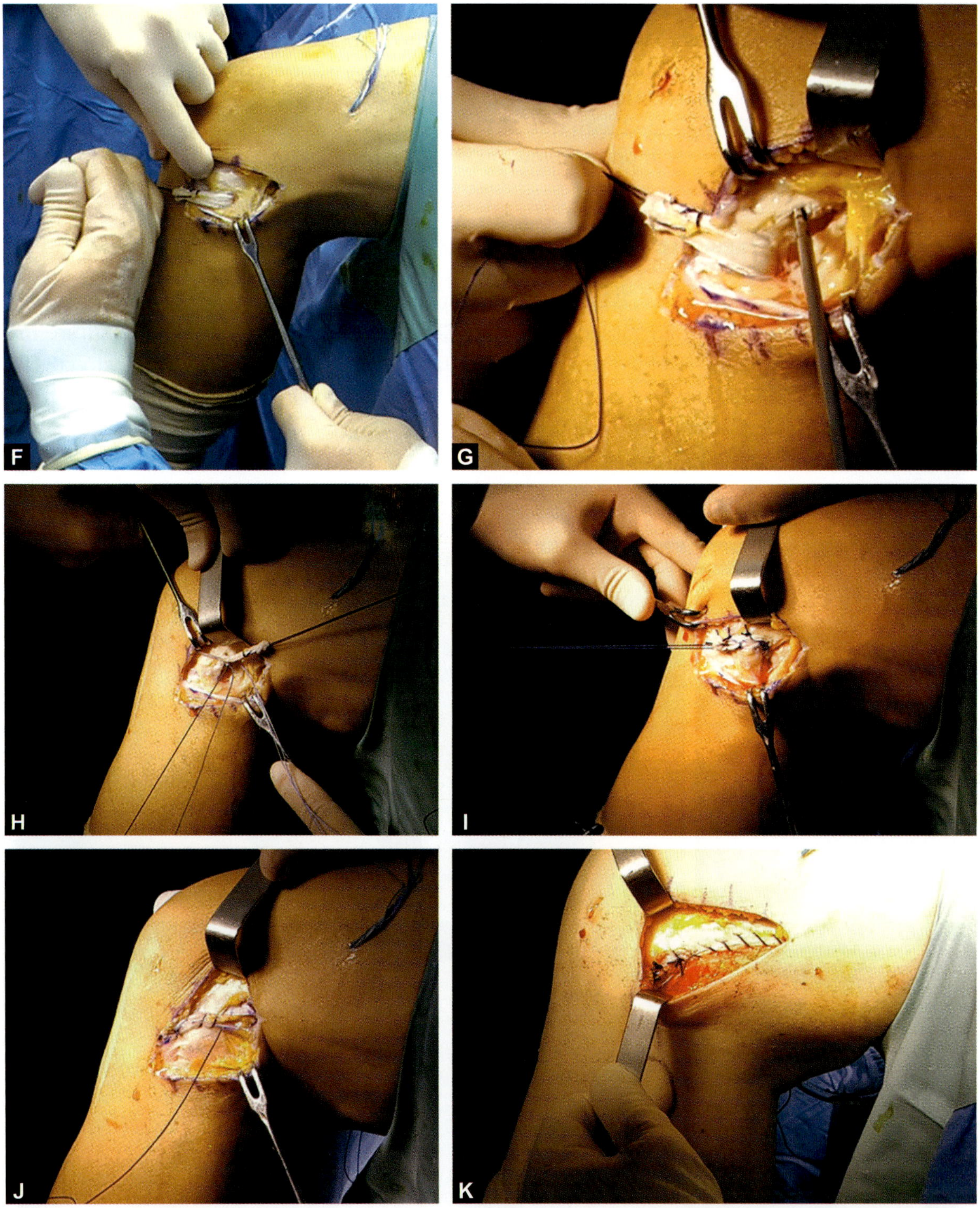

Figs. 29.5A to K: Lateral extra-articular tenodesis surgical steps: (A) skin landmarks after anterior cruciate ligament reconstruction [fibular head and lateral collateral ligament (LCL)]; (B) a 12-cm long and 1-cm wide iliotibial band (ITB) strip is marked on its inferior half and (C) then harvested and (D) loaded with sutures at its free end; (E) the graft is then passed underneath the LCL and (F) rerouted distally towards the Gerdy's tubercle; (G and H) a double-ended suture anchor is placed on the posterolateral aspect of the lateral femoral condyle and used to fix the proximal part of the graft at this point; (I) the remaining portion of the graft is then sutured back on itself and (J and K) the ITB is then closed without excessive tension in a continuous fashion.

Prior to performing a concomitant extra-articular anterolateral tenodesis, checking lateral compartment cartilage quality was highly recommended in the past, as the described old procedures for LET have proven to cause an overstrain to lateral compartment with consequent pain.[62] Increased incidence of patellofemoral crepitation or pain and reduction of knee flexion have been also associated with certain extra-articular techniques.[58] As a consequence of these problems and to the highly improved ACL intra-articular reconstructions, isolated extra-articular reconstruction must be considered obsolete nowadays.

With modern and more aggressive rehabilitation protocols and if performed concomitant to an intra-articular ACL reconstruction, over tensioning of an LET is less likely, therefore guarding against fixed subluxation is seen in isolated extra-articular reconstructions in the past.

It must be noted that the LET is tensioned with the tibia externally rotated in most of the described techniques, which may have an impact on overtightening the lateral side of the knee. Hence, Neyret has recommended tibial fixation of LET with the tibia in neutral rotation.

CONCLUSION

Even though several recent studies have shown the possible benefits of the addition of a lateral extra-articular reconstruction (LET), its indication is still far from receiving a unanimous vote in the literature. Lateral tenodesis has not yet shown to yield short- or long-term clinical improvements. Whether the incremental benefits in joint stability with a combined approach justifies the added surgery is still to be defined. Furthermore, reports showing residual instability after ACL reconstruction mostly are outdated, and consequently an old-fashioned vertical tunnel might be the origin of the high rate of reported residual rotational instability.[63-65]

Most extra-articular procedures described in the literature are non-anatomic. The unreliable results of LET in the past may partly be due to incomplete knowledge of the anatomy and biomechanics of this area. As understanding of the anatomy of the anterolateral compartment of the knee evolves and becomes clearer, the LET procedures may be modified to allow truly anatomic ALL reconstructions, which may improve results and minimize donor site morbidity. The exact site of femoral attachment and tension of the extra-articular reconstruction could be critical in determining the successful restoration of normal biomechanics. As more anatomically and biomechanically appropriate extra-articular reconstruction techniques are developed to be used in conjunction with anatomic intra-articular reconstruction in selected cases, failure and recurrence rates in ACL surgery will hopefully be reduced.[65]

Considering recent literature reviews, we are still not strongly convinced that ALL anatomical reconstruction can be considered the actual golden standard. Consequently, we believe the role of the ITB complex must not be forgotten and underestimated after the ALL discovery. ITB still contributes in controlling rotatory stability of the knee. We therefore prefer to perform an LET procedure with ITB reinforcement.

REFERENCES

1. Hewison CE, Tran MN, Kaniki N, et al. Lateral Extra-articular Tenodesis Reduces Rotational Laxity When Combined With Anterior Cruciate Ligament Reconstruction: A Systematic Review of the Literature. Arthroscopy. 2015;31(10):2022-34.
2. Mohtadi NG, Chan DS, Dainty KN, et al. Patellar tendon versus hamstring tendon autograft for anterior cruciate ligament rupture in adults. Cochrane Database Syst Rev. 2011(9):CD005960.
3. Magnussen RA, Lawrence JT, West RL, et al. Graft size and patient age are predictors of early revision after anterior cruciate ligament reconstruction with hamstring autograft. Arthroscopy. 2012;28(4):526-31.
4. Chouliaras V, Ristanis S, Moraiti C, et al. Effectiveness of reconstruction of the anterior cruciate ligament with quadrupled hamstrings and bone-patellar tendon-bone autografts: an in vivo study comparing tibial internal-external rotation. Am J Sports Med. 2007;35(2):189-96.
5. Goldman AB, Pavlov H, Rubenstein D. The Segond fracture of the proximal tibia: a small avulsion that reflects major ligamentous damage. AJR Am J Roentgenol. 1988;151(6):1163-7.

6. Segond P. Recherches cliniques et expe´rimentales sur les e´panchements sanguins du genou par entorse. Prog Med. 1879;7:297-341.
7. Vieira EL, Vieira EÁ, da Silva RT, et al. An anatomic study of the iliotibial tract. Arthroscopy. 2007;23(3):269-74.
8. Heygroves E. Operation for the repair of the crucial ligaments. Lancet. 1917;190(4914):674-6.
9. Slocum DB, Larson RL. Rotatory instability of the knee. J Bone Joint Surg Am. 2002;84(5):868.
10. Last RJ. Some anatomical details of the knee joint. J Bone Joint Surg Br. 1948;30B(4):683-8.
11. Hughston JC, Andrews JR, Cross MJ, et al. Classification of knee ligament instabilities. Part II. The lateral compartment. J Bone Joint Surg Am. 1976;58(2):173-9.
12. Johnson LL. Lateral capsular ligament complex: anatomical and surgical considerations. Am J Sports Med. 1979;7(3):156-60.
13. Fulkerson JP, Gossling HR. Anatomy of the knee joint lateral retinaculum. Clin Orthop Relat Res. 1980;153:183-8.
14. Terry GC, Hughston JC, Norwood LA. The anatomy of the iliopatellar band and iliotibial tract. Am J Sports Med. 1986;14(1):39-45.
15. Irvine G, Dias J, Finlay D. Segond fractures of the lateral tibial condyle: brief report. J Bone Joint Surg Br. 1987;69:613-4.
16. Vincent JP, Magnussen RA, Gezmez F, et al. The anterolateral ligament of the human knee: an anatomic and histologic study. Knee Surg Sports Traumatol Arthrosc. 2012;20(1):147-52.
17. Claes S, Vereecke E, Maes M, et al. Anatomy of the anterolateral ligament of the knee. J Anat. 2013;223(4):321-8.
18. Van der Watt L, Khan M, Rothrauff BB, et al. The structure and function of the anterolateral ligament of the knee: a systematic review. Arthroscopy. 2015;31(3):569-82.e3.
19. Lutz C, Sonnery-Cottet B, Niglis L, et al. Behavior of the anterolateral structures of the knee during internal rotation. Orthop Traumatol Surg Res. 2015;101(5):523-8.
20. Helito CP, Demange MK, Bonadio MB, et al. Radiographic landmarks for locating the femoral origin and tibial insertion of the knee anterolateral ligament. Am J Sports Med. 2014;42(10):2356-62.
21. Helito CP, Demange MK, Bonadio MB, et al. Anatomy and Histology of the Knee Anterolateral Ligament. Orthop J Sports Med. 2013;1(7):2325967113513546.
22. Helito CP, Bonadio MB, Soares TQ, et al. The meniscal insertion of the knee anterolateral ligament. Surg Radiol Anat. 2016;38(2):223-8.
23. Caterine S, Litchfield R, Johnson M, et al. A cadaveric study of the anterolateral ligament: re-introducing the lateral capsular ligament. Knee Surg Sports Traumatol Arthrosc. 2014;23(11):3186-95.
24. Dombrowski ME, Costello JM, Ohashi B, et al. Macroscopic anatomical, histological and magnetic resonance imaging correlation of the lateral capsule of the knee. Knee Surg Sports Traumatol Arthrosc. 2015;24(9):2854-60.
25. Helito CP, Helito PVP, Costa HP, et al. MRI evaluation of the anterolateral ligament of the knee: assessment in routine 1.5-T scans. Skeletal Radiol. 2014;43(10):1421-7.
26. LaPrade RF, Gilbert TJ, Bollom TS, et al. The magnetic resonance imaging appearance of individual structures of the posterolateral knee. A prospective study of normal knees and knees with surgically verified grade III injuries. Am J Sports Med. 2000;28:191-9.
27. Sonnery-Cottet B, Thaunat M, Freychet B, et al. Outcome of a Combined Anterior Cruciate Ligament and Anterolateral Ligament Reconstruction Technique With a Minimum 2-Year Follow-up. Am J Sports Med. 2015;43(7):1598-605.
28. Cianca J, John J, Pandit S, et al. Musculoskeletal ultrasound imaging of the recently described anterolateral ligament of the knee. Am J Phys Med Rehabil. 2014;93(2):186.
29. Monaco E, Ferretti A, Labianca L, et al. Navigated knee kinematics after cutting of the ACL and its secondary restraint. Knee Surg Sports Traumatol Arthrosc. 2012;20(5):870-7.
30. Yasuda K, Kondo E, Ichiyama H, et al. Anatomic reconstruction of the anteromedial and posterolateral bundles of the anterior cruciate ligament using hamstring tendon grafts. Arthroscopy. 2004;20(10):1015-25.
31. Bull AM, Amis AA. The pivot-shift phenomenon: a clinical and biomechanical perspective. Knee. 1998;5(3):141-58.
32. Matsumoto H, Seedhom BB. Treatment of the pivot-shift intraarticular versus extraarticular or combined reconstruction procedures: a biomechanical study. Clin Orthop Relat Res. 1994;299:298-304.
33. Norwood LA, Andrews JR, Meisterling RC, et al. Acute anterolateral rotatory instability of the knee. J Bone Joint Surg Am. 1979;61(5):704-9.
34. Fetto JF, Marshall JL. Injury to the anterior cruciate ligament producing the pivot-shift sign. J Bone Joint Surg Am. 1979;61(5):710-4.

35. Kennedy MI, Claes S, Fuso FA, et al. The Anterolateral Ligament. Am J Sports Med. 2015;43(7):1606-15.
36. Dodds AL, Halewood C, Gupte CM, et al. The anterolateral ligament: Anatomy, length changes and association with the Segond fracture. Bone Joint J. 2014;96-B(3):325-31.
37. Parsons EM, Gee AO, Spiekerman C, et al. The biomechanical function of the anterolateral ligament of the knee. Am J Sports Med. 2015;43(8):NP22.
38. Lemaire M. Rupture ancienne du ligament croise´ ante´rieur du genou. J Chir. 1967;93:311-20.
39. Yamaguchi S, Sasho T, Tsuchiya A, et al. Long term results of anterior cruciate ligament reconstruction with iliotibial tract: 6-, 13-, and 24-year longitudinal follow-up. Knee Surg Sports Traumatol Arthrosc. 2006;14(11):1094-100.
40. Saragaglia D, Pison A, Refaie R. Lateral tenodesis combined with anterior cruciate ligament reconstruction using a unique semitendinosus and gracilis transplant. Int Orthop. 2013;37(8): 1575-81.
41. VuMedi. Antwerp Monoloop procedure. [online] VuMedi website. Available from www.vumedi.com/video/the-antwerp-monoloop-for-reconstruction-of-the-anterolateral-ligament-all [Accessed March, 2017].
42. Roessler PP, Schüttler KF, Heyse TJ, et al. The anterolateral ligament (ALL) and its role in rotational extra-articular stability of the knee joint: a review of anatomy and surgical concepts. Arch Orthop Trauma Surg. 2016;136(3):305-13.
43. Marshall JL, Warren RF, Wickiewicz TL, et al. The anterior cruciate ligament: a technique of repair and reconstruction. Clin Orthop Relat Res. 1979;143:97-106.
44. Marcacci M, Zaffagnini S, Iacono F, et al. Arthroscopic intra- and extra-articular anterior cruciate ligament reconstruction with gracilis and semitendinosus tendons. Knee Surg Sports Traumatol Arthrosc. 1998;6(2):68-75.
45. Helito CP, Bonadio MB, Gobbi RG, et al. Combined Intra- and Extra-articular Reconstruction of the Anterior Cruciate Ligament: The Reconstruction of the Knee Anterolateral Ligament. Arthrosc Tech. 2015;4(3):e239-44.
46. Colombet PD. Navigated intra-articular ACL reconstruction with additional extra-articular tenodesis using the same hamstring graft. Knee Surg Sports Traumatol Arthrosc. 2010;19(3):384-9.
47. Dejour H, Walch G, Neyret P, et al. Results of surgically treated chronic anterior laxities. Apropos of 251 cases reviewed with a minimum follow-up of 3 years. Rev Chir Orthop Reparatrice Appar Mot. 1988;74(7):622-36.
48. Magnussen RA, Jacobi M, Demey G, et al. Lateral Extra-articular Augmentation of ACL Reconstruction. Tech Knee Surg. 2011;10(4):224-30.
49. Duthon VB, Magnussen RA, Servien E, et al. ACL reconstruction and extra-articular tenodesis. Clin Sports Med. 2013;32(1):141-53.
50. Monaco E, Labianca L, Conteduca F, et al. Double bundle or single bundle plus extraarticular tenodesis in ACL reconstruction? Knee Surg Sports Traumatol Arthrosc. 2007;15(10):1168-74.
51. Zaffagnini S, Signorelli C, Lopomo N, et al. Anatomic double-bundle and over-the-top single-bundle with additional extra-articular tenodesis: an in vivo quantitative assessment of knee laxity in two different ACL reconstructions. Knee Surg Sports Traumatol Arthrosc. 2011;20(1):153-9.
52. Monaco E, Maestri B, Conteduca F, et al. Extra-articular ACL Reconstruction and Pivot Shift. Am J Sports Med. 2014;42(7):1669-74.
53. Zaffagnini S, Marcacci M, Lo Presti M, et al. Prospective and randomized evaluation of ACL reconstruction with three techniques: a clinical and radiographic evaluation at 5 years follow-up. Knee Surg Sports Traumatol Arthrosc. 2006;14(11):1060-9.
54. Marcacci M, Zaffagnini S, Giordano G, et al. Anterior cruciate ligament reconstruction associated with extra-articular tenodesis: a prospective clinical and radiographic evaluation with 10- to 13-year follow-up. Am J Sports Med. 2009;37(4):707-14.
55. Dejour D, Vanconcelos W, Bonin N, et al. Comparative study between mono-bundle bone-patellar tendon-bone, double-bundle hamstring and mono-bundle bone-patellar tendon-bone combined with a modified Lemaire extra-articular procedure in anterior cruciate ligament reconstruction. Int Orthop. 2013;37(2):193-9.
56. Vadalà AP, Iorio R, De Carli A, et al. An extra-articular procedure improves the clinical outcome in anterior cruciate ligament reconstruction with hamstrings in female athletes. Int Orthop. 2012;37(2):187-92.
57. Engebretsen L, Lew WD, Lewis JL, et al. Knee mechanics after repair of the anterior cruciate ligament A cadaver study of ligament augmentation. Acta Orthop Scand. 1989;60(6):703-9.
58. Anderson A, Snyder R, Lipscomb AB Jr. Anterior cruciate ligament reconstruction: a prospective randomized study of three surgical methods. Am J Sports Med. 2001;29(3):272-9.

59. Rezende FC, de Moraes VY, Martimbianco AL, et al. Does Combined Intra- and Extraarticular ACL Reconstruction Improve Function and Stability? A Meta-analysis. Clin Orthop Relat Res. 2015;473(8):2609-18.
60. Song GY, Hong L, Zhang H, et al. Clinical Outcomes of Combined Lateral Extra-articular Tenodesis and Intra-articular Anterior Cruciate Ligament Reconstruction in Addressing High-Grade Pivot-Shift Phenomenon. Arthroscopy. 2016;32(5):898-905.
61. Bonasia DE, D'Amelio A, Pellegrino P, et al. Anterolateral ligament of the knee: back to the future in anterior cruciate ligament reconstruction. Orthop Rev. 2015;7(2):5773.
62. Imbert P, Belvedere C, Leardini A. Knee laxity modifications after ACL rupture and surgical intra- and extra-articular reconstructions: intra-operative measures in reconstructed and healthy knees. Knee Surg Sports Traumatol Arthrosc. 2015. [Epub ahead of print].
63. Logan MC, Williams A, Lavelle J, et al. Tibiofemoral kinematics following successful anterior cruciate ligament reconstruction using dynamic multiple resonance imaging. Am J Sports Med. 2004;32(4):984-92.
64. Ristanis S, Stergiou N, Patras K, et al. Excessive Tibial Rotation During High-Demand Activities Is Not Restored by Anterior Cruciate Ligament Reconstruction. Arthroscopy. 2005;21(11):1323-9.
65. Dodds AL, Gupte CM, Neyret P, et al. Extra-articular techniques in anterior cruciate ligament reconstruction: a literature review. J Bone Joint Surg Br. 2011;93(11):1440-8.

CHAPTER

30 Minimally Invasive Anterolateral Ligament Reconstruction

Sachin Tapasvi, Anshu Shekhar, Shantanu Patil

INTRODUCTION

Arthroscopic reconstruction of the anterior cruciate ligament (ACL) is an evolving science, with the aim of improving outcomes after the surgery. Some contentious issues like transportal versus transtibial technique for femoral tunnel placement have been largely sorted out.[1] There is a raging debate as to whether the ACL is actually made of two discreet bundles or a flat, ribbon like structure.[2-6] A new controversy which has literally divided the arthroscopy fraternity is the anterolateral ligament (ALL).[7] Questions like whether the ALL really exists, its role in the native and ACL deficient knee, scope of surgery for the ALL are still very much unanswered. In this chapter we briefly visit the controversy surrounding ALL and describe our surgical technique for reconstructing this ligament using a minimally invasive approach.

REVIEW OF LITERATURE

Does the Anterolateral Ligament Really Exist?

Paul Segond's description of "a pearly, resistant, fibrous band" attached to the anterolateral tibia is perhaps the earliest description of what is now known as the ALL.[8] Injury to this structure is classically called the Segond fracture and is pathognomonic of associated ACL tear.[9] Vieira et al. in their anatomic study of 10 human cadavers described the presence of a distinct ligamentous structure in the capsular-osseous layer of the iliotibial tract and called it the ALL, probably the first time this terminology appears in literature.[10] Vincent et al. subsequently described it as a flat structure with histological evidence of a fibrous core surrounded by synovium in 40 knees (10 cadavers and 30 undergoing a total knee replacement).[11] It was the detailed dissection of 41 unpaired knees by Claes et al. that characterized the qualitative and quantitative anatomy of the ALL in no uncertain terms. They described the femoral origin of the ALL as being present anterior to the attachment of the lateral collateral ligament (LCL) on the prominence of the lateral epicondyle. Tibial attachment was about 6.5 mm distal to the cartilage margin and described as being broad and almost midway between the Gerdy's tubercle (GT) and fibular head (FH), with some fibers attaching to the middle third of the lateral meniscus (Fig. 30.1).[12] The dual insertion onto the lateral meniscus and anterolateral tibia was confirmed by Helito later.[13] Kennedy et al. in their cadaveric study to delineate the ALL described the femoral attachment to be located 4.7 mm posterior and proximal to the fibular

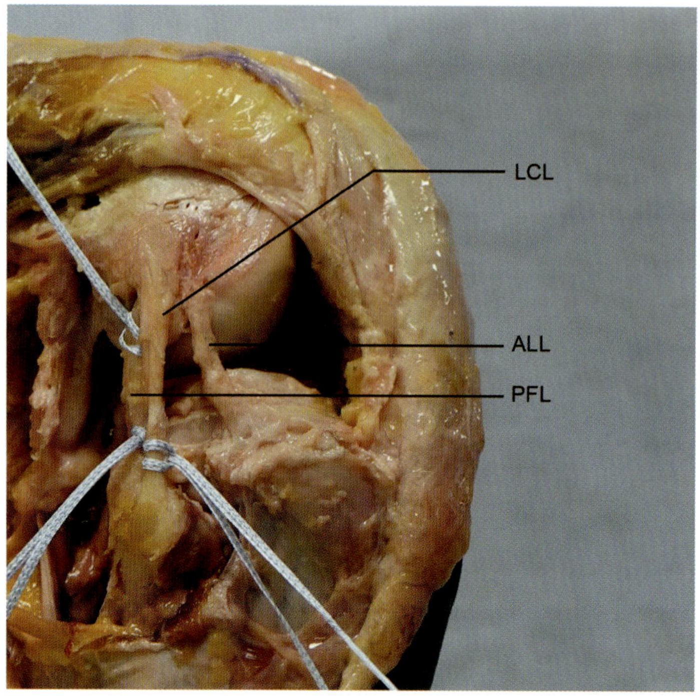

Fig. 30.1: Cadaveric dissection of the right knee seen from the lateral side. Note the ALL is attached on the femur in close proximity to the LCL and fans out distally at its tibial attachment.
(ALL: Anterolateral ligament; LCL: Lateral collateral ligament; PFL: Popliteofibular ligament).

collateral ligament attachment with an anterodistal course to its anterolateral tibial attachment, approximately midway between the center of the GT and the anterior margin of the FH, 13.1 mm distal to the lateral tibial plateau.[14] Daggett et al. described a detailed method of dissection to reliably locate the ALL. They described the femoral insertion as being slightly proximal and posterior to the lateral epicondyle. Distally, the insertion is in a fan-like fashion, with an anterior insertion just distal to the joint line and a posterior insertion slightly more distal, almost midway between the GT and FH and some fibers inserting onto the lateral meniscus.[15] There was quite some variation in the description of the ALL by various authors. To clarify this confusion, Helito published another cadaveric study where they described the ALL as having superficial and a deep layer. The superficial ALL presented a posterior and proximal origin to the center of the lateral epicondyle exhibiting no contact with the lateral meniscus. The deep ALL was located in the center of the lateral epicondyle and had a meniscal insertion. Both structures had a similar tibial insertion site; however, the insertion site of the deep ALL was located more posteriorly. The length of the superficial ALL increased on knee extension while the length of deep ALL increased on knee flexion.[16] Daggett et al. have also reported that the ALL is about two times thicker in males than females.[17]

Presence of the ALL and its injury on magnetic resonance imaging (MRI) scans have also been studied. The ALL can be visualized in routine 1.5-T MRI scans. Although some of the ligament could be depicted in nearly all of the scans (97.4%), it could only be observed in its entirety in about 71.7% of the tests with maximum visualization of the meniscal attachment followed by the femoral and tibial.[18] In another MRI study to assess ALL lesions with acute ACL injuries, the ALL could be visualized in

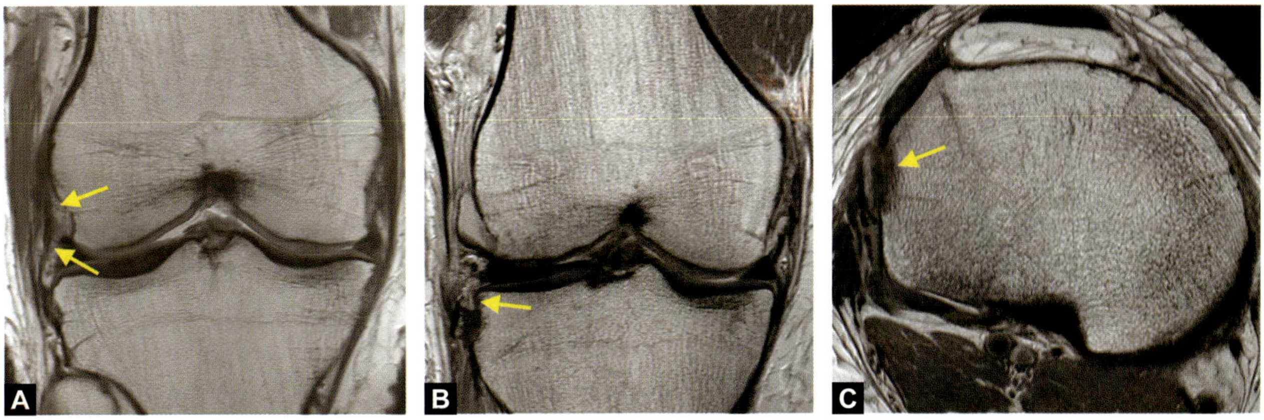

Figs. 30.2A to C: (A) Magnetic resonance imaging (MRI) scan showing the course of the anterolateral ligament in T2 weighted proton density (PD) coronal images. (B) A classical Segond's fracture or tibial avulsion of the anterolateral ligament as seen in T2 weighted PD coronal and (C) PD axial sections.

87.1% patients, a third of whom had injuries to this ligament. The most common site of injury was proximal (72%), while 21% showed distal lesions and 48% had abnormalities in the meniscal portion.[19] T2-weighted coronal sections with proton density fat-suppressed evaluation are the best for visualization of the ALL (Figs. 30.2A to C).[20] ACL injury history has also been reported to be associated with a higher incidence of sonographic abnormalities within the distal insertion of the anterolateral complex.[21]

In spite of the overwhelming evidence recently available, there are others who are still not convinced of the presence of the ALL. In their dissection of twenty one fetal knees, Sabzevari et al. could not prove the presence of a distinct capsular or extracapsular ligamentous structure in the anterolateral capsular complex area. Histological analysis also revealed a loose, hypocellular connective tissue with less organized collagen fibers compared with ligament and tendinous structures.[22] Guenther et al. found that the anterolateral capsule carries negligible forces in the longitudinal direction, and the forces transmitted between regions of the capsule were similar to the forces carried by the other structures at the knee, suggesting that it does not function as a traditional ligament. They believed that the anterolateral capsule should be considered a sheet of tissue as the force in the anterolateral capsule was significantly smaller than that in the other structures at all knee flexion angles for both loading conditions of anterior tibial load and internal tibial torque.[23]

What Role does the Anterolateral Ligament Play in Knee Joint Stability?

Those who believe that the ALL does indeed exist, attribute its key role in anterolateral stability of the knee. Monaco et al. analyzed the role of ACL and lateral capsular ligament in controlling knee stability using a navigation system. They found that cutting the PL bundle does not increase anterior translation and rotation, while cutting the anteromedial (AM) bundle significantly increased the anteroposterior (AP) translation at 30° and 60°, but does not increase rotation of the knee whereas cutting the lateral capsular ligament increased anterior translation at 60° ($p = 0.04$) and rotation at 30°, 45°, and 60°.[24] Parsons et al. assessed 11 cadaver knees which were subjected to 134 N of anterior drawer at flexion angles between 0° and 90° and separately to 5 Nm of internal rotation at the same flexion angles. They concluded that the ALL is an important stabilizer of internal rotation at flexion angles greater than 35° but not to anterior tibial translation at all flexion angles. The ACL on the other hand is the primary resister during anterior drawer at all flexion angles and during internal rotation at flexion angles less than 35°.[25] Sonnery-Cottet performed serial sectioning of ACL, ALL and iliotibial band (ITB) in one and in the reverse order in the contralateral cadaveric knee. Measurements of internal rotation at 20° and 90° of flexion and simulated pivot-shift test consisting of coupled axial rotation at 30° of flexion were collected using a surgical navigation system before and after each sectioning. They concluded that ALL is involved in rotational control of the knee at varying degrees of knee flexion and during a simulated pivot shift. Concomitant to an ACL or ITB transection, sectioning the ALL further increased rotational laxity.[26] Similarly, the study by Lutz et al. demonstrated two distinct anterolateral tissue planes that tightened during internal rotation of the tibia: a superficial plane represented by the iliotibial tract and the Kaplan fibers, which acts as a ligament structure, and a deep plane represented by a triangular capsular ligament complex within which the ALL and the anterolateral capsule are recruited.[27]

A contrary view was presented by Saiegh et al. who studied 14 cadaveric knees and recorded tibial translation and rotations using a navigation system. They found no changes in the magnitudes of translation or rotation after sectioning of the ALL compared to the ACL-deficient knee but concluded that it remains unclear whether injury to the ALL would result in substantial knee instability in the setting of ACL injury in vivo.[28] Stentz-Olesen also performed a cadaveric study on eight human knees to analyze the contribution of ALL in anterolateral laxity. They found that cutting the ALL in ACL-deficient knees increased the internal rotation at flexion angles of 0° (p = 0.04), 30° (p = 0.03) and 60° (p <0.01) by 1.0°, 1.6° and 2.5°, respectively. However, no decrease in laxity was found after reconstructing the ALL in ACL-reconstructed knees using a gracilis tendon autograft.[29] Noyes et al. studied rotational instability in 14 cadaveric ACL-deficient knees. They found with ACL sectioning, a positive pivot-shift anterior subluxation occurred even with intact ALL and ITB structures, indicating that these are not primary restraints but function together as anterolateral secondary restraints. With ACL deficiency, concurrent loss of the ALL and ITB resulted in conversion in a majority of knees (71%) to a Grade-3 pivot-shift subluxation, along with major increase of internal rotation in selected knees.[30]

The dilemma is that although cadaveric studies have made a very important contribution to our understanding of anatomy, their weakness lies in a difficulty in knowing whether extrapolating biomechanical findings from a laboratory study to the clinical scenario can be valid.[31] The consensus of ALL Expert was that the ALL acts as a restraint for internal rotation of the tibia and affects the pivot shift in the ACL-deficient knee. The mean stiffness is 31 N/mm and mean load to failure is about 180 N.[20]

Why Should the Anterolateral Ligament be Reconstructed?

The ALL provides restrain to anterolateral instability in ACL deficient knees. However, not all ACL injuries are associated with a pivot-shift phenomenon and display exaggerated anterior tibial translation only. Song et al. studied the correlation between pivot-shift test performed under anesthesia and prevalence of

ALL injury on MRI scans. They found that high-grade pivot-shift phenomenon showed higher prevalence of concomitant ALL injury compared to those with low-grade pivot-shift phenomenon after acute ACL injuries.[32] Some form of anterolateral reconstruction or tenodesis has been found to be effective in eliminating the high-grade pivot-shift phenomenon. For ACL injuries with high-grade pivot shift, lateral tenodesis performed along with ACL reconstruction (ACLR) provides a significant reduction in the prevalence of residual pivot shift but no differences in objective International Knee Documentation Committee (IKDC) scores and anterior knee stability compared with isolated ACLR at short-term follow-up has been found.[33] The same group performed a retrospective study to identify independent risk factors that were associated with grade 3 pivot shift in patients undergoing ACLRs using univariable and multivariable logistic regressions. The best set of predictors for a grade 3 pivot were pivoting sports involvement at the time of injury, abnormal lateral posterior-inferior tibial slope, anterolateral capsular ligament disruptions and combined lateral meniscal lesions. This provides firm guidelines for identifying and counseling patients at risk for residual laxity and graft rupture.[34]

A double-bundle ACLR has not been shown to be superior to a single bundle technique for controlling the pivot-shift phenomenon in cadaveric or clinical studies; both techniques provide similar knee kinematics and have similar graft failure rates.[35-37] Bonanzinga et al. showed in a cadaveric study that at 30° on knee flexion, single bundle ACLR with lateral plasty (SBLP) by the Marcacci technique allowed the greatest reduction of internal rotational laxity when compared to double-bundle reconstruction. With regards to the pivot-shift test, only SBLP procedure significantly decreased laxity considering the acceleration reached by the joint, when compared with the ACL + ALL deficient state when tested using a navigation system.[38,39] Sonnery-Cottet evaluated 83 patients who underwent a combined ACL and minimally invasive ALL reconstruction after a minimum of 2 years. Preoperatively 41 patients had a grade 1, 23 patients had a grade 2, and 19 patients had a grade 3 pivot shift according to the IKDC criteria which was eliminated in 76 patients while it was grade 1 is 7 patients after the reconstruction.[40]

Return to sports and graft rupture rates are important outcome measures of ACL surgery. A systematic review and meta-analysis reported that only 55% patients return to competitive sports following ACLR.[41] Lai et al. reviewed return to sports amongst elite athletes and found this rate to be 83% with 5.2% rate of graft rupture.[42] Sonnery-Cottet et al. reported the minimum 2-year outcomes of the Scientific ACL NeTwork International (SANTI) Study Group. Survivorship data from Kaplan-Meier analysis were analyzed in multivariate Cox regression models to identify the prognosticators of graft ruptures and return to sport following ACLR. They found that in a high-risk population of young patients participating in pivoting sports, the rate of graft failure following combined ACLR with hamstring tendon (HT) and ALL reconstruction was 2.5 times less than ACLR with bone-patella tendon-bone (BPTB) grafts and 3.1 times less than ACLR with 4HT grafts. The HT + ALL graft was also associated with greater odds of returning to preinjury levels of sport when compared with the 4HT graft but not compared with the BPTB grafts.[43] This is the largest study of combined ACL with ALL reconstruction reported till date and has encouraging results.

A decision algorithm as to who are the candidates for a concomitant ACL and ALL reconstruction has been provided by the ALL Expert Group in a consensus paper.[20] There are three decision-making points:

(1) *patient history* (revision surgery or contralateral ACL tear), (2) *clinical examination and imaging* (for assessment of laxity or Segond fracture or a deep lateral femoral notch sign), and (3) *patient profile* (age, hyperlaxity, and participation in pivoting sports). They described "decisive" and "secondary" criteria and recommended performance of a minimally invasive ALL reconstruction in patients who met at least one decisive and two secondary criteria (Fig. 30.3).

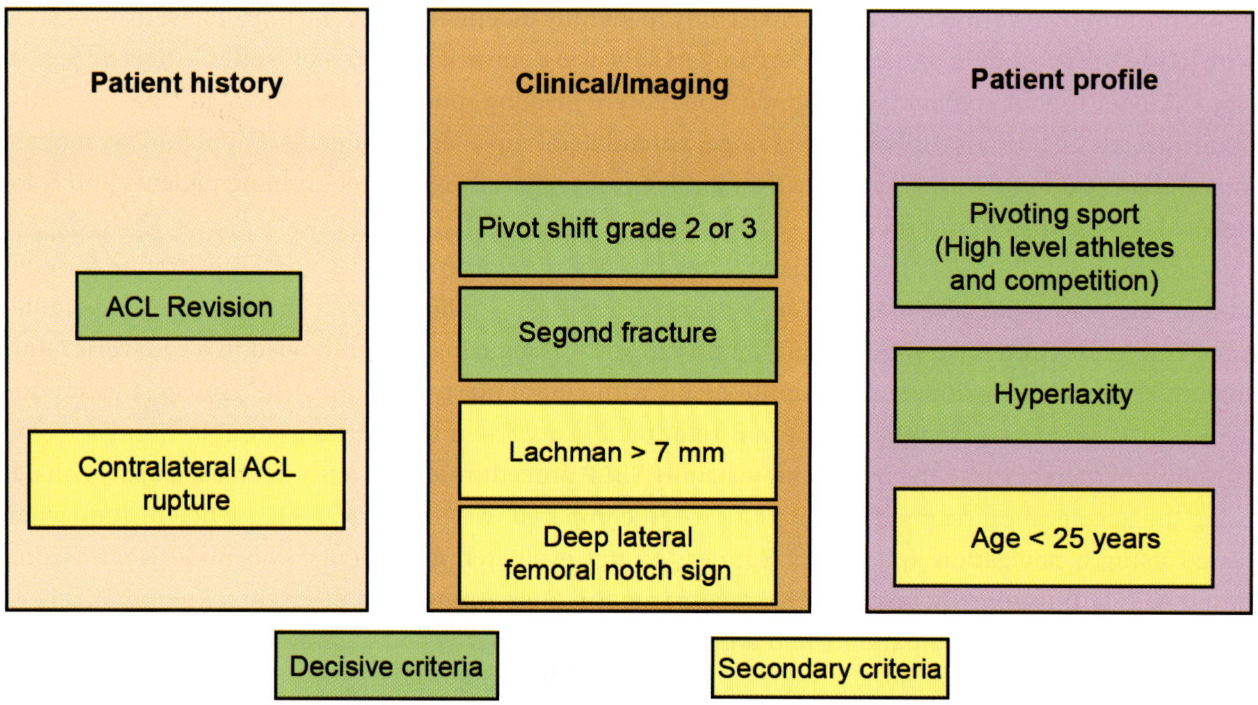

Fig. 30.3: Decision algorithm for performing a minimally invasive ALL reconstruction concomitant with ACL reconstruction. *Source:* Adapted from Sonnery-Cottet B, Daggett M, Fayard JM, et al. Anterolateral Ligament Expert Group consensus paper on the management of internal rotation and instability of the anterior cruciate ligament—deficient knee. J Orthop Traumatol. 2017;doi:10.1007/s10195-017-0449-8.

SURGICAL TECHNIQUE

The principles of performing an ALL reconstruction are as follows:

- Replication of anatomy
- Replication of isometry
- Respect of soft tissues
- Optimal graft tensioning and fixation.

We employ a minimally invasive technique of ALL reconstruction which is similar to the technique described by Sonnery-Cottet et al.[44,45] We would like to stress that compliance with the principles is more critical than minor variations of technique.

Setup and Preparation

The patient is positioned supine on a flat table and high thigh tourniquet is applied. A side support is place to support the proximal thigh while a foot support is fixed on the table to stabilize the foot in 90° of flexion. Prior to skin preparation, an examination under anesthesia is mandatory to assess the laxity by performing a Lachman, anterior drawer and pivot-shift tests. Skin is prepared and draped in a sterile fashion. Prior to embarking on a diagnostic arthroscopy, the following landmarks are drawn on the skin: lateral femoral epicondyle, fibula head, GT, joint line, and tibial tuberosity (Fig. 30.4). In obese patients, delineation of these landmarks maybe difficult and one would rather confirm them using an image intensifier or forego the plan to perform a minimally-invasive reconstruction.

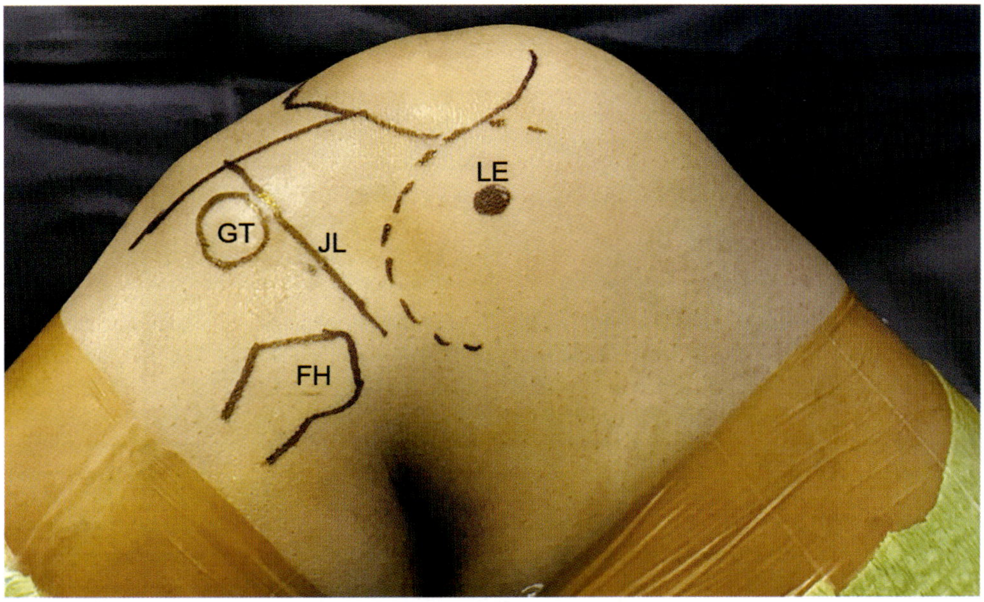

Fig. 30.4: Surface marking of important landmarks in performing an ALL reconstruction of the left knee. (LE: Lateral femoral epicondyle; GT: Gerdy's tubercle; FH: Fibula head; JL: Joint line).

A standard anatomic ACLR is then performed. This can be done using a semitendinosus graft using the all-inside technique or a bone-patella tendon-bone or central quadriceps tendon graft. In a revision scenario where the ipsilateral hamstring tendons are not available or when the same side medial collateral injury has been conservatively managed and hamstring harvest is not desirable, one may opt either for an allograft or to harvest the contralateral hamstring tendons. We have observed that in primary cases without concomitant hyperlaxity, a meniscus ramp lesion or lateral meniscus posterior root avulsion is present with the ACL tear and subsequent to repair of this injury, the pivot shift disappears.

After the ACL is reconstructed and other intra-articular pathologies are managed, we proceed with the ALL reconstruction. We perform this procedure using a gracilis autograft or an allograft, as a single loop of gracilis tendon has a strength of 838 N, which is adequate for the maximal load requirement for the ALL of 175 N.[46] The graft is placed in an inverted V layout to replicate the anatomy of the native ALL with a femoral insertion proximal and posterior to the lateral epicondyle and a fan-shaped broad tibial insertion between the GT and FH.[14,17]

Isometry Testing

The next step is identification of points where the sockets would need to be created. An incision is made slightly proximal and posterior to the lateral epicondyle and the ITB in cut-in line with the incision. A 2.4 mm drill-tip passing pin (Smith & Nephew, Andover, MA) is drilled starting at a point just proximal and posterior to the lateral epicondyle and directed superior-anterior to emerge out of the skin on the medial side.

The second incision is made at the center of the GT and FH. Blunt dissection is carried out to reach the bone. The second 2.4 mm drill-tip passing pin is drilled starting at a point midway between the center of GT and tip of FH, about 7–10 mm distal to the joint line and directed medially. A third 2.4 mm drill-tip passing pin is drilled at the superolateral margin of the GT and directed medially. Hence, we have three pins in position now (Fig. 30.5).

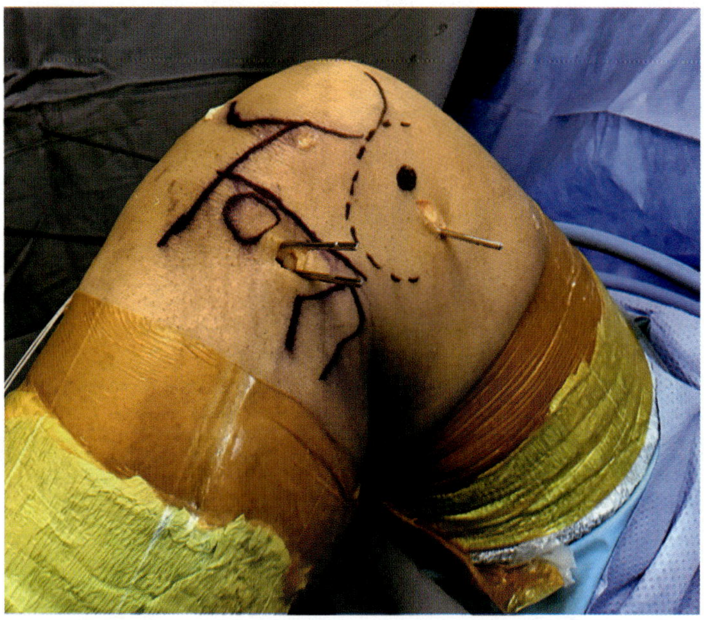

Fig. 30.5: Incision on the femur is placed proximal and posterior to the lateral epicondyle and the passing pin is drilled. Incision on the tibia is centered between the Gerdy's tubercle and fibular head and two passing pins are drilled.

Testing of the isometry of this configuration is done next. The ALL is taught in extension and slackens in flexion beyond 90°. The proximal-posterior to lateral epicondyle position on the femur has been shown to replicate the isometry of the ALL.[47-50] Ideally, an ALL reconstruction should control internal tibial rotation at around 20° of flexion without limitation of range of motion (ROM) during flexion and internal tibial rotation at 90°.[48] A long suture is wound around the femoral and tibial pins in full extension and clamped distally to maintain maximum tension in extension. The knee is then flexed to about 100–120°. It must be observed that the suture slackens when the knee flexes beyond 90°, which is similar to the isometric behavior of the ALL (Figs. 30.6A and B). If this does not happen or the suture tightens in flexion, the femoral pin position is wrong and must be readjusted till this phenomenon is observed. The distance between the femoral pin and each tibial pin is measured to prepare the graft.

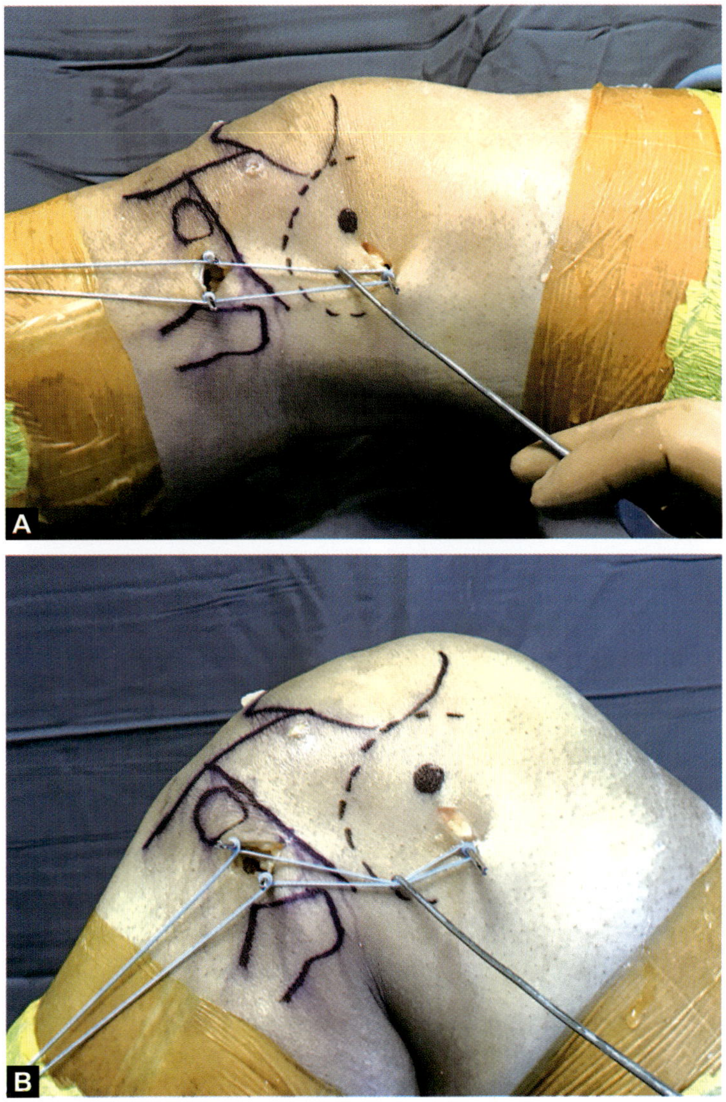

Figs. 30.6A and B: Isometry testing is done by passing a suture around the femoral and tibial pins. (A) The suture must be taut in extension. (B) Slackens when the knee is flexed to about 100°.

Graft Preparation

The free gracilis graft is doubled and marked at 23 mm at the loop end which would go into the femoral socket. This end is then whip-stitched using a FiberLoop® (Arthrex, Naples, FL) or #2 FiberWire® (Arthrex, Naples, FL) for a distance of 23 mm. Stitching this end prevents graft slippage within the socket and use of a high-strength suture material prevents graft laceration during fixation. The two free ends of the graft are measured from the distal end of first mark for a distance equal to the distance between the femur and tibial pins in full extension plus 23 mm and cut. These ends are then whip stitched in a similar manner for a distance of 23 mm. Hence we get a V-shaped graft which has been stitched at all the three corners (Figs. 30.7A to D). The prepared graft is then sized to prepare sockets of suitable diameter at all the three sites (Figs. 30.8A to C). One end of gracilis graft is usually thinner and this would be used in the anterior tibial socket.

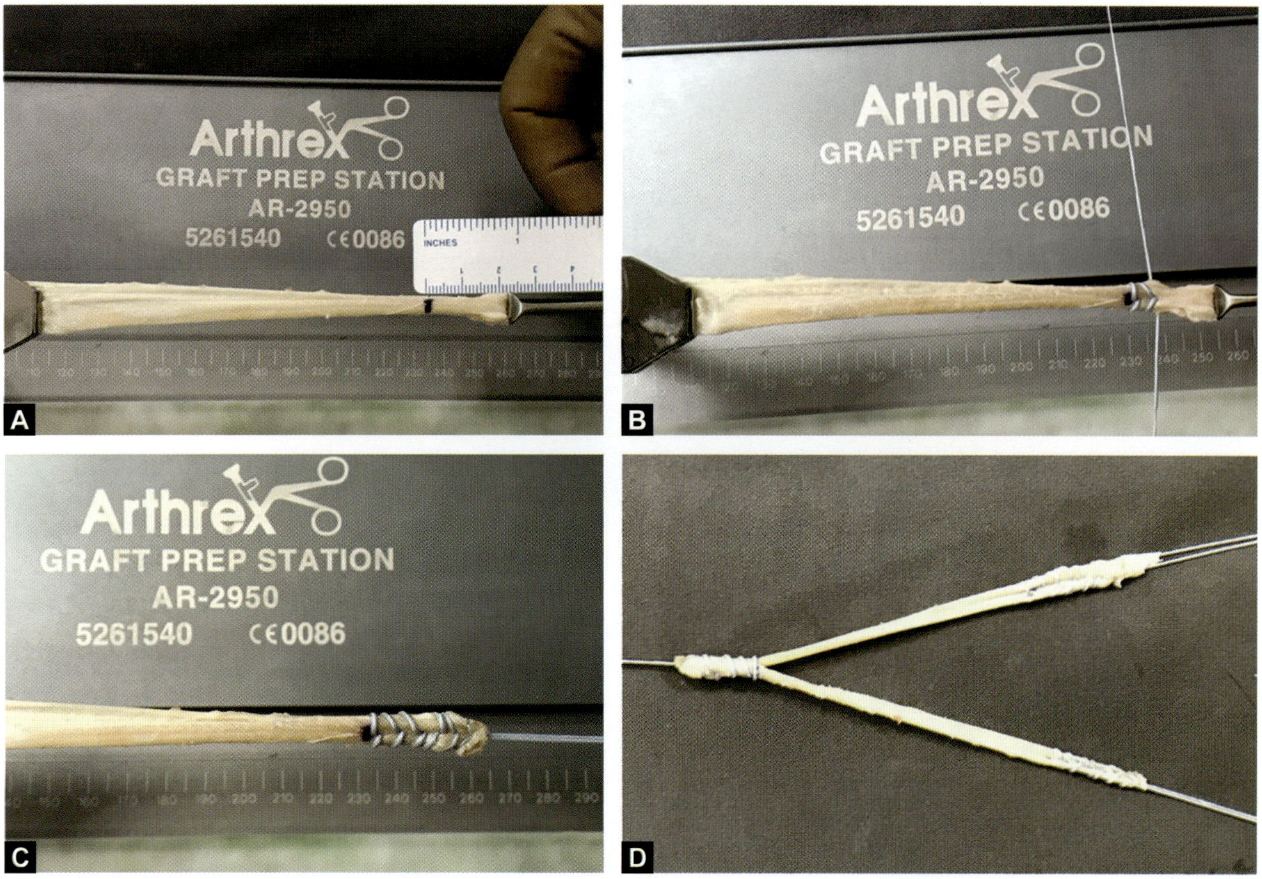

Figs. 30.7A to D: (A) Preparation for a gracilis graft is started by marking the looped end at 23 mm. (B and C) This end is stitched first using a FiberLoop® for a distance of 23 mm. (D) The two free ends are subsequently whip stitched using #2 FiberWire® to obtain a V-shaped graft construct with sutures at each end.

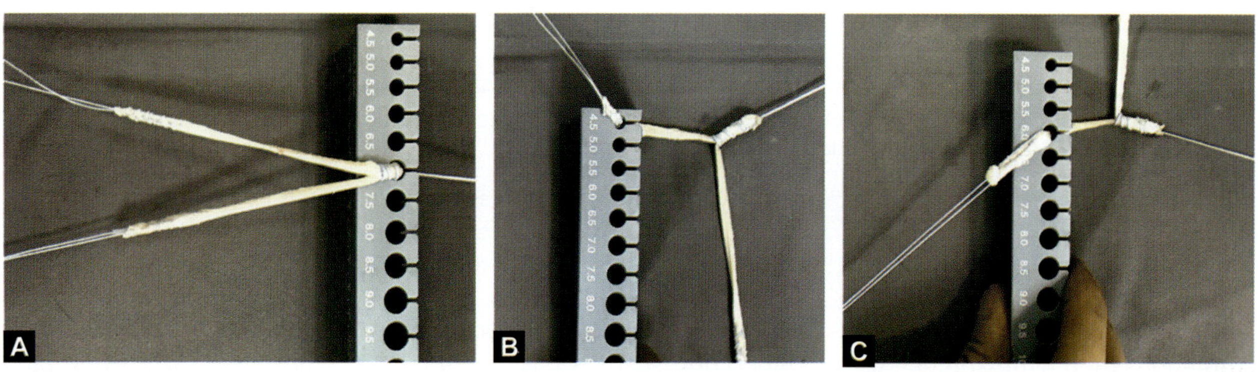

Figs. 30.8A to C: Sizing of the looped end and both free ends of the graft is done to prepare appropriate size sockets for graft placement.

Preparation of Graft Sockets

A 4.5 mm ENDOBUTTON™ drill bit (Smith & Nephew, Andover, MA) is used to drill both the cortices over the passing pins. This step facilitates suture passage and fixation later. The femoral socket is created first using an appropriate size Low Profile Reamer® (Arthrex, Naples,

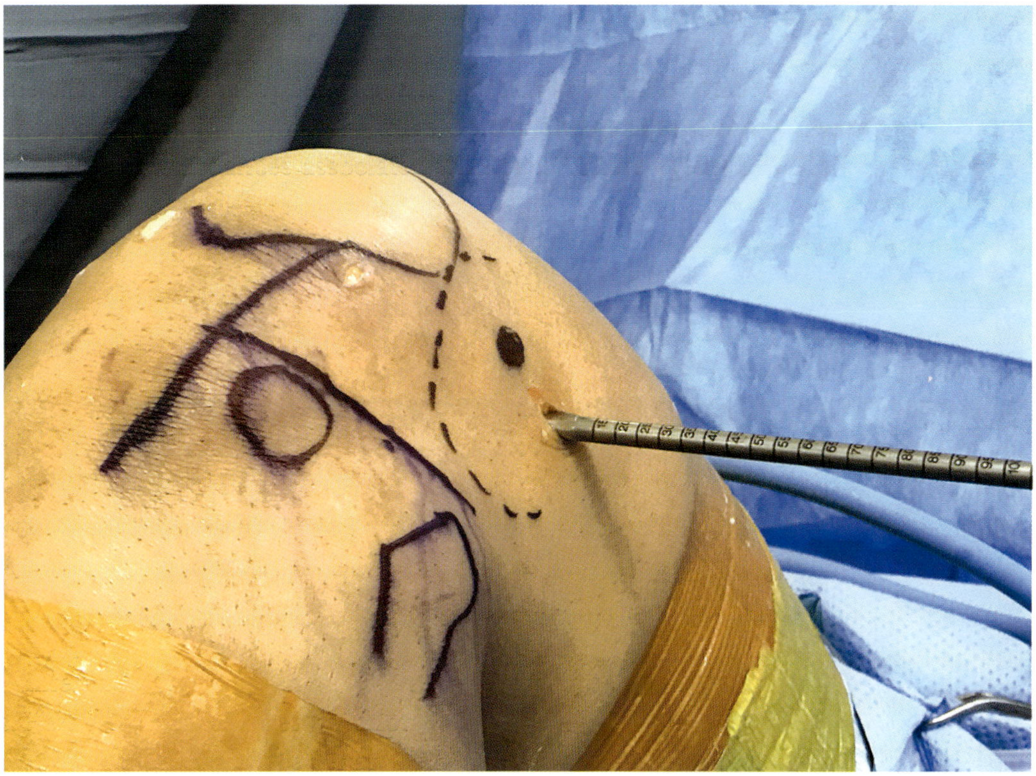

Fig. 30.9: Sockets are created using Low Profile Reamer® over the passing pin at all the three sites.

FL) over the passing pin (Fig. 30.9). Usually this is 7 mm in diameter. A socket of 25–28 mm is created. The anterior and posterior tibial sockets are similarly created using Low-Profile Reamer® (Arthrex, Naples, FL) over the passing pins for a depth of 25 mm. An arthroscopic curette is then used to clear the orifice of all the sockets of bone debris, which can cause graft abrasion and difficulty in passage.

Graft Passage and Fixation

An arthroscopic tissue grasper or hemostatic forceps is inserted from the proximal incision, passed deep to the ITB to emerge in the distal incision. The sutures of the looped end of the graft if held and pulled in so that the graft is positioned deep to the ITB. Care must be taken that the two distal tails are not twisted around each other and the thinner one lies anteriorly. Femoral side fixation is performed first. The suture ends are passed into the eyelet of the passing pin and a guide wire for BioComposite™ Interference screw (Arthrex, Naples, FL) is inserted into the socket. The guide is pulled out from the medial side and the sutures which emerge are then pulled to insert the graft into the socket till the marked end. Fixation is performed with a 23 mm BioComposite™ Interference screw (Arthrex, Naples, FL) of the same diameter as the socket, usually 7 mm (Figs. 30.10A to D).

The knee is brought in full extension. Sutures of the two ends distally are fed into the eyelets of the passing pins, screw guide wires inserted and then passing pins pulled out medially one by one. The sutures for the anterior and posterior graft ends are pulled medially and good tension in the graft in extension is confirmed using a hook probe. An assistant maintains the knee in full extension and neutral rotation while the second assistant pulls both the ends of the graft sutures in maximum tension. Tibial fixation is performed

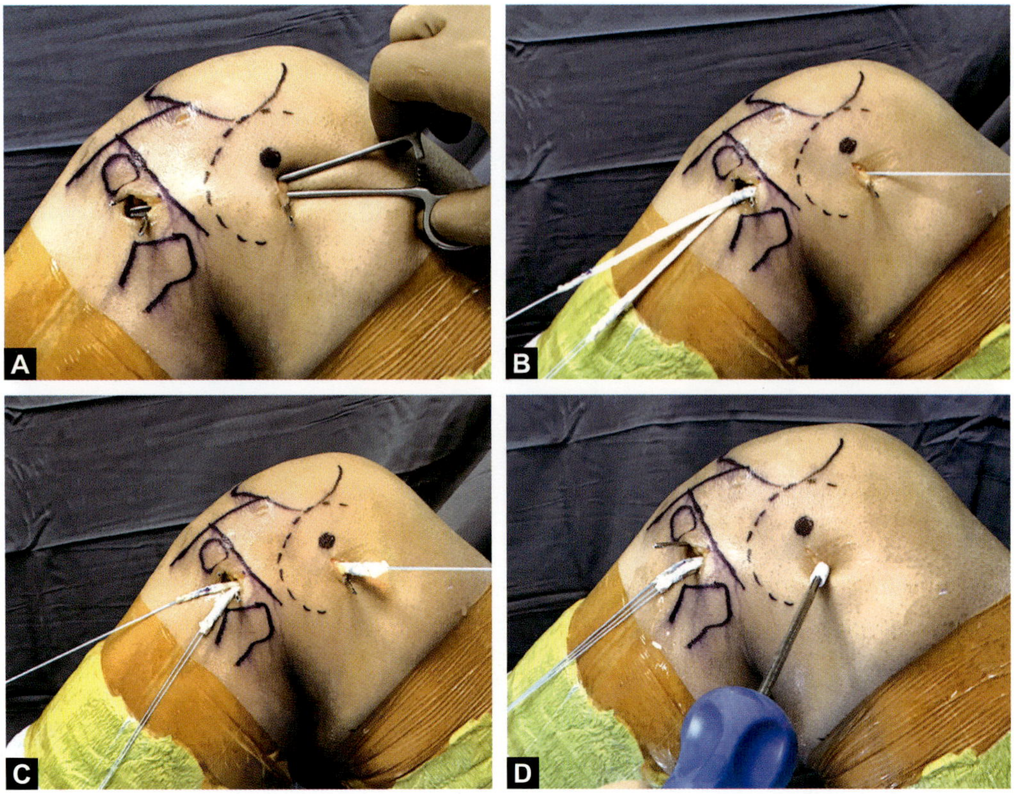

Figs. 30.10A to D: (A) A hemostat forceps is passed from the femoral incision, deep to the iliotibial band to emerge at the tibial incision. (B and C) The graft is pulled in and comes to lie extracapsular but deep to the iliotibial band. (D) Fixation of the femoral side is performed after the graft is inserted into the socket using a BioComposite® Interference screw.

using 23 mm BioComposite™ Interference screws (Arthrex, Naples, FL) of the same diameter as the sockets, usually 6 mm (Figs. 30.11A and B).

Pivot shift test is performed to confirm the stability of the reconstruction. ITB is sutured in the proximal incision and wound closure is performed in layers in the standard fashion.

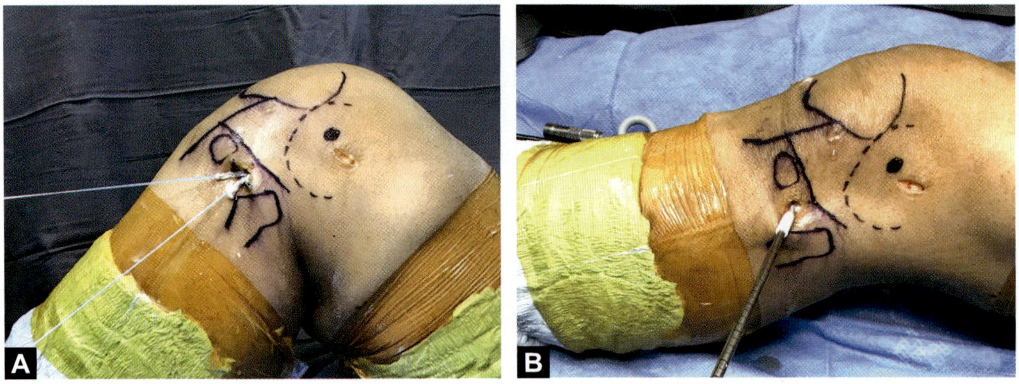

Figs. 30.11A and B: The graft ends on the tibial side are inserted into their respective sockets and fixation is performed with the knee in full extension and neutral rotation.

Rehabilitation

The rehabilitation protocol following an ACLR with ALL reconstruction is no different than that after a single-bundle anatomic ACLR. No restrictions of knee ROM or weight bearing apply. Protection in a brace in full extension for three weeks and subsequently in a hinge brace (FormFit® Knee ROM Brace, Össur, Reykjavik, Iceland) for 3 months is followed. Return to sport is between 6 months and 9 months, based on periodic assessment and fitness for the same.

PEARLS AND PITFALLS

- Recognition of the landmarks for graft fixation is crucial. In obese individuals where these cannot be palpated, one must not hesitate to take the aid of an image-intensifier rather than create non-anatomic tunnels.
- Testing of isometry must be done before socket creation. Sutures tied around passing pins should be tight in extension and loose in flexion beyond 90°.
- Utilizing an inverted V graft layout replicates the anatomy of the native ALL with a femoral insertion proximal and posterior to the lateral epicondyle and a fan-shaped broad tibial insertion between the GT and FH.
- Single looped gracilis graft provides good strength to the reconstruction.
- Precise graft measurement before and sizing after preparation allows a reconstruction in optimal tension and avoids problems in graft passage.
- The graft must be tunneled deep to the ITB and this must be sutured later.
- Graft fixation must be done in full extension and neutral rotation.

CONCLUSION

While the debate about the ALL rages on in scientific literature, one needs to objectively look at the controversy. While the jury is still out, some have emphasized that this phenomenon is similar to the controversy surrounding the medial patellofemoral ligament in the past.[20] We believe that ALL reconstruction definitely has a role in management of anterolateral instability of the knee. A minimally invasive technique preserves the integrity of the ITB which is an important anterolateral stabilizer, unlike a lateral extra-articular tenodesis procedure of some kind (*detailed in Chapter 29 "Lateral Extra-articular Tenodesis"*). Adherence to principles of ALL reconstruction is critical to the success of this procedure. Long-term follow-up studies will shape the future of this surgery even as new knowledge continues to improve our understanding of enigma of the pivot shift. The surgical skill sets required for this technique are very similar to those utilized during a soft tissue collateral ligament reconstruction. Hence, simplicity of this technique allows for easy reproducibility.

Acknowledgment

The authors are grateful to Dr Anupama Patil, Musculoskeletal Radiologist, Star Imaging and Research Center, Pune for providing the MRI images.

REFERENCES

1. Rahnemai-Azar AA, Sabzevari S, Irarrazaval S, et al. Restoring nature through individualized anatomic anterior cruciate ligament reconstruction surgery. Arch Bone Jt Surg. 2016;4:289-90.
2. Sonnery-Cottet B. Single or double bundle? In: Bonnin M, Amendola A, Bellemans J, et al. The Knee Joint. Paris: Springer Nature; 2012. pp. 227-34.
3. Ferretti M, Levicoff EA, Macpherson TA, et al. The fetal anterior cruciate ligament: an anatomic and histologic study. Arthroscopy. 2007;23:278-83.

4. Irarrázaval S, Albers M, Chao T, et al. Gross, arthroscopic, and radiographic anatomies of the anterior cruciate ligament: foundations for anterior cruciate ligament surgery. Clin Sports Med. 2017;36:9-23.
5. Siebold R. Flat ACL anatomy: fact no fiction. Knee Surg Sports Traumatol Arthrosc. 2015;23:3133-5.
6. Śmigielski R, Zdanowicz U, Drwięga M, et al. Ribbon like appearance of the midsubstance fibres of the anterior cruciate ligament close to its femoral insertion site: a cadaveric study including 111 knees. Knee Surg Sports Traumatol Arthrosc. 2015;23:3143-50.
7. Musahl V, Getgood A, Neyret P, et al. Contributions of the anterolateral complex and the anterolateral ligament to rotatory knee stability in the setting of ACL Injury: a roundtable discussion. Knee Surg Sports Traumatol Arthrosc. 2017;doi: 10.1007/s00167-017-4436-7.
8. Segond P. Recherches cliniques et expe´rimentales sur les e´panchements sanguins du genou par entorse. Prog Med. 1879;7:297-341.
9. Goldman AB, Pavlov H, Rubenstein D. The Segond fracture of the proximal tibia: a small avulsion that reflects major ligamentous damage. AJR Am J Roentgenol. 1988;151:1163-7.
10. Vieira EL, Vieira EÁ, da Silva RT, et al. An anatomic study of the iliotibial tract. Arthroscopy. 2007;23:269-74.
11. Vincent JP, Magnussen RA, Gezmez F, et al. The anterolateral ligament of the human knee: an anatomic and histologic study. Knee Surg Sports Traumatol Arthrosc. 2012;20:147-52.
12. Claes S, Vereecke E, Maes M, et al. Anatomy of the anterolateral ligament of the knee. J Anat. 2013;223:321-8.
13. Helito CP, Demange MK, Bonadio MB, et al. Radiographic landmarks for locating the femoral origin and tibial insertion of the knee anterolateral ligament. Am J Sports Med. 2014;42:2356-62.
14. Kennedy MI, Claes S, Fuso FA, et al. The anterolateral ligament: an anatomic, radiographic, and biomechanical analysis. Am J Sports Med. 2015;43:1606-15.
15. Daggett M, Busch K, Sonnery-Cottet B. Surgical dissection of the anterolateral ligament. Arthrosc Tech. 2016;5:e185-8.
16. Helito CP, do Amaral C Jr, Nakamichi YD, et al. Why do authors differ with regard to the femoral and meniscal anatomic parameters of the knee anterolateral ligament?: Dissection by layers and a description of its superficial and deep layers. Orthop J Sports Med. 2016;4:2325967116675604.
17. Daggett M, Helito C, Cullen M, et al. The anterolateral ligament: an anatomic study on sex-based differences. Orthop J Sports Med. 2017;5:2325967116689387.
18. Helito CP, Helito PV, Costa HP, et al. MRI evaluation of the anterolateral ligament of the knee: assessment in routine 1.5-T scans. Skeletal Radiol. 2014;43:1421-7.
19. Helito CP, Helito PV, Costa HP, et al. Assessment of the anterolateral ligament of the knee by magnetic resonance imaging in acute injuries of the anterior cruciate ligament. Arthroscopy. 2017;33:140-6.
20. Sonnery-Cottet B, Daggett M, Fayard JM, et al. Anterolateral ligament expert group consensus paper on the management of internal rotation and instability of the anterior cruciate ligament—deficient knee. J Orthop Traumatol. 2017;doi: 10.1007/s10195-017-0449-8.
21. Yoshida M, Herbst E, Albers M, et al. The anterolateral complex in anterior cruciate ligament deficient knees demonstrate sonographic abnormalities on high-resolution sonography. Knee Surg Sports Traumatol Arthrosc. 2017.
22. Sabzevari S, Rahnemai-Azar AA, Albers M, et al. Anatomic and histological investigation of the anterolateral capsular complex in the fetal knee. Am J Sports Med. 2017:363546517692534.
23. Guenther D, Rahnemai-Azar AA, Bell KM, et al. The anterolateral capsule of the knee behaves like a sheet of fibrous tissue. Am J Sports Med. 2017;45:849-55.
24. Monaco E, Ferretti A, Labianca L, et al. Navigated knee kinematics after cutting of the ACL and its secondary restraint. Knee Surg Sports Traumatol Arthrosc. 2011;20:870-7.
25. Parsons EM, Gee AO, Spiekerman C, et al. The biomechanical function of the anterolateral ligament of the knee. Am J Sports Med. 2015;43:669-74.
26. Sonnery-Cottet B, Lutz C, Daggett M, et al. The involvement of the anterolateral ligament in rotational control of the knee. Am J Sports Med. 2016;44:1209-14.

27. Lutz C, Sonnery-Cottet B, Niglis L, et al. Behavior of the anterolateral structures of the knee during internal rotation. Orthop Traumatol Surg Res. 2015;101:523-8.
28. Saiegh YA, Suero EM, Guenther D, et al. Sectioning the anterolateral ligament did not increase tibiofemoral translation or rotation in an ACL-deficient cadaveric model. Knee Surg Sports Traumatol Arthrosc. 2015.
29. Stentz-Olesen K, Nielsen ET, de Raedt S, et al. Reconstructing the anterolateral ligament does not decrease rotational knee laxity in ACL-reconstructed knees. Knee Surg Sports Traumatol Arthrosc. 2017;doi: 10.1007/s00167-017-4500-3.
30. Noyes FR, Huser LE, Levy MS. Rotational knee instability in ACL-deficient knees: role of the anterolateral ligament and iliotibial band as defined by tibiofemoral compartment translations and rotations. J Bone Joint Surg Am. 2017;99: 305-14.
31. Sonnery-Cottet B. Editorial Commentary: studying the anterolateral ligament of the knee-have we lost track of our main focus? Arthroscopy. 2017;33:605-7.
32. Song GY, Zhang H, Wu G, et al. Patients with high-grade pivot-shift phenomenon are associated with higher prevalence of anterolateral ligament injury after acute anterior cruciate ligament injuries. Knee Surg Sports Traumatol Arthrosc. 2017:doi: 10.1007/s00167-017-4492-z.
33. Song GY, Hong L, Zhang H, et al. Clinical outcomes of combined lateral extra-articular tenodesis and intra-articular anterior cruciate ligament reconstruction in addressing high-grade pivot-shift phenomenon. Arthroscopy. 2016;32: 898-905.
34. Song GY, Zhang H, Wang QQ, et al. Risk factors associated with grade 3 pivot shift after acute anterior cruciate ligament injuries. Am J Sports Med. 2016;44:362-9.
35. Liu Y, Cui G, Yan H, et al. Comparison between single- and double-bundle anterior cruciate ligament reconstruction with 6- to 8-stranded hamstring autograft: a prospective, randomized clinical trial. Am J Sports Med. 2016;44:2314-22.
36. Herbort M, Domnick C, Raschke MJ, et al. Comparison of knee kinematics after single-bundle anterior cruciate ligament reconstruction via the medial portal technique with a central femoral tunnel and an eccentric femoral tunnel and after anatomic double-bundle reconstruction. Am J Sports Med. 2016;44:126-32.
37. Song EK, Seon JK, Yim JH, et al. Progression of osteoarthritis after double- and single-bundle anterior cruciate ligament reconstruction. Am J Sports Med. 2013;41:2340-6.
38. Marcacci M, Zaffagnini S, Iacono F, et al. Arthroscopic intra- and extra-articular anterior cruciate ligament reconstruction with gracilis and semitendinosus tendons. Knee Surg Sports Traumatol Arthrosc. 1998;6:68-75.
39. Bonanzinga T, Signorelli C, Grassi A, et al. Kinematics of ACL and anterolateral ligament. Part II: anterolateral and anterior cruciate ligament reconstruction. Knee Surg Sports Traumatol Arthrosc. 2017;doi: 10.1007/s00167-017-4496-8.
40. Sonnery-Cottet B, Thaunat M, Freychet B, et al. Outcome of a combined anterior cruciate ligament and anterolateral ligament reconstruction technique with a minimum 2-year follow-up. Am J Sports Med. 2015;43:1598-605.
41. Ardern CL, Taylor NF, Feller JA, et al. Fifty-five per cent return to competitive sport following anterior cruciate ligament reconstruction surgery: an updated systematic review and meta-analysis including aspects of physical functioning and contextual factors. Br J Sports Med. 2014;48:1543-52.
42. Lai CCH, Ardern CL, Feller JA, et al. Eighty-three per cent of elite athletes return to preinjury sport after anterior cruciate ligament reconstruction: a systematic review with meta-analysis of return to sport rates, graft rupture rates and performance outcomes. Br J Sports Med. 2017:bjsports-2016-096836.
43. Sonnery-Cottet B, Saithna A, Cavalier M, et al. Anterolateral ligament reconstruction is associated with significantly reduced ACL graft rupture rates at a minimum follow-up of 2 years. Am J Sports Med. 2017:036354651668605.
44. Sonnery-Cottet B, Barbosa NC, Tuteja S, et al. Minimally invasive anterolateral ligament reconstruction in the setting of anterior cruciate ligament injury. Arthrosc Tech. 2016;5:e211-5.
45. Sonnery-Cottet B, Daggett M, Helito CP, et al. Combined anterior cruciate ligament and anterolateral ligament reconstruction. Arthrosc Tech. 2016;5:e1253-9.

46. Sonnery-Cottet B, Archbold P, Rezende FC, et al. Arthroscopic identification of the anterolateral ligament of the knee. Arthrosc Tech. 2014;3:e389-92.
47. Wieser K, Fürnstahl P, Carrillo F, et al. Assessment of the isometry of the anterolateral ligament in a 3-dimensional weight-bearing computed tomography simulation. Arthroscopy. 2017;pii: S0749-8063(16)30910-0. doi: 10.1016/j.arthro.2016.11.005.
48. Imbert P, Lutz C, Daggett M, et al. Isometric characteristics of the anterolateral ligament of the knee: a cadaveric navigation study. Arthroscopy. 2016;32:2017-24.
49. Kittl C, Halewood C, Stephen JM, et al. Length change patterns in the lateral extra-articular structures of the knee and related reconstructions. Am J Sports Med. 2015;43:354-62.
50. Dodds AL, Halewood C, Gupte CM, et al. The anterolateral ligament: Anatomy, length changes and association with the Segond fracture. Bone Joint J. 2014;96-B:325-31.

CHAPTER

31 Double Bundle Anterior Cruciate Ligament Reconstruction

Deepak Chaudhary, Deepak Joshi, Ankit Goyal

INTRODUCTION

Anterior cruciate ligament (ACL) reconstruction is one of the most common procedures performed by orthopedic surgeons, with approximately 100,000 such procedures being performed per year in the United States alone.[1] With the current trend of participation in organized sports at a younger age, this number will continue to increase.[2] Because of its high prevalence of injury, the ACL continues to be intensively studied, and outcomes of ACL surgery receive considerable attention. Traditional ACL reconstruction techniques have focused on reconstruction of one portion of the ACL—the anteromedial (AM) bundle. Single-bundle ACL reconstruction is the criterion standard and has provided good to excellent results, with many athletes being able to return to sports.[3,4] However, recently, other authors have noted persistent instability with functional testing and degenerative radiographic changes after single-bundle ACL reconstruction.[5-10] As a result, many surgeons have attempted to improve upon the single-bundle technique by reconstructing both the AM and posterolateral (PL) bundles of the ACL, the so-called anatomic double-bundle ACL reconstruction technique.

The earliest published discussions of double-bundle ACL reconstruction are from the 1980s. However, by the time Mott[11] published his surgical technique of a "double-bundle" reconstruction in 1983, he had been using the technique for 5 years. As this was a surgical technique only, he did not include follow-up, treatment group descriptions, or outcome measures. His reconstruction described using a semitendinosus autograft through two tunnels in both the femur and tibia. Soon after, Zaricznyj[12] published a similar technique, using two tibial tunnels and one femoral tunnel. He followed 14 patients for 2 years and noted that 12 of the 14 patients scored good-excellent by the Hospital for Special Surgery (HSS) knee score. Zaricznyj also noted that none of the patients had a pivot shift following reconstruction, but three knees had a 1+ anterior drawer test. No mention was made of whether these patients were able to resume their previous activity levels or their previous occupations. Several years after these published techniques, Radford and Amis reported their biomechanical assessment of double- versus single-bundle reconstruction. In this study, the investigators tested the flexion stability of six ACL intact cadaveric knees at both 20° and 90°. The native ACL was then removed, and testing was repeated with an over-the-top reconstruction method simulating the AM bundle, and then a trans-lateral femoral-condyle reconstruction simulating the posteromedial (PM) bundle. A double-bundle construct was also simulated by the combination of the two. Of note, the reconstructed bundles were synthetic, created with polyester tape instead of biological components. The grafts were tensioned according to the investigators' estimation of the laxity of the native ACL before sectioning. They reported that the AM bundle simulation stabilized best at 90° of flexion, and the PM bundle simulation stabilized best at 20° of flexion. The addition of both bundles replicated the stability of the native knee before disruption of the native ACL. They concluded that double-bundle reconstruction most closely reproduced the stability of a native knee.

ANATOMY

Anterior cruciate ligament consists of two distinct anatomic bundles, AM and PL. The size and length of each bundle are also unique. In addition, throughout the normal range of motion, a complex relation exists between the two bundles. In extension, the two bundles are oriented in parallel to the sagittal plane; however, as the knee is flexed, the PL bundle becomes crossed with respect to the AM bundle. Furthermore, other authors have attempted to replicate this twisting pattern simply by twisting the ACL graft 90° before fixation.[13-15]

Anteromedial bundle has isometric behavior. Anteromedial bundle tightens in flexion while the PL bundle relaxes in flexion. Anteromedial bundle limits anterior translation of the tibia on the femur with the knee in flexion and its absence may produce anterolateral (AL) instability.[13-15]

Posterolateral bundle provides more rotational control than AM bundle and is taut in full extension. The digitized origin and insertion of the AM and PL bundles occupies approximately 50% of the total femoral origin, with cross-sectional areas of 47 ± 13 mm^2 and 49 ± 13 mm^2 for the AM and PL bundles, respectively.[16,17]

AUTHORS' EXPERIENCE AND TECHNIQUE

Patient Selection

Inclusion criteria are primary ACL reconstruction with no combined posterior cruciate ligament injury, lateral collateral ligament injury, PL rotary instability or fracture around knee. All cases with previous knee ligament surgery, arthritic changes, subtotal or total meniscectomy, malalignment and articular cartilage lesions exceeding grade III and patients with open physis are excluded.

SURGICAL TECHNIQUE

Setup and Portal Establishment

All patients are operated under spinal anesthesia. Examination under anesthesia is done prior to the commencement of surgical procedure and tourniquet is used in all cases. Patient is made to lie supine with the knee hanging by the side of the table with a thigh support. A diagnostic arthroscopy is performed through the standard anterolateral and AM portals and the tear of ACL is confirmed and concomitant meniscal injuries are managed. Arthroscopic scale or any measurement device is inserted to measure tibial and femur footprints. Minimal length of stump should be 14 millimeter. We take minimum graft diameter for AM bundle as 7 mm and for PL bundle as 6 mm with 2 mm distance between the two bundles; it makes a total of 15 mm.

Graft Harvest

Semitendinosus and gracilis tendon are harvested using a vertical 3 cm incision on the AM aspect of the upper tibia and stripped of muscle fibers. The semitendinosus (for the AM bundle) is doubled and gracilis tendon (for the PL bundle) is doubled. The ends of tendons are stitched with No 5 Ethibond® (Ethicon Inc.) suture using a whip stitch technique and the grafts were pre-tensioned on a graft board. The prepared average doubled semitendinosus tendon graft for the AM bundle is usually 7 mm in diameter and prepared doubled gracilis tendon for the PL bundle is usually 6 mm in diameter. At times the diameter of PL is less than 6 mm. In this situation, we reinforce the graft with FiberTape® (Arthrex, Naples, FL). If AM bundle graft is less than 7 mm then it is tripled or reinforced with FiberTape®.

Preparation of Tunnels

The soft tissue remnants of the ACL are identified on the tibia and the femur as a guide for the insertion sites of AM and PL bundles. The tibial and femoral footprints of both AM and PL bundles were carefully defined. PL bundle inserts on posterolateral half of the stump and AM on the anteromedial half (Fig. 31.1). When the remnants of the ACL were not visualized, the bony landmarks (lateral intercondylar ridge and lateral bifurcate ridge) are visualized to delineate the attachment on the femoral side (Fig. 31.2). Tibial guide is used for making the tibial tunnels. The PL tibial tunnel is drilled first with the jig set at 65° at the center of PL bundle footprint with the knee at 90° flexion. The AM tibial tunnel is drilled next with the jig set at 55° about 1 cm anterior and medial to the PL tibial tunnel at the center of the footprint of AM bundle. AM tibial tunnel is then reamed according to the graft size of the bundle. *The PL bundle is not reamed as it avoids the saline outflow and thus maintains the pressure inside the joint.* Both tunnels are blocked with a tunnel plug to prevent saline outflow. *The tibial tunnels, since they are being drilled at different angles are divergent and thus, even if they meet at the mouth of the tunnels in the joint, it does not hamper aperture fixation at tibia.* The AM

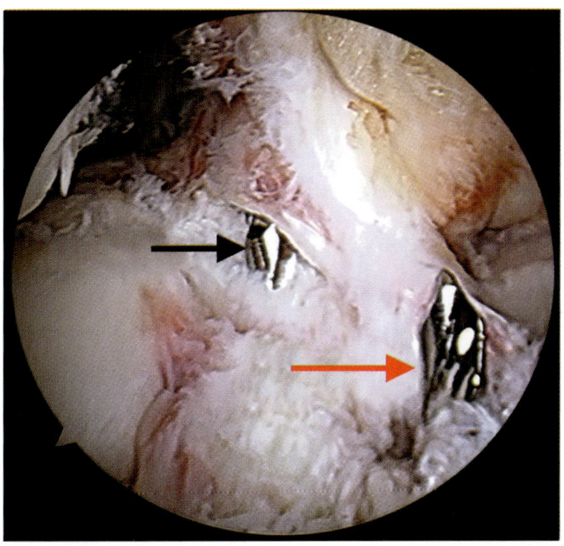

Fig. 31.1: Tibial ACL footprints AM (red arrow) and PL (black arrow).
(ACL: Anterior cruciate ligament; AM: Anteromedial; PL: Posterolateral).

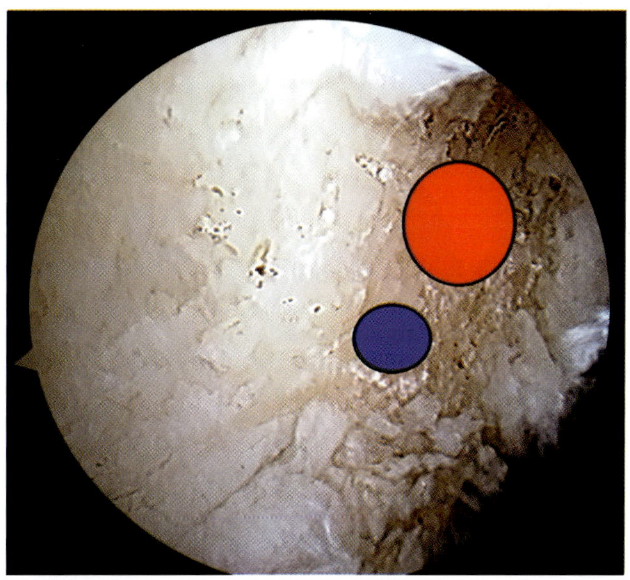

Fig. 31.2: Lateral femoral wall with resident ridge anteromedial (AM) (red circle) and posterolateral (PL) (blue circle).

femoral tunnel is drilled next using the transtibial 6 mm femoral offset through the AM portal with the knee in 90° flexion (Fig. 31.3). By using an offset for reaming the femoral tunnels, we are able to drill the tunnel at the exact position on the condyle at the ACL footprint so that there is no blowout of the posterior wall. The tunnel is drilled at the previous AM femoral footprint leaving at least 2 mm of posterior wall intact (Figs. 31.4 and 31.5). The length of the AM femoral tunnel is kept between 20 mm and 25 mm. For the PL bundle, femoral tunnel is made with knee in hyperflexion, using 5 mm transtibial femoral offset at PL footprint with a drill bit via AM portal and brought out through the skin (Fig. 31.6). By using this offset we are able to make the PL tunnel lower and anterior on the lateral femoral condyle and also avoid confluence of tunnels. PL femoral

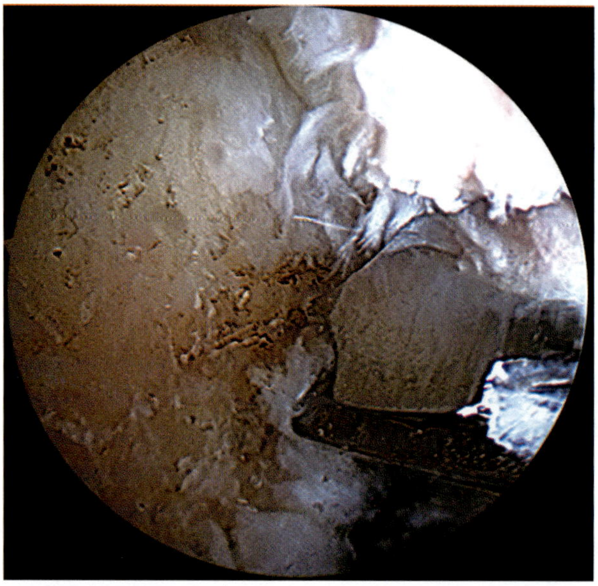
Fig. 31.3: Anteromedial (AM) femoral tunnel with 6 mm offset.

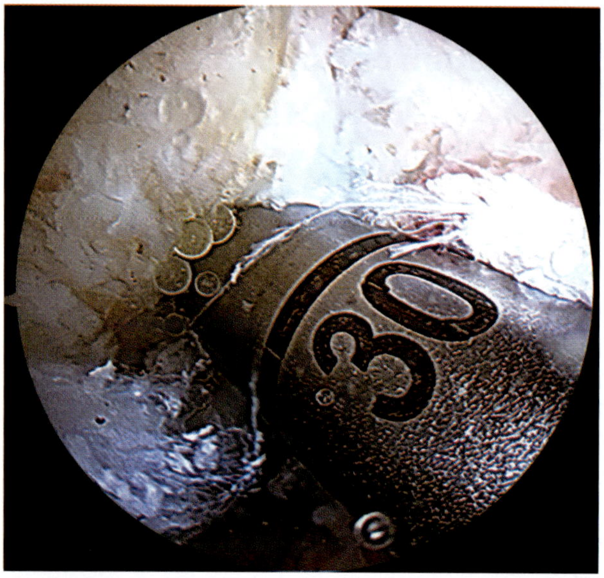
Fig. 31.4: Reaming of the femoral tunnel as per tunnel size.

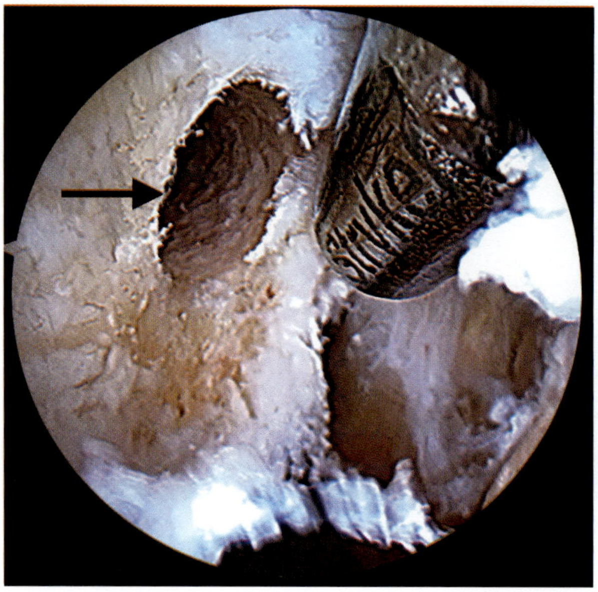
Fig. 31.5: Anteromedial (AM) femoral tunnel (black arrow).

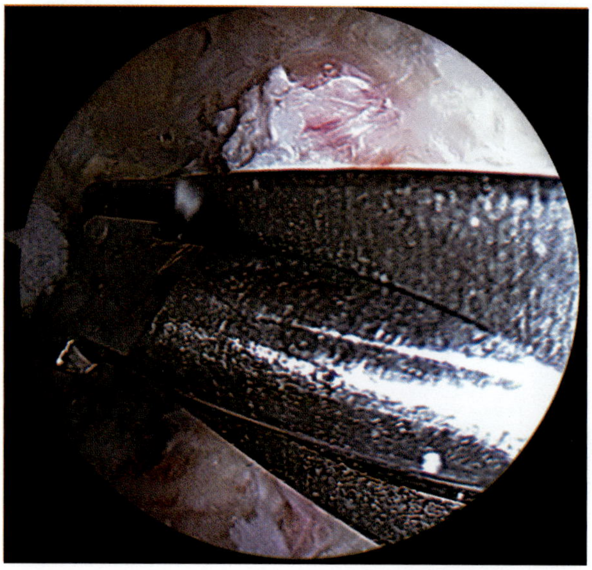
Fig. 31.6: Posterolateral (PL) femoral tunnel with 5 mm offset.

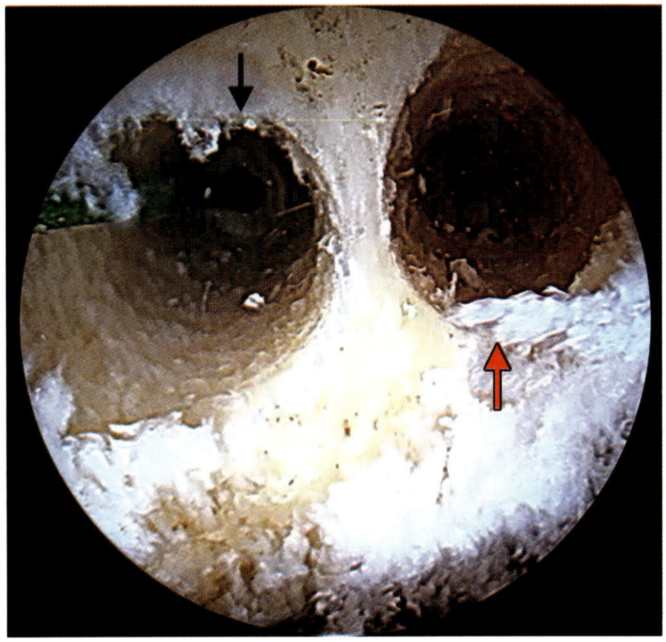

Fig. 31.7: Anteromedial (AM) (red arrow) and posterolateral (PL) (black arrow) femoral tunnels.

tunnel is subsequently reamed according to graft size up to 15–25 mm with a reamer. This helps us in keeping 2 mm wall intact (Fig. 31.7). By hyperflexing, the posterior portion of lateral condyle comes anteriorly and thus the tunnel drilled in anterior and lower as compared to AM.

Graft Passage and Fixation

The gracilis graft for the PL bundle is first railroaded through the AM portal into the femoral tunnel and fixed at the femoral side using a suspensory fixation device (TightRope® RT, Arthrex). AM bundle graft is then passed and fixed on the femoral side using another suspensory fixation device (TightRope® RT, Arthrex) (Fig. 31.8). The knee is then cycled several times through the range of motion and the PL graft

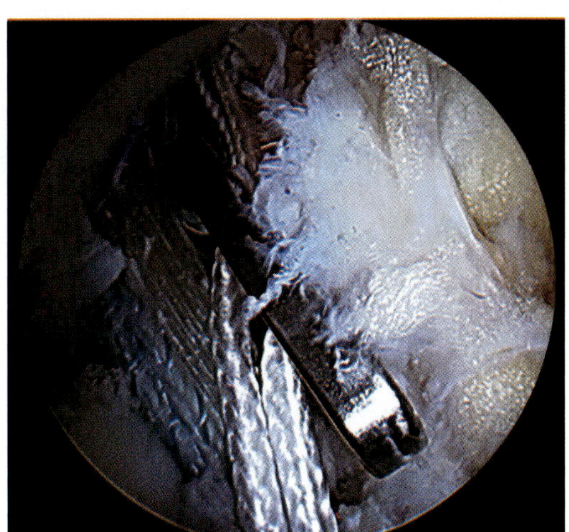

Fig. 31.8: Railroading of anteromedial (AM) graft.

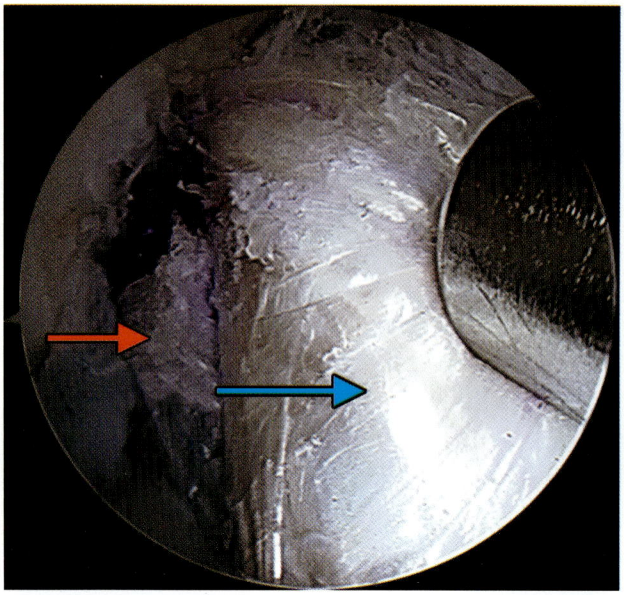

Fig. 31.9: Final double-bundle ACL AM (blue arrow) and PL (red arrow).
(ACL: Anterior cruciate ligament; AM: Anteromedial; PL: Posterolateral.

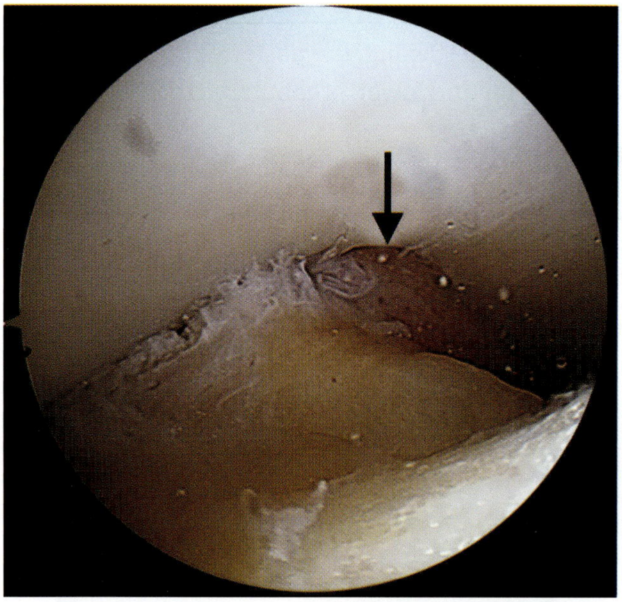

Fig. 31.10: Knee checked in extension to check notch impingement (black arrow).

is fixed on the tibial side at 0–15° of knee flexion whereas AM graft is fixed at 45° of knee flexion using biointerference screw (Fig. 31.9). The graft is assessed for any impingement in full extension and if present, notchplasty is done (Fig. 31.10).

At the end of reaming of tunnels there is 2 mm bony wall between two tunnels. It covers the entire stump of ACL and one can appreciate different tension in the grafts of two bundles at different flexion angles through range of motion.

Rehabilitation

Ice packs and static quadriceps exercises along with ankle pumps were started on the day of surgery. Patients were allowed weight bearing within the limits of pain with the help of crutches from the first post-operative day. A long leg knee extension immobilizer was kept for the next 2 weeks.

PEARLS AND PITFALLS

Graft Harvesting
- All the bands attached to the semitendinosus and gracilis graft should be cut before harvesting the graft.
- In case of slippage of the graft we can harvest the graft by giving a small incision on the PM portion of the thigh. This can be done with the help of arthroscope which is put through the graft harvesting site.
- Small sized grafts: Triple/augment with FiberTape® to minimum graft size of 7 mm/6 mm.

Portal Establishment
- Anteromedial portal should be made directly under vision with the help of 18-G spinal needle.
- The 11 No blade should always be tied with vicryl to avoid its breakage in the joint.

Drilling of Tunnels
- The PL tibial tunnel should be drilled first just at the level of PCL. Care should be taken to avoid lateral meniscal root or PCL injury while drilling. A shaver wash cannula or a curette should be kept at the tip of the drill pin while reaming to avoid such injury.
- Anteromedial tibial tunnel should be drilled in reference of the PL bundle. After drilling it, one should extend the knee before reaming to check for notch impingement. Also care should be taken to avoid anterior blowout.
- Anteromedial femoral tunnel is drilled with the help of an offset keeping minimum of 2 mm of posterior wall with minimum length of the tunnel being 30–35 mm. If there is a posterior blowout of the tunnel one should revise it by either making the tunnel a little higher than the previous tunnel or hyperflexing the knee.
- Posterolateral tunnel should be drilled last with the help of an offset. One should keep at least 2 mm wall between the two tunnels. If there is confluence of the two tunnels, it should be revised by changing the flexion of the knee.

Graft Passage and Fixation
- The same knee flexion angles should be kept which passing the graft as they were during drilling it.
- A notcher can be used while doing tibial screw fixation to avoid graft damage.

TAKE HOME MESSAGE

The double-bundle ACL technique performed at the Sports Injury Centre, Safdarjung Hospital, New Delhi, currently takes into account four fundamental principles. As implied already, the first and most important is the anatomy. The ACL is composed of two functional bundles, the AM bundle and the PL bundle. The AM bundle primarily controls anteroposterior stability, and the PL bundle primarily functions to control rotation. The second principle is the replication of the native ACL insertion site anatomy to restore normal kinematics of the knee. The third principle, which is line with the second principle, is to restore the tension of each bundle. The PL bundle tightens in extension and loosens in flexion whereas AM bundle is relatively taut throughout the range of motion of the knee. The fourth principle is to individualize ACL surgery to each patient. At the end, we may say that there may be a thousand ways to reconstruct ACL but by reconstructing two bundles we are relatively closer to anatomy. A long-term follow-up of 15–20 years is required to see if these patients do better than single bundle. However in large knees and patients involved in contact sports, double-bundle reconstruction has shown better results.

REFERENCES

1. Griffin LY, Agel J, Albohm MJ, et al. Noncontact anterior cruciate ligament injuries: risk factors and prevention strategies. J Am Acad Orthop Surg. 2000;8(3):141-50.
2. Stern HP, Bradley RH, Prince MT, et al. Young children in recreational sports: participation motivation. Clin Pediatr. 1990;29(2):89-94.
3. Cooley VJ, Deffner KT, Rosenberg TD. Quadrupled semitendinosus anterior cruciate ligament reconstruction: 5-year results in patients without meniscus loss. Arthroscopy. 2001;17(8):795-800.
4. Freedman K, D'amato M, Nedeff D, et al. Arthroscopic anterior cruciate ligament reconstruction: a metaanalysis comparing patellar tendon and hamstring tendon autografts. Am J Sports Med. 2003;31(1):2-11.
5. Jarvela T, Paakkala T, Kannus P, et al. The incidence of patellofemoral osteoarthritis and associated findings 7 years after anterior cruciate ligament reconstruction with a bone-patellar tendon-bone autograft. Am J Sports Med. 2001;29(1):18-24.
6. Ristanis S, Giakas G, Papageorgiou CD, et al. The effects of anterior cruciate ligament reconstruction on tibial rotation during pivoting after descending stairs. Knee Surg Sports Traumatol Arthrosc. 2003;11(6):360-5.
7. Tashman S, Collon D, Anderson K, et al. Abnormal rotational knee motion during running after anterior cruciate ligament reconstruction. Am J Sports Med. 2004;32(4):975-83.
8. Ristanis S, Stergiou N, Patras K, et al. Excessive tibial rotation during high-demand activities is not restored by anterior cruciate ligament reconstruction. Arthroscopy. 2005;21(11):1323-9.
9. Fithian DC. Prospective trial of a treatment algorithm for the management of the anterior cruciate ligament-injured knee. Am J Sports Med. 2005;33(3):335-46.
10. Roe J, Pinczewski LA, Russell VJ, et al. A 7-year follow-up of patellar tendon and hamstring tendon grafts for arthroscopic anterior cruciate ligament reconstruction: differences and similarities. Am J Sports Med. 2005;33(9):1337-45.
11. Mott HW. Semitendinosus anatomic reconstruction for cruciate ligament insufficiency. Clin Orthop Relat Res. 1983;172:90-2.
12. Zaricznyj B. Reconstruction of the anterior cruciate ligament of the knee using a doubled tendon graft. Clin Orthop Relat Res. 1987;220:162-75.
13. Mochizuki T, Muneta T, Nagase T, et al. Cadaveric knee observation study for describing anatomic femoral tunnel placement for two-bundle anterior cruciate ligament reconstruction. Arthroscopy. 2006;22(4):356-61.
14. Amis AA, Jakob RP. Anterior cruciate ligament graft positioning, tensioning and twisting. Knee Surg Sports Traumatol Arthrosc. 1998;6(1):S2-S12.
15. Diduch DR, Mann J, Geary SP, et al. The effect of pretwisting the ACL autograft on knee laxity. Am J Knee Surg. 1998;11(1):15-9.
16. Harner CD, Baek GH, Vogrin TM, et al. Quantitative analysis of human cruciate ligament insertions. Arthroscopy. 1999;15(7):741-9.
17. Takahashi M, Doi M, Abe M, et al. Anatomical study of the femoral and tibial insertions of the anteromedial and posterolateral bundles of human anterior cruciate ligament. Am J Sports Med. 2005;34(5):787-92.

CHAPTER 32

Anterior Cruciate Ligament Reconstruction Bone Tunnel Placement Using Intraoperative Fluoroscopy

Thomas Harlem, Eivind Inderhaug, Charles H Brown Jr

INTRODUCTION

Intraoperative fluoroscopy offers the knee surgeon a simple, noninvasive, cost-effective, accurate and reproducible method to achieve anatomic bone tunnel placement when performing an anterior cruciate ligament (ACL) reconstruction.[1-8] Image intensifiers are routinely available in most operating rooms so this method requires no additional equipment costs. Use of intraoperative fluoroscopy can provide real time, accurate and reproducible results and can help the surgeon decrease variability in the placement of the ACL bone tunnels (Figs. 32.1A and B).[6,7] Furthermore, this method allows the surgeon to objectively measure and document where the ACL bone tunnels are being placed during surgery. The immediate objective

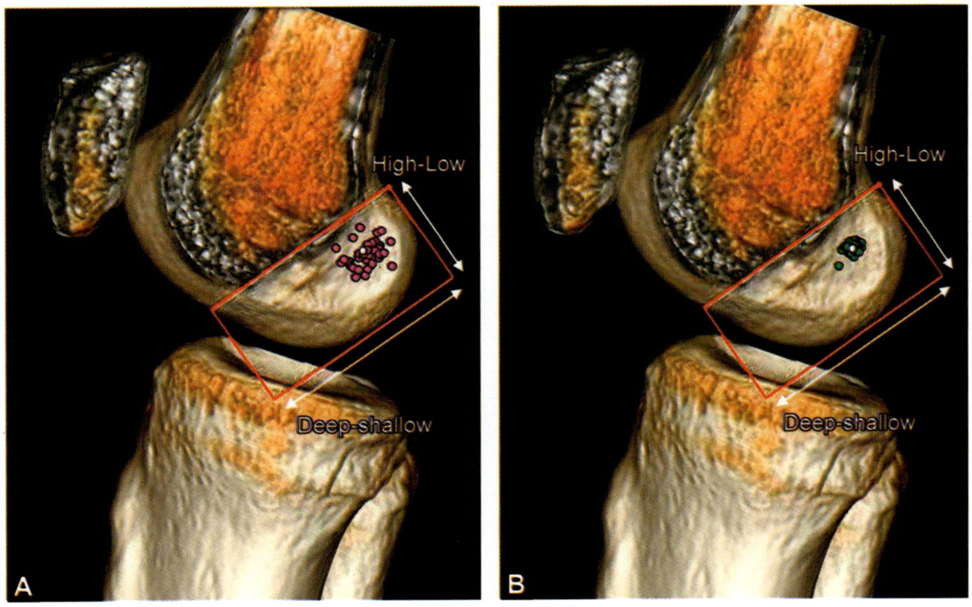

Figs. 32.1A and B: Anterior cruciate ligament (ACL) femoral tunnel position evaluated by postoperative 3D computed tomography (CT) scan. (A) ACL femoral tunnel placements for the last 50 ACL reconstructions performed by a single experienced knee surgeon before using intraoperative fluoroscopy to check the ACL femoral tunnel position. The white data point represents the weighted average position based on data from published radiographic anatomic studies of the ACL femoral attachment site.[9-25] (B) ACL femoral tunnel placements for the first 50 ACL reconstructions performed by the same surgeon after using intraoperative fluoroscopy to check the ACL femoral tunnel position. The use of intraoperative fluoroscopy resulted in more consistent placement of the ACL femoral tunnel. The ACL femoral tunnel positions are centered around the radiographic weighted average center position.[9-25]

feedback given to the surgeon allows unacceptable ACL bone tunnel positions to be detected and changed during the procedure. Intraoperative fluoroscopy is particularly useful during revision ACL surgery where it is often the case that the native ACL footprint has been removed and the bony anatomy of the ACL attachment sites has been altered by the previous ACL bone tunnels, notchplasty or bone grafting of the original bone tunnels. In the revision situation, fluoroscopy can be used to guide placement of new anatomic femoral and tibial bone tunnels based on preoperative radiographs or lateral computed tomography (CT) scans using published radiographic anatomy data of the native ACL attachment sites (Figs. 32.2A to E).[9-31] Fluoroscopy is also extremely useful when performing an augmentation technique for a partial ACL tear or a remnant sparing technique. In these situations, the native ACL footprint and the bony ACL anatomy cannot be used to guide placement of the ACL bone tunnels since exposing these anatomic landmarks would require resection of the intact ACL fibers. Using fluoroscopy, anatomic placement of the ACL bone

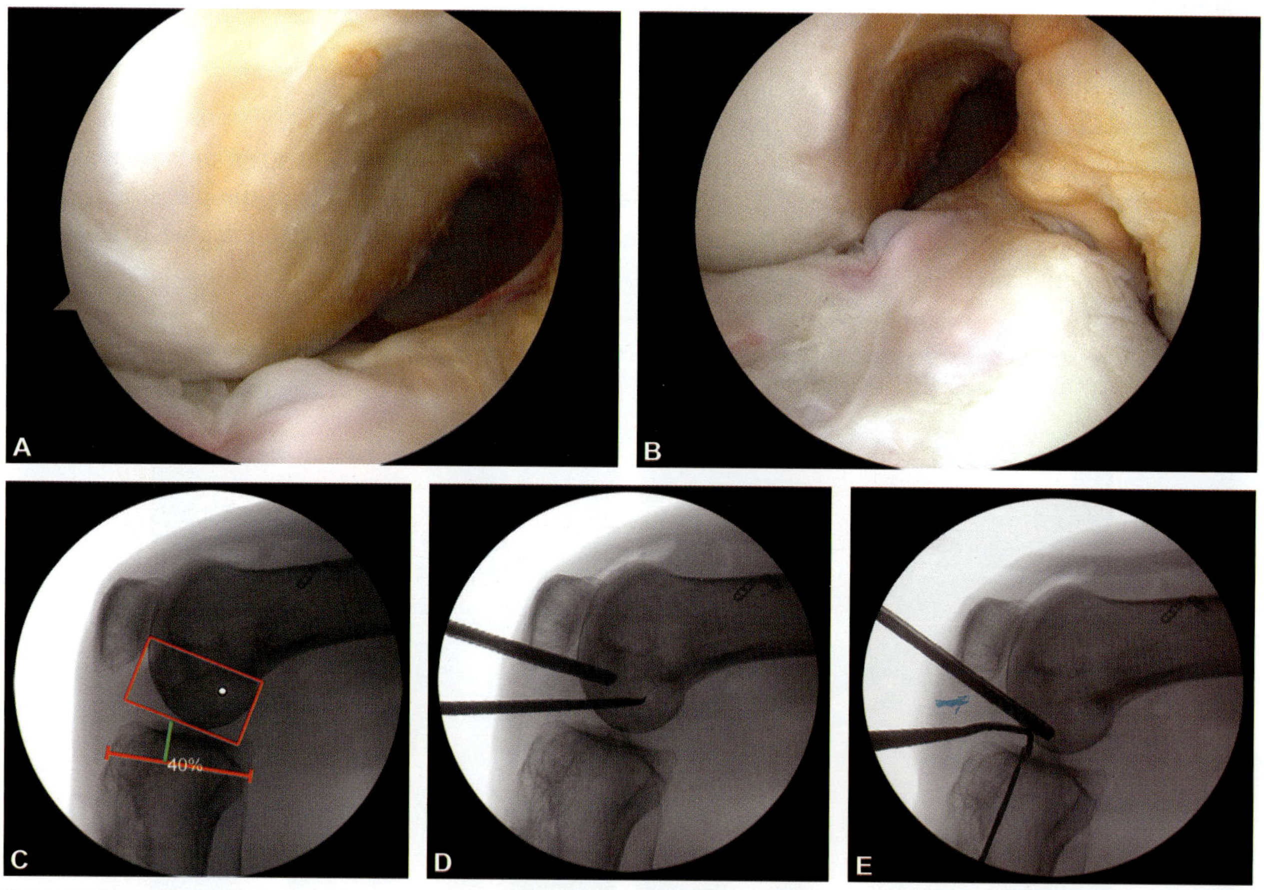

Figs. 32.2A to E: (A) 2-stage revision anterior cruciate ligament (ACL) reconstruction. Anteromedial portal view at 90°. The bony and soft tissue landmarks have been removed by bone grafting of the original ACL femoral and tibial tunnels, resulting in a "naked" lateral wall of the intercondylar notch. (B) Bony and soft tissue landmarks for the ACL tibial attachment site have been removed by bone grafting of the original tibial tunnel. (C) Preoperative planning of new anatomic ACL femoral and tibial tunnels. The white circle represents the weighted average center position of the ACL femoral attachment based on published radiographic studies of the native ACL femoral attachment site.[9-25] The green line is positioned at 40% along the Amis-Jakob line, which is the weighted average location of the center of the ACL tibial attachment site based on radiographic studies of the native ACL tibial attachment site.[12,13,18,27,29] (D) Intraoperative fluoroscopic image. The tip of the microfracture awl is located at the center of the preoperatively planned ACL femoral tunnel. (E) The tip of the tibial aimer and guide pin are located at the position of the preoperatively planned ACL tibial tunnel.

tunnels can be accomplished without the need to resect intact ACL fibers (Figs. 32.3A to H). Potential disadvantages of fluoroscopy include the extra operating time required and the radiation exposure to the patient and the operating room staff. When properly performed, intraoperative fluoroscopy adds only an

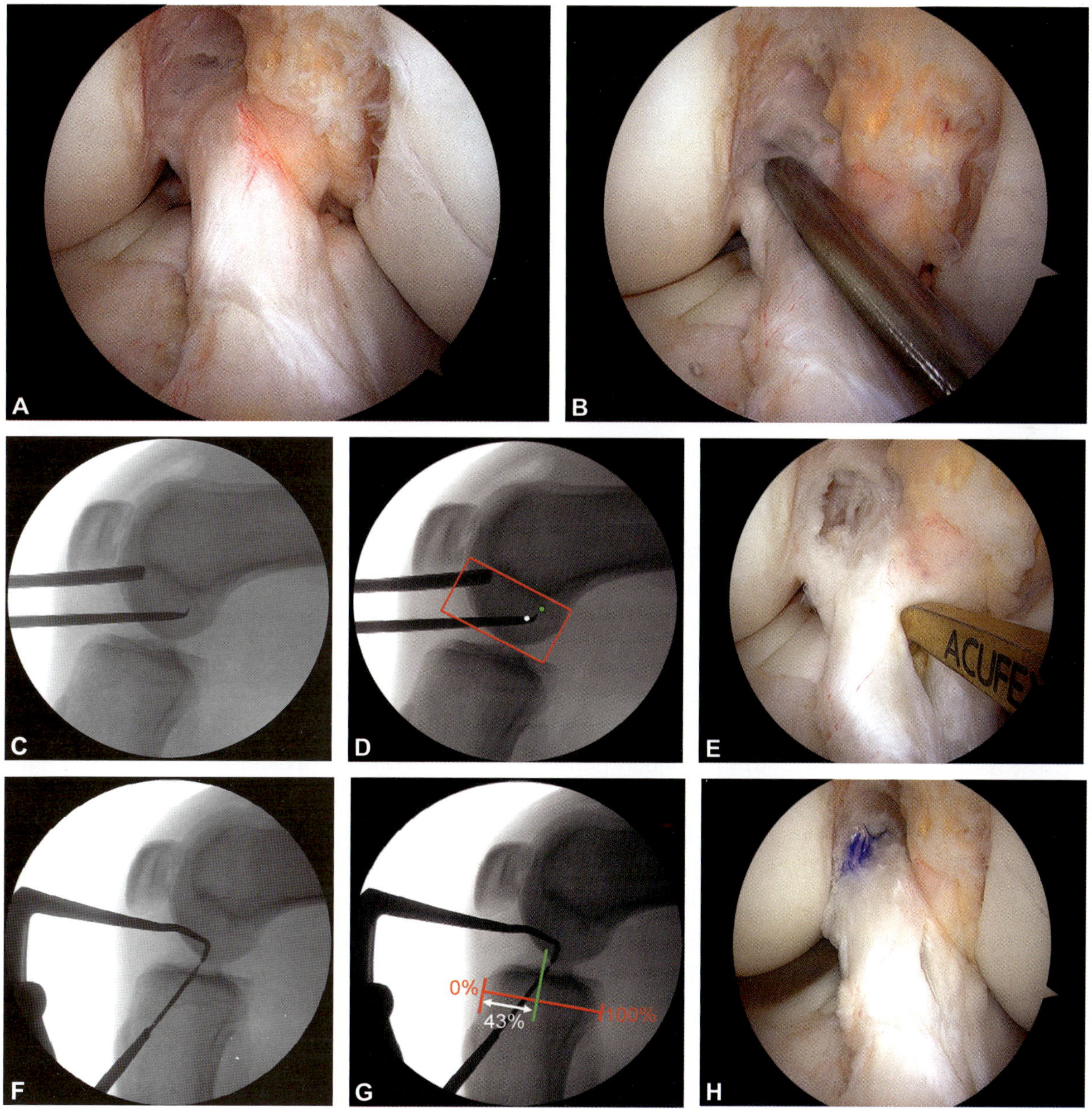

Figs. 32.3A to H: ACL augmentation procedure. (A) Intact AM bundle. (B) Tip of the 45° microfracture awl is placed at the proposed location for the center of the ACL femoral tunnel. (C) Fluoroscopic image of the proposed position for the center of the ACL femoral tunnel. (D) Fluoroscopic image demonstrates that the tip of the microfracture awl is located midway between the weighted average position of the center of the PL bundle (white circle) and the AM bundle (green circle). (E) ACL tibial aimer is inserted into a slit in the ACL tibial remnant and the tibial guide pin is drilled into the knee joint. (F) Fluoroscopic image of the tibial guide pin. (G) Fluoroscopy reveals that the tip of the tibial guide pin is positioned at 43% along the Amis-Jakob line. (H) 5-strand (8 mm) hamstring ACL augmentation graft.
(ACL: Anterior cruciate ligament; AM: Anteromedial; PL: Posteromedial).

additional few minutes to the total operating time. Chitnavis et al.[32] reported that the effective dose of radiation during the use of intraoperative fluoroscopy for ACL reconstruction was 0.001 mSv per patient, making the lifetime risk of developing cancer less than 0.0001%. The radiation exposure using intraoperative fluoroscopy during an ACL reconstruction was amongst the lowest of all fluoroscopic procedures and was less than that associated with common imaging such as plain limb radiographs. Some authors have criticized using averaged data from radiographic anatomical studies to guide placement of the ACL bone tunnels in an individual patient.[23] An individualized anatomic ACL reconstruction is best performed by identifying the native ACL footprint or bony anatomic ACL landmarks in each patient. However, this approach also has limitations since the native ACL footprint and anatomic bony landmarks may not always be present or be correctly identified by the surgeon. The goal of using intraoperative fluoroscopy is not necessarily to place the ACL bone tunnels in the same location in every patient, but rather to avoid unintended tunnel placements or unrecognized deviation in tunnel placements that might lead to failure of the ACL reconstruction.[33-42]

OPERATING ROOM SETUP

Successful use of intraoperative fluoroscopy is dependent on the ability to obtain true lateral radiographs of the knee. To obtain true intraoperative lateral radiographs it is important to control abduction-adduction and internal-external rotation of the leg. Positional control of the operative leg is best accomplished by keeping the operating room table flat and using a padded thigh post and hip positioner placed at the level of the patient's pelvis. The thigh post and hip positioner stabilize the patient's leg and pelvis and prevent the hip from abducting and the leg from externally rotating. A padded L-shaped foot support is applied to the side rail at the end of the operating table and adjusted, so the knee is maintained at 90° of flexion when the foot is placed on the support.[2,5] Prepositioning and adjusting the C-arm before prepping and draping the patient can help reduce the time required to obtain acceptable images. The operative leg is flexed to 90°, the foot of the patient is placed on the foot support and the C-arm positioned at the level of the knee joint. The X-ray beam of the C-arm is aligned parallel to the epicondylar axis of the knee. A trial lateral image is taken and the position of the C-arm and the knee are adjusted until the proximal, posterior and distal borders of the medial and lateral femoral condyles overlap (Fig. 32.4).

The proximal borders of the femoral condyles are lined up by rotating the C-arm in the plane parallel to the floor or by abducting or adducting the leg. The posterior borders are lined up by internally or externally rotating the knee. This is achieved by moving the patient's foot on the foot support. Moving the foot away from the midline internally rotates the femur, while moving the foot toward the midline externally rotates the femur. Due to the size difference between the medial and lateral femoral condyles, it is sometimes difficult to achieve a perfect overlap of the distal borders of the lateral femoral condyles. However, this is not necessary for plotting the Bernard-Hertel grid on the images.[9] After obtaining a satisfactory lateral image, the C-arm position is locked and the location of the wheels marked on the floor with wide adhesive tape (Fig. 32.5). The C-arm is moved out of the operative field and sterilely draped for later use during the procedure. When radiographic images are required, the C-arm is moved back into the operative field and the wheels are positioned at the previously marked locations on the floor. This method can help decrease the number of C-arm adjustments and the number of X-ray exposures required to obtain satisfactory images during surgery.

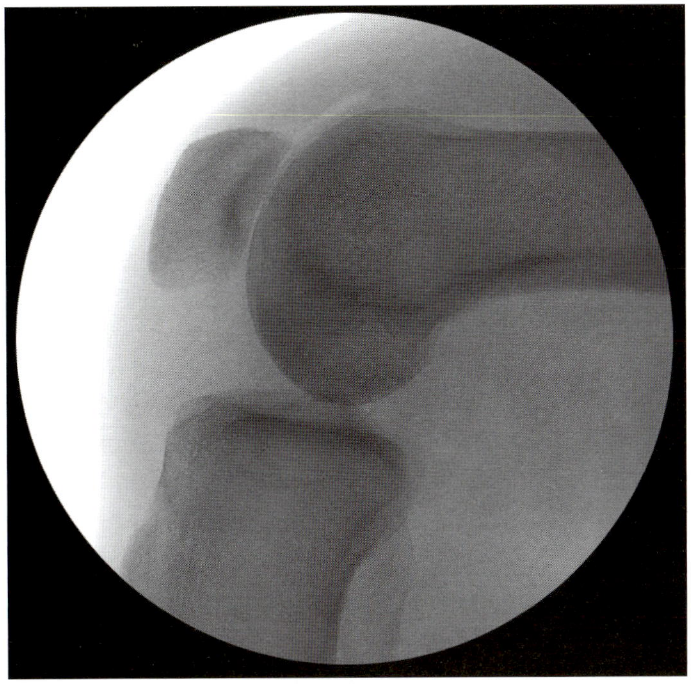

Fig. 32.4: Perfect lateral image of the knee. The proximal, distal, anterior and posterior borders of the medial and lateral femoral condyles overlap.

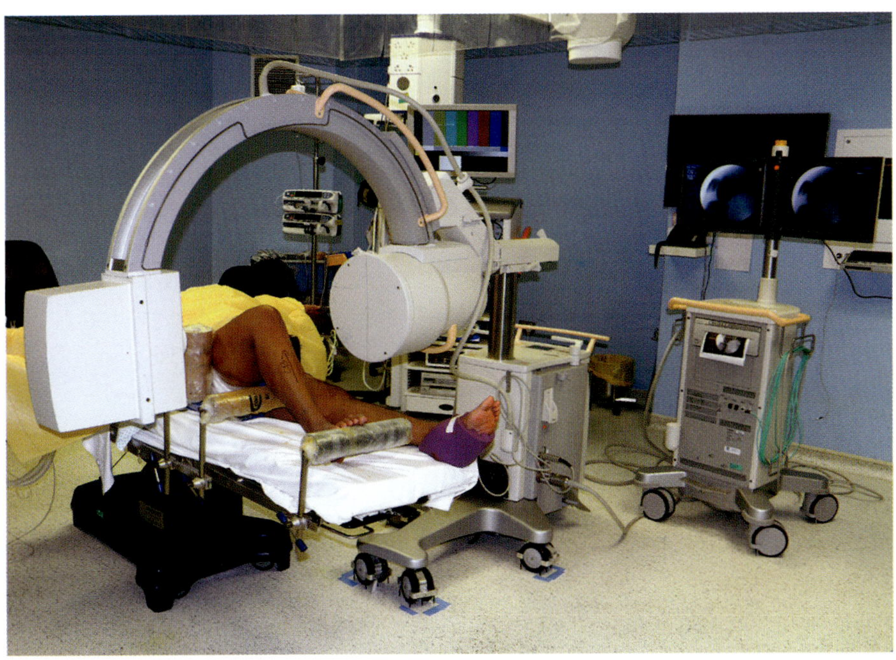

Fig. 32.5: A padded round thigh post and an L-shaped foot support positioned near the end of the operating room table are used to stabilize the knee at 90° of flexion. A second foot support is used to maintain the knee in hyperflexion when drilling the anterior cruciate ligament (ACL) femoral tunnel through a medial portal. The X-ray beam of the C-arm is aligned parallel to the epicondylar axis of the knee. After obtaining an acceptable image, the position of the C-arm wheels are marked on the floor with tape.

ANTERIOR CRUCIATE LIGAMENT FEMORAL TUNNEL PLACEMENT

Placement of the ACL bone tunnel using fluoroscopy does not depend on identifying the native ACL footprint or the bony anatomy of the ACL femoral attachment site, so only minimum preparation of the lateral wall of the intercondylar notch is required. The knee is placed at 70–90° of flexion and maintained at this position until the desired ACL femoral tunnel position has been achieved. The sterilely draped C-arm is moved into the operative field and a lateral image of the knee is taken. Adjustments in the C-arm position and the position of the knee are made until a true lateral image is obtained. Under arthroscopic visualization, the tip of a 45° angled microfracture awl is positioned against the lateral wall of the intercondylar notch at the proposed location for the ACL femoral tunnel. When identified, anatomic landmarks such as the native ACL footprint and the bony ACL ridges can be used as references to help position the ACL femoral tunnel. A lateral C-arm image of the knee is taken and the initial position of the tip of the microfracture awl evaluated. The microfracture awl should be rotated, so that the tip is clearly visible on the C-arm image (Figs. 32.6A to C). The location of the tip of the

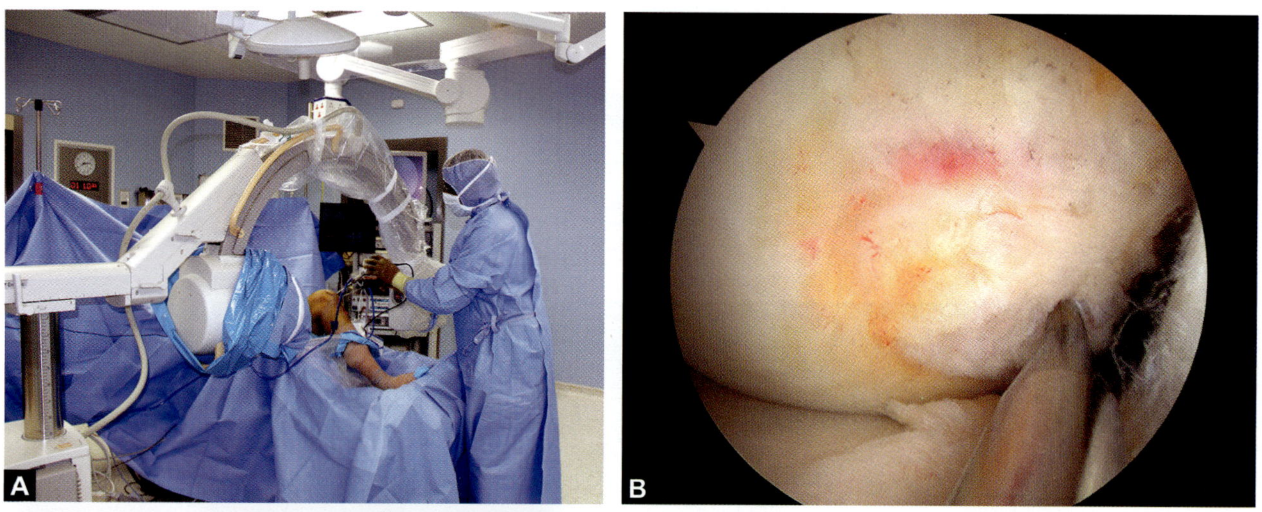

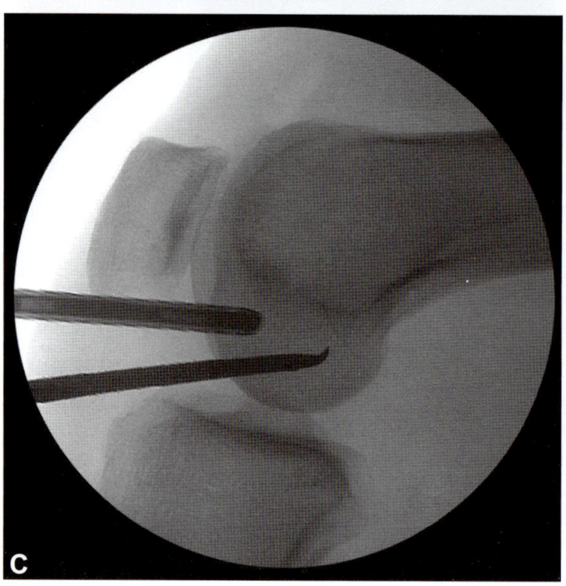

Figs. 32.6A to C: (A) The anterior cruciate ligament (ACL) femoral tunnel position is located using fluoroscopic guidance. (B) Anteromedial portal view of the ACL femoral attachment site. The tip of a 45° microfracture awl is placed at the site of the proposed ACL femoral tunnel. Since fluoroscopic placement of the ACL femoral tunnel does not rely on identifying specific ACL anatomic landmarks there is no need for extensive removal of soft tissue from the ACL femoral insertion site. (C) Intraoperative fluoroscopic image. The tip of the microfracture awl marks the location of the center of the proposed ACL femoral tunnel.

microfracture awl can be compared to a preoperatively planned ideal ACL femoral tunnel position or alternatively compared to data from published radiographic anatomic studies of the native ACL femoral attachment site.[9-25] Under arthroscopic and fluoroscopic control, the tip of the microfracture awl is adjusted until the desired ACL femoral tunnel position is achieved.

MEASURING THE ANTERIOR CRUCIATE LIGAMENT FEMORAL TUNNEL POSITION

The Bernard and Hertel grid is the most commonly used method to measure the position of the ACL femoral tunnel in cadaveric anatomic radiographic studies of the native ACL femoral attachment site and in clinical studies.[9-25] This rectangular grid is applied to an image of the lateral femoral condyle and allows any position along the inner wall of the lateral femoral condyle to be measured in the shallow (distal)—deep (proximal) direction (X-axis) and the high (anterior)—low (posterior) direction (Y-axis). The method is easy to use and has been shown to be independent of the knee size, shape and the distance between the X-ray tube and the patient.[9] This measurement method is versatile and can be plotted on plain lateral knee radiographs, lateral C-arm images and CT images. Intra- and inter-observer reliability of ACL femoral tunnel measurements on lateral CT images using the Bernard-Hertel grid has been found to be reliable.[43] In a study evaluating postoperative ACL femoral tunnel placement in 31 knees, the inter-observer intraclass correlation coefficient (ICC) was 0.999 for depth and 0.993 for height measurements along the lateral femoral condyle.[43] The intraobserver ICC ranged from 0.992 to 0.998 for depth and 0.995 to 0.963 for height.

The Bernard-Hertel grid is drawn on a lateral knee radiographic image in the following way:

- Draw a tangent to the roof of the intercondylar notch (Blumensaat's line).
- Draw two lines perpendicular to the first-line, one at the intersection of the tangent line with the shallow (distal) border of the lateral femoral condyle and the other with the intersection of the tangent line and the deep (proximal) border of the lateral femoral condyle. The lateral femoral condyle can be identified by an indentation at the distal margin (Grant's notch) and the fact that the medial femoral condyle extends more distally.
- Draw another line parallel to Blumensaat's line and tangent to the inferior (posterior) border of the lateral femoral condyle.

The inter- and intraobserver reliability in drawing the Bernard-Hertel grid on a lateral radiographic image has been reported to be 0.99.[19] Measurements of the ACL femoral tunnel position are made as percentages along Blumensaat's line (d), which represents the maximum sagittal diameter of the lateral femoral condyle, and line (h), which represents the maximum intercondylar notch height (Figs. 32.7A to E).

The Bernard-Hertel grid method has been used to measure the location of the center of the posterolateral (PL) and anteromedial (AM) bundles in human cadaveric specimens.[9-25] Using data from these published studies, a weighted average position for the center of the PL and AM bundles can be calculated (Table 32.1). Although, the position of the center of the ACL femoral attachment site was directly measured in only a few of the studies, it is possible to perform a linear extrapolation of the location of the center position by assuming that the center of the ACL femoral attachment site lies halfway between the center of the PL and AM bundle attachment sites. The weighted average extrapolated position for the center of the ACL femoral attachment site is calculated as follows:

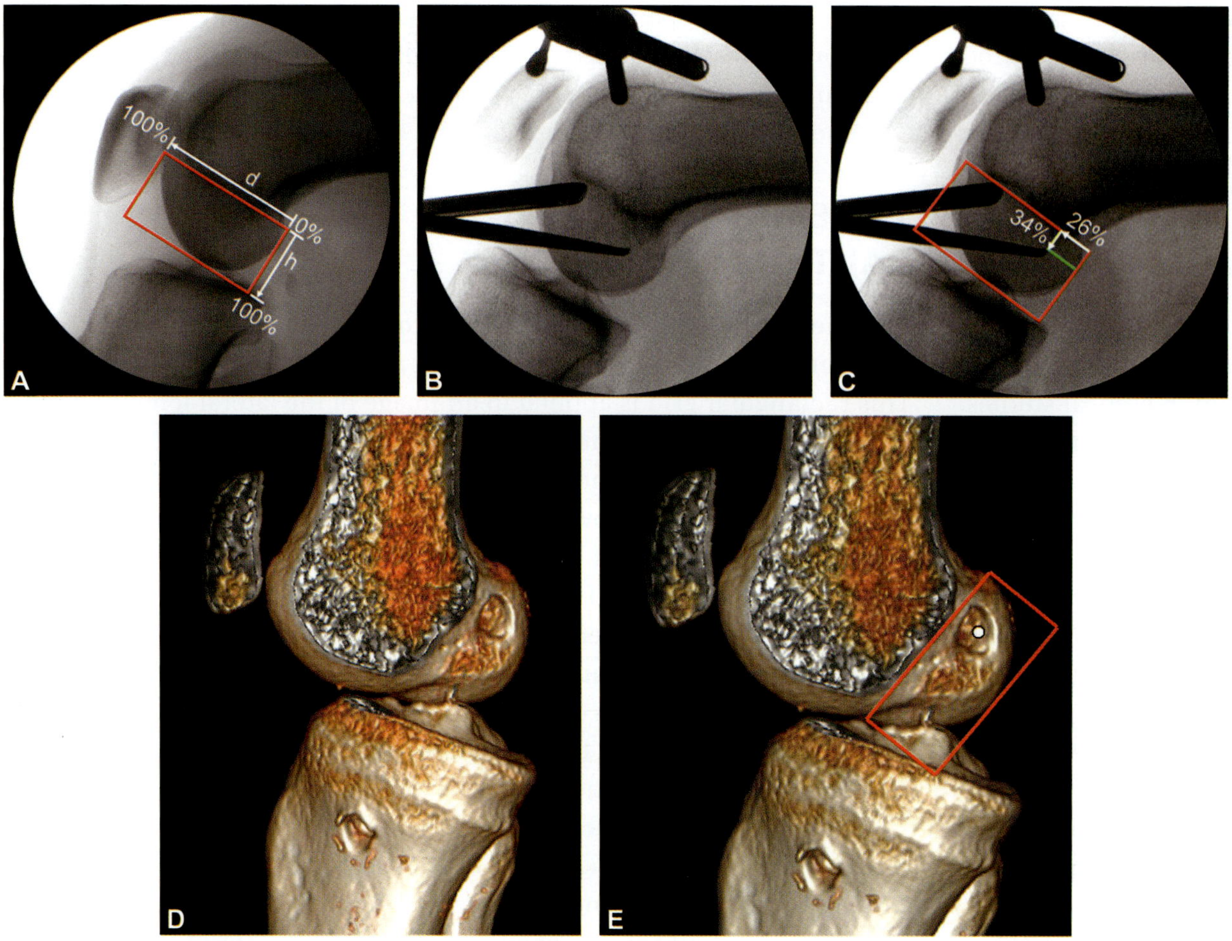

Figs. 32.7A to E: (A) Bernard-Hertel grid. The depth of the anterior cruciate ligament (ACL) femoral tunnel position is measured parallel to Blumensaat's line (d), and the height (h) along a line perpendicular to Blumensaat's line. (B) Intraoperative C-arm image. The tip of the microfracture awl is located at the center of proposed ACL femoral tunnel. (C) Bernard-Hertel grid plotted on the intraoperative C-arm image. The tip of the microfracture awl is positioned at a point 26% of the depth of the lateral femoral condyle and 34% of the height of the lateral femoral condyle. (D) Postoperative 3D computed tomography (CT) scan demonstrating the location of the ACL femoral tunnel. (E) Applying the Bernard-Hertel grid to the postoperative 3D CT scan demonstrates that the center of the ACL femoral tunnel is located at the weighted average center of the ACL femoral attachment site (white circle).[9-25]

Depth of the center position = [Posterolateral bundle (PLB) depth + anteromedial bundle (AMB) depth]/2

Height of the center position = (PLB height + AMB height)/2.

The calculation for the extrapolated weighted average for the center of the ACL femoral attachment site across all the included studies reveals that the center of the ACL femoral attachment site is located at a point which is 28% along Blumensaat's line and 34% along the height of the intercondylar notch. The weighted average location for the center of the PL and AM bundles and the extrapolated center of the ACL femoral attachment site can be plotted on a preoperative lateral radiograph or C-arm image and these images can be used as a reference to guide placement of the ACL femoral tunnel during surgery (Figs. 32.8A and B). Having identified the desired ACL femoral tunnel location, the ACL femoral tunnel can be drilled through an AM portal or using outside-in drilling (Figs. 32.9A to D).

Table 32.1: Radiographic measurements of the anterior cruciate ligament (ACL) femoral attachment site.

Author	*N*	*AMB depth (%)*	*PLB Depth (%)*	*Average center depth (%)*	*AMB height (%)*	*PLB height (%)*	*Average center height (%)*
Bernard-Hertel[9] (1997)	10			24.8			28.5
Luites[23](2015)	29	21.0	26.6	23.5	19.2	42.2	32.3
Musahl[10] (2003)	8			27			28
Yamamoto[11] (2004)	10	25	29	27	16	42	29
Colombet[12] (2006)	7	26.4	32.3	29.4	25.3	47.6	36.5
Zantop[13] (2008)	20	18.5	29.3	23.9	22.3	53.6	38.0
Tsukada[14] (2008)	36	25.9	34.8	30.4	17.8	42.1	30.0
Lorenz[15] (2009)	12	21	27	24	22	45	34
Forsythe[16] (2010)	8	21.7	35.1	28.4	33.2	55.3	44.3
Iriuchishima[17] (2010)	15	15	32	23.5	26	52	39
Pietrini[18] (2011)	12	21.6	28.9	25.3	14.6	42.3	28.5
Moloney[19] (2013)	20			33.7			32.0
deAbreu-e-Silva[20] (2015)	8			30.0			35.3
Lee[21] (2015)	15	33.5	38.3	35.9	27.6	55.1	41.4
Luites[23] (2015)	12	23.2	25.2	24.9	15.1	38.1	31.9
Davis[24] (2016)	12	27.1	39.3	32.9	24.1	49.3	36.6
Weighted average	**234**	**23.2**	**31.4**	**27.8**	**21.1**	**46.3**	**33.7**

(AMB: Anteromedial bundle; PLB: Posteromedial bundle).

ANTERIOR CRUCIATE LIGAMENT TIBIAL TUNNEL PLACEMENT

At the present time there is a lack of agreement on what anatomic landmarks to use to guide placement of the ACL tibial tunnel. The lack of agreement on anatomic landmarks makes placement of the ACL tibial tunnel challenging. Behrend et al.[44] reported that 36% of the ACL tibial tunnels compared to 22% of the ACL femoral tunnels were incorrectly positioned by surgeons performing ACL reconstruction at a Swiss teaching hospital. In this study, there was no correlation between the surgeon's experience and placement of the ACL tibial tunnel. Werner et al.[45] reported that using the posterior border of the anterior horn of lateral meniscus as a landmark resulted in inconsistent placement of the ACL tibial tunnel. In this study, only 18% of the tibial tunnels were located between 40% and 44.9% of the sagittal width of the tibia. Intraoperative lateral C-arm images of the knee allow the surgeon to accurately measure the position of the center of the ACL tibial tunnel in the sagittal plane.

The knee is placed between 70° and 90° of flexion and the tibial guide pin is drilled at the desired location in the ACL tibial attachment site using a standard ACL tibial aimer. In general the tibial guide pin is placed approximately 2–3 mm anterior to the posterior margin of the anterior horn of the lateral meniscus and just lateral to the medial border of the ACL tibial footprint (medial intercondylar ridge of the tibia) in the medial-lateral direction (Fig. 32.10). The position of the tibial guide pin in the sagittal

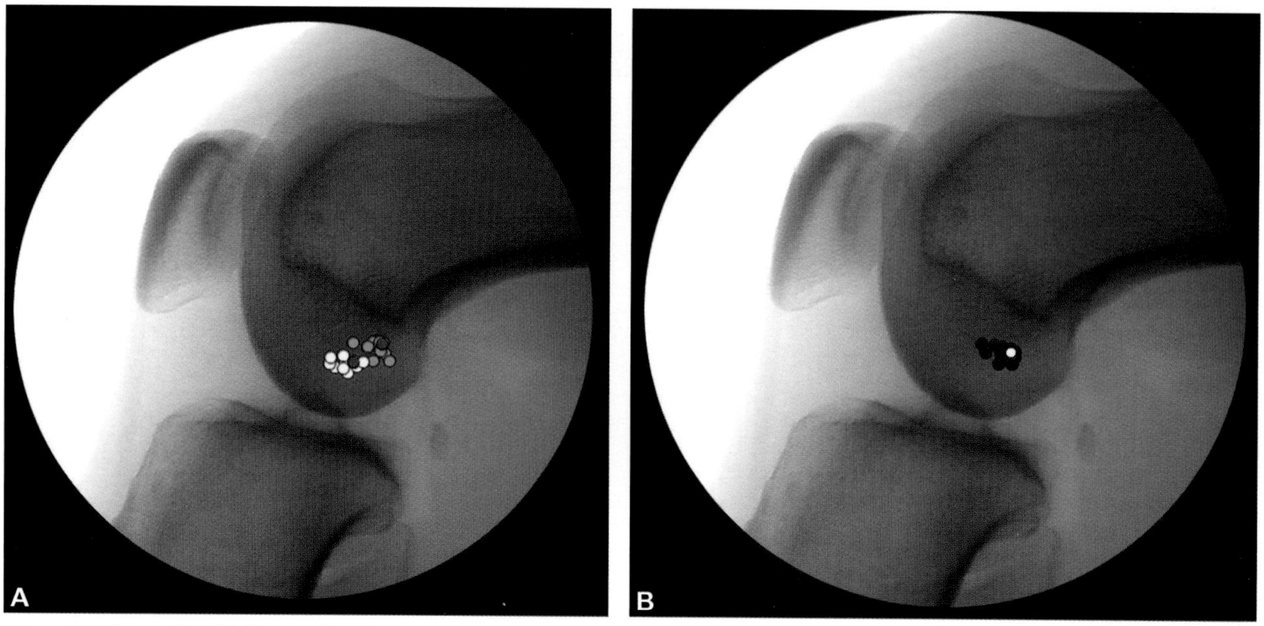

Figs. 32.8A and B: (A) Data points for the center of the posterolateral (PL) (white circles) and the anteromedial (AM) bundle (green circles) from published radiographic anatomic studies of the anterior cruciate ligament (ACL) femoral attachment site.[9-25] The red circles represent the weighted average position for the center of the PL and AM bundles. (B) Data points (blue circles) for the center of the ACL femoral attachment site using data from published radiographic anatomic studies of the ACL femoral attachment site.[9-25] The white circle represents the weighted average position for the center of the ACL femoral attachment site.

plane is measured by taking a lateral C-arm image of the knee in maximum extension or at 90° of flexion as described earlier for the ACL femoral tunnel. One advantage of evaluating the tibial guide pin position in maximum extension is that the guide pin position can be accessed for roof impingement by checking the relationship of the guide pin to Blumensaat's line. The knee is held in maximum extension and a lateral image of the knee is taken. The goal is to obtain a lateral view of the tibia with the posterior borders of the medial and lateral tibial condyles overlapping (Figs. 32.11A and B). Internally or externally rotating the knee will adjust the overlap of the posterior borders of the medial and lateral tibial and femoral condyles, while abducting and adducting the knee affects the overlap of the medial and lateral joint lines and the proximal borders of the medial and lateral tibial condyles. Although one should aim to obtain a perfect image with complete overlap of the posterior borders of the tibial condyles, small amounts of malrotation can be accepted. Haasper et al.[46] demonstrated that 20° of external rotation resulted in only a 3.3% difference in the ACL tibial tunnel position measured along the Amis-Jakob line.

An alternative method for checking the position of the tibial guide pin is to insert the tip of the ACL tibial aimer at the desired location in the ACL tibial attachment site and take a lateral C-arm image with the knee at 70–90° of flexion. Typical, the tip of the ACL tibial aimer is placed on the upslope of the medial tibial spine, which can be easily seen on the C-arm image. The desired position for the tibial tunnel can be plotted on a preoperative lateral X-ray or C-arm image and this position can be referred to a location along the medial tibial spine. An advantage of this method is the tip of the ACL tibial aimer can be adjusted under fluoroscopic control until the desired sagittal position of the ACL tibial tunnel is achieved. Once the desired position is achieved, the guide pin is then drilled into position (Figs. 32.12A

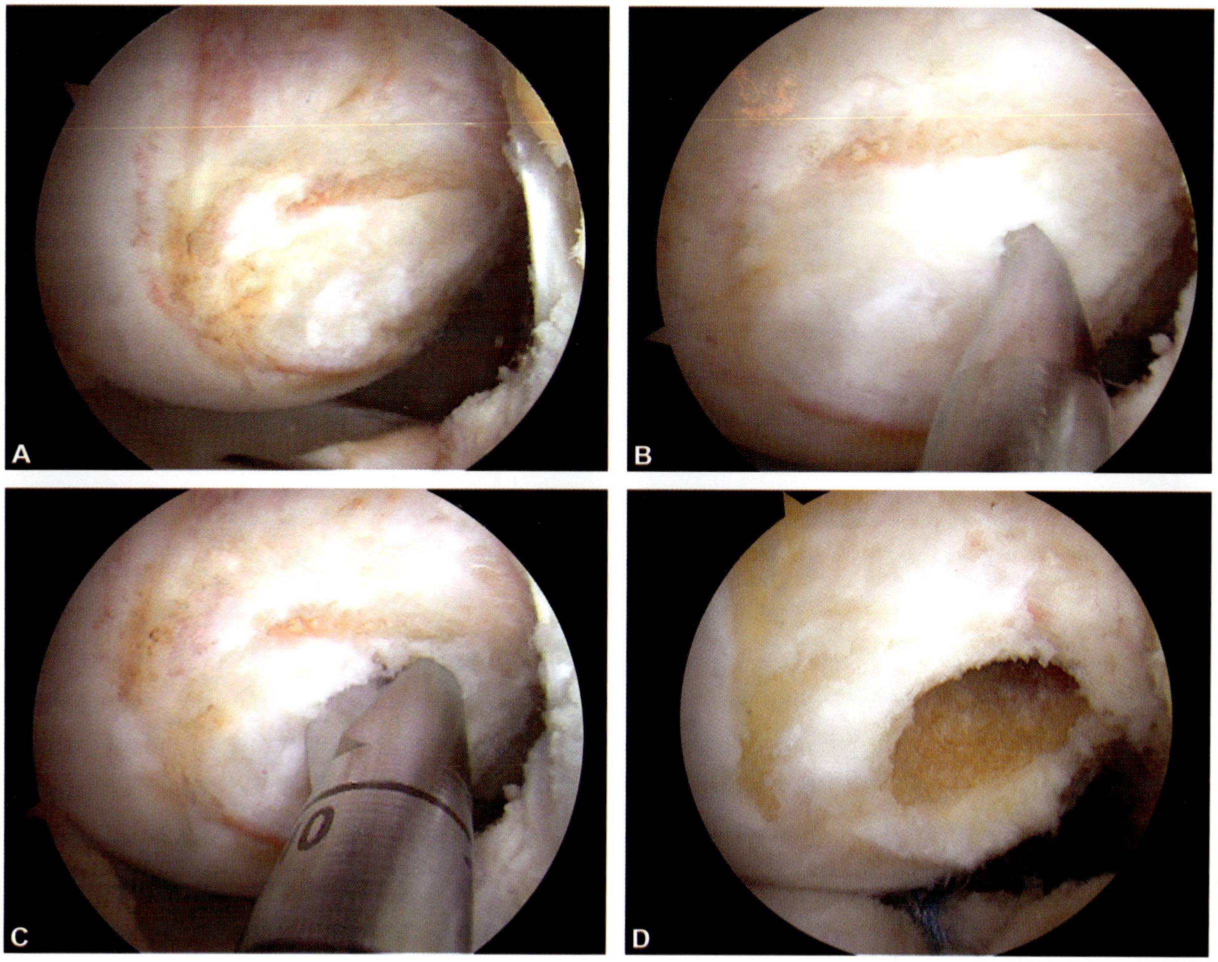

Figs. 32.9A to D: Anteromedial portal view at 90° flexion. (A) Native anterior cruciate ligament (ACL) femoral attachment site. (B) Microfracture awl marking the proposed location for the ACL femoral tunnel. (C) Drilling ACL femoral through a low accessory anteromedial portal. Viewing the ACL femoral attachment site through the anteromedial portal and drilling the tunnel through a low accessory anteromedial portal allows the surgeon to see exactly where the femoral tunnel will be positioned within the native ACL femoral attachment site. (D) ACL femoral tunnel. The tunnel is seen to lie completely within the native ACL femoral attachment site.

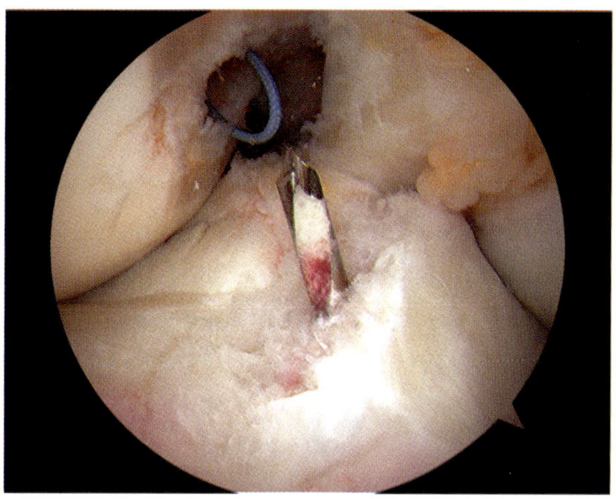

Fig. 32.10: Tibial guide pin. The tibial guide pin is positioned 2–3 mm anterior to the posterior margin of the anterior horn of the lateral meniscus and just lateral to the medial intercondylar ridge of the tibia.

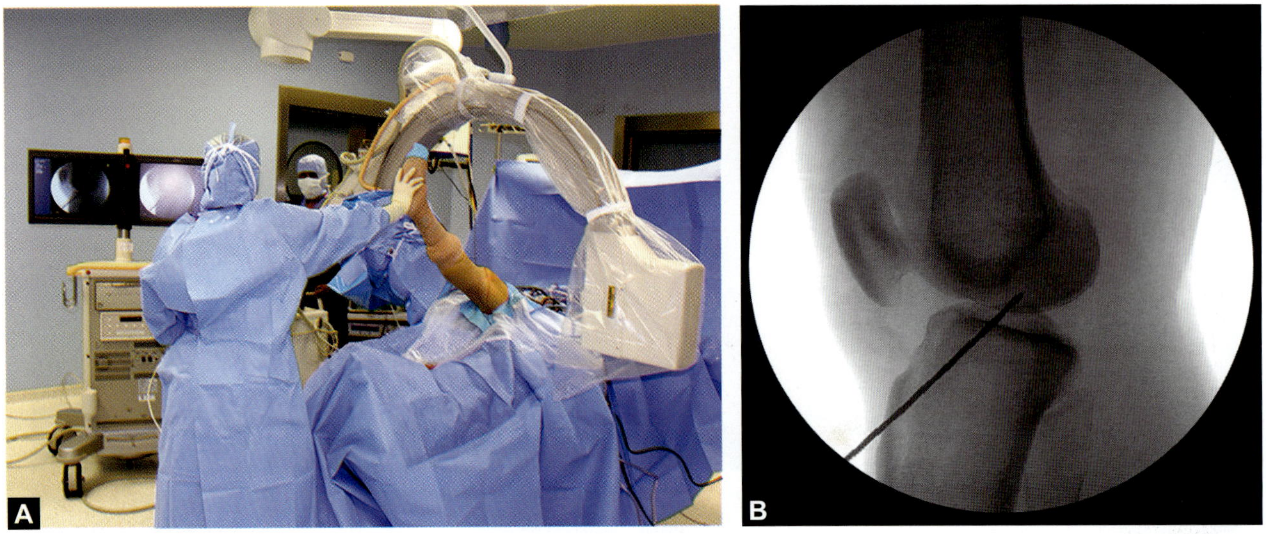

Figs. 32.11A and B: (A) The knee is held in maximum extension and a lateral C-arm image taken. (B) Lateral C-arm image. The tibial guide pin is located parallel and posterior to Blumensaat's line (impingement free tibial tunnel).

and B). This method eliminates the possibility of drilling an errant tibial guide pin and having to reposition the pin. This technique is particularly useful when preserving an ACL tibial remnant. A small slit is made in the ACL tibial remnant and the tip of the tip ACL aimer is inserted into the slit. The tip of the ACL tibial aimer can be adjusted under fluoroscopic control until the desired sagittal position of the guide pin is achieved. One disadvantage of this method is that the relationship of the guide pin to Blumensaat's line cannot be established with the knee at 90° of flexion. If this information is desired, then the knee will need to be placed in maximum extension and a new lateral C-arm image taken. It is possible to use intraoperative fluoroscopy to check the medial-lateral position of the tibial guide pin (Fig. 32.13). However, this will require rotating the C-arm to take an anterior-posterior image of the knee. In our experience, the medial-lateral position of the tibial guide pin can be reliably assessed arthroscopically.

MEASURING THE ANTERIOR CRUCIATE LIGAMENT TIBIAL TUNNEL POSITION

The position of the tibial guide pin is measured using the method of Amis and Jakob.[47] In this method, a line is drawn from the highest point of the anterior aspect of the medial tibial joint line to the highest point of the posterior aspect of the medial tibial joint line. The medial tibial condyle and medial joint line are identified by the fact that the medial tibial condyle is concave, while the lateral tibial condyle is convex. The Amis-Jakob line is drawn from the anterior aspect of the tibia to the posterior corner of the widest part of the medial tibial condyle parallel to the previously placed line marking the medial joint line. The posterior aspect of the medial tibial condyle is indentified by the fact that the posterior contour is squared off, while the posterior aspect of the lateral tibial condyle has a downward slope. The anterior tibial cortex represents 0% and the posterior tibial cortex 100% of the sagittal width of the tibia. The tibial guide pin position is cal-

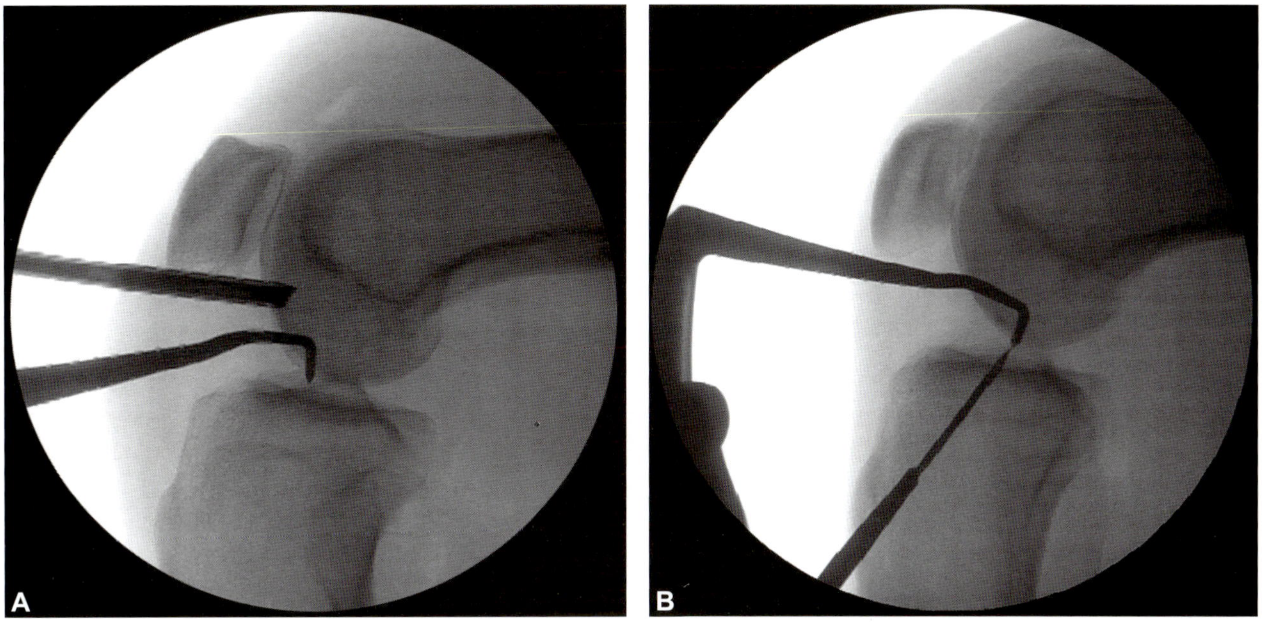

Figs. 32.12A and B: (A) Tip of the anterior cruciate ligament (ACL) tibial aimer is adjusted under fluoroscopic control until the desired position for the center of the tibial tunnel is achieved. (B) Tibial guide pin is drilled into position.

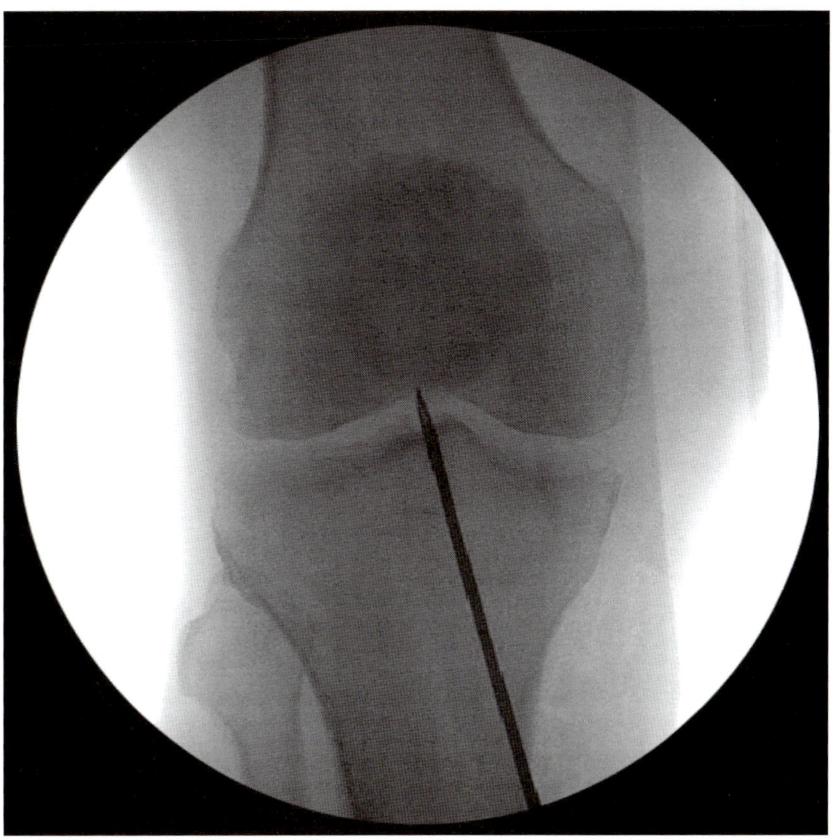

Fig. 32.13: The medial-lateral placement of the tibial guide pin can be determined by taking an anteroposterior (AP) C-arm image.

culated by dropping an orthogonal line from the point where the tibial guide pin crosses the medial joint line onto the Amis-Jakob line. The distance from the anterior tibial cortex (0%) to the orthogonal projection onto the Amis-Jakob line is represented as a percentage of the total length of the Amis-Jakob (Fig. 32.14). The location of the centers of the AM and PL bundles and the center of the ACL tibial attachment site has been measured using the Amis-Jakob line and the anterior-posterior diameter of the tibia on cadavers, on patients undergoing surgery and on the normal population using radiographs, CT and MRI (Table 32.2). The weighted average position of the center of the ACL using published X-ray studies that used the Amis-Jakob line as the measurement method is 40% (Table 32.3). Using fluoroscopy, the goal is to place the tibial guide pin between 40% and 44% along the Amis-Jakob line. Having located the desired ACL tibial tunnel position, the tibial tunnel is drilled in the conventional fashion (Figs. 32.15A to C).

CONCLUSION

Intraoperative fluoroscopy is an easy, noninvasive, cost-effective, accurate and reproducible method for evaluating bone tunnel placement during ACL surgery. Intraoperative fluoroscopy allows the surgeon in real time to objectively measure and document where the ACL bone tunnels are being placed during ACL surgery. It provides immediate feedback to the surgeon and allows undesirable tunnel positions to be detected and changed during the procedure.

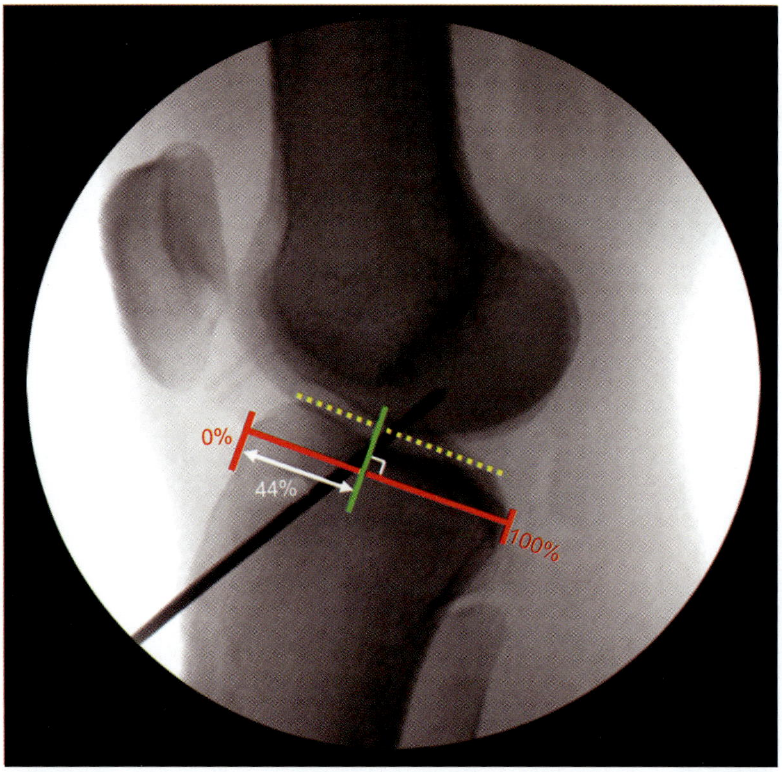

Fig. 32.14: Amis-Jakob line. The medial joint line is marked by the dotted yellow line. The Amis-Jakob line (red line) passes through the posterior corner of the widest part of the medial tibial plateau (square posterior border) parallel to the medial joint line. The anterior tibial cortex represents 0%, and the posterior tibial cortex 100% of the sagittal width of the tibia. The tibial guide pin position is calculated by dropping an orthogonal line (green line) from the point where the tibial guide pin crosses the medial joint line onto the Amis-Jakob line. The distance from the anterior tibial cortex (0%) to the orthogonal projection onto the Amis-Jakob line (white line with arrowheads) is represented as a percentage of the total length of the Amis-Jakob line. The tibial guide pin in this case is located at 44% along the Amis-Jakob line.

Table 32.2: Radiographic measurements of the anterior cruciate ligament (ACL) tibial attachment site.

Author	*Methods*	*N*	*Evaluation method*	*Average AMB center*	*Average PLB center*	*Average ACL center*
Staubli[26] (1994)	Cadaver Cyrosection MRI (male) MRI (female)	10 5 23 12	AP width tibia			41.2% 43.3% 44.1% 43.7%
Musahl[10] (2003)	Cadaver: Radiograph Cadaver: CT scan	8 8	AP width tibia AP width tibia			46.2% 45.4%
Colombet[12] (2006)	Cadaver: Radiograph	7	Amis-Jakob line	36%	52%	
Zantop[13] (2008)	Cadaver: Radiograph	20	Amis-Jakob line	30%	44%	
Doi[27] (2008)	Cadaver: Radiograph	31	Amis-Jakob line	34.6%	38.4%	
Lorenz[15] (2009)	Cadaver: CT scan	12	AP width tibia	41%	52%	
Forsythe[16] (2010)	Cadaver: CT scan	8	AP width tibia	25%	46.4%	
Iriuchishima[17] (2010)	Cadaver: Radiograph	15	AP width tibia	31%	50%	
Frank[28] (2010)	Normal population: MRI	100	AP width tibia			46%
Kasten[29] (2010)	Surgery: C-arm	67	Amis-Jakob line	35%	48%	41%
Pietrini[18] (2011)	Cadaver: Radiograph	12	Amis-Jakob line	36.3%	51.0%	
Scheffel[30] (2012)	Normal population: MRI	138	AP width tibia			44.1%
de Abreau-e-Silva[20] (2015)	Cadaver: CT scan	8	AP width tibia			40.5%
Lee[21] (2015)	Cadaver: Dissection Cadaver: Radiograph Cadaver: CT scan	8	AP width tibia	37.6% 36.3% 36.7%	43.8% 43.4% 42.2%	
Parkinson[31] (2015)	Normal population: MRI Normal population: CT	76 26	Amis-Jakob line			39% 38%

(AMB: Anteromedial bundle; PLB: Posteromedial bundle; MRI: Magnetic resonance imaging; CT: Computed tomography; AP: Anteroposterior).

Table 32.3: Radiographic measurements of the anterior cruciate ligament (ACL) tibial attachment site using the Amis-Jakob line.

Author	*Methods*	*N*	*Evaluation method*	*Average AMB center*	*Average PLB center*	*Average ACL center*
Colombet[12] (2006)	Cadaver: Radiograph	7	Amis-Jakob line	36%	52%	44%
Zantop[13] (2008)	Cadaver: Radiograph	20	Amis-Jakob line	30%	44%	37%
Doi[27] (2009)	Cadaver: Radiograph	31	Amis-Jakob line	34.6%	38.4%	36.5%
Kasten[29] (2010)	Surgery: C-arm	67	Amis-Jakob line	35%	48%	41.5%
Pietrini[18] (2011)	Cadaver: Radiograph	12	Amis-Jakob line	36.3%	51.0%	43.6%
Weighted average		**137**		**34.3%**	**45.7%**	**40.2%**

(AMB: Anteromedial bundle; PLB: Posteromedial bundle).

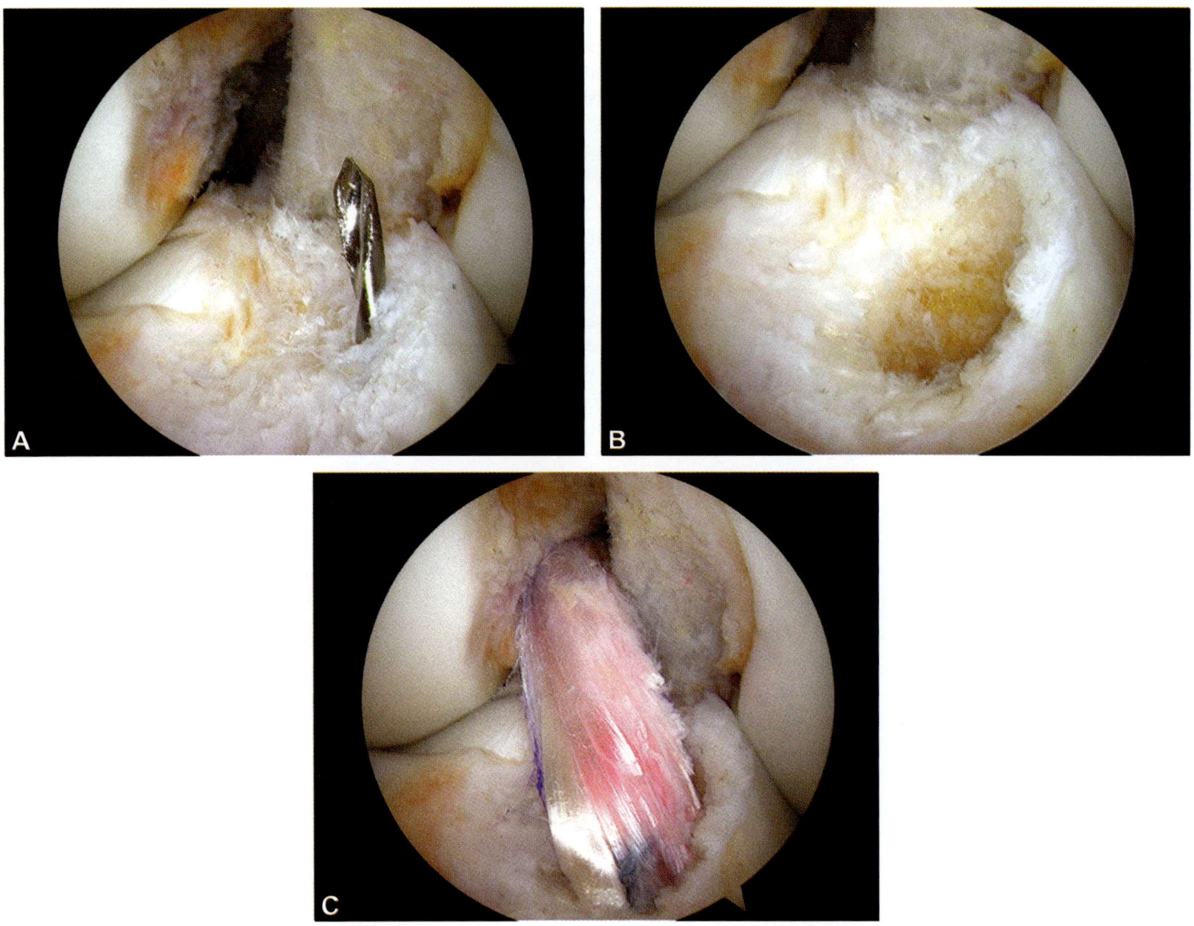

Figs. 32.15A to C: (A) Tibial guide pin. (B) Eccentric reaming was performed using progressively larger drill bits to create an elliptically shaped tibial tunnel. The tibial tunnel is positioned as medially as possible in the native anterior cruciate ligament (ACL) tibial attachment site to avoid having the reamers damage the root attachment of the anterior horn of the lateral meniscus. (C) 6-strand hamstring tendon ACL reconstruction.

REFERENCES

1. Singh AP, Singh BK. The use of intra-operative image intensifier control for the ACL surgeon. The Knee. 2011; 18: 379-81.
2. Brown CH, Spalding T, Robb C. Medial portal technique for single-bundle anatomical anterior cruciate (ACL) reconstruction. Int Ortho. 2013;37:253-69.
3. Hulet C, Rochcongar G, Chapus V. Tibial bone tunnel placement (arthroscopically and fluoroscopy). In: Siebold R, Dejour D, Zaffagnini S, eds. Anterior Cruciate Ligament Reconstruction: A Practical Surgical Guide. Heidelberg New York Dordrecht London: Springer, 2014;147-58.
4. Siebold R, Passler HH. Fluroscopy for bone tunnel placement. In: Siebold R, Dejour D, Zaffagnini S, eds. Anterior Cruciate Ligament Reconstruction: A Practical Surgical Guide. Heidelberg New York Dordrecht London: Springer, 2014;181-4.
5. Spalding T, Robb C, Brown CH. Femoral bone tunnel placement (arthroscopically and with fluoroscopy). In: Siebold R, Dejour D, Zaffagnini S, eds. Anterior Cruciate Ligament Reconstruction: A Practical Surgical Guide. Heidelberg New York Dordrecht London: Springer, 2014;159-79.
6. Sven S, Maurice B, Hocher J, et al. Variability of tunnel positioning in fluoroscopic-assisted ACL reconstruction. Knee Surg Sports Traumatol Arthros. 2015; 23:2269-77.
7. Inderhaug et al. The effect of intraoperative fluoroscopy on the accuracy of femoral tunnel placement in single-bundle anatomic ACL reconstruction. Knee Surg Sports Traumatol Arthros. 2015 (in press)
8. Dhawan A, Gallo RA, Lynch SA. Anatomic tunnel placement in anterior cruciate ligament reconstruction. J Am Acad Orthop Surg. 2016;24:443-54.
9. Bernard M, Hertel P, Hornung H, et al. Femoral insertion of the ACL. Radiographic quadrant method. Am J Knee Surg. 1997;10:14-22.
10. Musahl V, Burkart A, Debski RE, et al. Anterior cruciate ligament tunnel placement: comparison of insertion site anatomy with the guidelines of a computer-assisted surgical system. Arthroscopy. 2003;19:154-60.
11. Yamamoto Y, Hsu WH, Woo SL, et al. Knee stability and graft function after anterior cruciate ligament reconstruction: a comparison of a lateral and an anatomical femoral tunnel placement. Am J Sports Med. 2004;32:1825-32.
12. Columbet P, Robinson J, Christel P, et al. Morphology of anterior cruciate ligament attachments for anatomic reconstruction: a cadaveric dissection and radiographic study. Arthroscopy. 2006;22:984-92.
13. Zantop T, Wellman M, Fu FH, et al. Tunnel positioning of anteromedial and posterolateral bundles in anatomic anterior cruciate ligament reconstruction. Anatomic and radiographic findings. Am J Sports Med 2008;36:65-72.
14. Tsukada H, Ishibashi Y, Tsuda E, et al. Anatomical analysis of the anterior cruciate ligament femoral and tibial footprints. J Ortho Sci. 2008;13:122-9.
15. Lorenz S, Elser F, Mitterer M, et al. Radiographic evaluation of the insertion sites of the 2 functional bundles of the anterior cruciate ligament using 3-dimensional computed tomography. Am J Sports Med. 2009;37:2368-76.
16. Forsythe B, Kopf S, Wong AK, et al. The location of femoral and tibial tunnels in anatomic double-bundle anterior cruciate ligament reconstruction analyzed by three-dimensional computed tomography models. J Bone Joint Surg Am. 2010;92-A:1418-29.
17. Iriuchishima T, Ingham SJM, Tajima G, et al. Evaluation of the tunnel placement in the anatomical double-bundle ACL reconstruction: a cadaver study. Knee Surg Sports Traumatol Arthrosc. 2010;18:1226-31.
18. Pietrini SD, Ziegler CG, Anderson CJ, et al. Radiographic landmarks for tunnel positioning in double-bundle ACL reconstructions. Knee Surg Sports Traumatol Arthrosc 2011;19:792-800.
19. Moloney G, Araujo P, Rabuck S, et al. Use of a fluoroscopic overlay to assist arthroscopic anterior cruciate ligament reconstruction. Am J Sports Med. 2013;41:1794-1800.
20. Abreu-e-Silva GM, Oliveira MHGCN, Maranhao GS, et al. Three-dimensional computed tomography evaluation of anterior cruciate ligament reconstruction footprint for anatomic single-bundle reconstruction. Knee Surg Sports Traumatol Arthros. 2015;23:770-6.

21. Lee JK, Lee S, Seong SC, et al. Anatomy of the anterior cruciate ligament insertion sites: comparison of plain radiography and three-dimensional computed tomographic imaging to anatomic dissection. Knee Surg Sports Traumatol Arthrosc. 2015;23:2297-2305.
22. Sullivan JP, Cook S, Gao Y, et al. Radiographic anatomy of the native anterior cruciate ligament: a systematic review. HSSJ. 2015;11:154-65.
23. Luites WH, Verdonschot N. Radiographic positions of femoral ACL, AM and PL centres: accuracy of guideline based on the lateral quadrant method. Knee Surg Sports Traumatol Arthros 2015 (in press)
24. Davis AD, Manaqibwala MI, Brown CH, et al. Height and depth guidelines for anatomic femoral tunnels in anterior cruciate reconstruction. Arthroscopy. 2016;32:1098-1105.
25. Parkar AP, Adriaensen M, Vinfeld S, et al. The anatomic centers of the femoral and tibial insertions of the anterior cruciate ligament. A systematic review of imaging and cadaveric studies reporting normal center location. Am J Sports Med. 2017 (in press)
26. Staubli HU, Rauschning W. Tibial attachment area of the anterior cruciate ligament in the extended knee position. Anatomy and cryosections in vitro complemented by magnetic resonance arthrography in vivo. Knee Surg Sports Traumatol Arthrosc. 1994; 2:138-46.
27. Doi M, Takahashi M, Abe M, et al. Lateral radiographic study of the tibial insertions of the anteromedial and posterolateral bundles of human anterior cruciate ligament. Knee Surg Sport Traumatol Arthrosc. 2009;17: 347-51.
28. Frank RM, Seroyer ST, Lewis PB, et al. MRI analysis of tibial position of the anterior cruciate ligament. Knee Surg Sports Traumatol Arthrosc. 2010;18:1607-11.
29. Kasten P, Szczodry M, Irrgang J, et al. What is the role of intra-operative fluoroscopic measurement to determine tibial tunnel placement in anatomical anterior cruciate ligament reconstruction. Knee Surg Sports Traumatol Arthros. 2010;18:1169-75.
30. Scheffel PT, Henninger HB, Burks RT. Relationship of the intercondylar roof and the tibial footprint of the ACL. Implications for ACL reconstruction. Am J Sports Med. 2012;41:396-401.
31. Parkinson B, Gogna R, Robb C, et al. Anatomic ACL reconstruction: the normal central tibia footprint position and a standardized technique for measuring tibial tunnel location on 3D CT. Knee Surg Sports Traumatol Arthrosc. Published on-line: 01 July 2015-08-31
32. Chitnavis JP, Karthikesaligam A, Macdonald A, et al. Radiation risk from fluoroscopically-assisted anterior cruciate ligament reconstruction. Ann R Coll Surg Engl. 2010;92:330-4.
33. Carson EW, Anisko EM, Restrepo C, et al. Revision anterior cruciate ligament reconstruction: etiology of failures and clinical results. J Knee Surg. 2004;17:127-32.
34. Lee MC, Seong SC, Lee S, et al. Vertical femoral tunnel placement results in rotational knee laxity after anterior cruciate ligament reconstruction. Arthroscopy. 2007;23:771-78.
35. Marchant BG, Noyes FR, Barber-Westin SD, et al. Prevalence of nonanatomical graft placement in a series of failed anterior cruciate ligament reconstruction. Am J Sports Med. 2010;38:1987-96.
36. MARS group. Descriptive epidemiology of the multicenter ACL revision study (MARS) cohort. Am J Sports Med. 2010;38:1979-86.
37. Kamath GV, Redfern JC, Greis PE, et al. Revision anterior cruciate ligament reconstruction. Am J Sports Med. 2011;39:1999-2017.
38. Sadoghi P, Kropfl A, Jansson V, et al. Impact of tibial and femoral tunnel position on clinical results after anterior cruciate ligament reconstruction. Arthroscopy. 2011;27:355-64.
39. Trojani C, Sbihi A, Dijan P, et al. Causes for failure of ACL reconstruction and influence of meniscectomies after revision. Knee Surg Sports Traumatol Arthrosc. 2011;19:196–201.

40. Morgan JA, Dahm D, Levy B, et al. Femoral tunnel malposition in ACL revision reconstruction. J Knee Surg. 2012;25: 361-68.
41. Fernandez TL, Fregni F, Weaver K, et al. The influence of femoral tunnel position on functional outcomes and return to sports. Knee Surg Sports Tramatol Arthrosc. 2014;22:97-103.
42. MARS Group. Radiographic findings in revision anterior cruciate ligament reconstructions from the MARS cohort. J Knee Surg. 2013;26:239-48.
43. Lertwanich P, Martins CAQ, Asai S, et al. Anterior cruciate ligament tunnel position measurement reliability on 3-dimensional reconstructed computed tomography. Arthroscopy. 2011;27:391-98.
44. Behrend H, Stutz G, Kessler MA, et al. Tunnel placement in anterior cruciate ligament (ACL) reconstructions: quality control in a teaching hospital. Knee Surg Sports Traumatol Arthros. 2006;14:1159-65.
45. Werner BC, Burrus MT, Gwathmey FW, et al. A prospective evaluation of the anterior horn of the lateral meniscus as a landmark for tibial tunnel placement in anterior cruciate ligament (ACL) reconstruction. Knee. 2015 (in press).
46. Haasper C, Kopf S, Lorenz S, et al. Influence of tibial rotation on tibial tunnel position measurement using lateral fluoroscopy in anterior cruciate ligament reconstruction. Knee Surg Sports Traumatol Arthros. 2015;23: 649-54.
47. Amis A, Jakob R. Anterior cruciate ligament graft positioning, tensioning and twisting. Knee Surg Sports Traumatol Arthros. 1998;6:S2-S12 (Suppl 1).

CHAPTER

33

Rehabilitation after Anterior Cruciate Ligament Reconstruction: Optimizing Outcomes by Restoring Dynamic Knee Stability

John Nyland, Jun Matsuno

INTRODUCTION

The key focus of rehabilitation following anterior cruciate ligament (ACL) reconstruction or repair is the restoration of functional, dynamic knee stability.[1] Incorporated in this is the minimization of translational and pivot shift tibiofemoral joint laxity. To date, a high percentage of individuals who undergo ACL reconstruction and rehabilitation do not return to sports at their previous intensity or frequency level.[2,3] Both surgeons and rehabilitation clinicians need to remember that the native ACL, in addition to serving a key biomechanical restraint role, is a neurosensory organ that functions in close synchrony with the posterior cruciate ligament and menisci, sending afferent signals to the spinal cord and brain, activating precise neuromuscular responses and influencing muscle spindle receptor sensitivity (Fig. 33.1).[4-8] The purpose

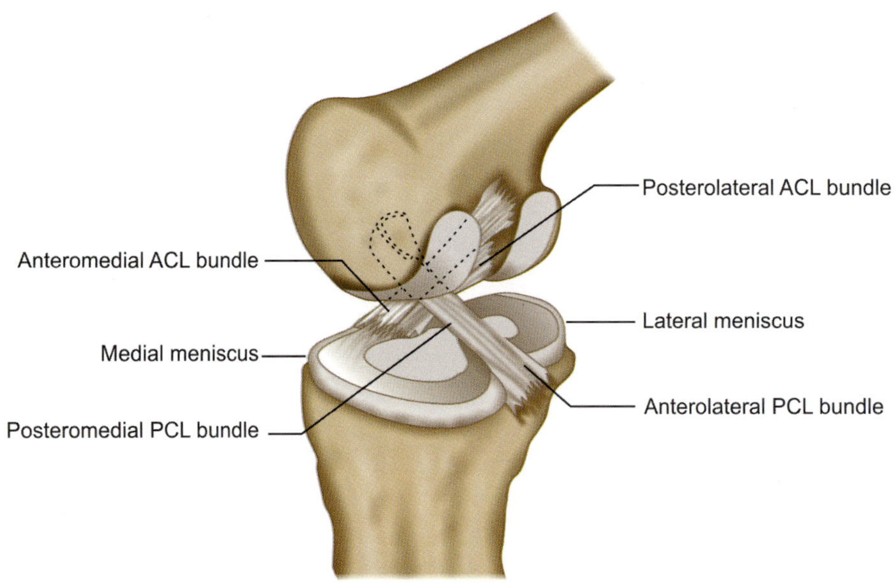

Fig. 33.1: Native anterior cruciate and posterior cruciate bundles function in close synergy with adjacent knee structures. (ACL: Anterior cruciate ligament; PCL: Posterior cruciate ligament).

of this chapter is to present a supplemental ACL rehabilitation progression based on restoration of normal active knee and hip range of motion, nonimpaired locomotor capabilities, lower extremity strength, power, and agility. Special consideration is placed on biologic, biomechanical, and psychobehavioral[9,10] healing factors, in addition to sport- and position-specific neuromuscular control. Early patient outcomes following 5 years of experience using this program are discussed.

MORE SURGICAL METHOD AND REHABILITATION TIMELINE OPTIONS

Today's knee surgeons and rehabilitation clinicians have an increasing number of treatment options.[8] With careful evaluation, some patients may not require immediate surgical intervention following ACL injury provided they display the coping characteristics deemed essential to continued safe function.[11] Similarly, with a growing appreciation for preserving native ACL characteristics such as mechanoreceptor dense regions, natural entheses, and remaining ligament viability postpartial tears, the surgeon may place greater attention on the possibility of ACL repair, associated biological and physiological healing time-frames,[12-14] and restoration, or at least significant recovery of premorbid neurosensory function.[8]

Over time, arthroscopic ACL reconstruction techniques have evolved from historical sole use of the bone-patellar tendon-bone autograft to an ever growing use of other autograft, allograft, xenograft, and synthetic graft options.[1,8,15,16] The multitude of graft options speaks to the inability of any current option to achieve a positive outcome that always satisfies the patient, the rehabilitation team, or the knee surgeon.[17] Additionally, autograft harvest is known to weaken structures adjacent to the graft harvest site and to negatively influence knee function.[18-20] Whichever option is being used, they are now being implanted with a greater appreciation for anatomical placement, minimization of further impairment associated with graft harvest or surgical method, and closer replication of double bundle, ribbon, or strand function.[8,21] Surgeons continue to seek the most efficacious procedure that minimizes the need for autogenous graft harvest, and preserves existing neurosensory proprioceptive structures when possible. Neurogenic mechanisms induce bone mineral density reduction from hip to heel on the side of ACL injury. Despite improvements in post-ACL reconstruction and rehabilitation, to date, it has not been firmly established that this key indicator of osseous function and health ever returns to its preinjury condition.[22] As ACL repair[12-14] becomes more efficacious for a growing number of patients, the surgical and rehabilitation team will be further challenged to identify the most effective rehabilitation progression and tissue loading timelines.

BE PROGRESSIVE AS NEEDED TO BUILD STRONG TISSUE, BUT DO NO HARM

Although the primary focus of postoperative ACL rehabilitation guidelines changes over time (Fig. 33.2), key principles exist over the entire continuum. These include:

- Creation of a rehabilitation environment that facilitates biologic, biomechanical, and psychobehavioral healing, while simultaneously using therapeutic exercise movement experiences to educate patients
- Do no harm

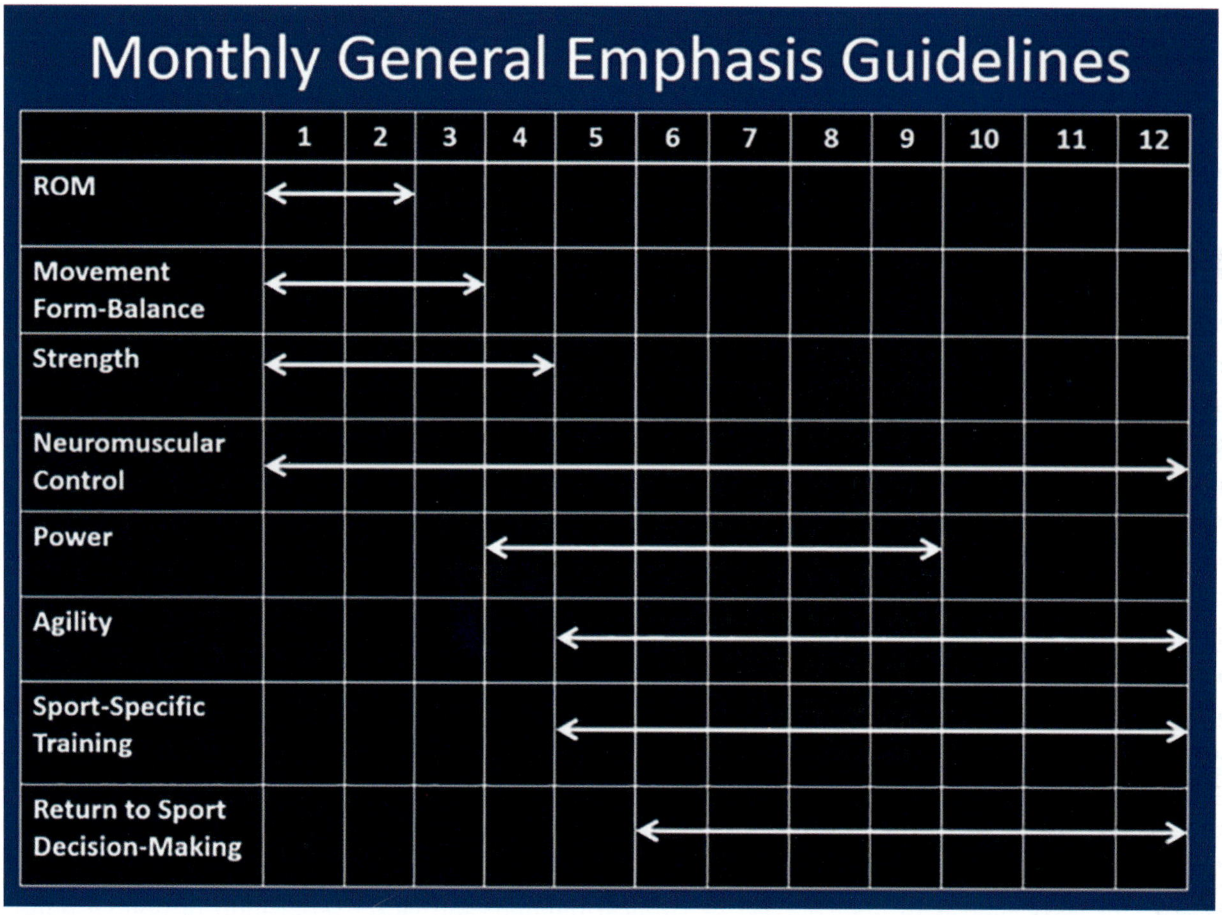

Fig. 33.2: Monthly general rehabilitation emphasis guidelines following anterior cruciate ligament reconstruction.

- Develop patient self-efficacy, cognitive appraisal, and resilience skills (multidimensional coping)
- Focus more on functional movement quality, only increasing total exercise volume, frequency, or load when appropriate movement form is consistent, and sufficient neuromuscular control is reestablished.

The program we describe has been used as a supplementary program for patients who desire to return to sports participation following ACL reconstruction. The 8-week program consists of weekly 2-hour duration functional exercise training supplemented by weekly progressive resistance single leg press exercises and baseline 2 mile jog/run (≤20 min/mile pace) to sport-specific sprinting requirement repeats. All patients that have participated in this program were status-post standard acute care physical therapy program participation. The program focused on the following weekly themes with each week adding unique nuances to the exercise program:

- Week 1: Basic functional movement instruction
- Week 2: Functional movement performance with resistance applied through a weighted vest (10% to 20% bodyweight load)
- Week 3: Double leg hops and jumps
- Week 4: Single leg hops and jumps

- Week 5: Agility maneuvers
- Week 6–8: Focus on weak points such as anaerobic capacity, single leg power, form, or general fatigue tolerance.

The patient completes the Knee Outcome Survey—Sports Activity Scale prior to beginning this program to obtain baseline information regarding perceived knee sports function capabilities.[23]

PROGRAM ENTRY

Postphysical therapy, most patients reported moderately perceived sports readiness levels of approximately 80% in response to the following question: "How would you rate the current function of your knee during sports activities on a scale from 0 to 100 with 100 being your level of knee function prior to your injury and 0 being the inability to perform any sports activities?"[23] However, when asked this question again just after completing the initial session of this more intensive supplemental training program, subjects reported a global score of approximately 50%. We surmise that this sudden drop in perceived function was related to the patient not having had experienced therapeutic exercises with similar intensity, or sports movement and metabolic energy system specificity during conventional physical therapy sessions. Based on this finding, we recommend that clinicians be extremely careful when using perceived function data to assist with return to play decision making. The patient's sports capability perceptions are loaded with bias, and less rigorous, early rehabilitation exercises performed in climate controlled environments with favorable rest: work ratios likely leads to an over estimation of their true sports capabilities. Self-efficacy measurements are only as valid as the relevance of the functional movement tasks they are linked with. If these measurements are linked solely with less intense, single repetition movement tasks performed in isolation from the abundant environmental, psychological, and physiological stressors associated with their sport, the patient may develop a false sense of confidence regarding their true sports capability readiness. This first element of the program we describe is re-setting the patient's perception of their actual readiness for returning to their sport.

RESTORE FULL FUNCTIONAL HIP, KNEE, AND ANKLE RANGE OF MOTION

An essential component of early rehabilitation following ACL injury and surgery is restoring full functional hip, knee, and ankle range of motion. In general, this progression smoothly transitions from pain-free active knee range of motion (with earlier reestablishment of knee extension) to balanced composite lower extremity movements, strength, power, agility, and sport-specific function. The priority of reestablishing proper neuromuscular control is an overarching programmatic goal.[1] Each of these factors should be restored prior to finalizing return to sport decision-making plans. Return to sports decision-making represents a multitiered, complex process which will be discussed in detail later in this chapter.

Typically, post-ACL reconstruction, the first priority is the reestablishment of nonimpaired passive and active terminal knee extension by quadriceps femoris muscle activation facilitation. This is essential to set the stage for neuromuscular control normalization during gait and to avoid early use of maladaptive overdependence on compensatory neuromuscular activation through the hip and ankle/subtalar joint musculature. Closely following restoration of nonimpaired active terminal knee extension in importance is reestablishing pain-free passive and active knee flexion in positions of function (with the hip positioned in degrees of extension). Rehabilitation clinicians are advised to avoid placing functional relevance on knee flexion range of motion or strength measurements performed with the hip in flexion (seated) or neutral (supine) as this may provide misleading measurements of true functional range of motion or strength. When posterior horn or root meniscal tears have been repaired, the rehabilitation clinician should delay knee flexion greater than 90° for several weeks to enable sufficient meniscal healing to occur. Nonimpaired, pain-free active knee extension and flexion range of motion is essential to prevent patellofemoral region irritation and knee extensor mechanism dysfunction. Even after early knee range of motion goals have been achieved, the rehabilitation clinician should re-check this essential foundational element to overall knee health on a regular basis, particularly as strength, power, agility, and sport-specific training task intensity increases. Decreased musculotendinous extensibility and increased stiffness are common maladaptive compensations for effective neuromuscular function.[24]

Some examples of essential hip-knee stretch maneuvers to achieve a more balanced hip-knee function following ACL reconstruction include:

- Prone high knee flexion with hip extension. This concurrently stretches the iliopsoas and hip portion of rectus femoris muscles in addition to stretching the vasti muscles (Fig. 33.3).
- Crossed knee to chest ("piriformis stretch") stretch (Fig. 33.4).
- Back-step, butt-kick with upright trunk (Fig. 33.5).
- Frontal plane side lunge with upright trunk and level pelvis (Fig. 33.6).[1]

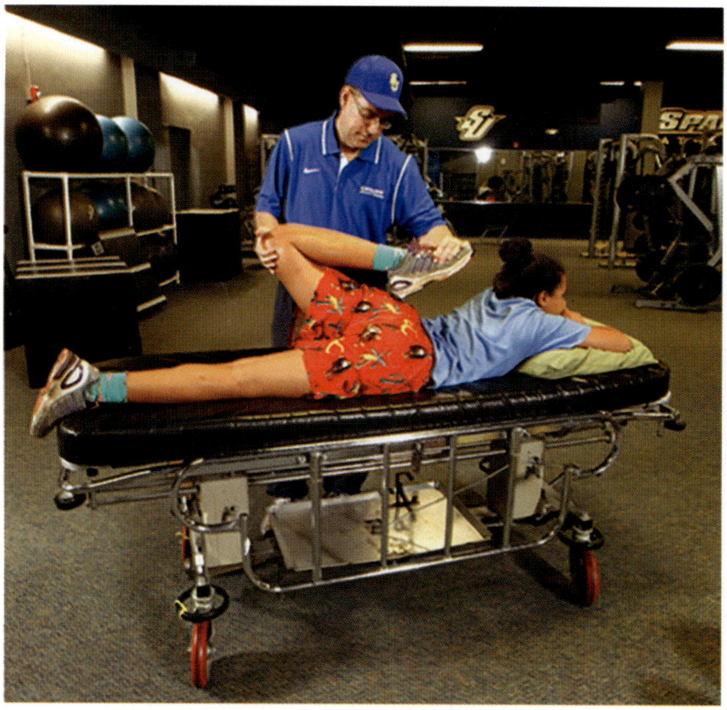

Fig. 33.3: Prone quadriceps femoris stretch (high knee flexion) and hip flexor stretch (with hip extension). It is important to confirm that musculotendinous extensibility has been restored and maintained in positions of sports function prior to adding resistance or otherwise increasing exercise intensity.

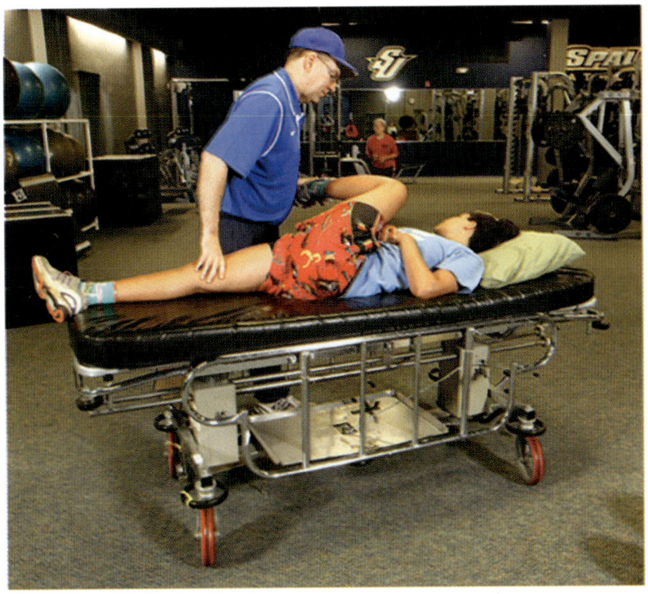

Fig. 33.4: Crossed knee to chest (piriformis stretch) to increase extensibility of hip extensor, abductor, and external rotator musculature.

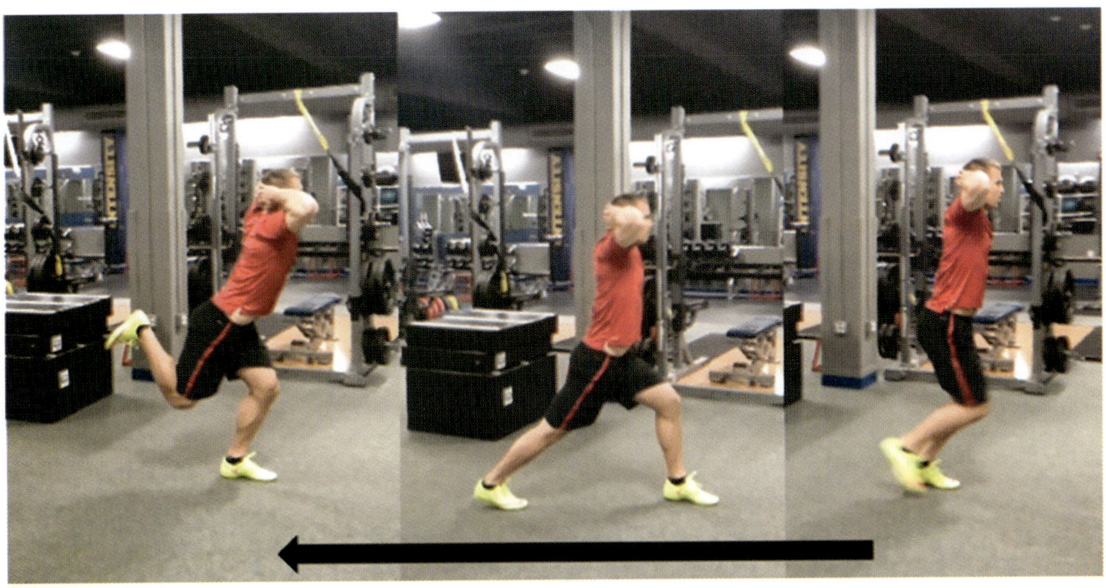

Fig. 33.5: Backstep-Butt kick. Dynamic high knee flexion with the hip and trunk extended. This maneuver dynamically stretches the hip flexors and rectus femoris, while active hamstring activation attempts to restore normal high end knee flexion. This movement is performed as the patient takes a series of slow, full backward steps while maintaining balance on the contralateral lower extremity.

The forward lunge with ipsilateral trunk rotation helps increase functional mobilization of the trunk and hips (Fig. 33.7). Two to three static stretch repetitions for each side held for 20–30 seconds are essential to restoring more balanced hip and knee joint mobility. Performance enhancing ballistic stretching is also performed during quicker performance tasks. Both static and dynamic stretching methods have unique benefits when appropriately placed within the rehabilitation program.[25]

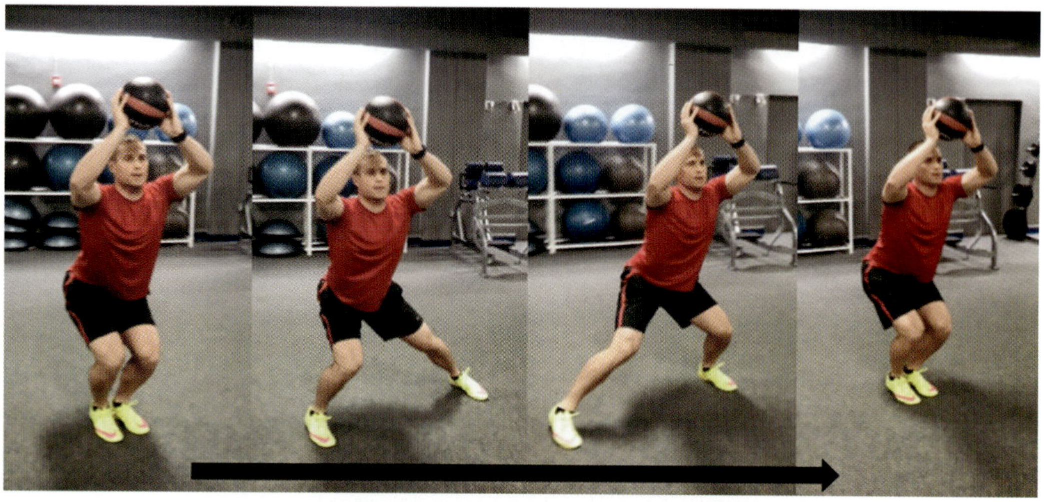

Fig. 33.6: Frontal plane side lunge with erect trunk, and level pelvis holding a medicine ball overhead. A dynamic movement intended to increase frontal plane hip muscle extensibility and strength while challenging knee extensor muscle function with knees maintained in approximately 30–40° of flexion.

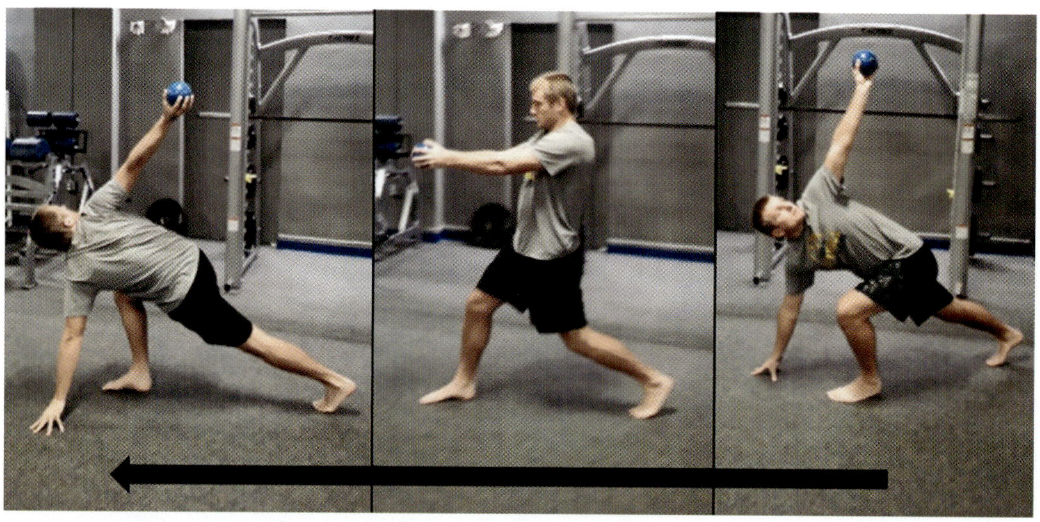

Fig. 33.7: Forward lunge with ipsilateral trunk rotation helps increase functional mobility of the trunk and hips.

MULTIPLANAR LOCOMOTION

Some examples of early locomotion form maneuvers that integrate hip-knee-ankle muscle function include:

- The imposed "knee wobble" progression (Figs. 33.8A to D)[26]
- Multidirectional matrix movement stepping (Fig. 33.9)
- Form run simulation (Fig. 33.10)
- Single leg "speed skater" maneuvers (Fig. 33.11).

Each of these tasks focuses on restoration of local knee range of motion objectives within the context of balanced knee-hip-ankle/subtalar joint mobility and maintenance of a level pelvis and upright trunk. These movements are performed slowly, with rehabilitation clinician feedback as needed to ensure

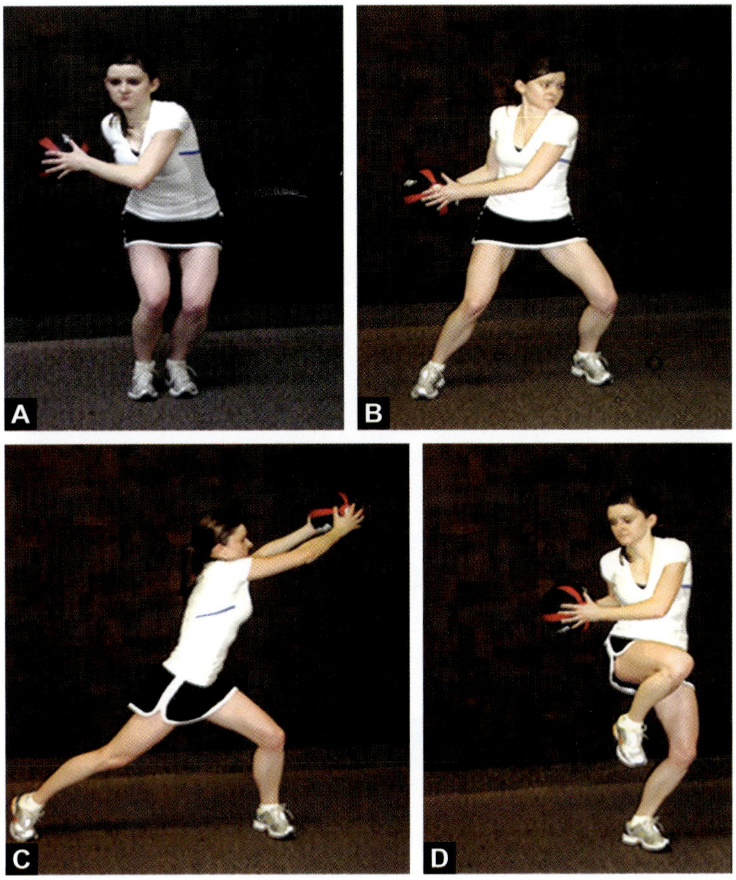

Figs. 33.8A to D: Side lunge with long axis rotation. This movement induces a "knee wobble". Steps "C" and "D" are repeated three times before the patient takes another side lunge and repeats the movement sequence.

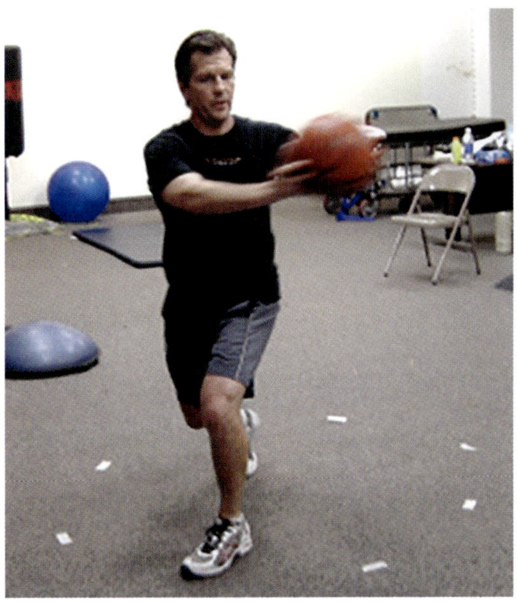

Fig. 33.9: Multiplanar "Matrix" stepping. This exercise sequence effectively integrates trunk long axis rotation with bilateral hip-knee-ankle function. The patient performs this movement slowly for a 3-minute set duration.

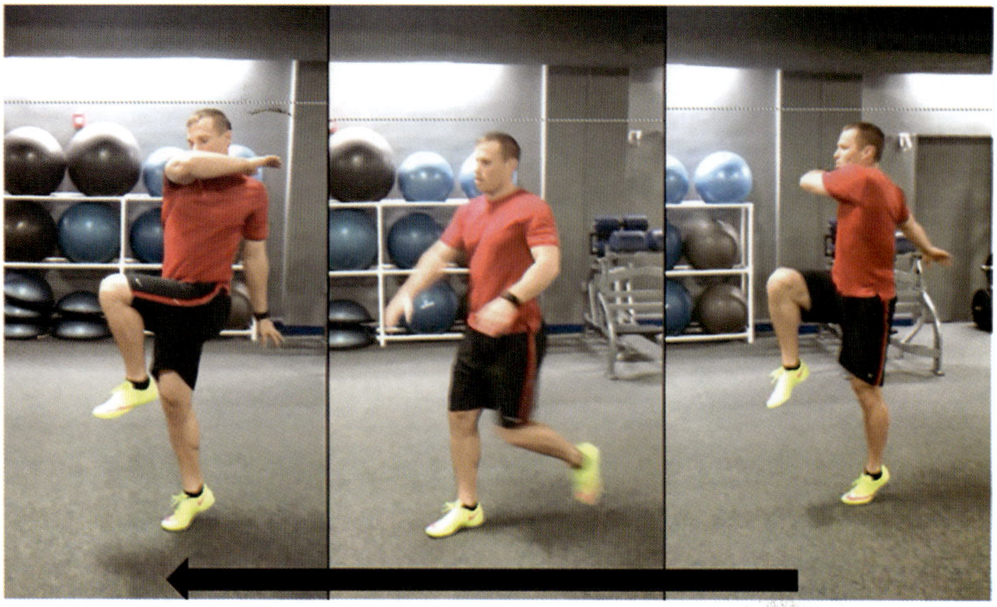

Fig. 33.10: Form run simulation. A slow speed simulation of running during which the patient rotates their upper body in the opposite direction of the lower body and holds a single leg support balance position for approximately 2–3 seconds.

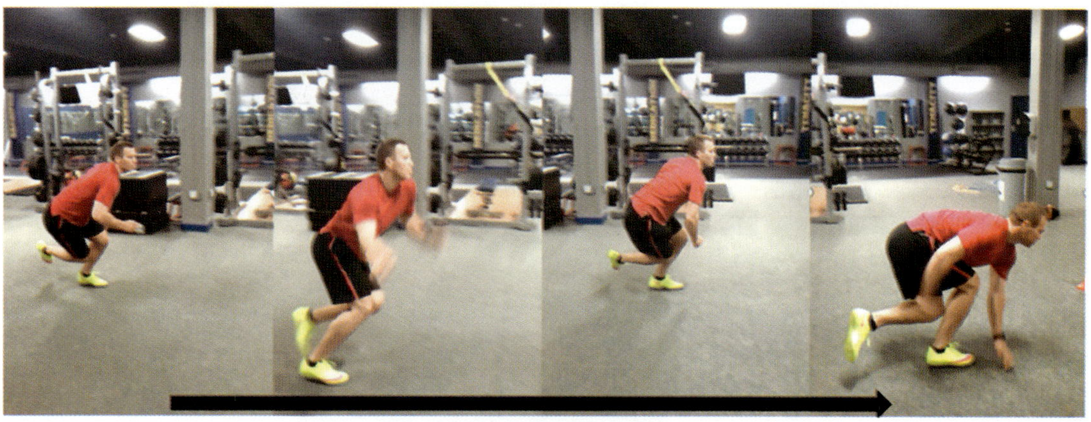

Fig. 33.11: Single leg "speed skater" movement. Beginning and finishing on the surgical lower extremity, the patient performs a quick diagonal side step toward the surgical side, followed by a similar movement to the nonsurgical side, before finishing on the surgical side and maintaining appropriate trunk and lower extremity posture for approximately 2–3 seconds with approximately 20–30° of knee flexion.

patient education of proper technique. By moving slowly, the presence of any underlying lower extremity or trunk strength, range of motion, or balance impairments or significant side-to-side asymmetries can be more easily identified and corrected.

STRENGTH TRAINING, NEUROMUSCULAR CONTROL, AND BALANCE TRAINING INTEGRATION

In addition to normalizing pain-free passive and active knee mobility prior to transitioning too quickly into the functional training realm (particularly with single leg hopping progressions), it is also essential to restore adequate foundational strength throughout the involved lower extremity, particularly at the quadriceps femoris, hip abductors-extensors-external rotators, and ankle plantar flexors.[1] In addition to restoring full range terminal knee extension, rehabilitation clinicians should be cognizant of restoring high knee flexion function (greater than 110°) with the hip in slight to moderate extension. This important sports movement requirement is often lacking long after ACL reconstruction, particularly when bone-patellar tendon-bone or quadriceps tendons (knee extensor healing stiffness), or hamstring autograft (knee flexor weakness) are used.[20] In addition to progressive resistance single leg presses with a focus on a 12-12-10-10-8-8 repetition (progressively handling resistance greater than or equal to bodyweight), patients also perform single leg lateral step-up movements with an upright trunk and a ball held overhead (Figs. 33.12A and B), and lateral "scissor" planks (Fig. 33.13). This plank movement facilitates isometric or eccentric "negative" neuromuscular activation at the floor side lower extremity and concentric "positive" neuromuscular activation at the top side lower extremity. This helps prepare the lower extremity and core for integrated hip-knee function during single leg jump landings.[27] During lateral "scissor" plank performance, the patient is instructed to generate "length before lift", and to raise the top side lower extremity in an "up and back" diagonal path to optimize hip abductor-extensor-external rotator function. With weight bearing or closed kinetic chain type movements such as single leg squats (Figs. 33.14A to C), single leg flexed knee "deadlifts", and supine heel walking, the focus is placed on restoring dynamic mid-range knee stability, particularly if the patient displays positive lower extremity Beighton sign scores.[28] Identification of positive Beighton joint hypermobility scores as evidenced by hyperextension laxity, or soft and lax joint end feels with valgus-varus stress testing suggests less than ideal capsuloligamentous contributions to dynamic knee stability. Individuals with this predisposition should focus rehabilitation attention almost exclusively on restoring mid-range neuromuscular control of dynamic knee stability, avoiding

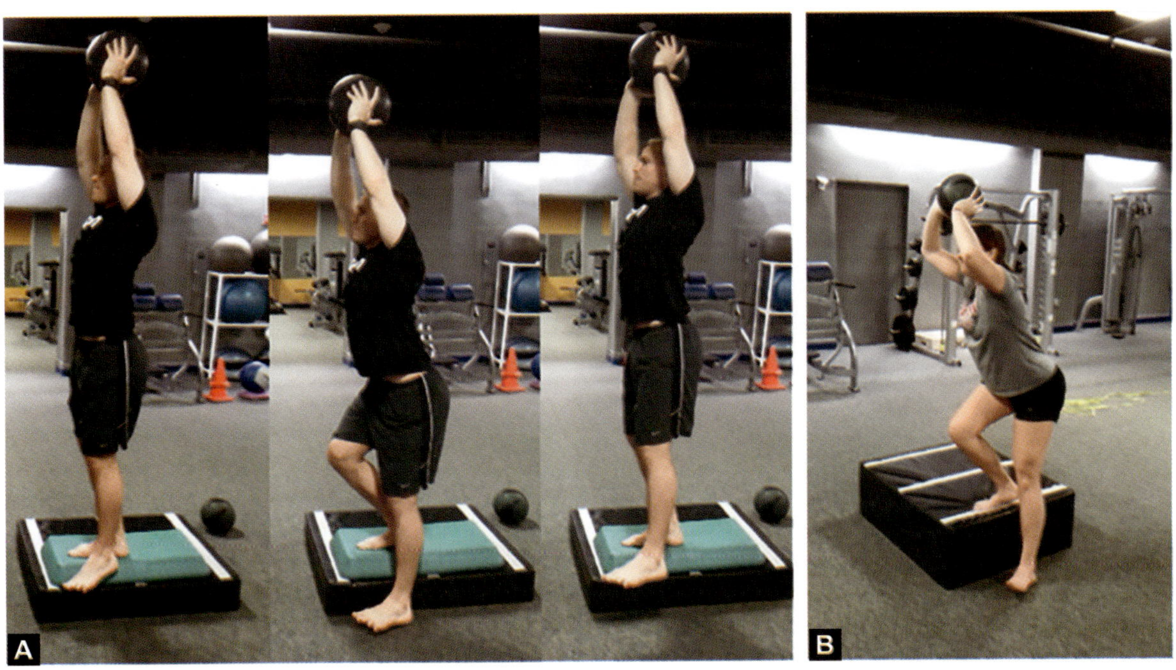

Figs. 33.12A and B: Single leg lateral step-ups with appropriate trunk alignment indicating balanced use of hip, knee, and ankle extensors (A), and with inappropriate trunk alignment signifying compensatory hip extensor use substituting for quadriceps femoris function (B).

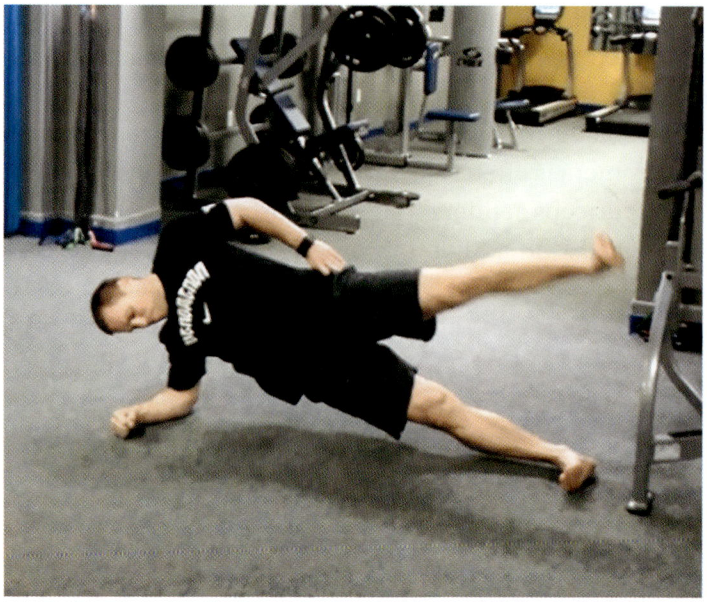

Fig. 33.13: Lateral scissor planks. An excellent method of integrating sagittal plane knee extensor function with frontal plane hip abductor-extensor-external rotator, and trunk strength. This integration is vital to multiplanar control of the knee during single leg jump landing performance.

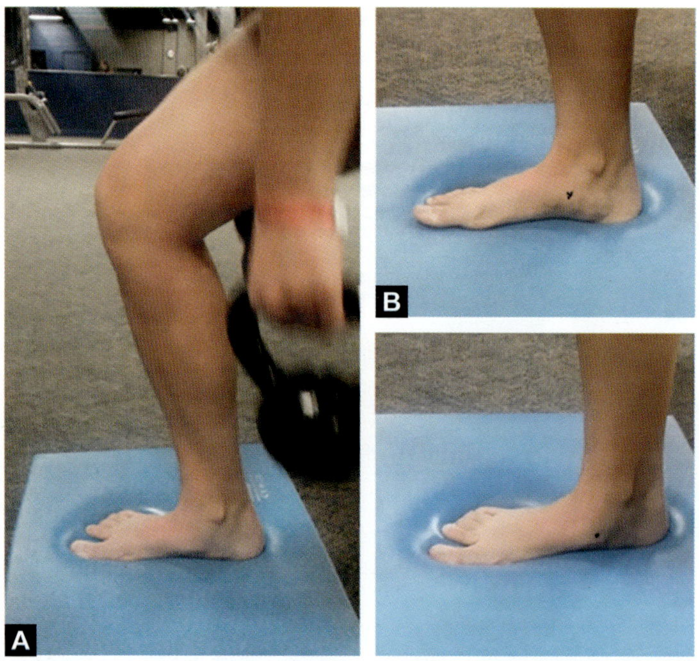

Figs. 33.14A to C: Single leg squats performed without shoes or socks on an AirEx balance pad (AirEx AG, Switzerland) (A). Barefoot training enables focused neuromuscular control training of ankle and subtalar joint musculature (B and C). The black dot signifies tarsal navicular movement.

repetitious end range during therapeutic exercise activities that further increases knee laxity. Use of soft tissue autografts or allografts for ACL reconstruction among patients with these predispositions may be contraindicated for fear of graft elongation or tunnel pullout. Should they be used, back-up fixation should be considered and the rehabilitation progression should be delayed with increased focus placed on proper lower extremity biomechanical alignment and neuromuscular control during single leg hop and jump landings.[29]

It is essential that the rehabilitation clinician helps the patient learn to move more effectively from the "athletic ready position" to the postures assumed during the performance of planned and unplanned sport specific movements, as well as recovery from falls, near falls, and collisions.[1] This becomes particularly important as the patient advances toward release from care and return to unrestricted sports participation. The rehabilitation clinician needs to evaluate the patient for consistent use of appropriate, safe technique without favoring the surgical side lower extremity. This is an excellent opportunity to facilitate enhanced somatosensory system recovery by denying vision (decreased exteroceptive input) during select, double to single leg low impact or no impact stepping movements.[1,26]

RESTORING SUFFICIENT LOWER EXTREMITY POWER TO PREVENT REINJURY

In addition to improving mid-range dynamic knee stability, more advanced lower extremity neuromuscular control exercise activities help the patient prepare for double or single leg hopping progressions.[30-33] Maneuvers performed at this time include: Chop-step–single leg hop stabilization (Fig. 33.15), squatting on a full sphere Bosu ball with bumper protection (Fig. 33.16), and group dual task performance such as tossing and catching a ball, medicine ball handoffs on paired Bosu balls (Fig. 33.17). Prior to initiating a double-to-single leg hopping task progression, the rehabilitation clinician evaluates movement quality of slower, small amplitude movements both with and without athletic footwear use. Removal of the foot cushioning and arch control characteristics of athletic footwear can enable the rehabilitation clinician

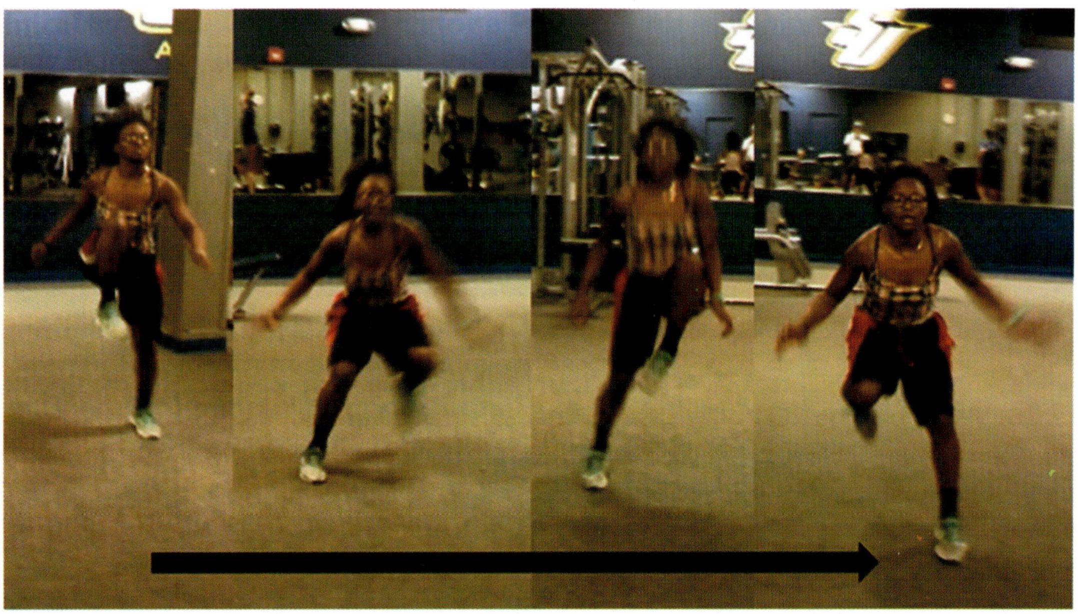

Fig. 33.15: Chop-step-single leg stabilization. From an athletic ready position, the patient does alternating high knee to chest movements for five repetitions before hopping diagonally to stabilize on a single lower extremity and holding for 2–3 seconds with appropriate trunk, and lower extremity alignment and with the knee maintained in 20–30° of flexion.

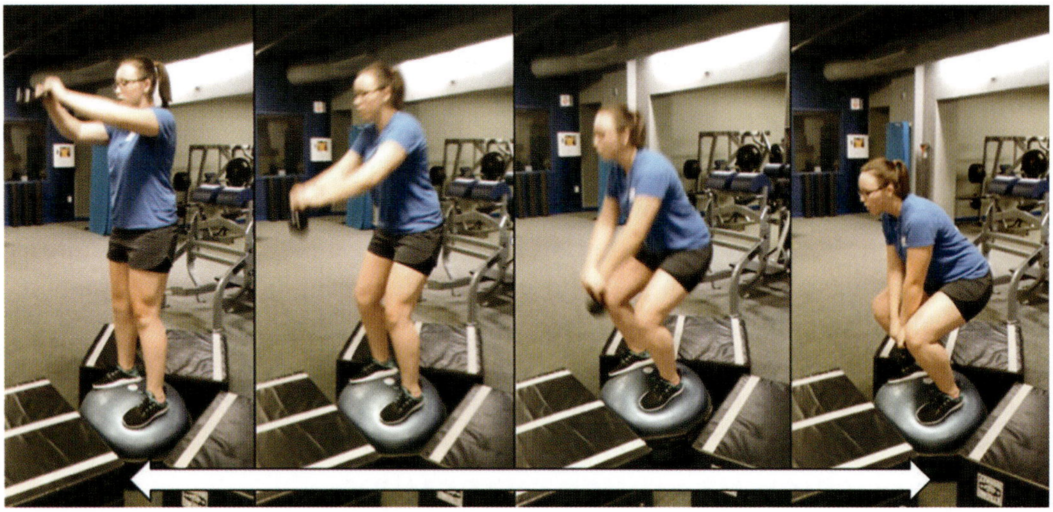

Fig. 33.16: Squatting on a whole sphere Bosu ball with bumper protection. This movement while performing kettle bell swings creates a dynamic postural control challenge as the patient moves from the athletic ready position to a squat position.

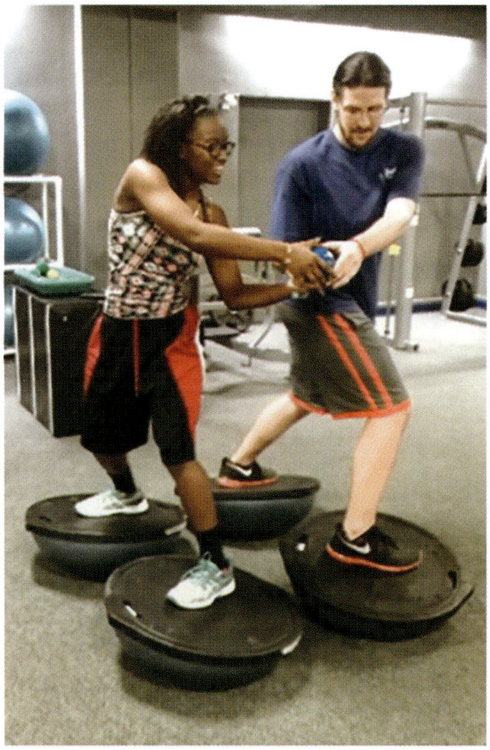

Fig. 33.17: Side-to-side passing of a medicine ball on paired Bosu balls.

to more easily identify functional movement impairments. Since bone mineral density is likely reduced throughout the involved lower extremity following ACL injury, surgery, and rehabilitation,[22] athletic footwear (albeit with reduced heel height to more functionally tension the Achilles tendon and increase soleus extensibility)[24] should be worn during higher intensity, higher volume plyometric movement task performance to avoid exacerbation of bone stress reactions.

During plyometric task performance, the rehabilitation clinician should be vigilant in establishing that involved side lower extremity favoring is not evident and that single leg propulsion and landing movements and postures are near symmetrical. As mentioned earlier, but of particular importance during higher impact task performance is the need for high-quality movement technique, with evidence of appropriate knee flexion, and balanced use of the hips, knees, and ankle/subtalar joints without excessive anterior or lateral trunk lean. Excessive or poorly controlled trunk lean is directly associated with impaired hip and/or knee strength or neuromuscular control.[27] An essential purpose for plyometric task performance is to better facilitate fast twitch muscle fiber contributions to both negative (lengthening eccentric) and positive (shortening concentric) neuromuscular activation.[34,35] For this to occur the entire lower extremity (hip-knee-ankle), but particularly the knee must move from relative extension to controlled composite lower extremity flexion, and then back to extension (stretch-shortening cycle) in a quick, efficient manner. This optimizes the amortization phase of eccentric-concentric neuromuscular activation with maximal fast twitch muscle fiber contributions occurring in <0.2 seconds. During the performance of multiplanar plyometric tasks, the patient experiences the functional dilemma of attempting to move with powerful, near maximal or maximal effort single or double leg propulsion while also displaying soft, controlled landings. The plyometric progression includes bilateral kangaroo hops (Fig. 33.18), frog hops (Fig. 33.19), double and single leg crossover hopping over a tape (Fig. 33.20), two-leg lateral hops with one leg landing, retro-hop movements, sagittal and frontal plane mini-trampoline depth hops (Fig. 33.21).[1,26,36]

Ultimately, to safely return to sports, the patient needs to resume the "athlete role" and leave the "patient role",[37,38] not letting knee joint-related thoughts drive negative behaviors associated with fear, lack of confidence, or depression.[39] One way that we support this concept is to let patients get a drink or take a rest at any time during early program stages. However, when they are ready to go, the expectation is that the task will be completed with high attention to detail. The performance objective is to successfully complete the task effectively no matter its intensity level or duration, just like when stepping onto the field to compete in a sport.

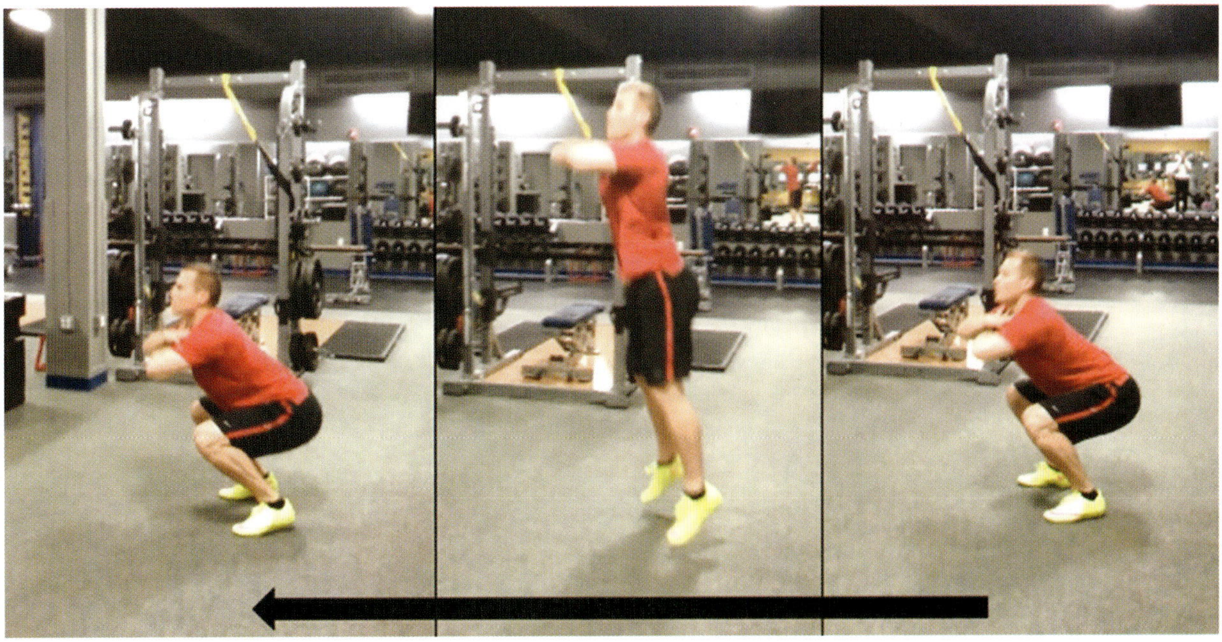

Fig. 33.18: Kangaroo hopping to initiate simple, symmetrical bilateral stretch-shortening neuromuscular activation.

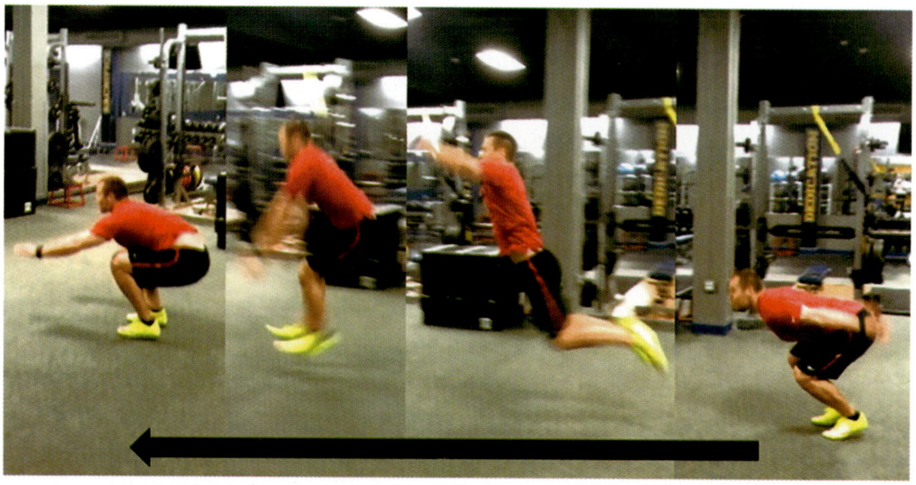

Fig. 33.19: Frog hopping to initiate balanced, explosive symmetrical bilateral stretch-shortening neuromuscular activation.

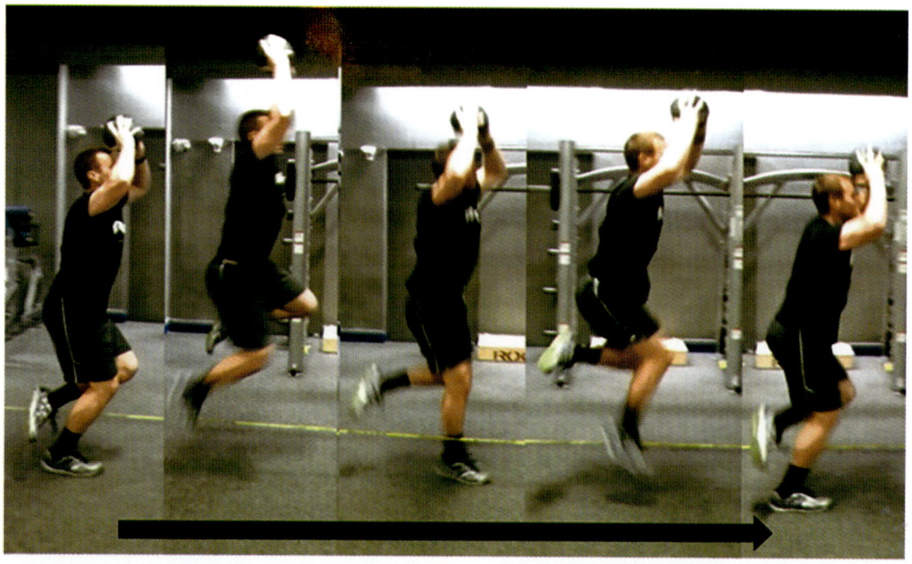

Fig. 33.20: Single leg crossover hopping. A demanding test of single lower extremity dynamic power and sudden knee stability readiness.

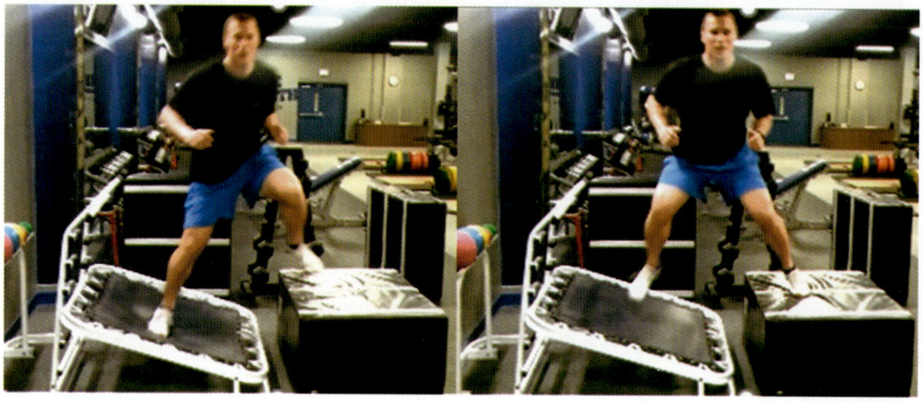

Fig. 33.21: Frontal plane mini-trampoline depth hops. An explosive method of training high intensity, integrated trunk-lower extremity neuromuscular control.

RESTORING FUNCTIONAL AGILITY

When single leg plyometric tasks reveal approximately 70% bilateral power equivalence and acceptable form, agility maneuvers are initiated moving from slow-to-fast velocities, from small-to-large amplitude tasks, from more exploratory to more performatory movements, from more planned to progressively less planned and more chaotic movements, while always focusing on movement quality over specific time, distance, or total volume performance metrics. During all functional movements, it is important that the patient attempt to perform high-quality movements, but not be afraid to make mistakes. Attempting to be perfect in performance tends to decrease the creativity, natural movement variability, and the educational and coping process development needed to better assure return to play readiness. Additionally, constrained lower extremity movement patterns post-ACL injury, surgery, and rehabilitation are believed to contribute to the more focal articular cartilage contact pressures that precede knee osteoarthritis development. Examples of agility tasks include the 3-cone agility drill (short-ball-tall) (Fig. 33.22), and the 10-meter (m) circuit board progression (Figs. 33.23A and B).

FUNCTIONAL TRAINING FOR SPECIFIC SPORTS, SPORT POSITIONS, AND METABOLIC ENERGY SYSTEM NEEDS

The rehabilitation clinician is encouraged to have a sound understanding of the patients' anaerobic and aerobic metabolic capacity and the requirements of their sport, position within that sport, and role in the team. Eventually the patient will indeed need to practice themselves into sports shape. However, if they are allowed to return to sport-specific training while deconditioned, they are at greater risk of knee reinjury or injury to their contralateral knee. For example, short (<10 second) duration, high-intensity tasks require efficient anaerobic adenosine-triphosphate/creatine phosphate system function and recovery. To develop this capacity, the athlete needs to perform multiple

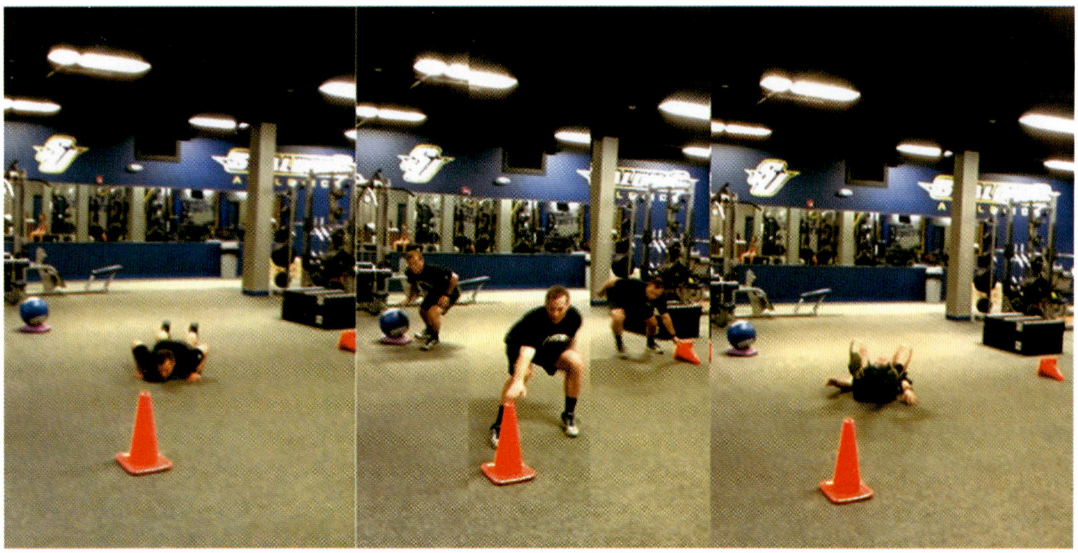

Fig. 33.22: Three cone agility drill (short-ball-tall). This exercise trains and evaluates quick multidirectional movement capability, the ability to get up and down from the ground quickly, and cue responsiveness for 30 seconds duration repeats.

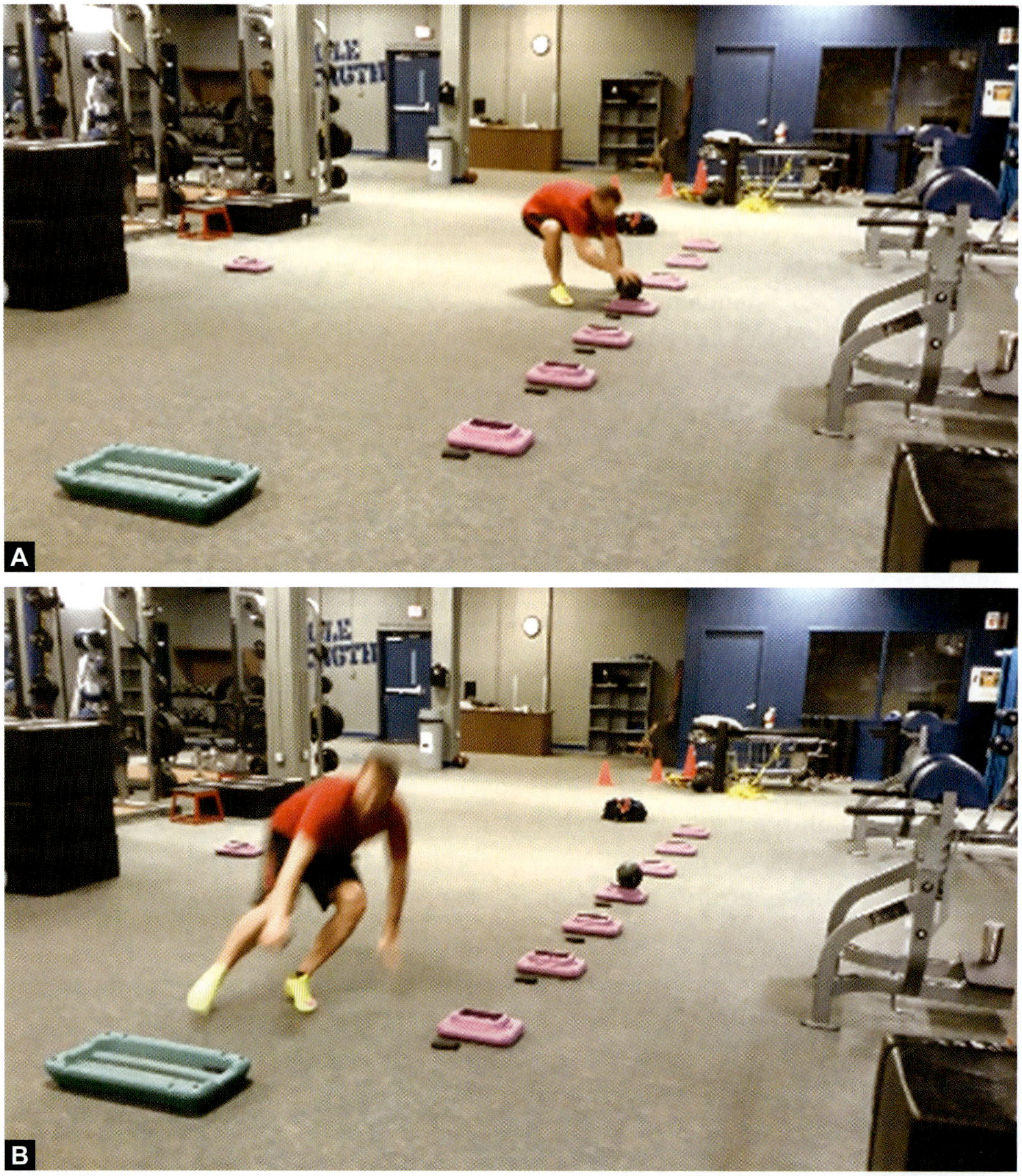

Figs. 33.23A and B: Circuit board directional change progression. This exercise trains and evaluates quick, repeated cutting movements while moving a 4 pound (1.8 kg) medicine ball (A) from socket to socket to transfer a small soft weight (1 pound = 0.45 kg) to scoring bins (B).

≤10 second duration task repetitions with a 3:1 rest to work ratio to facilitate recovery. Athletes such as soccer midfielders and basketball guards make greater use of anaerobic glycolysis with continuous high-intensity task durations of up to 2 minutes. Athletes such as these need to train using a series of ≥2 minute task duration repeats and closer to a 2:1 rest to work ratio. All sports have at least a baseline aerobic energy system requirement which generally gets addressed earlier in the rehabilitation progression. Even for sports that display predominantly anaerobic energy system needs, establishing a minimum aerobic conditioning base is important. Determining the ease with which a recovering athlete can run a 2-3 mile distance following ACL reconstruction can provide useful information about baseline aerobic conditioning. This activity also provides essential information about knee shock absorber system robustness, and pain sensitivity at the knee joint line, patellofemoral joint, and ACL reconstruction tunnel regions. Greater attention to the rehabilitating athlete's anaerobic and aerobic metabolic energy system needs earlier during rehabilitation program development can pay huge dividends later when they advance to sport-specific training.

KNEE BRACING

Just as surgeons and rehabilitation clinicians have more options to consider regarding surgical or nonsurgical approaches following ACL injury, the options are similarly abundant regarding the use of functional knee braces. Surgical and rehabilitation approaches have evolved from nonanatomic, single strand reconstruction for all patients to greater consideration of physiological native ACL functional preservation, anatomic partial or complete single or double bundle reconstruction in certain cases, and nonsurgical approaches in other cases. The philosophical rationale behind functional brace use needs to similarly evolve. While functional brace use following ACL reconstruction using soft tissue grafts in a patient with significantly positive Beighton laxity signs would seem prudent,[40,41] it must be understood that this type of bracing also tends to alter lower extremity running kinematics, muscle activation patterns, and knee joint range of motion. The transition from solely mechanocentric ACL reconstruction approaches to greater consideration of native ACL neurosensory contributions to function and biological tissue healing suggests the need for greater consideration for the different brace use purposes. This may be an ideal time for manufacturers to develop braces that more prescriptively ensure the tissue loading and off-loading needed to both prevent reinjury and to facilitate effective tissue remodeling. Given the increasing use of biological tissue growth and healing factors derived from platelet rich plasma, stem cells, and amniotic membrane tissue, it seems logical that bracing should similarly transition from providing more rigid, consistent restrictions to enabling progressively greater tissue loading while not adversely affecting knee joint and lower extremity neuromuscular function. Perhaps bracing systems might evolve to better support the suture, tape, and tissue-based internal scaffolding and bracing systems that are increasingly in use.

RETURN TO PLAY READINESS EVALUATION

The evaluation process that we use includes five categories: (1) movement form, (2) dynamic knee stability, (3) lower extremity power, (3) agility-reaction time, and (5) endurant skill performance.[29,36] Some examples of form movements include the form run simulation, lateral shuffles, and forward lunge-trunk rotations. Dynamic knee stability tests include the 20 m single-leg timed crossover hop and a triple hop for distance (Fig. 33.24). Lower extremity power tasks include 20 m frog hops and 20 m kangaroo hops, and 40 m sprints with directional change cutting for three repetitions. An example of an agility-reaction time activity is the previously described 3-cone triangle agility maneuver. Endurant skill tasks are very sport and position-specific. Some examples include dribble-drive lay-up and three-point shot repeats by basketball players and ball control, touch pass, cross, cross return, goal strike repeats for soccer players. A total of 3–5 tasks are selected for each category. At this time the patient also completes the Knee Outcome Survey–Sports Activity Scale a second time to obtain more current perceived knee sports function capability information.[23]

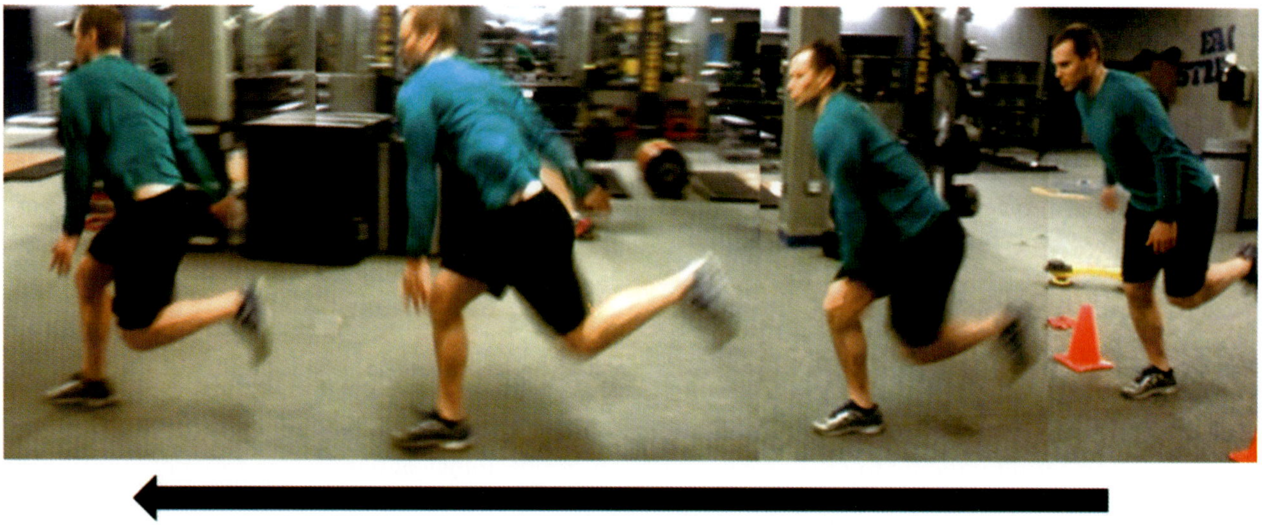

Fig. 33.24: Single leg triple hop for distance test. A dynamic test that challenges stretch-shortening cycle power and ability to dynamically stabilize on the flexed surgical knee while maintaining appropriate trunk and lower extremity neuromuscular alignment for 2–3 seconds.

RETURN TO PLAY DECISION-MAKING

The decision for when it is safe to return a patient back to unrestricted sports participation following ACL injury and surgery is both difficult and complex. This should include a blend of objective with subjective physical and psychobehavioral function measurements. To improve both measurement validity and generalizability, these tests should display elements of peripheral or central neuromuscular fatigue, unexpected, somewhat chaotic movement requirements, and/or spontaneous combined movement task-cognitive challenges. Having a solid understanding of how the recovering athlete performs under less than ideal physical, mental, and environmental conditions greatly improves the likelihood of obtaining the meaningful data needed to make such an important decision. Even after it has been decided that an athlete is ready to return to sports practice activities, this in itself represents another level of decision-making. Sports practices usually represent a combination of general conditioning drills, general skill development drills, individual position-specific skill and tactical development drills, and team skill development and tactical strategy drills unique to particular sports and styles of play within a given sport. Related to the knee reinjury risk from contact mechanisms is the number of players that are located in close proximity to each other. The likelihood that sudden contact, collisions, falling to the ground or upon one another will occur when players are in close proximity adds another element of risk to these decisions. For this reason, we recommend a multitiered and variably-paced return to practice approach. This begins with performing more isolated conditioning activities at practice, followed by full team conditioning activities, individual general skill development drills, individual position-specific skill development drills, small group (2–3 players) general skill development drills, and small group position-specific skill development drills prior to returning to full team skill and tactical development drills, intrasquad scrimmaging, and full competition. These tiers provide an opportunity for the rehabilitation clinician to observe the athlete under progressively more intense activities, with progressively greater physical contact. This provides an important transition zone and time period for the athlete to truly become cognitively aware of their competitive readiness. This progression may occur over 2 to 4 weeks or it may be more condensed into a shorter timeframe provided the athlete displays evidence of moving normally with sufficient dynamic knee stability, does not favor his/her injured lower extremity and does not display any evidence of knee effusion.

Even following successful release to full competition, we ask that athletes include specific therapeutic exercises in a regular neuromuscular control training maintenance program. This is based on perceived need for continued work on neuromuscular control of the hip and trunk, single leg standing balance, stretching to maintain hip and low back region range of motion, or any other characteristic that suggests that further improvement may be achieved. In following this program over the last 5 years, we have experienced quite low reinjury rates from noncontact mechanisms, significantly higher perceived sports function, and generally comparable bilateral functional performance test results.[36]

POST-PROGRAM PARTICIPATION OUTCOMES

Based on reset baseline perceived knee sports function values, Knee Outcome Survey—Sports Activity Scale scores improved approximately 80% following program participation. Objective field testing revealed no difference for 20 m single leg timed crossover hop performance. A statistically significant mean difference of 0.2 second was observed for the 20 m single leg timed hop, with slower speeds using the surgical side; however, 96% bilateral equivalence was restored. Triple hop for distance also revealed a statistically significant mean difference of 0.18 m; however, 95% bilateral equivalence was restored. Measurements such as these were not performed at program-entry, as our perception was that many patients could not withstand such rigorous tests without considerable reinjury or new injury risk.

Patients were also asked: "How would you rate the overall function of your knee during sports activities?" (Please check the one response that best describes you.) Response options included severely abnormal, abnormal, nearly normal, or normal. Seventy percent of the patients improved by two levels, moving from abnormal to normal. This was a highly significant finding and in combination with the objective test results it provides compelling evidence for the efficacy of this program.

REINJURY STATUS

All 80 patients returned to sports at their previous sports intensity level. At 5 years following program participation, only two subjects had reinjured their knee. Both of these injuries were related to direct contact. One occurred while the athlete was playing American college football and the other was from an off-road motorcycle racing accident. The overall ACL reinjury rate was 2.5%. Given the level of sports function to which the athletes returned, this is considered an excellent outcome.[42]

SUMMARY

Following ACL injury and surgery we recommend early correction or minimization of the influence of both knee and associated impairments and conditions such as hip weakness, and the development of an active neuromuscular control learning environment. Within this context, the physical therapist and athletic trainer carefully guide clients through difficult

Contd...

Contd...

neuromusculoskeletal functional performance recovery, coping behaviors, and cognitive appraisal experiences. The combination of evidence-based objective clinical and field testing with perceived function assessment data collected during valid test conditions greatly improves the meaningfulness of these data. This factor greatly helps the rehabilitation clinician advise, advocate for, and administer the return to sports participation plan. Criterion-based return to play assessments are evolving rapidly.[43-45] With a growing understanding of central nervous system and bilateral lower extremity compensations and impairments following ACL injury and appreciation for psychobehavioral factors such as self-efficacy, kinesiophobia, and depression, researchers are developing criterion-based inventories that will further strengthen the decision-making process.

REFERENCES

1. Nyland J, Mattocks A, Kibbe S, et al. Anterior cruciate ligament reconstruction, rehabilitation, and return to play: 2015 update. Open Access J Sports Med. 2016;7:21-32.
2. Ardern CL, Webster KE, Taylor NF, et al. Return to sport following anterior cruciate ligament reconstruction surgery: a systematic review and meta-analysis of the state of play. Br J Sports Med. 2011;45:596-606.
3. Ardern CL, Webster KE, Taylor NF, et al. Return to the preinjury level of competitive sport after anterior cruciate ligament reconstruction surgery. Two-thirds of patients have not returned by 12 months after surgery. Am J Sports Med. 2011;39:538-43.
4. Swanik C. Brains and sprains: the brain's role in noncontact anterior cruciate ligament injuries. J Athl Train. 2015;50:1100-2.
5. Lepley AS, Gribble PA, Thomas AC, et al. Quadriceps neural alterations in anterior cruciate ligament reconstructed patients: a 6-month longitudinal investigation. Scan J Med Sci Sports. 2015;25:828-39.
6. Grooms D, Appelbaum G, Onate J. Neuroplasticity following anterior cruciate ligament injury: A framework for visual-motor training approaches to rehabilitation. J Orthop Sports Phys Ther. 2015;5:381-93.
7. Windhorst U. Muscle spindles are multi-functional. Brain Res Bull. 2008;28;75(5):507-8.
8. Nyland J, Gamble C, Franklin T, et al. Permanent knee sensorimotor system changes following ACL injury and surgery. Knee Surg Sports Traumatol Arthrosc. 2017 Feb 2. doi: 10.1007/s00167-017-4432-y.
9. Langford JL, Webster KE, Feller JA. A prospective longitudinal study to assess psychological changes following anterior cruciate ligament reconstruction surgery. Br J Sports Med. 2009;43:377-81.
10. Kvist J, Ek A, Sporrstedt K, et al. Fear of re-injury: a hindrance for returning to sports after anterior cruciate ligament reconstruction. Knee Surg Sports Traumatol Arthrosc. 2005;13:393-7.
11. Rudolph KS, Axe MJ, Snyder-Mackler L. Dynamic stability after ACL injury: who can hop? Knee Surg Sports Traumatol Arthrosc. 2000;8(5):262-9.
12. Vavken P, Fleming BC, Mastrangelo AN, et al. Biomechanical outcomes after bioenhanced anterior cruciate ligament repair and anterior cruciate ligament reconstruction are equal in a porcine model. Arthroscopy. 2012;28:672-680.
13. Vavken P, Murray MM. The potential for primary repair of the ACL. Sports Med Arthrosc. 2011;19:44-9.
14. Farraro KF, Sasaki N, Woo SL, et al. Magnesium ring device to restore function of a transected anterior cruciate ligament in the goat stifle joint. J Orthop Res. 2016;34:2001-8.
15. Wei J, Yang HB, Qin JB, et al. A meta-analysis of anterior cruciate ligament reconstruction with autograft compared with nonirradiated allograft. Knee. 2015;22:372-9.
16. Chahal J, Lee A, Heard W, et al. A retrospective review of anterior cruciate ligament reconstruction using patellar tendon: 25 years of experience. Orthop J Sports Med. 2013;1(3):2325967113501789.
17. Foster TE, Wolfe BL, Ryan S, et al. Does the graft source really matter in the outcome of patients undergoing anterior cruciate ligament reconstruction? An evaluation of autograft versus allograft reconstruction results: a systematic review. Am J Sports Med. 2010;38:189-99.
18. Inderhaug E, Strand T, Solheim E. The impact of sensory deficits after harvesting hamstrings autograft for ACL reconstruction. Knee Surg Sports Traumatol Arthrosc. 2015;23:1060-4.
19. Li S, Chen Y, Lin Z, et al. A systematic review of randomized controlled clinical trials comparing hamstring autografts versus bone-patellar tendon-bone autografts for the reconstruction of the anterior cruciate ligament. Arch Orthop Trauma Surg. 2012;132:1287-97.

20. Elmlinger BS, Nyland JA, Tillett ED. Knee flexor function 2 years after anterior cruciate ligament reconstruction with semitendinous-gracilis autografts. Arthroscopy. 2006;22:650-5.
21. Śmigielski R, Zdanowicz U, Drwięga M, et al. The anatomy of the anterior cruciate ligament and its relevance to the technique of reconstruction. Bone Joint J. 2016;98B:1020-6.
22. Nyland J, Fisher B, Brand E, et al. Osseous deficits after anterior cruciate ligament injury and reconstruction: A systematic review with suggestions to improve osseous homeostasis. Arthroscopy. 2010;26:1248-57.
23. Ross MD, Irrgang JJ, Denegar CR, et al. The relationship between participation restrictions and selected clinical measures following anterior cruciate ligament reconstruction. Knee Surg Sports Traumatol Arthrosc. 2002;10:10-19.
24. Nyland J, Klein S, Caborn DN. Lower extremity compensatory neuromuscular and biomechanical adaptations 2 to 11 years after anterior cruciate ligament reconstruction. Arthroscopy. 2010;26:1212-25.
25. Mahieu NN, McNair P, De Muynck M, et al. Effect of static and ballistic stretching on the muscle-tendon tissue properties. Med Sci Sports Exerc. 2007;39:494-501.
26. Nyland JA. Therapeutic strategies for developing neuromuscular control in the kinetic chain. In: Hughes C (Ed). Independent Study Course 22.1: Education and Intervention for Musculoskeletal Injuries: A Biomechanical Approach. La Crosse, WI: Orthopaedic Section of American Physical Therapy Association; 2012.
27. Hewett TE, Myer GD. The mechanistic connection between the trunk, hip, knee, and anterior cruciate ligament injury. Exerc Sport Sci Rev. 2011;39:161-6.
28. Beighton P, Solmon L, Soskolne CL. Articular mobility in an African population. Ann Rheum Dis. 973;32:413-8.
29. Nyland J, Proniewicz A. Rehabilitation of ACL reconstruction. ESSKA Academy 2014;58981.
30. Fitzgerald GK, Lephart SM, Hwang JH, et al. Hop tests as predictors of dynamic knee stability. J Orthop Sports Phys Ther. 2001;31:588-97.
31. Paterno MV, Ford KR, Myer GD, et al. Limb asymmetries in landing and jumping 2 years following anterior cruciate ligament reconstruction. Clin J Sports Med. 2007;17:258-62.
32. Paterno MV, Schmitt LC, Ford KR, et al. Biomechanical measures during landing and postural stability predict second anterior cruciate ligament injury after anterior cruciate ligament reconstruction and return to sport. Am J Sports Med. 2010;38:1968-78.
33. Thomee R, Kaplan Y, Kvist J, et al. Muscle strength and hop performance criteria prior to return to sports after ACL reconstruction. Knee Surg Sports Traumatol Arthrosc. 2011;19:1798-805.
34. Angelozzi M, Madama M, Corsica C, et al. Rate of force development as an adjunctive outcome measure for return-to-sport decisions after anterior cruciate ligament reconstruction. J Orthop Sports Phys Ther. 2012;42:772-80.
35. Gerber JP, Marcus RL, Dibble LE, et al. Effects of early progressive eccentric exercise on muscle structure after anterior cruciate ligament reconstruction. J Bone Joint Surg Am. 2007;89:559-70.
36. Nyland J, Krupp R, Caborn DNM. Knee re-injury prevention program following rehabilitation improves sports performance and patient outcomes. Abstract #866, 60th ACSM Annual Meeting and 4th World Congress on Exercise is Medicine. Indianapolis, IN, USA, 2013, May 28-June 1.
37. Brewer BW, Cornelius AE. Self-protective changes in athletic identity following anterior cruciate ligament reconstruction. Psychol Sport Exerc. 2010;11:1-5.
38. Brewer BW, Van Raalte JL, Linder DE. Athletic identity: Hercules' muscles or Achilles Heel? Int J Sport Psychol. 1993;24:237-54.
39. Chmielewski TL, Jones D, Day T, et al. The association of pain and fear of movement/reinjury with function during anterior cruciate ligament reconstruction rehabilitation. J Orthop Sports Phys Ther. 2008;38:746-53.
40. Giotis D, Tsiaras V, Ristanis S, et al. Knee braces can decrease tibial rotation during pivoting that occurs in high demanding activities. Knee Surg Sports Traumatol Arthrosc. 2011;19:1347-54.
41. Wright RW, Preston E, Fleming BC, et al. A systematic review of anterior cruciate ligament reconstruction rehabilitation: Part I: continuous passive motion, early weight bearing, postoperative bracing, and home-based rehabilitation. J Knee Surg. 2008;21:217-24.
42. Yabroudi MA, Björnsson H, Lynch AD, et al. Predictors of revision surgery after primary anterior cruciate ligament reconstruction. Orthop J Sports Med. 2016;4:2325967116666039.
43. Myer GD, Martin L Jr., Ford KR, et al. No association of time from surgery with functional deficits in athletes after anterior cruciate ligament reconstruction: evidence for objective return-to-sport criteria. Am J Sports Med. 2012;40:2256-63.
44. Myer GD, Paterno MV, Ford KR, et al. Rehabilitation after anterior cruciate ligament reconstruction: Criteria-based progression through the return-to-sport phase. J Orthop Sports Phys Ther. 2006;36:385-402.
45. Smith FW, Rosenlund EA, Aune AK, et al. Subjective functional assessments and the return to competitive sport after anterior cruciate ligament reconstruction. Br J Sports Med. 2004;38:279-84.

CHAPTER

34

Improving Outcomes of ACL Reconstruction: Pharmacological Measures

Anshu Shekhar, Sachin Tapasvi

INTRODUCTION

Anterior cruciate ligament (ACL) injury is a common clinical problem encountered in orthopedic practice. ACL tear could be the result of traumatic injuries, sport injuries, accidents or occupational injuries. Accidents and occupational trauma are the common causes of ACL tear in Indian patients.[1] Though strong epidemiological data is not available from India, ACL injury is more commonly seen in adult male patients compared to females, probably due to their nature of work and occupation. ACL injuries represent a significant economic burden.[2]

Ligament reconstruction is the standard of care for patients with ACL injury. It is also important to reconstruct the ligament at the earliest to reduce the risk of meniscal tears. An Indian study has shown that delay in surgery is associated with meniscal pathology.[1] With advance of technology, patient's expectations and economic benefits, trend of performing ACL reconstructions (ACLRs) as outpatient is increasing globally[3] and also in India.

Anterior cruciate ligament reconstruction may be associated with development of knee osteoarthritis (OA). A retrospective study involving 249 patients undergoing ACLR showed radiological signs of OA in 39% patients after about 7.8 years. The patients undergoing ACLR have higher risk of knee OA compared to the general population, especially in obese patients and in those with severe chondrosis in the medial compartment.[4] Optimal management of patients post ACLR is important to improve short-term as well as long-term outcomes. The goals of treatment include relief from pain, and swelling, improving range of motion, strength and neuromuscular control.[5]

Different approaches have been evaluated in improving the outcomes of ACLR. The approaches can be broadly divided into nonpharmacological and pharmacological interventions. Ice compression, muscle strengthening exercises and neuromuscular training are very commonly employed nonpharmacological methods. The other nonpharmacological approaches include cryotherapy and electrical muscle (EM) stimulation. The pharmacological management options include use of anti-inflammatory medicines to reduce pain, anabolic steroids to increase muscle mass, multivitamins and use of intra-articular injections in the form of platelet-rich plasma (PRP) and hyaluronic acid (HA) preparations.

Rehabilitation after ACLR is very important in determining the successful outcome of the procedure.[6] There has been significant improvement in the rehabilitation process during last many years.[7] The rehabilitation procedures may differ based on the patient's occupation and level of commitment. Broadly, the rehabilitation procedure is decided based on the level of impairment and need of the person to return to play.[8]

In this chapter, we discuss the pharmacological measures to improve the outcomes after ACLR.

PHARMACOLOGICAL MANAGEMENT

Broadly, the pharmacological options used in patients with ACLR include agents used for reducing pain, such as nonsteroidal anti-inflammatory drugs, opioids and gabapentin. Agents, such as zolpidem, are used for improving sleep disturbances associated with pain.[9] These agents provide symptomatic relief. Intra-articular injections are becoming more popular and are also being used in the management of patients with ACLR. We review evidence on the use of two "novel" approaches, i.e. intra-articular HA and PRP for improving clinical outcomes in patients undergoing ACL repair.

Viscosupplementation

Hyaluronic acid is an important component of synovial fluid in humans which provides rheological properties, i.e. elasticity and viscosity to the healthy synovial fluid. In the absence of sufficient synovial fluid with normal rheological properties, functions of the joint (lubrication and shock absorption) are greatly hampered.[10]

Currently, there are several HA preparations available in the market which differ based on their source, manufacturing process, molecular properties, molecular weight, dosage schedule, elasticity and viscocity.[11] These preparations are either extracted from rooster combs, or are fermentative or synthetic in origin.[12] The differences in physiochemical properties of viscosupplements may result in different clinical outcomes. Hence, all viscosupplementation should not be considered similar in efficacy.

Use of viscosupplementation after arthroscopy procedures is gaining acceptance among surgeons. In arthroscopic practice, intra-articular HA administration has been studied for its efficacy and safety after arthroscopic levage,[13] following arthroscopic meniscectomy[14] and after ACLR.[15,16]

Intra-articular HA has been tested for its efficacy after arthroscopic knee joint lavage in patients with OA having persistent knee pain. In this study of 80 patients, after joint lavage they were administered 0.5% sodium hyaluronate. The results of this 2-year study show that postarthroscopic administration of HA helps in pain and function improvement. In a prospective, open-label study, Huskin and colleagues[14] evaluated efficacy and safety of Hylan G-F 20, a high molecular weight, cross-linked supplementation in patients with mild-to-moderate knee OA with persistent pain 4–12 weeks postarthroscopic meniscectomy. Hylan G-F 20 significantly reduced the pain showing favorable risk benefit profile for use in these patients.

Intra-articular HA also known as viscosupplement or synovial fluid replacement therapy (SFRT) is increasingly being accepted as one of the treatment modalities for improving outcomes of ACLR. Patients undergoing ACLR are benefited with intra-articular HA due to several properties, such as anti-inflammatory, anabolic, and pain-relieving actions.[17,18] Hylan G-F 20, a high molecular weight, cross-linked viscosupplementation is prepared from two hylan polymers: Hylan A (80%) and Hylan B (20%) with different rheological properties. The formulation is significantly different compared to unmodified hyaluronan.[11] HA products have different molecular weights (500 KD to >90 million D). Hylans have a higher molecular weight due to cross-linking of HA. Similarly, they also have higher elastoviscous properties.[12,19] The molecular weight and elasticity of hylan G-F 20 closely resembles to that of healthy young synovial fluid.[20]

Raman and Day[21] have also studied use of hylan G-F 20 in patients with knee pain and mechanical symptoms after arthroscopic debridement and/or minimal trimming of the cartilage. Hylan G-F 20 given after 6 weeks, resulted in significant pain relief and improvement in functions of OA patients. In another prospective study, Raman and colleagues[22] evaluated effects of hylan G-F 20 after chondral surgery and ligament reconstruction of the knee joint among 326 patients (ACLR, n = 139). Overall, at 26 weeks, there was significant pain reduction in the study group. The authors postulated that chondroprotective properties of hylan G-F 20 may be useful in chondral repair and pain relief. Huang and colleagues[16] in a randomized, controlled clinical trial showed that use of HA therapy results in more functional and muscle peak torque improvement in ACL rehabilitation.

Timing of HA administration after arthroscopy is a debatable topic with some using it immediately after the arthroscopic surgery[15] to reduce pain or facilitate muscle rehabilitation while others administering it after few weeks. In one study, HA was administered on 4, 8 and 12 weeks of surgery in patients who underwent ACLR.[16]

A randomized trial (n = 32) compared use of arthroscopic ACLR followed by intra-articular HA versus arthroscopic ACLR alone. On day 1 and 2 of surgery, the improvements in pain and activities of daily living were significantly better in the patients who received HA. From 2 weeks onwards, improvement in pain was similar in both groups. On day 1 and 2, patients in HA group had significantly less knee swelling (p = 0.009). The results of this trial showed improvement of pain and swelling with intra-articular HA as early as day 1.[15]

Huang and colleagues[16] also evaluated comparative outcomes of HA administration when it was initiated at 4, 8 and 12 weeks after the arthroscopic ACLR. All the patients (n = 120) who were divided into four arms of 30 each (Group I: HA started at 4 weeks after surgery; Group II: HA started at 8 weeks; Group III: HA started at 12 weeks; Group IV: normal saline at 4 weeks after surgery) received regular rehabilitation for 16 weeks. The results of this study indicate administration of HA after 8 weeks of surgery provides best outcome. The healing process involves several steps of which early inflammatory phase could be useful for early vascularity. Anti-inflammatory response provided by HA during the proliferation and migration phase may explain the best response with HA administration after 8 weeks of procedure, according to the authors.

Overall, HA preparations are well tolerated. Those obtained from rooster combs are contraindicated in egg allergy or allergy to chicken.[12] Intra-articular injection of hylan G-F 20 is well tolerated. Minor side effects, such as arthralgia, joint effusion and pain at the site of injection, are some of the reported side effects with use of intra-articular injections of HA.[19]

Currently available evidence for use of intra-articular viscosupplementation after ACLR is promising. There is no robust data from either systematic reviews or meta-analysis comparing effects of HAs versus standard therapies. Similarly, there are no head-to-head comparative trials between different HA preparations after arthroscopic ACLR.

Platelet-Rich Plasma

Platelets play an important role in the normal healing process via secretion of growth factors.[23] PRP is a biological therapy containing several growth factors prepared from autologous centrifuged blood.[23,24] The preparation contains threefold to fivefold higher level of growth factors compared to whole blood.[24]

Platelet-rich plasma and growth factors [e.g. vascular endothelial growth factor (VEGF), platelet-derived growth factor (PDGF), transforming growth factor-beta (TGF-β)] are being studied in the orthopedic practice and their popularity is also increasing,[2,25,26] especially in ligament healing. It may have benefits in some patients undergoing ACL surgery,[27] but it is important to critically analyze the evidence supporting its use in patients with ACLR.

A randomized study (n = 98) demonstrated faster remodeling of patellar tendon grafts on magnetic resonance imaging (MRI). Compared to patients without PRP, those who received it had better remodeling at 4 months ($p = 0.003$). The effect was consistent at 6 months ($p = 0.0001$), and 1 year ($p = 0.354$).[28] The MRI findings also show reduced edema, enhanced blood supply and microvessel permeability in the proximal tibial tunnel.[29] Application of PRP results in better cortical bone formation around, but is not seen before 1 month after ACLR. Another study showed improved cortical bone formation around the tibial tunnel at two and half months after ACLR.[30]

A randomized, prospective comparative study (n = 100) in patients with arthroscopic patellar tendon allograft did not show significant difference in regards to clinical scores, inflammatory changes or MRI appearance of the graft between two groups, i.e. using PDGF or no PDGF.[31] Another prospective comparative study (n = 40) comparing single-bundle hamstring reconstruction with or without PRP showed that PRP does not result in enhancement of graft remodeling.[32] In a small Indian study (n = 11), Dhillon and colleagues[33] studied ACL remnants of patients undergoing ACLR which were treated with PRP. Analysis of cultured cell indicated that PRP may assist in improving ACL cell viability and proliferation. In the tibial tunnel, PRP may result in improvement of vascularization but does not have much effect in the femoral tunnels.[2] In patients undergoing ACLR, PRP has no significant effect on prevention of tunnel widening.[26]

A recent systematic review of 11 clinical studies suggested a promising evidence for the use of PRP as an adjuvant therapy in achieving faster maturity of the graft in patients undergoing ACLR (n = 266) compared to no PRP (n = 250). However, there was no significant benefit for tunnel healing with PRP therapy.[34] The use of PRP and growth factors is currently a subject of investigation for use in patients with ACLR.[2,35]

It is also important to understand the limitations for use of PRP. The practical limitation is its heterogeneous nature and several confounding parameters affecting the clinical outcomes.[27] A study compared effects of double-spinning platelet-enriched gel (PRP) with leukocytes, no gel and a platelet-rich preparation from a single-spinning procedure (PRGF) without leukocytes. The third arm resulted in significant improvement in swelling and inflammatory parameters after 24 hours of surgery ($p < 0.05$). However, there was no significant difference between three groups in terms of MRI and clinical effects.[36] Current evidence does not support the notion of improvement in clinical outcomes with the use of PRP in patients undergoing ACL repair.[27]

It seems that use of specific growth factors: VEGF, PDGF and TGF-β may be better compared to generic PRP for graft healing.[2] Use of PRP is common in sports medicine.[37] In the absence of strong data, it is difficult to provide conclusive remarks in favor of either PRP or growth factors.

The challenges for use of PRP include absence of ideal concentration, differences in commercial preparations, differences in the amount of platelet, type of anticoagulant used[23] and absence of well-deigned larger controlled clinical trials. More studies with good design and large sample size are required before a definitive conclusion can be reached.

SUMMARY

Anterior cruciate ligament tear is a common clinical problem, especially in adult male patients, commonly because of the sports injury, road traffic accident or occupational injury. Several measures are employed for improving short-term and long-term outcomes of ACLR. Cryotherapy and exercises are important and well-established nonpharmacological methods for the rehabilitation of patients after ACL repair. Among the pharmacological therapy, intra-articular HA administration is gaining acceptance for improving long-term outcomes. HA preparations differ in their rheological properties, i.e. elasticity and viscosity. Hylan G-F 20 has been shown to provide beneficial effects post ACLR. Adherence to rehabilitation is of prime importance in optimizing the outcomes of ACLR.

REFERENCES

1. Jacob KM, Oommen AT. A retrospective analysis of risk factors for meniscal co-morbidities in anterior cruciate ligament injuries. Indian J Orthop. 2012;46(5):566-9.
2. Bissell L, Tibrewal S, Sahni V, et al. Growth factors and platelet rich plasma in anterior cruciate ligament reconstruction. Curr Stem Cell Res Ther. 2015;10(1):19-25.
3. Baverel L, Cucurulo T, Lutz C, et al. Anesthesia and analgesia methods for outpatient anterior cruciate ligament reconstruction. Orthop Traumatol Surg Res. 2016;102(8S):S251-5.
4. Li RT, Lorenz S, Xu Y, et al. Predictors of radiographic knee osteoarthritis after anterior cruciate ligament reconstruction. Am J Sports Med. 2011;39(12):2595-603.
5. van Grinsven S, van Cingel RE, Holla CJ, et al. Evidence-based rehabilitation following anterior cruciate ligament reconstruction. Knee Surg Sports Traumatol Arthrosc. 2010;18(8):1128-44.
6. Ruffilli A, Buda R, Castagnini F, et al. Temperature-controlled continuous cold flow device versus traditional icing regimen following anterior cruciate ligament reconstruction: a prospective randomized comparative trial. Arch Orthop Trauma Surg. 2015;135(10):1405-10.
7. Biggs A, Jenkins WL, Urch SE, et al. Rehabilitation for patients following ACL reconstruction: A knee symmetry model. N Am J Sports Phys Ther. 2009;4(1):2-12.
8. van Melick N, van Cingel RE, Brooijmans F, et al. Evidence-based clinical practice update: practice guidelines for anterior cruciate ligament rehabilitation based on a systematic review and multidisciplinary consensus. Br J Sports Med. 2016;50(24):1506-15.
9. Secrist ES, Freedman KB, Ciccotti MG, et al. Pain management after outpatient anterior cruciate ligament reconstruction: A systematic review of randomized controlled trials. Am J Sports Med. 2016;44(9):2435-47.
10. Agerup B, Berg P, Akermark C. Non-animal stabilized hyaluronic acid: a new formulation for the treatment of osteoarthritis. BioDrugs. 2005;19(1):23-30.
11. Migliore A, Giovannangeli F, Granata M, et al. Hylan G-F 20: Review of its safety and efficacy in the management of joint pain in osteoarthritis. Clin Med Insights: Arthritis Musculoskelet Disord. 2010;3:55-68.
12. Migliore A, Granata M. Intra-articular use of hyaluronic acid in the treatment of osteoarthritis. Clin Interv Aging. 2008;3(2):365-9.
13. Hempfling H. Intra-articular hyaluronic acid after knee arthroscopy: a two-year study. Knee Surg Sports Traumatol Arthrosc. 2007;15(5):537-46.
14. Huskin JP, Vandekerckhove B, Delince P, et al. Multicentre, prospective, open study to evaluate the safety and efficacy of hylan G-F 20 in knee osteoarthritis subjects presenting with pain following arthroscopic meniscectomy. Knee Surg Sports Traumatol Arthrosc. 2008;16(8):747-52.
15. Chau JY, Chan WL, Woo SB, et al. Hyaluronic acid instillation following arthroscopic anterior cruciate ligament reconstruction: a double-blinded, randomised controlled study. J Orthop Surg (Hong Kong). 2012;20(2):162-5.
16. Huang MH, Yang RC, Chou PH. Preliminary effects of hyaluronic acid on early rehabilitation of patients with isolated anterior cruciate ligament reconstruction. Clin J Sport Med. 2007;17(4):242-50.
17. Axe JM, Snyder-Mackler L, Axe MJ. The role of viscosupplementation. Sports Med Arthrosc. 2013;21(1):18-22.
18. Marshall KW. Intra-articular hyaluronan therapy. Curr Opin Rheumatol. 2000;12(5):468-74.
19. Frampton JE. Hylan G-F 20 single-injection formulation. Drugs Aging. 2010;27(1):77-85.
20. Synvisc One Science. Hylan G-F 20. [online] Available from www.synvisconehcp.com/science. [Accessed March, 2017].
21. Raman R, Day N. (2013). Viscosupplementation after arthroscopic surgery of the knee: Safety and efficacy compared to arthritic knee. Abstract number 34541. SICOT 2013. [online] Available from lhcnews.sicot.org/resources/File/Hyderabad/Hyderabad%20Abstract%20Book%20-%20Poster% 20Presentations%20final.pdf. [Accessed March, 2017].
22. Raman R, Shaw C, Johnson G, et al. (2013). Safety and efficacy of viscosupplementation following chondral surgery and ligament reconstruction of the knee. Abstract number 34538. SICOT 2013. [online] Available from lhcnews.sicot.org/resources/File/Hyderabad/Hyderabad%20Abstract%20Book%20-%20Poster%20Presentations%20final.pdf. [Accessed March, 2017].
23. Willits K, Kaniki N, Bryant D. The use of platelet-rich plasma in orthopedic injuries. Sports Med Arthrosc. 2013;21(4):225-30.
24. Figueroa PD, Figueroa BF, Ahumada PX, et al. [Use of platelet rich plasma in knee ligament surgery]. Rev Med Chil. 2013;141(10):1315-20.
25. Braun HJ, Wasterlain AS, Dragoo JL. The use of PRP in ligament and meniscal healing. Sports Med Arthrosc. 2013;21(4):206-12.

26. Mirzatolooei F, Alamdari MT, Khalkhali HR. The impact of platelet-rich plasma on the prevention of tunnel widening in anterior cruciate ligament reconstruction using quadrupled autologous hamstring tendon: a randomised clinical trial. Bone Joint J. 2013;95-B(1):65-9.
27. Lubowitz JH. Editorial commentary: platelet-rich plasma in ACL surgery. Arthroscopy. 2015;31(5):989.
28. Seijas R, Ares O, Catala J, et al. Magnetic resonance imaging evaluation of patellar tendon graft remodelling after anterior cruciate ligament reconstruction with or without platelet-rich plasma. J Orthop Sur (Hong Kong). 2013;21: 10-4.
29. Rupreht M, Jevtic V, Sersa I, et al. Evaluation of the tibial tunnel after intraoperatively administered platelet-rich plasma gel during anterior cruciate ligament reconstruction using diffusion weighted and dynamic contrast-enhanced MRI. J Magn Reson Imaging. 2013;37:928-35.
30. Rupreht M, Vogrin M, Hussein M. MRI evaluation of tibial tunnel wall cortical bone formation after platelet-rich plasma applied during anterior cruciate ligament reconstruction. Radiol Oncol. 2013;47(2):119-24.
31. Nin JR, Gasque GM, Azcarate AV, et al. Has platelet-rich plasma any role in anterior cruciate ligament allograft healing? Arthroscopy. 2009;25(11):1206-13.
32. Komzak M, Hart R, Smid P, et al. [The effect of platelet-rich plasma on graft healing in reconstruction of the anterior cruciate ligament of the knee joint: prospective study]. Acta Chir Orthop Traumatol Cech. 2015;82(2):135-9.
33. Dhillon MS, Karna SK, Dhatt SS, et al. Can platelet rich plasma stimulate human ACL growth in culture? A preliminary experience. Muscles Ligaments Tendons J. 2015;5(3):156-61.
34. Figueroa D, Figueroa F, Calvo R, et al. Platelet-rich plasma use in anterior cruciate ligament surgery: systematic review of the literature. Arthroscopy. 2015;31(5):981-8.
35. Hutchinson ID, Rodeo SA, Perrone GS, et al. Can platelet-rich plasma enhance anterior cruciate ligament and meniscal repair? J Knee Surg. 2015;28(1):19-28.
36. Valenti AA, Lamo-Espinosa J, Aquerreta BJ, et al. Comparison between two different platelet-rich plasma preparations and control applied during anterior cruciate ligament reconstruction. Is there any evidence to support their use? Injury. 2014;(Suppl 4):S36-41.
37. Nourissat G, Mainard D, Kelberine F, et al. Current concept for the use of PRP in arthroscopic surgery. Orthop Traumatol Surg Res. 2013;99(8 Suppl):S407-10.

Index

Page numbers followed by *t* refer to table.

A

B

C

D

E

F

G

H

I

K

L

M

T

V

W